Occupational Therapy and Physical Dysfunction

For Churchill Livingstone

Editorial Director: Mary Law
Project Editor: Dinah Thom
Copy Editor: Carrie Walker
Indexer: Nina Boyd
Project Manager: Valerie Burgess
Design Direction: Judith Wright
Sales Promotion Executive: Maria O'Connor

Occupational Therapy and Physical Dysfunction

Principles, Skills and Practice

Edited by

Ann Turner TDipCOT MA
Course Leader, St Andrew's School of Occupational Therapy, Nene College, Northampton

Margaret Foster TDipCOT CertEd MMedSci
Senior Lecturer, School of Health and Community Studies, University of Derby, Derby

Sybil E. Johnson TDipCOT DMS CertHSM FETC
Senior Practitioner Occupational Therapist, Dorset Social Services. Formerly District Occupational Therapist, Sheffield

Foreword by

Averil M. Stewart TDipCOT FCOT BA
Professor and Head of Department of Occupational Therapy, Queen Margaret College, Edinburgh

FOURTH EDITION

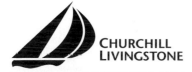
CHURCHILL
LIVINGSTONE

NEW YORK. EDINBURGH LONDON MADRID MELBOURNE SAN FRANCISCO AND TOKYO 1996

CHURCHILL LIVINGSTONE
Medical Division of Pearson Professional Limited

Distributed in the United States of America by Churchill
Livingstone Inc., 650 Avenue of the Americas, New York,
N. Y. 10011, and by associated companies, branches and
representatives throughout the world.

First edition 1981
Second edition 1987
Third edition 1992
Fourth edition 1996

ISBN 0 443 05177 1

British Library of Cataloguing in Publication Data
A catalogue record for this book is available from the British
Library.

Library of Congress Cataloging in Publication Data
A catalogue record for this book is available from the
Library of Congress

9609119
WB 555

The
publisher's
policy is to use
**paper manufactured
from sustainable forests**

Produced by Longman Malaysia
Printed in Singapore

Contents

Contributors

Theresa Baxter DipCOT MEd
Lecturer, School of Health and Community
Studies, University of Derby, Derby

Alison J. Beattie DipCOT
Consultant Occupational Therapist, Parkinson's
Disease Society, London

Susan Beresford DipCOT
Head Occupational Therapist, Northampton
General Hospital NHS Trust, Northampton

Patricia M. Church DipCOT
Occupational Therapy Manager, Queen's
Medical Centre, University Hospital,
Nottingham

Laura Ann Cicinelli OTR BSc
Formerly Senior Occupational Therapist,
Wolfson Medical Rehabilitation Centre, Copse
Hill, Wimbledon

Jean Colburn DipCOT BOT MSc
Formerly Senior Lecturer, Dorset House School
of Occupational Therapy, Oxford, and Senior
Lecturer, School of Health Care Studies, Oxford
Brookes University, Oxford

Maryanne Cook DipCOT CertEd
Senior Lecturer in Occupational Therapy, School
of Health and Social Sciences, Coventry
University, Coventry

Rosemary Cooper DipCOT
Occupational Therapy Manager, Pinderfields
Hospital NHS Trust, Wakefield, West Yorkshire

Elizabeth Cracknell TDipCOT BSc(Hons) MA
Head of Occupational Therapy Division, Nene
College. Formerly Principal of St Andrew's
School of Occupational Therapy, Northampton

Louise Cusack DipCOT
Head Occupational Therapist, HIV/AIDS
Specialist, HIV Services, Chelsea and
Westminster Hospital, London

Margaret Foster TDipCOT CertEd MMedSci
Senior Lecturer, School of Health and
Community Studies, University of Derby, Derby

Alison Hammond DipCOT BSc(Hons) MSc PhD
Senior Lecturer, School of Health and
Community Studies, University of Derby, Derby

Jane Henshaw DipCOT CertHSM
Independent Rehabilitation Consultant working
in the medico-legal field. Formerly Head
Occupational Therapist, Duke of Cornwall
Spinal Treatment Centre, Salisbury District
Hospital, Salisbury, Wiltshire

Glynis L. Hill DipCOT CertEd BA MA
Senior Lecturer, St Andrew's School of
Occupational Therapy, Nene College,
Northampton

Vivienne Ibbotson DipCOT
Senior Occupational Therapist, Disablement
Services Centre, Northern General Hospital
NHS Trust, Sheffield

Sue Jackson DipCOT
Senior Occupational Therapist, Northern
General Hospital NHS Trust, Sheffield

Jane James DipCOT DMS
Team Manager (Adult Resources), Leicestershire Social Services

Sybil E. Johnson TDipCOT DMS CertHSM FETC
Senior Practitioner Occupational Therapist, Dorset Social Services. Formerly District Occupational Therapist, Sheffield

Jenny C. King DipCOT MSc
Senior Lecturer, London School of Occupational Therapy, Department of Health Studies, Brunel University College, Isleworth, Middlesex. Formerly Head Occupational Therapist (Cardiology), Charing Cross Hospital, London

Annette C. Leveridge DipCOT
Head Occupational Therapist, Specialist Occupational Therapist, Plastic Surgery and Burns, Mount Vernon and Watford Hospital Trust, Northwood, Middlesex

Charlotte V. MacCaul DipCOT BSc MSc
Head Occupational Therapist, Swale Day Hospital, Keycol Hospital, Sittingbourne, Kent

Steve McWilliams DipCOT BA(Hons)
Independent Head Injury Case Manager and

Senior Occupational Therapist, Royal Manchester Children's Hospital, Manchester

Louise Phillips DipCOT
Senior Occupational Therapist, St Pancras Hospital, London. Formerly Senior Occupational Therapist, HIV/AIDS, Riverside Health Authority, London

Pauline Rowe DipCOT CertEd MEd
Senior Lecturer, School of Health and Community Studies, University of Derby, Derby

Liz Tipping DipCOT
Senior Practitioner Occupational Therapist, Dorset Social Services

Ann Turner TDipCOT MA
Course Leader, St Andrew's School of Occupational Therapy, Nene College, Northampton

Jenny Wilsdon DipCOT BSc(Hons)
Senior Lecturer in Biological Sciences and Professional Studies (Paediatrics), St Andrew's School of Occupational Therapy, Nene College, Northampton

Foreword

Many, many students and therapists will, I am sure, be joining me in congratulating this stalwart team of co-editors for having produced the Fourth Edition of this popular and invaluable text. It is warmly commended.

It is but four years since the last edition. Changes in the delivery of health and social services have been considerable, with resulting changes in the practice of occupational therapy. In addition, much has been written on both sides of the Atlantic about the theoretical underpinnings of the profession, and there are increasing signs of the evidence of research findings and their influences on practice.

First, let's look at the team: I call them 'stalwart' for they have remained together as a strong trio for the past 17 years. They have been courageous in setting down beliefs and principles with a resoluteness and determination that does not lend itself to complacency. This updated Fourth Edition is based on a critical awareness of change and a constant seeking for improvements and even greater relevance in the application of knowledge. The team has demonstrated a hardiness which in Kobasa's terminology (see p. 771 of this textbook) reflects challenge, commitment and control. As editors they have taken control of over 20 authors, of whom 5 are new to the Fourth Edition. This edition shows a commitment to the identification of the theoretical basis for occupational therapy, and presents new challenges for its readers, students and practitioners alike.

Of the changes, these are to be found in relation to both content and structure. The latter, while still based on the three parts — Foundations for practice, Skills and Practice — contains prefaces to each part which set them in context with a logical progression from understanding to actual application. Combining philosophy and history into one chapter and introducing a chapter on theoretical frameworks in Part 1 give evidence of the critical and logical thinking which the editors have applied throughout, shifting components to obtain greater clarity and to demonstrate progression in thinking. In Part 2, the chapter on management takes up a more logical position at the end rather than at the beginning. The previous descriptive chapter on workshop activities has been cut and an excellent and welcome chapter on the therapeutic use of activity introduced. This is welcome in the the sense that it adopts a more global analytical stance, challenging the use of exercise regimes and pseudo activity which often draw on the techniques of others rather than promoting real activities, no matter how mundane, which are fundamental to the practice of occupational therapy. In many chapters this more reflective rather than descriptive approach can be found.

In relation to content, the psychology of learning as a particular frame of reference is developed further than previously, and new models include Cynkin & Robinson's Activities Health Model (1990) and Reed & Sanderson's Personal Adaptation through Occupation Model (1992). There is an emphasis on theoretical frameworks within each chapter related to practice with different groups of clients, and numerous case studies will give a reality to the theory. In addition, the authors have tackled the semantic debate which has previously led to confusing overlaps where the frames of reference of one theorist are the models of another. Adherence to rigid terminology can lead to narrow and automatic acceptance. Sections of this new edition challenge the reader to think critically and not absorb blindly.

A number of chapters, particularly where new authors have been involved, have had a major rewrite, emphasising psychological theories as well as practical interventions. In addition, the findings of recent research have been incorporated and many up-to-date references added. The introductory chapters, such as those on neurology and cardiac rehabilitation, reflect the new trend. Other new and welcome components relate to more on sexuality, euthanasia, legislation on lifting, post-traumatic stress, work assessment, complementary therapies and team work.

Changes there are, but the overall shape and content will strike most as being familiar. Useful diagrams, photographs and tables have been retained. As with other texts by Churchill Livingstone, there is the helpful inclusion of many headings and subheadings resulting in a user-friendly book.

As an educator I look for texts which will inform and challenge students, texts that are not prescriptive but present alternative points of view and, just as importantly, other sources of up-to-date information. As members of the profession in the UK gain higher qualifications and develop research skills, so one would expect to find in a future edition ever more citing of such references thereby enhancing the book's Britishness. In conclusion, this Fourth Edition reflects the dynamic context of occupational therapy. Occupational therapy is essentially a practical profession. It is about doing and enabling others to do, but without thought the actions can be meaningless. The authors convey their conviction and expertise with enthusiasm. May the stalwart co-editors' aspirations for constant review and updating be taken as examples of good professional practice, for none of us should ever stand still. To Annie, Margaret and Sybil, thank you for helping to lead the way.

Edinburgh, 1996   A.M.S.

Preface

Since the last edition of this book was published, there has been a period of tremendous change within occupational therapy. This change has been brought about by external and internal forces acting upon the profession and its practitioners, affecting both the way we think and the way we practise.

Externally, the predominant changes have been dictated by recent legislation, which has resulted in very significant philosophical and cultural changes in health and social care provision. In practice, this means that the NHS, social services departments, housing authorities and other, familiar public institutions have become 'purchasing' and/or 'providing' organisations. These changes have produced many far-reaching outcomes, including faster throughput from hospital-based services, greater emphasis on care in the community and, for occupational therapists, an increasing interest in, and move towards, private practice. Significantly, these changes have rocked the thinking, attitudes, day-to-day practice and, on occasions, the very culture in which occupational therapists function.

Internally, the profession has been through a period of looking to its laurels and evaluating its practice in the light of current and future need. Therapists have been required to justify their practice, to identify the outcomes of their intervention and to define the boundaries of their professional practice. This has been a demanding task, sometimes requiring the acquisition of new skills and language.

Partly, therefore, as a reaction to the changing culture of health and social care in the UK, and partly as a natural growth process, occupational therapy has developed a far more overt theory base, founded on the fundamental beliefs of the profession. The 'new' overtness continues to develop and offers us a constantly developing base upon which its members think, practise, evaluate and communicate.

As part of these changes, the education of occupational therapists has not stood still. The validation of occupational therapy courses at first degree level, and the consequent shift of location from primarily independent status to inclusion in the network of higher education, has found courses relocated within universities and colleges of higher education. Students are now seen as a small cohort within a large and diverse group of undergraduates, with consequent advantages and disadvantages for the student therapists. This change has inevitably led to altered attitudes, values and confidence among newly qualifying therapists, who now see themselves as equal members in academically and business-dominated cultures.

Mirroring this academic change is the continuing evidence of success and confidence among practitioners as they undertake an increasingly wide range of studies, many at first and higher degree levels.

Despite these changes in attitude, confidence and knowledge, however, it is essential that we, as a profession, do not lose sight of what is required of us by service users. Our increasing ability to produce strategies, business plans and dissertations must not detract us from the fundamental beliefs and skills upon which our profession functions. It is good that we have a language with which to define our profession and its practice, but we must not lose sight of our ability to enable an elderly person to function as he wishes within his abilities. It is essential that we have a clear framework of theory that helps us plan our intervention, but we must not become so engrossed in academia and technique that we forget how to enable people to address the everyday problems caused by their dysfunctions. Equally, our ability to present strategic plans and address committees must never preclude us from working in partnership with service users and their carers, understanding their needs, problems and strengths, and focusing on their goals, while operating within the all-too-real constraints of health, social care and financial resources.

Occupational therapy practice today demands many qualities and skills. It demands enthusiasm, energy and independence from its practitioners, whose sights must include service purchasers and providers, and users and carers. Compiling a text that is both proactive and reactive in this era of change has called for much re-thinking and re-writing.

While still in three parts, Foundations for practice, Skills and Practice, the emphasis and content of these parts have undergone considerable change. Part 1 Foundations for practice, sees an increase in the exploration of the theoretical underpinning of the profession. Part 2, Skills, reflects the changing needs and culture of our practice, and aims not only to discuss, but also to evaluate our skills base.

Reflecting on Practice in Part 3 has called upon senior practitioners within the profession to make concrete use of the emerging theoretical frameworks to underpin their current and future practice.

However, the editors have endeavoured not to throw out the baby with the bathwater. The text remains user-friendly, with a clear layout and copious illustrations. The language aims to remain accessible but also profession-specific.

The three editors have continued to enjoy working as a team. Despite geographic distance, tasks and responsibilities have been shared, experience, knowledge and frustrations exchanged and many good lunches eaten! Our thanks go especially to our contributors, our colleagues at work and our long-suffering families. We also particularly thank staff at Churchill Livingstone, especially Dinah Thom, who has guided us once again through this monumental task with patience and calm. We hope to have produced between us a text that will assist and challenge the occupational therapist approaching practice in the 21st century.

Northampton, 1996   A.T.
                                                         M.F.
                                                         S.E.J.

Foundations for practice

Any structure based on a firm foundation is most likely to survive the ravages of time: boats with a sturdy keel sail steadily in choppy seas; the house built upon the rock stands the battering of storms and winds.

Thus it is with a profession. Any profession founded on a firm base of philosophy and theory will find that these act as a tether for its practitioners. If a profession's practice is based on a strong foundation, it will stand firm against the batterings of fashion, re-structuring, legislation, finance and other external forces that bring pressure to bear upon it.

A profession with a firm foundation will produce practitioners with the ability to develop and evaluate their practice and its skills, techniques and interventions. They will be able critically to analyse new and established media and techniques to determine how appropriate they are and how they may be adapted to meet changing needs. A profession's theoretical heritage enables its practitioners and researchers to explore the roots of its beliefs, so that these may be used not only to inform current practice, but also to act as a conceptual framework for the development of the profession.

Occupational therapists are by nature practical, pragmatic people. Their professional strength lies in their ability to relate to people and work with them to help address the functional difficulties that affect their daily lives. Occupational therapists generally see themselves as active and creative. Their professional activity, however, demands that they understand the nature of their 'doing'. Knowledge of people, how they normally function; how to discover what is important to them, and how to help them address their difficulties is fundamental to the work of the occupational therapist. For intervention to be successful, the therapist must understand how to identify a person's need and be able to make an informed choice of intervention strategies from the range she has available to her.

This first part of the book, therefore, describes and explores the theoretical foundations that underpin the practice of the occupational therapy profession. It explores the roots of the thinking behind occupational therapists' beliefs, and presents and evaluates a range of assessment and intervention tools that may be used by the practitioner. Knowledge of these foundations will enable the practitioner to offer the best of professional intervention and to evaluate and justify the skills, media and techniques of her profession.

1

The philosophy and history of occupational therapy

Ann Turner

INTRODUCTION

In 1962 Mary Reilly, an American professor of occupational therapy, wrote an article entitled 'Occupational therapy can be one of the great ideas of the twentieth century'. This was published at a time when the status of scientific research heralded the race to put a man on the moon, when technology was creating new materials, splitting atoms and putting colour onto television screens, and medical science was advancing its knowledge, success and fields of practice at such a rate that drugs, surgery and the use of technology were seen as the universal way forward in the treatment of all areas of disease. In this time of scientific advancement and status a small, relatively newly formed profession was expounding the idea that, for many people with dysfunction or disability, the way to restore well-being was not only within their own power but also possible by non-invasive means. In contrast to the use of scientific equipment, designer drugs and other advancing invasive techniques, occupational therapists began articulating a belief that, in certain circumstances in which such means were inappropriate or of limited success, a person might increase his* well-being by learning or relearning to do things important to him, and that this process could be achieved using ideas and activities that interested him. To help restore

---

*Throughout the text, and purely for the sake of ease, 'he/his' is used to refer to the person receiving occupational therapy and 'she/her' is used to refer to the therapist.

3

abilities, occupational therapists proposed the use of activities as diverse as gardening, cookery, pottery, car maintenance and singing. They also showed that where there remained a shortfall in ability, normal function could be restored by adapting the activity to suit the person, rather than trying to make the person cope with an inappropriate environment, attitude or piece of equipment. They showed that the choice of activity should be made in accordance with principles and theories based on a knowledge of how healthy people function.

In contrast to the objectivity and scientific proof upon which medical practice was developing, occupational therapy appeared subjective, unproven and 'homely'. Its practice, while able to be observed qualitatively, was not scrutinised quantifiably. Its use of everyday equipment and activities as media for treatment, and its belief in people as individuals who should be encouraged to decide what they wished to achieve and how they wished to achieve it, meant that occupational therapy was not a concept that was readily understood, especially by those used to looking for quantifiable proof of the effectiveness of practice.

The concept of occupational therapy, for both its practitioners and others, is fundamental to the successful practice of the profession, and in order for therapists to gain a firm foundation for practice and a strong professional identity, it is important for them to understand both the underlying philosophy of the profession and the historic foundations from which it arises.

This chapter looks at the philosophical assumptions underpinning the practice of occupational therapy, i.e. the profession's view of the nature of its existence. This philosophy, which guides and informs occupational therapists' professional practice, is a set of core beliefs, values and principles — a creed that shapes the thinking and actions of the profession. The chapter looks at the evidence through history for the existence of ideas and concepts which underpin the profession, and traces these through to modern-day practice. In conclusion the chapter looks forward to the 21st century to visualise the way in which the profession will develop.

DEFINITIONS OF OCCUPATIONAL THERAPY

While occupational therapy has been established in the United Kingdom only since the Second World War, some of its basic principles are rooted in the medical practice of ancient times. More than 100 years before Christ, Aesclepiades was reputed to recommend activity for his patients. In AD 172, Galen maintained that 'Employment is nature's best physician and is essential to human happiness' (cited in MacDonald et al 1970). In modern times, definitions of occupational therapy have echoed this idea, while, at the same time, expanding the thinking that underlies the profession's holistic ideas.

One of the earliest definitions of occupational therapy came from the Board of Control in England in a 1933 memorandum, which stated that 'Occupational therapy is the treatment, under medical direction, of physical or mental disorders, by the application of occupation and recreation, with the object of promoting recovery, of creating new habits and of preventing deterioration.'

In 1945 J. H. C. Colson, author of *The Rehabilitation of the Injured,* defined occupational therapy as 'the use of any occupation which is prescribed and guided for the purpose of contributing to, and hastening the rehabilitation of the unfit'. In 1946, Howarth and MacDonald, early pioneers of occupational therapy in Britain, published *The Theory of Occupational Therapy,* in which they defined occupational therapy as 'any work or recreational activity, mental or physical, definitely prescribed and guided, for the distinct purpose of contributing to, and hastening recovery from, disease or injury'.

'An active method of treatment with a profound psychological justification' was the definition put forward by Clark in 1952, followed, in 1955, by O'Sullivan, an English doctor specialising in physical medicine, who wrote in *The Textbook of Occupational Therapy* that he favoured the definition that occupational therapy was 'the treatment, under expert medical supervision, of mental or physical disease, by means of suitable occupation, whether mental, physical, social or recreational'.

As occupational therapy practice continued to expand and gain credibility, various definitions of the profession appeared in order to explain and consolidate the basis upon which occupational therapists practised. More modern definitions have endeavoured to either give a fully comprehensive idea of the scope of occupational therapy — namely, this Definition for Licensure from the Minutes of the 1981 AOTA Representative Assembly: 'Occupational therapy is the use of purposeful activity with individuals who are limited by physical injury or illness, psychosocial dysfunction, developmental or learning disabilities, poverty and cultural differences or the aging process in order to maximise independence, prevent disability and maintain health'; and this, written in *Current Occupational Therapy Practice* by a group of occupational therapists working in the North East Thames Regional Health Authority in 1987: 'Occupational therapy is the assessment and treatment of people of all ages with physical and mental health problems, through specifically selected and graded activities in order to help them reach their maximum level of functioning and independence in all aspects of daily life. These aspects will include their personal independence, employment, social, recreational and leisure pursuits and their interpersonal relationships.'

Alternatively, the profession has tried to provide a short, readily understood and easily remembered definition such as this European definition published in the *British Journal of Occupational Therapy* in May 1989: 'Occupational therapists assess and treat people using purposeful activity to prevent disability and develop independent function'; or this World Federation of Occupational Therapy definition (also May 1989): 'Occupational therapy is the treatment of physical and psychiatric conditions through specific activities in order to help people reach their maximum level of function and independence in all aspects of daily life.'

FUNDAMENTAL BELIEFS

While none of these statements would probably claim to be definitive they serve as excellent starting points for an examination of the underlying beliefs or philosophy of occupational therapy. The philosophy of the profession is concerned with the fundamental beliefs upon which the therapist bases her professional practice. The philosophy forms a basis for practice and for the acquisition of knowledge, skills, principles and methods.

Throughout the definitions there appear to run several thoughts and common links. These are defined below and examined to show how they may form the basic philosophy of professional occupational therapy practice (Box 1.1).

Box 1.1   A philosophy for occupational therapy

- People are individuals of worth and inherently different from one another
- Activity is fundamental to well-being
- Where occupational performance has been interrupted a person can:
  — through the medium of activity develop the adaptive skills required to restore, maintain or acquire function, and/or
  — modify activity in order to facilitate occupational performance

---

1. People as individuals

The basis for this element of the philosophy, that people are individuals of worth and inherently different from each other, is found in the development of Moral Treatment, a movement which began in England in the 18th century. This movement was based on the fundamental belief of the essential worth of each individual and the right of each person to humane care when ill. In 1791, moved by their spiritual and humanistic beliefs, the Society of Friends, a Quaker group, felt the need to establish its own institution 'in which a milder and more appropriate system of treatment than that usually practised, might be adopted' (Tuke 1813, p. 23). The Society believed that existing treatment 'was too frequently calculated to depress and degrade, rather than to awaken the slumbering reason'. Their institution, The Retreat, near York, was established in 1796 under

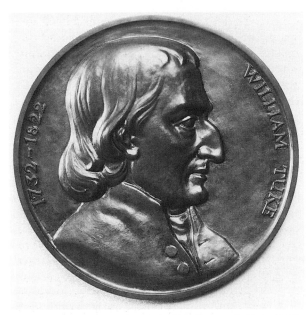

Fig. 1.1 William Tuke, founder of The Retreat in York, 1796. (Reproduced by kind permission of The Retreat, York.)

the charge of a Quaker physician, William Tuke (1732–1822) (Fig. 1.1).

Tuke, whose work linked closely with that of the French physician Philippe Pinel, believed that Moral Treatment should be considered in three parts:

By what means the power of the patient to control the disorder, is strengthened and assisted,
What modes of coercion are employed when restraint is absolutely necessary,
By what means the general comfort of the insane is promoted.

(Tuke 1813, p. 102)

He therefore established a regime within The Retreat which reflected these beliefs.

First, he looked at the importance of the person's self-esteem. He saw that 'much advantage [was] found . . . from treating the patient as much in the manner of a rational being' and that 'considerable advantage may certainly be derived . . . from an acquaintance with the previous habits, manners and prejudices of the individual' (Tuke 1813, p. 158). Contrary to existing regimes of treatment for the sick, Tuke placed great confidence in what his patients said, and respected their opinions. In showing the results of this attitude he talks

of 'One of the worst patients in the house who, previously to his indisposition, had been a considerable grazier, give very sensible directions for the treatment of a diseased cow' (Tuke 1813, p. 159).

In reflecting the worth of individuals, getting to know them as people and respecting their opinions, Tuke established an atmosphere in which staff began to see patients as people of equal worth, rather than a group of lesser beings to be punished and derided for their misfortunes. Such respect, he saw, raised people's self-esteem, thus encouraging and motivating them towards wellness.

Second, Tuke believed that 'the patient, feeling himself of some consequence, is induced to support it by exertion' (Tuke 1813, p. 143). Thus, while he saw that staff had a responsibility to respect patients and increase their feelings of self-worth, the patients themselves also had a responsibility to conduct themselves in an appropriate manner. He sites examples of people who were able to be released from their shackles and those able to participate in tea parties as a result of this mutual consideration. He also writes of explaining to a 'maniac . . . of almost Herculean size and figure' his anxious wish to make every inhabitant of The Retreat as comfortable as possible, and that the person 'so completely succeeded that, during his stay, no coercive means were ever employed towards him . . . and in about four months he was discharged perfectly recovered' (Tuke 1813, p. 147).

Thus, Tuke's fundamental beliefs in people's individuality and worth were reflected through his treatment of them with respect and kindness, and also by giving them responsibility for their own actions and behaviour, such that both staff and patients had a part to play in the person's recovery. He reflected, 'I can truly declare that by gentleness of manner, and kindness of treatment, I have seldom failed to obtain the confidence and conciliate the esteem [of people]' (Tuke 1813, p. 135).

Humanism

These early ideas were further developed through

the ideas of humanists in the early part of this century, and their belief in the concepts of personal freedom, self-determination and creativity. Two important exponents of this theory, Abraham Maslow and Carl Rogers, expanded our understanding of, and belief in, treating people as individuals.

Maslow saw that the essence of Being was that we are whole, free, healthy and purposeful. He studied healthy, well-functioning people and saw their motivations as a core concept to their well-being. He placed these motivations in a hierarchy (see Ch. 32) with self-actualisation, i.e. the full use and exploration of talents, capacities and potentials, at the top. He concluded that there is, in all individuals, a drive towards actualisation of inherent potentials, thus enhancing life, and a desire to satisfy needs which ensure physical and psychological survival and well-being, thus maintaining life. Maslow felt that a person could only strive towards actualisation once survival needs had been satisfied. In everyday terms this could mean, for example, that a person could not enjoy the challenge of mastering a new computer program (esteem and self-esteem) if he had an unresolved argument with a partner (love and belonging), nor settle to complete some embroidery (self-actualisation) if she needed to visit the toilet (physiological needs)!

Carl Rogers also studied individuals' abilities to maintain their health and well-being. He believed that people are free, normally capable of dealing with the limitations of life and able to be in charge of their own destiny and make choices concerning their future. He saw people as having the capacity to change and grow, and, like Maslow, believed that a desire for self-actualisation underlies their actions. From these beliefs came the idea that people should exercise their capacity to develop and change, and indeed had a responsibility to do so.

Rogers, like Tuke, saw self-esteem as an important element in the way in which people function and their ability to do so. He said that people had a need for unconditional positive regard, i.e. the need for other people to treat them with respect as a person of worth, regardless of their circumstances. Because people have a need for

positive regard they are aware of, and hold important, attitudes towards them of those whom they see as significant in their lives. As people aim to gain positive regard and become aware of others' approval or disapproval of them, they will develop a sense of themselves — a self-concept. This idea of self is seen to underpin the direction in which self-actualisation is manifest. For example, a person who is seen to be a competent artist, parent, mathematician or cook will see such an image as part of himself. This concept will therefore underpin his ideas, and thus his behaviour, as he strives towards self-actualisation.

Humanism also stressed the importance of a person's own subjective and individual view of himself and his world. Barris et al (1983) saw subjectivity (the way in which an individual sees a situation or event) and intuition (a person's natural instinctive feeling for something) as vital and important elements in the way people experience things. Therefore, an individual's own view of a situation is valid and important for him.

Beliefs as an influence on practice

Such beliefs, as a fundamental element in the philosophy of occupational therapy, are reflected in the attitudes that therapists have towards the people they work with, and the ways in which they work with them.

First, occupational therapists believe that people are individuals. They do not treat all people alike, nor see some opinions as being of lesser value. They should, as a result, get to know the person and help him to identify his needs in order to be able to organise appropriate intervention strategies. A belief that people are different from each other should lead to tolerance of those who do not conform to social norms, and the therapist must therefore be aware of accommodating differing ideas and attitudes. She should not be led in her decisions primarily by the person's diagnosis, nor by the values, fashions and pressures of the service or system in which she works — an element that is sometimes difficult to identify and overcome. Thus, the therapist's belief in humanism gives rise to a person-centred approach.

Second, occupational therapists believe that

the way in which a person views something is important and should be treated as reality for that individual. She shows this belief through expressing an understanding of the person's feeling an acceptance of its validity for him. For example, if a person has undergone trauma which has affected coordination in all four limbs, the therapist should not dismiss the fact that his primary concern is that he cannot hold a newspaper simply because she feels his overriding difficulty is that he cannot walk. Related to this is the therapist's belief in the worth of individuals. If she believes people are of worth, her action must be to respect their opinions and build their self-esteem. Where, for instance, a decision has to be made about a discharge destination for an elderly person, or where assessment is being made for a piece of equipment, the person's opinions and expectations are of equal importance and value to those of the therapist or other care workers. The therapist's knowledge of motivation, coupled with her respect for people's opinions, leads her to believe that a decision made primarily by a person himself is more likely to be upheld than one made by others on his behalf. How many occupational therapists, with the wisdom of hindsight, can remember occasions on which they ordered equipment or advised on different strategies, only to discover, some time later, that the equipment is still wrapped in brown paper or that old ways are still adhered to, because the person had not been sufficiently involved in the decision-making process and therefore did not incorporate another's suggestions into his life-style.

Such beliefs also affect and dictate the relationship developed with an individual, which should be one based on mutual respect and cooperation. The therapist, in believing that an individual is responsible for his own life and in charge of his destiny, will work with a person to facilitate his ability to make treatment decisions and to develop skills he sees as appropriate.

Occupational therapists also believe that a person has the ability to adapt to unforeseen circumstances so that he can carry on with his life in a way that is meaningful to him. While not everyone will adapt to a similar circumstance in the same way (for example one person whose car fails to start on the way to work in the morning may ask for a lift from a neighbour, another may fetch his toolkit and tackle the job himself, a third may call a taxi, while another may telephone a motoring organisation or perhaps phone in sick to work!), each person will be able to alter his behaviour in order to deal effectively with the unforeseen circumstance. The therapist is optimistic about the person's ability to shape his own life. In believing that he has a responsibility for his life the therapist will not encourage him passively to accept what has happened as an act of fate that cannot be addressed, but will encourage him to strive actively to reshape his life. She may discover, of course, that some people's religious and/or cultural beliefs may make such action difficult or impossible. Where this happens it is the therapist's responsibility, through her understanding of such values, to ensure that any decisions made are compatible with the person's underlying beliefs. She will, therefore, use only strategies that will actively involve the person in achieving his own aims and will not use media which require him to be passive or to act in a way contrary to his value system. The occupational therapist should not, therefore, encourage the person to strive to achieve what she, or the service providers, feels is 'best' for the person, nor perhaps should she consider, without thorough evaluation, the use of media such as massage, vibration, aromatherapy or reflexology unless these are used specifically to increase active participation.

Last, in believing that actualisation is the prime motivator for action the occupational therapist should work with the person in order to identify the areas he sees as important and in which he wishes to fulfil his potential. Intervention should be based on activities which have meaning for that person, as these will then act as inherent motivators and reflect a positive self-concept. For example, for an elderly person aiming to regain upper limb function, activities related to grandchildren (making cakes for the school fête or a rack to hold CDs) may be more meaningful, whereas for a young person with similar difficulties activities incorporating their interest in sport or music may help them towards regaining skills.

Having a knowledge of, and a respect for, the people she is working with is of prime importance to the occupational therapist. Treating people as individuals, accepting their view of events, encouraging them to take responsibility for the way their life progresses, and believing in their ability to do so, are the main ways in which the occupational therapist's belief in people as individuals is translated into her everyday professional practice.

2. Activity as fundamental to well-being

'To do is to be' (Mill, cited in Cracknell 1993). If we watch people going about their daily business it is easy to concur with the idea that humans are occupational by nature. If we observe a toddler's day we see that he is busy from dawn until dusk (with the possible exception of a few hours sleep), in an endless round of exploring, climbing, playing with water, pulling toys, building bricks, bouncing on the bed, banging objects together, eating and drinking. His day is full of activities, each fulfilling a purpose (quenching thirst, developing his ability to explore his world or making a noise) and each helping him to learn and develop. Piaget (1969), indeed, states that all our knowledge of the world comes from engagement in activity.

Activity continues to occur spontaneously throughout the life of healthy individuals. As a person grows older the nature of his 'doing' will change. This change, and the content of the person's activities, will be determined in part by his perceived roles and responsibilities, and influenced by the culture and society in which he lives. Deviation from the boundaries of activity set by the group within which he lives is often not acceptable, and can lead to negative feedback and lowered self-esteem.

Activities will, therefore, reflect a person's view of himself and his occupation. Occupation is that which defines and organises a sphere of action (a range of activity) over a period of time, and is perceived by the individual as part of his identity, i.e. as something that he 'owns'. Occupation may

be related to a role title, such as 'farmer' or 'dancer', or may organise a sphere of activity reflecting the person's self-identity but bringing no particular role with the title, such as the image of oneself as an independent person or one who believes in helping the welfare of others. Thus a person's occupations are reflected in the activities he performs. A young adult, for example, may spend his day in personal care activities, eating, travelling to work or college, meeting and talking with friends, working, playing in a band or organising a charity event, and each of his occupations will reflect the image he holds of himself as, for example, independent person, student, musician and charity worker. As a person progresses through life, activities, as reflected by occupations, roles and beliefs, will vary, as also do the number and pace of activities, as his life stage and abilities alter.

People in a state of well-being, therefore, are active and occupational by nature. The need for activity is central to human existence, as any being must work in order to survive. All living organisms, no matter how simple or complex, must locate and absorb food, maintain themselves in a suitable environment and reproduce. As humans developed more efficient ways of ensuring their own survival, societies were established in which labour was divided between its members. Thus individuals had the opportunity not only to develop particular skills within their area of concern, but also to fulfil their need for creativity and to enjoy periods of leisure.

It can be seen, therefore, that to maintain a state of occupational well-being people require a balance of the activities and occupations that our complex societies have created, and this balance is reflected in the habits and routines which control the rhythm of our lives. Routines and habits balanced between success in activities of productivity (which may be related to maintaining our environment and/or acquiring sustenance), self-care (related to maintenance of the individual) and leisure (in which the person has the opportunity to fulfil his own creative, aesthetic, physical, social or intellectual pursuits) will maintain a state of well-being. Cynkin & Robinson (1990) show that healthy individuals

---

Box 1.2 Basic assumptions in occupational therapy (based on Meyer 1922)

- A fundamental link exists between health and occupation
- Healthy occupation maintains a balance between existing, thinking and acting
- A unity exists between mind and body
- When participation in occupation is interrupted mind and body deteriorate
- As occupation maintains mind and body it is suited to the restoration of functional ability

---

have flexible and adaptable routines which reflect their abilities, responsibilities and potentials.

Five fundamental assumptions

In looking at the occupational nature of people Meyer, writing in *The Archives of Occupational Therapy* in 1922, explored five fundamental assumptions (Box 1.2). First, he linked occupation and health, suggesting that occupation was linked to both physical and psychological well-being. We know, for example, that our body and its functions deteriorate if not regularly used, joints stiffen and muscles weaken if under-exercised, and vital capacity and coronary function suffer if lungs and heart are not regularly challenged. We know also that we suffer disorientation if we are deprived of sensory stimulation. Similarly people require to be socially and cognitively active to maintain psychological health. Memory, language, thinking and other psychological skills will ultimately diminish if not used.

Second, Meyer proposed that healthy occupation maintains a balance between existing, thinking and acting. If we reflect upon our own lives we know that we do not spend our time in a constant round of physical action. Our 'doing' is indeed balanced between existing (eating, drinking, visiting the toilet, sleeping, resting, making love), thinking (which may include studying, remembering loved ones, problem-solving, writing a shopping list or creative thinking such as designing, writing or computer programming) and action (which may include any form of physical activity). It is determined by our roles, occupa-

tions and interests, and is usually organised into habits and routines which control our 'being'.

Third, Meyer assumed an invisible link between mind and body. He saw that morale and will are maintained by participation in activity, and that a synergy exists between physical and mental activity. Individuals, by nature, are likely to strive for function, acceptance and well-being. Our need for activity, however, comes from an intrinsic desire to explore and master our environment. Through this underlying need we can gain information about both ourselves and our surroundings, and, in endeavouring to achieve mastery, we gain the skills, confidence and abilities by which we measure our self-worth and enhance our well-being. Thus, activities we are personally motivated to do bring their own rewards. These rewards, known as intrinsic motivators, reflect the link between our thinking and doing (mind and body) and are the prime motivators of our actions. If we reflect on the activities and tasks into which we put most effort, we can see that our desire for mastery and the successful participation in an activity is its own reward. By our nature we are attracted towards novel situations, particularly those that have particular meaning for us. Edmund Hillary, for example, climbed Mount Everest 'because it was there'; the effort we put into learning to play an instrument or drive a car reflects our desire for mastery, a need for self-worth, a feeling of well-being and an intrinsic reward from the outcome of our efforts. The gain from repairing a radio bought for a few pence at a boot sale, or from planning a surprise party for a friend, shows us that mastery and activity of our own choosing brings its own reward. Therefore, when a person participates in an activity that has meaning for him, he is more likely to put effort into it and to continue it for a longer period, and one can sympathise, perhaps, with the anonymous patient who wrote:

Here I sit at this great big loom,
Making God knows what for God knows whom.

Perhaps the principles of intrinsic motivation were not fully understood nor put to use by his occupational therapist!

Extrinsic motivators, i.e. those coming from

outside or being imposed, may in the short term engage a person in activity, but will not ultimately lead to well-being.

Fourth, Meyer related that the inability to participate in activity, for whatever reason, resulted in a breakdown of habits and routines and in physical and psychological deterioration. Any 'enforced idleness' which results in a lack of occupation can lead to the person's inability to live his life competently. Our experience shows us this is so. Accounts of the behaviours of prisoners, and more recently hostages, have highlighted the difficulties that lack of activity can create. Studies of animals kept in captivity show negative changes in behaviour, and our anecdotal sayings, such as 'The less you do the less you want to do' and 'To rest is to rust', reflect our awareness that inactivity changes behaviour and affects self-worth, ability and motivation. Similarly we can imagine that, should a return to meaningful activity not be encouraged in a person with a dysfunction, a downward spiral of non-participation, non-mastery, lowered self-esteem and lack of motivation will ensue. Fidler & Fidler (1978) summarised this process by stating that 'A reduction in doing generates pathology'.

Such a state is known as occupational dysfunction and is the primary area of concern of the occupational therapist. Because of the occupational therapist's belief in individuals, this state must be viewed in the light of how important a particular area of occupational dysfunction is to that person. Loss of a lower limb, for example, while in no way a trivial dysfunction, may be regarded by one individual, because of his outlook, roles and occupations, as a tragic but surmountable situation, whereas for another individual the same situation may appear utterly insurmountable. We can, therefore, see the concept upon which the World Health Organization based its 1980 definition of health and loss of healthy functioning:

● *Impairment* is any loss or abnormality of psychological, physiological or anatomical structure or function.
● *Disability* is any restriction or lack (resulting from an impairment) of ability to perform an activity in the manner or within the range considered normal for a human being.
● *Handicap* is the disadvantage for a given individual resulting from an impairment or disability that limits or prevents the fulfilment of a role that is normal (depending on age, sex, social and cultural factors) for that individual.

(Jeffrey 1993)

Such definitions show a growing understanding that the effect of dysfunction is determined by a person's attitudes and life-style and the society in which he lives, rather than by his diagnosis. While the definitions have been challenged because of the way in which 'ownership' of the handicap is placed upon the individual rather than society, they do show an understanding that the way in which a person functions is not mainly determined by diagnosis.

Finally, Meyer postulated that since occupation was the key component in the maintenance of well-being, it could also be used as the medium to restore and acquire functional ability (occupational performance).

This belief that occupation is fundamental to health is reflected in the principles and practice of occupational therapy. Clark (1979), in stating that 'Man's ability to direct and effect his own purpose in life may be seen as a most unique and primary indicator of his general well-being or health', reflects our belief that, in a healthy state, a person is able to adapt and achieve a satisfying life, function adequately in chosen roles and enjoy a sense of well-being, which in turn directs the thinking and action of occupational therapy practice.

The therapist sees her area of concern as being primarily the restoration or acquisition of occupational well-being in a person who is in a state of occupational dysfunction. In being aware of the need for balance in occupations the therapist will address dysfunctions in all areas of the person's life, and, where necessary, encourage the restoration or acquisition of a balance of activities related to his daily living skills, productivity and leisure. The therapist, in believing that activity brings its own reward, will use, either as a therapeutic medium or as an aim for the restoration of occupational well-being, those activities which hold particular interest and meaning for the individual, and will therefore act as prime motivators. In carrying forward this belief into practice the therapist will be able to assess the person's need and use, or facilitate, meaningful activity in order to help the person acquire occupational well-being.

3. Use of activity to restore occupational performance

Where occupational performance has been interrupted a person can:

a. through the medium of activity develop the adaptive skills required to restore, maintain or acquire function, and/or
b. modify activity in order to facilitate occupational performance.

Within the philosophy of Moral Treatment was the belief that mental illness occurred when people failed to adapt successfully to external pressures. As a result they were seen to adopt either faulty coping strategies or indeed no alternative strategies at all. These early assumptions have formed the basis of the belief that occupational dysfunction in any aspect of a person's life can occur as a result of the person's inability to acquire the ability to adapt (adaptive skills). This may occur for a variety of reasons.

First, a child may fail to develop adaptive skills as a result of dysfunction manifest at birth or in early childhood. A child, for example, who cannot explore the environment as a result of motor or sensory dysfunction, and possibly also because of overprotection by his parents, will be unable to develop the normal movement patterns or motor skills required to participate in everyday physical activities. His inability to move normally will not only prevent him developing adaptive motor and sensory skills (so that he can learn, for example, not to lose his balance while playing on his rocking horse or not to put his hand too near to the teapot because it is hot), but will also impede his development of social, language and other global skills because of his inability to participate in everyday experiences and relationships.

Alternatively, physical dysfunction as a result of an acquired illness, such as a neurological, metabolic or vascular condition, may inhibit or curtail a person's ability to use existing adaptive skills. His situation can appear so overwhelming that he cannot, on his own, acquire the necessary new adaptive skills that he needs for successful occupational performance. For example, an adult who has suffered a head injury will need assistance to acquire adaptive skills such as improving motor and cognitive function in order to regain his ability to look after his garden, drive his car or return to his job. Additionally he will need help in modifying activities in order to restore occupational performance. He may, for example, need to learn strategies to assist with shortfall in memory, or need help to adapt his telephone to compensate for poor speech.

However, it may be felt that maladaptive performance can be the cause, as well as the outcome, of some physical dysfunctions. Circumstances in which a person fails to adapt successfully to external stresses and adopts maladaptive coping strategies may lead to physical or psychological disorders. Yerxa (1983) felt that 'a person's level of health and their ability to adapt within occupational performance are interrelated'. Research indicates, for example, (see Ch. 29) that the origin of certain types of coronary dysfunction can be traced to poor coping strategies, and similar schools of thought have been postulated for conditions such as irritable bowel syndrome and certain skin and respiratory conditions.

a. Developing adaptive skills

It can be seen, therefore, that when successful adaptation (i.e. any change in function that promotes survival and self-actualisation [AOTA 1979]) is impaired for whatever reason, occupational performance will be interrupted. It is this interruption of occupational performance that is the prime concern of the occupational therapist, and the impact that a dysfunction has on a person, rather than the dysfunction itself, that is the focus of occupational therapy. For an occupational therapist, for example, working with a person who has an amputation of a lower limb, the main focus of intervention of occupational therapy is not the state of the remaining part of the limb, nor primarily the way in which he uses his prosthetic limb, but rather the impact that this change, and the related loss of adaptive skills, has on those activities he wishes to perform in his everyday life. It could be said that the occupational therapist focuses on handicap, rather than on impairment or disability.

Occupational therapists, because of their belief in individuals' abilities and responsibility to influence their environment and their health, see that a person's way forward in gaining or regaining adaptive skills is through his own efforts, i.e. through active participation in treatment. Such active participation may take many forms, and occupational therapists develop and encourage this by facilitating the person to make decisions, solve problems, develop new behaviours and habits and determine priorities in order to help him gain control over his dysfunction. Such a belief gives rise to Mary Reilly's (1962) influential and evocative words which state that:

Man, through the use of his hands, as they are energised by his mind and will, can influence the state of his own health.

In facilitating change in a person with dysfunction occupational therapists, believing that occupation is fundamental to health, also believe that activity can be used as the medium through which a person can acquire adaptive skills. When establishing the culture of moral treatment at The Retreat Tuke (1813, p. 156) wrote 'of all the modes by which patients may be reduced to restrain themselves, regular employment is perhaps the most generally efficacious'. Tuke not only saw that activity changed the person's focus from disability to activity, but also believed that 'those kinds of employment are doubtless to be preferred . . . that are most agreeable to the patient' (p. 156). Thus activities that are meaningful to the person and relate to his personal functional goals are those most successful in helping him to develop adaptive skills. For example, an occupational therapist may, through the use of activity analysis, know that working with wood will assist a man who has a hemiplegia to develop

adaptive motor and sensory skills. The use of this activity will therefore be considered as part of his programme. In order to facilitate his active participation in the activity the occupational therapist will understand that encouraging the man to produce a hobby horse for his grandson or a plant trough for his wife is more likely to provide intrinsic motivation than asking him to make a transfer board to add to the pile in the stock cupboard. By contrast a young woman with a hemiplegia as a result of a road traffic accident is perhaps more likely to be motivated by making a bedside lamp or a mobile for her niece. Equally the therapist may realise that, while woodwork may be functionally appropriate, an alternative medium such as gardening, computing or cookery may prove more purposeful for one or both of these people. Research has shown that where people are engaged in activity that is meaningful for them they are more likely to put more effort and time into the task.

b. Modifying activity

Where occupational performance has been limited by dysfunction and the occupational therapist considers that intervention to restore adaptive skills is not feasible, she may feel that the most appropriate method of restoring that performance is through adaptation not of the person's skills but of the way in which the activity is performed. For example, where a person has limited respiratory function because of a chronic respiratory condition, activities to restore his abilities to their previous level would seem to be inappropriate. In this instance, therefore, the occupational therapist would endeavour not to change the person's capacities to fit the existing activity but to adapt the activity so that he can then perform it within his existing level of performance. She may, for example, modify the activity of climbing upstairs to visit the bathroom or bedroom by discussing the installation of a stair lift, the creation of a comparable downstairs facility, or even the possibility of moving to a flat or bungalow. It is interesting to note that with current demographic, medical and legislative changes this area of adapting activities and environments to facilitate occupational performance in the chronically disabled is forming an ever-increasing part of the occupational therapist's role.

Activities used should therefore be person centred and directed through a task towards a meaningful goal, in order to bring their own rewards.

The fundamental concept related to the use of activity as the medium for restoring occupational behaviour is based on the belief that people have the ability to learn and change throughout life and thus affect their behaviour. Llorens (cited in Clark 1979) indeed referred to occupational therapists as 'change agents'. Any intervention undertaken by the therapist is founded on the basic understanding that the person, in order to change his behaviour, has the capacity to learn. It is important, therefore, when facilitating the acquisition of new skills, that the therapist has a sound knowledge of the styles and theories of learning. For some, such as a young person who loses part of his hand and has to relearn to drive his car, the process of learning to adapt his skill may be relatively quick and painless. However for others, maybe an elderly woman who has lost the ability to drive her car following a cerebrovascular accident, the adaptive processes involved in reorganising her life may take a long time to complete. Her capacity to learn will still remain, but may be tempered by lowered energy levels, long-term use of now inappropriate habits, a lack of immediate family support and her grief at her loss of capacity and the independence afforded by her car.

THE HISTORY OF OCCUPATIONAL THERAPY

As can be seen from the previous discussion, occupational therapy aims to help people with occupational dysfunction gain, regain or maintain the most appropriate pattern of occupational performance through the medium of purposeful activity. Although the profession itself is relatively young, the idea of using activity as a means of helping the 'sick' is by no means new.

ROOTS FROM ANCIENT TIMES

While there is no historical reference to occupational therapy as such until the present century, Egyptian writings dating from as long ago as 2000 BC tell of temples where 'melancholics' congregated in large numbers to seek relief. 'Games and recreations' were instituted, and everyone's time 'was taken up by some pleasurable occupation' (Pinel 1803, cited in Howarth & MacDonald 1946). The classical god of healing, Aesculapius, was reputed to have quietened delirium 'with songs, farces and music' (Le Clerc 1699, cited in MacDonald et al 1970). Aulus Cornelius Celsus (AD 14–37), a Roman encyclopaedist whose writings included an account of surgical practice, also recommended 'music, conversation, reading, exercise to the point of fatigue, travel and a change of scenery' to ease troubled minds (Licht 1948). The celebrated Greek physician, Galen (AD c. 130–200) advocated treatment by occupation, suggesting digging, fishing, housebuilding and shipbuilding. Galen also felt that 'Employment is nature's best physician and is essential to human happiness' (cited in MacDonald et al 1970).

Little development of the idea of using occupation therapeutically seems to have been recorded in the Dark Ages, although the 5th century author, Martianus Capella, recommended music for the treatment of 'disturbance of the mind and disease of the body' (Licht 1948) and Caelius Aurelianus, a physician whose writings date from the 4th or 5th century, emphasised that the patient should share the effort of rehabilitating himself.

THE 18TH AND 19TH CENTURIES

Our modern understanding of the nature and treatment of disease has its roots in the 19th century. Prior to that time, it was felt that the key to the treatment (of lunatics) lay in fear, and that the best means of producing fear was by punishment. Deriving from the practices of the Dark Ages, many forms of cruel and torturous 'treatments' were devised. Lunatics were not regarded as having rights and needs, but as deserving only ridicule, confinement and punishment. The French physician, Philippe Pinel (1745–1826),

---

Box 1.3 An outline of the historical concepts underpinning occupational therapy and the milestones in the development of the British profession

2600 BC	The Chinese thought that disease resulted from organic inactivity, so used physical training as therapy
2000 BC	The Egyptians dedicated temples for the treatment of melancholics. Here patients' time was spent in pleasurable activity such as games and recreation
1000 BC	The Persians used physical therapy to train their youth
600 BC	Aesculapius, the Greek classical god of healing, soothed delirium with songs, farces and music
600 BC–200 AD	Pythagorus, Thales and Orpheus used music to sooth troubled minds. Hippocrates emphasised the link between mind and body and recommended wrestling, riding, labour and vigorous exercise. Cornelius Celcus, who studied anatomy and medicine, recommended sailing, hunting, handling of arms, ball games, running and walking for their therapeutic benefits
1250–1700	Leonardo da Vinci, Decartes and Francis Bacon studied anatomy, movement, rhythm, posture and energy expenditure. Ramazzini, Professor of Practical Medicine, stressed the importance of the prevention of illness. He observed his patient-workers in his workshop and placed high value on weaving, cobbling, tailoring and pottery as exercise. This was early movement analysis
1780	Tissot used occupational exercise for the treatment of the mentally ill. He advocated sewing, playing the violin, sweeping, sawing, bell ringing, hammering, chopping wood, riding and swimming
1786	Philipe Pinel used work as therapy in Paris. His name is one associated with the concept of Moral Treatment
1786	William Cowper, in a letter to Lady Hesketh, dated 16 January 1786, described the malady which had seized him and how he improved his own state of mind by the use of carpentry, gardening, writing and poetry. This may be the first recorded account of a patient's own experience in English literature
1792	The Quaker William Tuke opened The Retreat in York. Tuke's name is very much associated with Moral Treatment
1850	The Crimean War enabled many women to take up careers. The nursing profession began to develop under Florence Nightingale
1914–1918	The First World War — physiotherapy began to develop

The development of occupational therapy as a profession

End of 19th century	An increasing awareness of the value of occupation as a treatment. The term 'occupational therapy' began to evolve. The emphasis was still very much on the use of occupation within the psychiatric field
1924	Dr Elizabeth Casson introduced occupational therapy into her nursing home in Clifton, Bristol, after attending a conference by Professor Sir David Henderson and visiting a newly established occupational therapy school in Philadelphia, USA
1925	Margaret Fulton, the first qualified occupational therapist to work in this country (after training in Philadelphia) established an occupational therapy department at the Royal Cornhill Hospital, Aberdeen. Dr Elizabeth Casson sent Constance Tebbit to train in the USA. She returned to work in the Dorset House Psychiatric Nursing Home in Bristol
1930	Dr Casson established the first British occupational training school at Dorset House, with Constance Tebbit as principal
1932	In Scotland the first professional association was formed. It had 30 members
1936	The Astley Ainslie school was established in Edinburgh. The Association of Occupational Therapists (AOT) was formed in England
1938	The first public examinations were held
1939–1945	The AOT set up short courses for occupational therapy auxilliaries. This could be upgraded to full professional status with further study. The War Emergency Diploma allowed professionals with previous qualifications, e.g. teachers and nurses, to qualify as occupational therapists
1941	St Andrews School of Occupational Therapy in Northampton was established as the second English school
1943	AOT included England, Wales and Northern Ireland
1947	The National Health Service Act. Occupational therapy schools were privately funded at this time
1950s	A Joint Council was formed to look at matters common to the AOT and Scottish AOT
1951	First International Congress run by the AOT
1952	World Federation of Occupational Therapists was inaugurated, with Margaret Fulton as president and Constance Glyn-Owens (née Tebbit) as secretary
1954	First World Congress, held in Edinburgh
1960/1	The establishment of the Council for the Professions Supplementary to Medicine leads to State Registration
1974	The British Association of Occupational Therapists was formed from a merger between AOT and SAOT
1977	First European Congress
1978	The Association divided into: The College of Occupational Therapists (which deals with professional and educational matters) and The British Association of Occupational Therapists (the trade union)
1990s	Training to first degree level is established on all pre-registration courses

took a more enlightened view and instituted reforms in the treatment of the mentally ill, the most famous of which was to release asylum inmates from their shackles. He 'prescribed physical exercises and manual occupations', believing that 'rigorously executed manual labour is the best method of securing good morale and discipline' (Pinel 1806, cited in Licht 1948). He wrote of a Spanish hospital which received patients of all ranks, pointing out that the recovery rate was higher among the lower classes, who were employed in the work of the hospital, than amongst the 'idle grandees'. But the idea of patients being 'put to work' met with resistance in private hospitals, where it was thought that those who paid for treatment should not be expected to work.

In this same period Tuke established The Retreat. Many physicians followed Tuke, and the 19th century saw more widespread acceptance of occupation and activity for the treatment of the mentally ill in particular. A Dr Cleaton of Liverpool, in a report to the Lunacy Commission, said: 'The most important recent improvement . . . is the extent to which occupation is adopted' (cited in Licht 1948).

THE 20TH CENTURY

By the beginning of the 20th century the idea of using activity, occupation or work in the treatment of the mentally ill had become quite widely established. At this time, it was becoming more socially acceptable for women to take up careers and to join the professions. Their traditional role, therefore, as carers of the sick, could now incorporate the expanding knowledge related to that care, and this role became more 'respectable'.

The term 'occupational therapy' was first coined in the 19th century by George Barton, an American doctor. The first English training school for occupational therapists was set up at Dorset House, Bristol, a treatment centre for neurotic and early psychotic patients, by Dr Elizabeth Casson in 1930 (Fig. 1.2) and the first English conference on occupational therapy was held in 1934. Shortly thereafter, in 1936, the English Association of Occupational Therapists was formed (its active membership rising to 120 by 1944) and in 1938 the first public exams in occupational therapy were held (Box 1.4).

The Second World War has often been seen as the herald of the expansion of occupational therapy, especially in the field of treatment of the physically injured. Many young men who suffered appalling physical and psychological trauma during the war needed rehabilitation, particularly in relation to their 'occupational' or work needs (Fig. 1.3).

The influence of the medical model

Occupational therapy at this time was firmly established within the medical model. For whatever reason, be it a desire to gain respectability, recognition or confidence, or a lack of adequate resources to carry out its 'holistic' philosophy independently, occupational therapy became firmly linked to the medical model. Early texts reflect this position. In *An approach to Occupational Therapy* (1960) Mary S. Jones writes: 'On admission the occupational therapist stresses to the patient that "the work is planned to fulfil the doctor's aims of treatment"' and that 'It is the medical officer's responsibility to place the emphasis of treatment where it is of most value to the individual patient.' Howarth & MacDonald (1946) state that 'The occupational therapist carries out her treatment on prescription from the medical officer only. No case should be dealt with without this prescription.' The use of words such as 'patient', 'prescription' and 'case' signals that the setting is certainly a medical one. The implication of this, i.e. that the medical officer takes overall responsibility for the treatment, certainly reflects that both the therapist and patient were well and truly under the doctor's thumb and that the treatment prescribed wholly reflected the doctor's rather than the patient's view of his needs. How different from practice later, in which, as Bumphrey (1987) states, 'The emphasis is on the therapist working *with* the disabled person to achieve what he or she wants to do.' Colson, in 1945, defined the aims of occupational therapy in purely physical terms. He said that they were:

Conservation of muscular function,

A

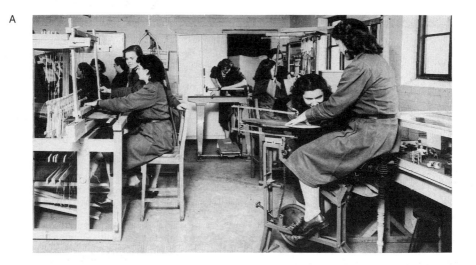

B

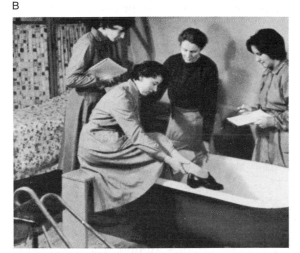

C

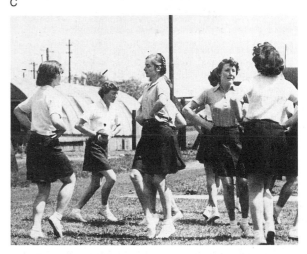

Fig. 1.2 Students training in the early days of the Dorset House School. (A) In the workshop. (B) In activities of daily living. (C) In recreational activities. (Reproduced by kind permission of the School of Occupational Therapy, Oxford Brookes University, Oxford.)

Strengthening of weak muscles,
Mobilising of stiff joints,
Re-education of neuromuscular co-ordination in the hand, and,
Teaching the normal use of the affected part.

In deference to the holistic approach buried deep within the philosophy of occupational therapy Colson did, lastly, say that it also aimed 'To encourage the patient' (Fig. 1.4).

A year later, in 1946, Howarth & MacDonald, in an effort to deal with the vastly increased numbers of people requiring the services of occu-

pational therapy, divided the discipline into two branches. These they defined as:

1. General: This was where some form of occupation was necessary, for example where a patient had to remain in bed for a long period, in order to prevent depression and to maintain his morale
2. Special: This, by contrast, was carefully selected and prescribed treatment which had some remedial purpose in view.

One can see the separation of occupational

Box 1.4 Case studies

The following case histories, published in the *Lancet*, were written in 1941 by Dr Elizabeth Casson, Medical Director of the Dorset House School of Occupational Therapy, to draw attention to occupational therapy. (Reproduced by kind permission of Oxford Brookes University, Oxford.)

Case 1

A woman of 23 with arthrodesis of a tuberculous hip. After operation she had developed a functional disease of the knee-joint. She was lacking in self-confidence and was too conscious of her disability. Her inability to sit at an ordinary table seemed the chief cause of her unhappiness and also her inability to return to her work as a shorthand-typist. She was taught to weave on a small loom with hand controls in order to interest her in the subject without referring to her leg. She was then promoted to a foot-power loom in which the warp was raised or lowered by flexing the knee-joint. While using the hand-loom she had become so keen on the texture and pattern of the material she was weaving that she was glad to perform the necessary movements, and was soon able to realise that her knee was quite capable of being bent to a more aesthetic posture. Her gait improved at the same time. She asked to stay on for a few weeks to finish the length of material she was weaving and then returned to her office work.

Case 2

A man of 53, suffering from the after-effects of acute infective polyneuritis. He had been completely paralysed for several months but had recovered sufficiently to walk, and by several trick movements he could feed himself. Treatment began with weaving a rug on a frame threaded with a warp of string. The patient's deltoid and extensor muscles were weak and could not bear the weight of his arms so his arms and hands were slung in canvas loops from brackets extended from the top of the frame. He had a spasmodic contraction of the shoulder muscles which relaxed when his arms were suspended. Improvement became evident in the first few days, since the patient enjoyed the work. The next stage was to support the wrists only on an adjustable slat placed across the frame, again leaving the fingers free to weave

and to push the threads into place, thus getting active extension of the fingers and wrists. As the muscles improved in tone and strength, new crafts were prescribed, such as knotting dog leads, stool-seating and woodwork. The dart-board for a few minutes each day helped in the cure.

Case 3

A man, aged 61, who had had a compound fracture of the radius from a conveyor-belt accident. His shoulder had been strained, and he had arthritis of shoulder, elbow and wrist with much residual disability of shoulder, arm and forearm. Mental depression was pronounced. Treatment was first given in the form of easy weaving on a small hand-loom; at this time the therapist was making friends with the patient and gaining his confidence. Later he made a warp on the 'mill', encouraged by the knowledge that the warp was needed for another patient's work. An occupation had to be chosen that could be carried out at a level which gave easy abduction of the upper arm to begin with; this was increased gradually by raising the height of the mill without the patient noticing that he was doing more. As soon as he realised that his angle of abduction had increased his confidence was aroused and he then willingly cooperated in carrying out the changes in his work that increased the effort needed. His recovery was completed by getting him to sand-paper and paint screens raised to a level above his shoulder and to drill holes in a solitaire board, which exercised flexion and extension of wrist. Finally he did weaving on a large foot-loom which enabled him to get larger movements; easy supination was achieved by throwing and catching the shuttle.

Case 4

A left-handed man with compound fracture of left proximal phalanx of the ring finger and simple fracture of the little finger. Even passive extension of these fingers was impossible. Treatment was by joinery, which was his hobby; first he did planing with fingers extended as far as possible on the plane, and then sawing and generalised movement, with various tools, to ensure complete movement and suppleness,. The patient was entirely cooperative and the fingers became almost normal.

---

therapy into 'diversional' (general) and 'therapeutic' (special) branches, a division which has plagued occupational therapists ever since. As 'special' occupational therapy was to be restricted to the 'curative workshops' and 'general' occupational therapy was to be restricted to long-term, bed-bound patients (Fig. 1.5), it is easy to see that the diversional side of occupational therapy is the one that was more on public view in the wards and, therefore, the one that became firmly

established as the main component of occupational therapy in the eyes of other patients and hospital staff. Additionally, as many conditions involved protracted bed treatment (two years bedrest was not exceptional for people with tuberculosis) and as, due to 'trade prejudice' it was not possible to use 'more realistic occupations' than crafts, 'the wrong emphasis [was given to] the occupational aspect of treatment' (MacDonald et al 1970). It is clear why present-

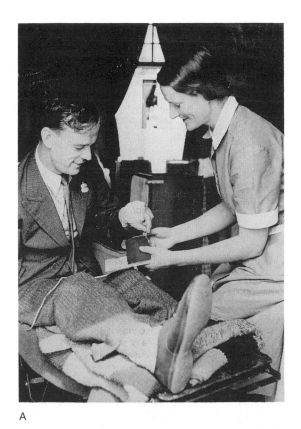

A

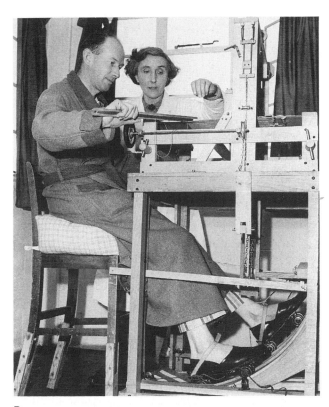

B

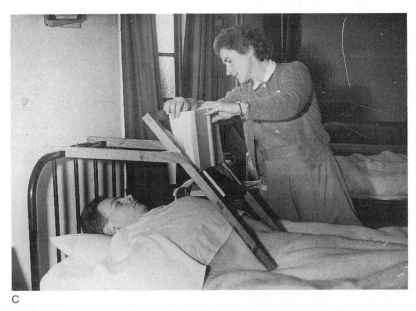

C

Fig. 1.3 Early days in physical occupational therapy. (A) A one-handed air-raid casualty learning to use his left hand. (B) Weaving on a loom adapted to encourage flexion and extension of the knees. (C) Providing a book to read for a tuberculosis sufferer on long-term bedrest. (Reproduced by kind permission of the School of Occupational Therapy, Oxford Brookes University, Oxford.)

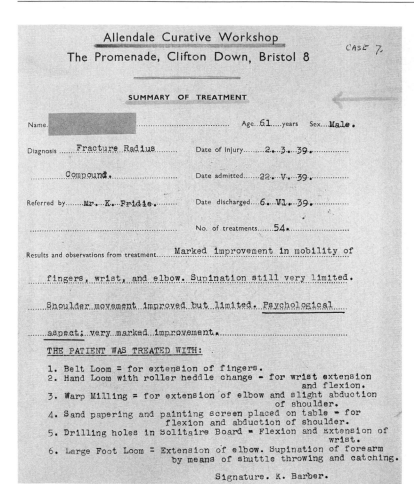

Allendale Curative Workshop
The Promenade, Clifton Down, Bristol 8

CASE 7.

SUMMARY OF TREATMENT

Name.. Age..61.....years Sex...Male.

Diagnosis ......Fracture Radius........ Date of Injury.........2..3..39..............

..........Compound........................ Date admitted.....22..V..39................

Referred by........Mr..K..Fridie........ Date discharged....6..V1..39................

.... No. of treatments.......54...................

Results and observations from treatment...... Marked improvement in mobility of

.......fingers, wrist, and elbow. Supination still very limited.

........Shoulder movement improved but limited. Psychological

........aspect: very marked improvement....................

THE PATIENT WAS TREATED WITH:

1. Belt Loom = for extension of fingers.
2. Hand Loom with roller heddle change - for wrist extension
                                          and flexion.
3. Warp Milling = for extension of elbow and slight abduction
                                          of shoulder.
4. Sand papering and painting screen placed on table - for
                                 flexion and abduction of shoulder.
5. Drilling holes in Solitaire Board - Flexion and Extension of
                                                          wrist.
6. Large Foot Loom = Extension of elbow. Supination of forearm
                        by means of shuttle throwing and catching.

Signature. K. Barber.

Fig. 1.4 Treatment report written in 1939. (Reproduced by kind permission of the School of Occupational Therapy, Oxford Brookes University, Oxford.)

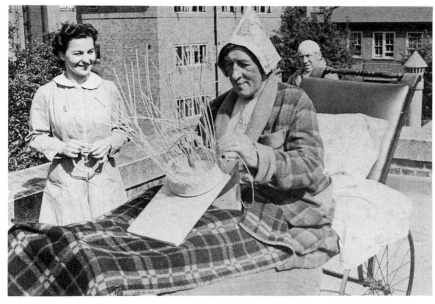

Fig. 1.5 Basketry (and sun hat!) for the long-term bed-bound patient, St John's and St Elizabeth Hospital, London, circa 1940. (Reproduced by kind permission of the School of Occupational Therapy, Oxford Brookes University, Oxford.)

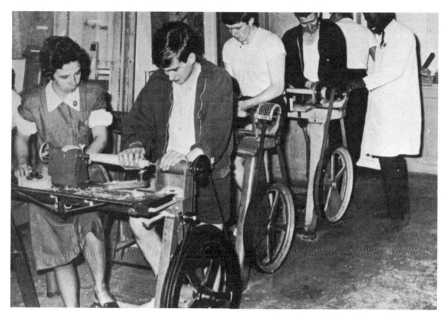

Fig. 1.6 Occupational therapy at Farnham Park Rehabilitation Centre, as depicted in the Association of Occupational Therapists' publicity brochure, 1960. (Reproduced by kind permission of the College of Occupational Therapists.)

day occupational therapists have had to work hard to dispel the idea that they are mainly involved in keeping people occupied with craft activities.

However, although we have inherited some negative legacies from the immediate post-war period we are also indebted to many active pioneers who set up excellent departments during this time, based on the specific therapeutic use of a wide range of both craft and non-craft activities. Jones (1960) describes the setting-up of the Farnham Park Rehabilitation Centre (Fig. 1.6). The occupational therapy department included in its treatment programmes the repair of old lawnmowers and other equipment which was then used for the benefit of the department. Tool-makers and engineers helped to work out 'Heath Robinson' ideas for the first specifically designed therapeutic machinery. Those requiring bricklaying as part of treatment built the wood-store and the occupational therapy office and 'bicycle fretsaws and filing machines [were] designed and made up in the OT workshops from angle iron'. Jones reflects that there was little difficulty in arousing cooperation, as almost all the patients had been in the services. One can envisage from her account the comradeship and military heritage inherent in the establishment and functioning of Farnham Park. It is also interesting to read that, where the occupational therapists were treating people with hemiplegia, they were advised to abandon treatment in order to make way for others if improvement did not make itself evident. Clearly this was the heyday of the biomechanical approach to treatment and the future of those who did not fit readily into this legacy of the Second World War was not given priority. The treatment of (basically) fit young men with orthopaedic or other biomechanical problems was the order of the day in the physical field.

Following this surge of occupational therapy practice came the establishment of the World Federation of Occupational Therapists (WFOT) in 1952. In 1960 occupational therapists became State Registered under the Professions Supplementary to Medicine Act. The Council for the Professions Supplementary to Medicine was established in 1961 and the Registration Board for occupational therapists in 1962.

In spite of this close alignment medicine and

Table 1.1 A comparison of the values underlying the practices of occupational therapy and medicine (from Kielhofner 1983)

Occupational therapy	Medicine
Essential humanity of patient, obligation to provide life satisfaction for severely disabled	Freedom from threat of death, responsibility limited to illness
Maintain and enhance health, support healthy aspects of person	Eradicate disease, pathology, confer the sick role
Self-directedness and responsibility of patient	Patient compliance to orders, moral authority
Generalist, integrated view of patient	Specialist, reductionistic emphasis on organ systems
Therapeutic relationship of mutual cooperation with patient; shared and sapiental authority of physician	Therapeutic relationship of activity of physician, passivity of patient; Aesculapian and sapiental authority of physician
Patient acts on environment rather than being determined by it	Patient as determined by environment and 'body machine'
Faith in patient's potential	Faith in science and healer's competence and charismatic authority
Patient productivity and participation	Patient relieved of all responsibilities except getting well
Play, leisure activities as essential components of balanced life	Recovery from illness, freedom from disease as major concern
Understand subjective perspectives of patient	Emphasis on objectivity, analysis, observation and diagnosis

occupational therapy have always been rather uneasy bedfellows (Table 1.1). Their beliefs are fundamentally different, even opposing, and while occupational therapy may have gained much in confidence and succour from medicine during its developmental years its status as a Profession Supplementary to Medicine is not one that rests entirely happily on its shoulders.

Re-establishing the basic philosophy

Around this period occupational therapy seemed to 'lose its way' somewhat. The basic philosophy, though unchanged, was battered by a change in expectations and attitudes, and by a vast increase in medical knowledge which left occupational therapists wondering exactly where their role lay and to which areas they should give priority. Treatment became somewhat recipe-like and occupational therapists appeared to jump on the bandwagon of whatever expanding body of knowledge was in fashion. Training schools crammed their syllabi full of 'essential' medical knowledge that the luckless student was obliged to take on board, and this academic emphasis often took place at the expense of the more practical 'activity' side of training, which was squeezed, somewhat, into second place. The basic philosophy of occupational therapy was rarely, if ever, mentioned and students, rather than being educated into the role of problem-solvers, were instructed in the use of rather rigid treatment programmes for differing diagnoses.

Despite changing demands, occupational therapists working in the physical field still saw the problems of their patients in mainly physical, medial and biomechanical terms. Most situations were treated using specifically designed or adapted equipment such that the complexity and importance of the adaptation or equipment frequently obscured the activity it was designed to perform. Equipment was, on occasion, used for its own sake entirely and the activity was forgotten, or felt to be unnecessary or too time-consuming to organise. Lip service was paid to 'psychological problems'. 'Boosting morale' or asking about leisure activities was felt to be important but the bulk of the treatment emphasis lay in the restoration of physical function. Occupational therapists were still being asked to 'occupy' patients. They complained of occupational therapy departments being used as 'dumping grounds' where bored or long-stay patients were sent to 'make something' or to 'occupy their minds'. Occupational therapists, who had an increasing lack of professional confidence and virtually no managerial expertise, did not know how to correct this appalling misuse of their services. They frequently tried to cover all requests on their time, spreading their skills so thinly that they became ineffectual. It became increasingly obvious that all was not well, that the profession had lost its way and that many occupational therapists, when challenged about what they actually did or what their philosophy was, found the question very hard to answer.

As a reaction to this, several people began hunting for a sound philosophical basis for the profession. Alongside this, the changing demands and treatments within the Health Service, the increased turnover of 'beds' within hospitals and the implementation of the Chronically Sick and Disabled Persons' Act in 1970, which heralded the influx of occupational therapists towards community care, forced occupational therapists to look back at their roots to discover and redefine the bases of their profession. From this re-examination sprang new concepts upon which occupational therapists began to be able to base their practice. These ideas, drawing upon the basic philosophy of occupational therapy, were conceptual representations aimed at organising the therapist's knowledge and making more effective and systematic her thinking and approach to the individual and his problems (see Ch. 2). 'Activities therapy', first presented by Anne Cronin Mosey in the early 1970s and the Model of Human Occupation developed by Gary Kielhofner in the 1970s and 80s are examples of such concepts.

Alongside these concepts, the first to be exclusive to occupational therapy, developed a series of approaches to specific functional problems. As previously mentioned, most intervention in the physical field was based upon the biomechanical approach. This approach viewed treatment in terms of strengthening muscles and increasing ranges of movement. As knowledge increased, however, there developed approaches to problems caused by neurological dysfunctions. Practitioners (not necessarily occupational therapists) such as Ayres, Bobath, Brunnstrom, Peto and Rood were instrumental in developing approaches to these particular problems, and their ideas were readily adopted in principle (and adapted in practice) by occupational therapists.

Additionally, occupational therapists worked increasingly in fields where preventative and prophylactic approaches were appropriate. These areas, which include coronary care, rheumatology and back care, are continually developing and implementing their approach and reflect the philosophy that the individual must take increased responsibility for his own health and well-being and work together with the therapist, who acts as a facilitator and teacher, in order to achieve this. Equally, as occupational therapists looked back to their professional roots and gained more confidence in their identity, they rediscovered the real meaning of a holistic approach to an individual and his problems. No longer are 'physical' occupational therapists averse to recognising that relaxation techniques, social skills training or behavioural regimes may be appropriate techniques to use with an individual that they are helping. Indeed, the use of educational and support groups and of perceptual and cognitive techniques are commonplace in what was once a rigid 'physical' approach to treatment.

CONCLUSION: THE FUTURE OF OCCUPATIONAL THERAPY

As practice, ideas and attitudes have developed and changed over the years, the underlying concepts and beliefs of the occupational therapist have held strong. Indeed they appear to be consolidating and emerging within professional practice as occupational therapists re-examine the basis of their profession, become more confident in their skills and beliefs, and understand more clearly their relationship with medical practice (Fig. 1.7).

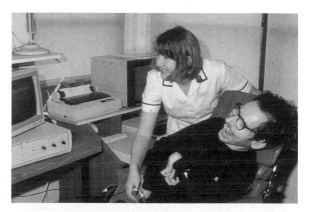

Fig. 1.7 Occupational therapy today.

With graduate and postgraduate education now widespread within the profession, therapists and students have relished the opportunity to develop their ability to reflect on their practice, to affirm their professional identity, to develop their clinical reasoning and to undertake research activities. More sure of the nature of their beliefs, and no longer feeling constrained to investigate their practice solely by producing statistical evidence of its effectiveness, occupational therapists are using both quantitative and qualitative research methods to explore their professional practice. In respecting the worth and opinions of individuals, occupational therapists find increasingly that the use of 'real world' research methods (those which use people's opinions, attitudes and ideas to understand and create theories about a situation) are often most appropriate in viewing attitudes and processes. Indeed, Yerxa (1991, p. 200) felt that 'qualitative research approaches have a goodness of fit with finding out what is worth knowing for occupational therapists'.

With new legislation constantly changing the structures, parameters and locations of occupational therapists' work, it is perhaps easy to believe that the only constant theme running throughout our practice is that what we learn and encompass today will be changed tomorrow. It would be easy, in this current climate of constant change, when new thinking creates a culture of purchasers and providers, and views sick people as consumers of services rather than passive patients and health care workers as service providers, to allow our professional practice to be buffeted and swayed entirely by fashions, finances, restructuring and the demands of those whose background is not based in caring. With occupational therapists increasingly working in situations in which they are unsupported by colleagues from their own profession, it seems even more imperative that their understanding of the roots and basis of their profession is not only firmly grasped but also effectively articulated. If we do not know who we are and what our aims are, how can we explain ourselves or be recognised by others?

As the 21st century awaits us we must be prepared to take our knowledge and beliefs forward to meet the changes and challenges of providing an effective, appropriate and efficient service for those we wish to help.

ACKNOWLEDGEMENT

Thanks go to Hilary Johnson, Senior Lecturer, St Andrew's School of Occupational Therapy, Nene College, Northampton, for compiling Box 1.3.

REFERENCES

American Occupational Therapy Association 1979 The Philosophical base of occupational therapy. American Journal of Occupational Therapy 33(12): 784–786

Barris R, Kielhofner G, Watts J H 1983 Psychosocial occupational therapy. Ramsco, Laurel, MD

British Journal of Occupational Therapy 1989 52(5): Occupational Therapy News

Bumphrey E 1987 Occupational therapy in the community. Woodhead-Faulkner, Cambridge

Clark P N 1979 Human development through occupation. Part 1, American Journal of Occupational Therapy 33(8): 505–514; Part 2, American Journal of Occupational Therapy 33(9): 577–585

Colson J H 1945 The rehabilitation of the injured. Cassell, London

Cynkin S, Robinson A M 1990 Occupational therapy and activities health: towards health through activity. Little, Brown, Boston

Fidler G S, Fidler J W 1978 Doing and becoming: purposeful action and self actualisation. Cited in Cynkin S, Robinson A M 1990 Occupational therapy and activities health: towards health through activity. Little, Brown, Boston

Howarth N A, MacDonald M 1946 The theory of occupational therapy. Baillière Tindall, London

Jeffrey L 1993 Aspects of selecting outcome measures to

demonstrate the effectiveness of comprehensive rehabilitation. Cited in Phillips J 1994 Disability and language: does it matter? British Journal of Occupational Therapy 57(11): 445–446

Jones M S 1960 An approach to occupational therapy. Butterworth, London

Kielhofner G 1985 A model of human occupation. Williams & Wilkins, Baltimore

Licht S 1948 The occupational therapy source book. Williams & Wilkins, Baltimore

MacDonald E M, MacCaul G, Murrey L 1970 Occupational therapy in rehabilitation, 3rd edn. Baillière Tindall, London

Meyer A 1922 A philosophy of occupational therapy. Cited in Kielhofner G 1992 Conceptual foundations of occupational therapy. F A Davis, Illinois

Mill J S. Cited in Cracknell E 1993 British Journal of Occupational Therapy 56(11): 391 (Lead article)

North East Thames Regional Health Authority 1987 Current occupational therapy practice

O'Sullivan E 1955 A textbook of occupational therapy. Lewis, London

Piaget J 1969 Psychology of the child. Cited in Cynkin S, Robinson A M 1990 Occupational therapy and activities health: towards health through activity. Little, Brown, Boston

Reilly M 1962 Occupational therapy can be one of the great ideas of twentieth century medicine. American Journal of Occupational Therapy 16: 1

Tuke S 1813 Description of The Retreat. Dawsons, London

World Federation of Occupational Therapy 1989 British Journal of Occupational Therapy 52(5): Occupational Therapy News

Yerxa E 1983 Audacious values: the energy source for occupational therapy practice. In: Kielhofner G 1983 Health through occupation. F A Davis, Philadelphia, Ch 6

Yerxa E 1991 Seeking a relevant, ethical and realistic way of knowing occupational therapy. American Journal of Occupational Therapy 45(3): 199–204

FURTHER READING

Glover M R 1984 The Retreat, York: an early experiment in the treatment of mental illness. Sessions, York

Hinojosa J, Sabari J, Pedretti L 1993 Position Paper 1 — Purposeful activity. American Journal of Occupational Therapy 47(12): 1081–1082

Kanny E 1993 Core values and attitudes of occupational therapy practice. American Journal of Occupational Therapy 47(12): 1085–1086

Kielhofner G 1992 Conceptual foundations of occupational therapy. F A Davis, Philadelphia

Kielhofner G 1983 Health through occupation. F A Davis, Philadelphia

Lycett R 1991 Well, what is occupational therapy? An examination of the definitions given by occupational therapists. British Journal of Occupational Therapy 54(11): 411–414

Maddi S R 1976 Personality theories. Dorsey, Illinois

Medcoj J, Roth J 1979 Approaches to psychology. Open University Press, Milton Keynes

Mocellin G 1992 An overview of occupational therapy in the context of the American influence on the profession. Part 1, British Journal of Occupational Therapy 55(1): 7–12; Part 2, British Journal of Occupational Therapy 55(2): 55–59

2

Theoretical frameworks

Margaret Foster

INTRODUCTION

Occupational therapy is a rapidly developing profession which is currently consolidating its theoretical basis in order to provide a solid foundation for research and evaluation and to more clearly explain its philosophy and practices to others.

For many years, occupational therapists have been using a variety of techniques in treatment and intervention, but in recent years there has been a reappraisal of the value of individual methods and practices, the basis on which these have developed, and the ways in which they interlink within the various branches of occupational therapy.

Competence in any profession depends upon an understanding of the theory that underlies it. 'Theory', in this general sense encompasses philosophical viewpoints, paradigms, frames of reference, models, approaches, and particular *theories*. The occupational therapist needs to be conversant with these elements of theory as they have developed within her own profession, so that she has a clear understanding of the principles of her discipline and a sound basis from which to plan, implement and justify her interventions.

While there are many texts available which present in-depth discussion of particular aspects of theory (see References and Further reading below), this chapter aims to provide an overview of the main aspects of occupational therapy theory which have application to the treatment of people with physical dysfunction.

The first sections of the chapter discuss the importance of theory to the profession of occupational therapy as a whole and to the individual therapist. Various terms used in the discussion of theory, such as 'paradigm', 'frame of reference', 'approach' and 'model', are defined. The interconnections between these areas of theory are then illustrated.

The next sections of the chapter turn to the application of theory to practice. First, specific theories that have had an important influence upon occupational therapy are discussed; these are the humanistic, occupations/activities, and psychosocial theories. The basic assumptions of each theory are outlined, and particular refinements on these theories as they have evolved within occupational therapy are described.

The remaining sections of the chapter are devoted to particular frames of reference that have had an important influence on the treatment of physical dysfunction, namely the developmental, biomechanical, compensatory and learning frames of reference. The merits and limitations of each frame of reference are set out, and their relevance to today's changing practice is discussed.

THE IMPORTANCE OF THEORY

PROFESSIONALISM

In today's competitive health care market, occupational therapy must have a sound theoretical framework by which it can define itself and justify its actions in order to maintain and enhance its professional standing. In 1989 the Report of a Commission of Inquiry, *Occupational Therapy, an Emerging Profession in Health Care*, recommended that therapists should 'seek to validate the profession's claim to professional status by devising ways of measuring and monitoring the effectiveness and efficiency of practices, procedures and organisational arrangements' (Blom Cooper 1989).

Before considering the nature and importance of the theoretical base, it is advantageous to consider the qualities essential to a profession.

What is a profession?

Professions do not come into existence by historical accident. Rather a complex interplay of forces over time ushers a profession into being. Internally there must be the vision and energy of those who found and develop the profession. Externally social movements provide ideas and support for its mission. Governmental systems legitimise and regulate the members' activities . . . underlying these factors is an implicit social contract . . . the profession meets a basic social need . . . Professions are able to provide their distinctive service because they have accumulated and developed a conceptual foundation that explains and directs their practical efforts.
(Kielhofner 1992)

No one definition exists that defines a profession, although various texts which outline the characteristics representative of a profession agree on a number of points. In addition to the social constructs of the profession the following points are considered to be fundamental to any profession (Wallis 1987):

- A unique body of knowledge which is pertinent to the practices and beliefs of the profession. Some knowledge may overlap with that of other professions, but the particular integration and utilisation of knowledge is unique to each profession
- A sound theory base on which to explain the profession's philosophies and values. Many texts state that this theory base should be proven by investigation and research
- Educational requirements in order to become a member of the profession; continuing education within the profession to maintain standards in the light of change
- Autonomy in determining the rules of the profession and maintaining standards
- Ethical responsibility to regulate the modes of behaviour of those within the profession and to protect the client
- Professional commitment within the membership to adhere to the practices and beliefs of the profession and to further its development.

The British Association of Occupational Therapists (1995) *Code of Ethics and Professional Conduct* defines the ways in which practitioners should meet professional obligations in relation to consumers in terms of responsibilities, relationships, professional integrity and standards of practice. Included in these are articles concerning professional demeanour, clinical competence, personal behaviour and professional development.

The College of Occupational Therapists, the Council for Professions Allied to Medicine and the Privy Council, together with the educational establishments, validate the educational programmes for entry into the profession.

Implications for occupational therapy

It is vital for occupational therapy to have a proven theory base if it is to continue to be recognised as a profession. Study of the theory base on which it is founded, and the basis on which its practices are carried out, should be an essential part of any profession's development. 'Although what they [occupational therapists] do looks simple, what they know is quite complex' (Mattingly et al 1994).

Skill as a 'doer' based on practice, repetition and experience reflects a technical level of competence. Professionalism, however, requires skill in thinking, in reflecting on previous experiences, and in linking these to theory and learning (Parham 1987) and to the presenting problem, in order to ensure that the choice of 'doing' is the most appropriate for the particular situation — clinical reasoning. Barnitt (1990) in a keynote paper to the WFOT 10th International Congress stressed the value of thinking. She outlined the structure of the profession as the 'shared body of knowledge, the skills practised by its members and the shared values and beliefs which underpin the ethics and motivation of the members'. She stated that 'the structure is dependent on the thinking which brought it into existence, which then propels it forward through change, progress and decline'; thinking is the means by which the structure is 'held together or separated out'. A high standard of thinking and clinical reasoning enhances not only the standing of the individual, but also the recognition of the profession as a whole. This may be reflected in academic credentials (diplomas, degrees or doctorates) and

through validated research, and should also be evident in the ways in which members of the profession are conversant with current theory, and reflect their theories and beliefs positively in their practice.

A sound understanding of the theoretical principles of her profession enhances the ability of the therapist to address issues confidently, make considered decisions and defend outcomes. The ability to justify actions is a vital component of today's health care provision, where there is increased demand for efficient, cost-effective practices. Clinical audit, contracting and litigation demand that professionals are able to explain or defend their practices to managers, purchasers and consumers. In order to maintain professionalism therapists should continue their own personal learning and development to ensure that their practice remains current, competent and ethical.

CLARITY OF PURPOSE

Theory is the lens through which we see reality more clearly.

(Kielhofner 1985)

The history of occupational therapy demonstrates the consequences of basing a profession on a weak theory base. Lacking a solid theoretical framework, the profession was, particularly in the 1960s, diverted from its original purpose and allied itself more closely to theories from other professions which appeared to have a sounder proven knowledge base, or which were particularly valued or fashionable at the time (see Ch. 1).

Since then, occupational therapists have begun both to question and to value their own basic philosophy. Through the development of conceptual models, the analysis of approaches and the evaluation of practices, they have been able to justify the basis on which therapy intervention is founded and more clearly explain the aims and goals of practice to themselves and to others.

Without a theoretical framework a profession is like a ship afloat without a compass in a sea of change. It is at the mercy of the waves and tides of fashion, regularly changing course according to their ebb and flow, without ever reaching its proper destination. It is at risk of washing up on an unknown shore, where its crew will be likely to modify their behaviour to match the customs or culture of the natives and thereby gain acceptance.

Theory is the compass which guides the profession's progress, keeping its direction true whatever storms or changes in tides it encounters. Theory sets the course (the therapy process) and guides the passage (the intervention) to ensure that the ship reaches its chosen shore.

Theory provides a means by which our professional practice can be explained and clarified — for our own benefit and in response to others. It is a framework in which we can explain the philosophy of our practice, justify the value of interventions, and measure the efficacy of treatment.

The move to increase community based services places more occupational therapists in multidisciplinary situations where they work with colleagues from disciplines other than their own. Sound professional knowledge and expertise is therefore essential to retain identity, educate others, and integrate occupational therapy practices into the multidisciplinary framework. The practitioner needs to be self-reliant within her discipline and demonstrate skills of independent thinking and clinical reasoning to meet people's needs and justify actions to others. In order to do this efficiently she needs a sound theoretical base to guide her judgements and develop practice expertise.

Theory is an integral part of competent professional practice (Fig. 2.1). Mont & Ross (cited in Black & Champion 1976) remind us that 'there is nothing impractical about good theory . . . Action divorced from theory is the random scurrying of a rat in a new maze. Good theory is the power to find the way to the goal with a minimum of lost motion and electric shock'.

COMMON UNDERSTANDING

In a profession which has such a broad spectrum of practice, it is essential to have a common understanding to retain professional identity within the membership, and in the perceptions of the purchasers and consumers.

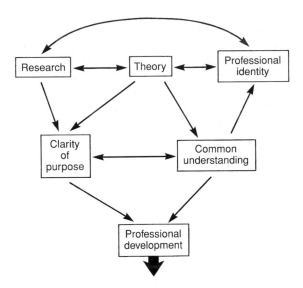

Fig. 2.1 The importance of theory to practice.

Clark et al (1991), in an article concerning occupational science, indicated the need for the profession to have 'a unified vision of what is at the heart of our practice'. In the 1960s the alliance of some areas of occupational therapy to the medical model led to a divergence in practice, with the development of specialist techniques based on medical factors rather than on individuals' occupational needs.

Such divergencies did nothing to enhance the understanding of the profession by consumers, clients, other professionals and employers. When individuals received different treatments and advice from different therapists there was understandably some confusion, often followed by a loss of respect for the methods used or the information given.

How can such a situation be explained? Much was due to the emphasis on competence in 'doing' rather than on the value of knowing the *why* behind the 'doing', or on clarity regarding the philosophy and process of intervention. The development of theory based on holism and humanism and the organisation of problem-based intervention strategies has enabled therapists to understand and explain more clearly the projected aims and goals of their practices and thereby justify the variations in the methods used to achieve specific outcomes to meet individual requirements.

The occupational therapist has been recognised for the unique breadth of her practice, but only at the risk of being considered a 'Jack of all trades and master of none'. Mastery *in combination with* breadth is increasingly important in the present climate of health care, in which there is more diversity in services and service delivery, and intervention is 'needs led'.

The clientele of occupational therapy has changed in recent years, and will change further in the future, to include more people with multiple and complex problems. This is occurring for various reasons, including:

- demographic changes, including an increase in the number of elderly people
- advances in surgical and survival techniques which enable people to survive longer following severe trauma and to live much longer with chronic medical conditions such as multiple sclerosis and cancer
- improved antenatal and neonatal care and diagnostic techniques which have enabled children with multiple handicaps to survive
- manpower demands which have led to simple orthopaedic conditions not being seen by occupational therapists in many areas because of the more pressing needs of those with chronic or more complex problems.

As a result of this shift in clientele, the narrow focus of earlier treatment techniques will be insufficient to meet people's needs. An increasing emphasis on a holistic understanding of the individual will be a spur to research into the merits of particular frames of reference and to investigation of how the many theories can be cohesively integrated to meet the complex needs of a changing clientele.

A BASIS FOR RESEARCH AND DEVELOPMENT

The interrelationship between theory and research in all areas of knowledge and development is well known. Theory forms the basis on which research is carried out, and research leads to the proving or disproving of theory.

The Concise Oxford Dictionary defines research as 'careful search or enquiry into a subject to discover facts by study or critical investigation'. Research is a question in search of an answer. In the present climate of therapy, as the professions re-examine their practices in order to justify them to employers, managers and other professions, and with a view to meeting changing patterns of need, research and investigation are vital. Occupational therapists need to investigate the premises on which their interventions are founded and prove the efficacy of those interventions to others.

While many therapists, and others, intuitively recognise the benefits of various occupational therapy practices, there is currently a dearth of research by which the effectiveness of these has been measured or proven. Reliance on intuition and face validity does not provide a sound basis on which to assess the value of a given practice or to build further developments.

Many people view research as something done by others from which they are able to gain information. This is quite true as far as it goes. However, this view is often linked to a hesitancy to personally embark on research because it is perceived to be specialist, complex, highly intellectual, remote or even 'detached from the real world'.

In the past, occupational therapists have gained recognition as 'doers'. They have been active in devising and utilising methods to facilitate patients' and clients' abilities as doers, and have been under pressure themselves to be doers as the number of people requiring their assistance has increased and the profession has expanded. This has inevitably been at the expense of time for research to qualify and quantify the results of the 'doing', or to promote new thinking.

Occupational therapists should all be involved in research in some aspect of their work, even if only to prove their own worth. This may be through the simplest form of evaluation of a particular practice or intervention, or through a more complex investigation of needs or modes of provision for future planning strategies. Research is also needed to develop more valid and reliable assessment instruments on which clinicians can confidently base their intervention strategies (Ellis 1981).

Investigation by Taylor & Mitchell (1990) reveals that many clinicians are not personally carrying out research because of the constraints of time, money, skills and caseload needs, but are in favour of clinical research and keen to collaborate with experienced researchers and to learn from their findings. This collaboration could raise the level of clinicians' involvement in research and in so doing raise the level of their interest, expertise and satisfaction, which could further lead to the instigation of personal research investigations. Taylor & Mitchell conclude that 'the profession needs to draw on clinicians' interest in research and develop strategies for increasing their involvement and productivity through mutual and supportive experiences'.

Lyons (1985) states that therapists have acquired a 'modest, but respectable body of knowledge' which should be 'defined, researched and systematised so that it becomes evident, definable, defensible and saleable'. The expansion of our knowledge base is vital to the maintenance and promotion of our professional identity.

No profession can stand still if it is to retain its credibility, but change should not occur just for the sake of change. While occupational therapy needs to keep pace with changing conditions, it should not lose sight of its original purpose.

Theory guides the attitudes and values of our profession. It forms the basis of our clinical reasoning (the questioning and determining of actions) and of our reflection on outcomes and the appropriateness of present practices. Theory based on sound reflection and proven findings makes a major contribution to the development of pro-active thinking for future needs (Parham 1987).

The history of the profession's divergence from its originating philosophy in the 1960s and 70s, when developments occurred without the support of a strong, defined and proven theory base, provides further argument for research and planned development based on sound theory.

DEFINING TERMS

Frequently there are slight differences among health care professionals in their understanding of theoretical terms. This may occur because some words are used differently between one profession and another. Additionally, the analysis of occupational therapy is a worldwide process and there are differences in the use and understanding of terms between nations and, depending on which source of information has been used, between individuals within one country. Therefore, definitions of terms as they are used in this text are given below.

PHILOSOPHY

A common use of the word 'philosophy' refers to a set of ultimate values, i.e. a view of the meaning of life and of the significance of the world we live in. Moral philosophy is the branch of knowledge which deals with the principles of human behaviour and ethics.

The philosophy of occupational therapy is based on the profession's view of what constitutes an acceptable or desirable quality of life. It determines the values, beliefs and practices of the profession, which are founded in what therapists consider is inherently good and provide a basis from which to approach theory and practice (Yerxa 1979).

One of the earliest philosophies for the profession, put forward by Adolph Meyer in 1922, identified occupational therapy as 'an awakening to the fullest meaning of time as the biggest wonder and asset of our lives and the valuation of opportunity and performance as the greatest measure of time'. The philosophy of occupational therapy is discussed in greater depth in Chapter 1.

PARADIGMS

The use of the word 'paradigm' became popular following the writings of the philosopher Thomas Kuhn in the 1960s (Kuhn 1970). Kielhofner (1983) uses the word 'paradigm' to refer to 'an agreed body of theory explaining and rationalising professional unity and practice, that incorporates all the profession's concerns, concepts and expertise, and guides values and commitments'.

A paradigm imposes a shape upon a science.

It derives from the values, principles and knowledge shared by members of a professional community, and determines the scope and boundaries of the profession, thus guiding practice, research and future development.

Paradigms are built by members of a profession. They are formulated to guide the development of theory and practice, and are eventually discarded as new findings and beliefs emerge to form a new paradigm. This is a natural process of development, which occurs in all areas of science. To take an historical example, after the explorations of Christopher Columbus and others the paradigm of a flat world was replaced by the paradigm of a round world. This shift in understanding further changed thinking and beliefs, and stimulated and guided new thinking and promoted other discoveries.

Paradigm developments have occurred in occupational therapy. The profession's initial paradigm was based on a view of man's need to be 'occupied'. This was replaced by a reductionist paradigm which emphasised body and mind mechanisms as discrete parts of a whole. The present paradigm combines elements from the previous two into a new whole reflecting occupational behaviour and performance. This paradigm has led to the development of new models, for example the Human Occupation Model (Reed & Sanderson 1983), the Model of Human Occupation (Kielhofner 1985) and the Activities Health Model (Cynkin & Robinson 1990).

THEORIES

The Heinemann English Dictionary (1987) defines 'theory' as:

- 'a systematically organised group of general propositions used to analyse, predict or explain facts or events'
- 'the whole collection of ideas, methods and theorems associated with a study, e.g. "the number theory"'
- 'an explanation of the principles of a subject, such as art, as distinct from the practice of it'
- 'a conjecture or opinion — "that's your theory but I disagree."'

In the present text, 'theory' might be used in any of the first three senses listed above. Thus, 'a theory' is an organised and systematic set of principles by which phenomena can be predicted and explained; these principles may be more or less comprehensive, and may constitute a methodology. Theory as 'conjecture or opinion' is less relevant to our purposes, although it should be remembered that particular theories that are regarded as sound may have elements of conjecture within them; indeed, they may be found, in the light of later experience, to be untrue.

In the introductory sections of this chapter, 'theory' has been used in the third, general sense given above to refer to the discussion of the 'principles' of our profession as opposed to its 'practice'. It should be borne in mind, however, that just as our practice should be firmly grounded in theory, our theory should never be far removed from practice. A theory that is not readily applicable to and verified by practice may have to be revised or discarded.

The reader will also notice the slight shift in meaning that occurs when we move from the discussion of 'theory' in its widest sense (i.e. a type of discourse, as in: 'The subject of this chapter is occupational therapy theory') to the discussion of 'a theory' or 'theories' (e.g. Piaget's theory of intellectual development). Thus, within the philosophy and paradigm of occupational therapy *theory*, various particular *theories* come into play, some of which are unique to our profession, and some of which have been borrowed and adapted from other disciplines.

FRAMES OF REFERENCE

A frame of reference is an organised body of knowledge, principles and research findings which forms the conceptual basis of a particular aspect of practice. Mosey (1981) defined a frame of reference as a 'set of inter-related internally consistant concepts, definitions and postulates that provide a systematic description of, and prescription for, a practitioner's interaction with a particular aspect of a profession's domain of concern'.

Unlike a paradigm, which provides a general structure for thought, a frame of reference rationalises and explains a particular facet of practice. It consists of a 'group of compatable theories that can be applied within a particular field of practice' (Creek & Feaver 1993). Young & Quinn (1992) define frames of reference as 'those aspects which influence our perceptions, decisions and practice'. They form a basis for clinical reasoning (Rogers 1983).

Occupational therapy models have evolved partly through experienced individuals using frames of reference to develop structures for practice. They have built on their own theories, values, knowledge, practice and research findings to develop patterns and processes which may be used by many members of the profession.

Frames of reference are therefore important to the professional development of the individual therapist and of the discipline as a whole. They lead to the use of 'a standard set of facts to judge, control or direct some action or expression' (Reed & Sanderson 1983) and to clarity in the explanation, evaluation and evolution of professional theory.

As Mosey (1981) writes:

A frame of reference delineates a particular aspect of a profession and provides a central theme to which to refer for decisions regarding the appropriateness of the programme design and content . . . It influences the practitioner's choices and approach to treatment and thus gives unity, balance and direction to the treatment programme.

However, confusion occurs because of the different labels given to frames of reference by different practitioners, according to their thinking and interlinking of ideas (Box 2.1). Variations occur between American theorists. Mosey (1981) named three frames of reference — 'analytical, acquisitional and developmental' — while Hopkins & Smith (1988) outline nine — 'behavioural, biomechanical, cognitive, developmental, neurodevelopmental, sensorimotor, occupational behaviour, rehabilitation and psychoanalytic'. These different labels indicate differences in thinking in what actually constitutes a 'frame of reference'. Mosey uses broader terms to reflect modes of progress than do Hopkins & Smith,

---

Box 2.1 Different authors' representations and terminology for occupational therapy frames of reference

Authors	Frames of reference
Mosey (1981)	Analytical, acquisitional, developmental
Hopkins & Smith (1988)	Behavioural, biomechanical, cognitive, developmental, neurodevelopmental, sensorimotor, occupational behaviour, rehabilitation, psychoanalytic
Creek (1990)	Psychoanalytic, developmental, learning, humanistic
Young & Quinn (1992)	Adaptive performance, developmental, sensorimotor, cognitive, role performance, rehabilitation
Hagedorn (1992)	Physiological, behavioural, cognitive, psychodynamic, humanist
Turner et al (1996) (this volume)	Phenomenological, developmental, biomechanical, learning, compensatory

---

whose titles are more allied to particular intervention strategies.

Variations also occur in Britain. Young & Quinn (1992) identified six frames of reference: 'adaptive performance, developmental, sensory motor, cognitive, role performance and rehabilitation'. In the same year Hagedorn (1992) cited five — 'physiological, behavioural, cognitive, psychodynamic and humanist'. Creek (1990), when considering occupational therapy in the field of mental health, identified four 'frames of reference', which she considered to be 'approaches derived from theories' of psychoanalysis, human development, learning and humanism.

Kielhofner (1992) challenges the title 'frames of reference', stating that he prefers to label them as conceptual models for practice. Other authors argue that a model is a diagrammatic representation, whereas a frame of reference is an interlinking of compatible ideas and themes to explain particular similarities in practices and occurrences.

The authors of this text agree with the term frame of reference as an interlinking of compatible ideas and themes which may be used to direct the thinking for methods of intervention, once goals and priorities have been established. The confusion and conflict has been addressed by identifying five fundamental frames of reference which guide occupational therapy for physical dysfunction, based on discussion with practitioners and the writings of others. These are the phenomenological frame of reference, founded in humanistic thinking, together with developmental, biomechanical, learning and compensatory frames of reference to reflect theories which influence therapeutic intervention. In some instances one primary frame of reference may be used to address a number of problems. In other cases a number of different frames of reference may be used to treat different problem areas. Similarly a number of frames of reference may be used to address one area at different stages of intervention; for example it may be advisable to use a biomechanical or developmental frame of reference to guide intervention in the recovery stages, but this may have less value in addressing problems resulting from residual impairment once improvement has reached a plateau, when a compensatory frame of reference may be more appropriate.

APPROACHES

Approaches are the *ways and means of 'doing'*, i.e. of implementing frames of reference. An approach consists of the rationale behind a specific technique and the way in which it is used in practice. An approach may be used singly, or in combination with others, to achieve an aim or goal. For example, the adaptive approach, which is based on the compensatory frame of reference — the belief that a problem can best be overcome by compensating for it, rather than through biomechanical or developmental means to improve anatomical or physiological functioning — may be used exclusively to treat a permanent impairment. However, where the impairment is likely to be temporary the adaptive approach may only be used for a short time, to be phased out in favour of another approach as recovery commences.

An approach determines *how* an activity may be used. Within the adaptive approach the therapist will assist a keen gardener to devise different techniques to continue his hobby, for example placing seed trays on the bench to prick out seedlings to avoid stooping and bending. Within the neurodevelopmental approach, gardening activities involving stooping and bending may be encouraged to promote balance and weight transfer. A heavy gardening activity, such as digging, may be used in the biomechanical approach to improve muscle strength and activity tolerance in the lower limbs.

MODELS

According to the Shorter Oxford English Dictionary (1993) a model is 'a simplified description of a system or process put forward as a basis for theoretical or empirical understanding; a conceptual or mental representation of something showing the arrangement of its component parts'. A *conceptual practice* model has been described as 'an abstract representation of practice' (Hopkins & Smith 1988, p. 383). It presents *theories* or ideas in schematic form, for example through charts, plans, pictures or flow diagrams, often showing the inter-relationship between the parts in the whole.

A conceptual model for professional practice represents the basic concepts or theories behind intervention in diagram or chart form, delineating a framework for professional action and thinking. This is based on professional values and beliefs, and displays the links between theory and practice. Such a model may be used to promote clearer understanding of professional actions, to clarify the boundaries and roles of intervention, to determine tasks within the intervention process, and to deduce anticipated outcomes.

A professional practice model may apply to various aspects of the profession, providing a framework for a number of areas of intervention in a variety of realms of practice. It may be used as a diagrammatic tool to explain the application of complex theories.

Models occur at different levels, depending on what they depict. Some models show the inter-linking of frames of reference with theory — for example the Model of Human Occupation portraying Kielhofner's interpretation of occupational behaviour theory. Reed & Sanderson (1983) refer to this type of model as a 'generic' model, because it can be applied across a number of areas of practice with a number of approaches. Other models are designed at a more specific level to delineate the process of application of a particular approach. Reed & Sanderson (1983) call these 'descriptive' models. Examples of these are the neurodevelopmental and sensorimotor models, which reflect the sequence of stages of particular aspects of development within the developmental frame of reference. Generic models may be used to determine the overall picture of a particular situation, whereas descriptive models may guide the application of particular frames of reference in intervention (Fig. 2.2).

Confusion occurs between authors on the use of the term model. Kielhofner (1992) prefers to use the term 'model' to describe what others refer to as a frame of reference. Hagedorn (1992) refers to a rehabilitation model, which some other authors would describe as a process. Within the context of this text, the terms generic and descriptive model, as described by Reed & Sanderson (1983) will be used. The definition of a conceptual practice model suggested by Creek, Hagedorn, Turner and others in 1993 is 'a simplified representation of the structure and content of a phenomenon or system, that describes or explains the complex relationships between concepts within the system and integrates elements of theory and practice'.

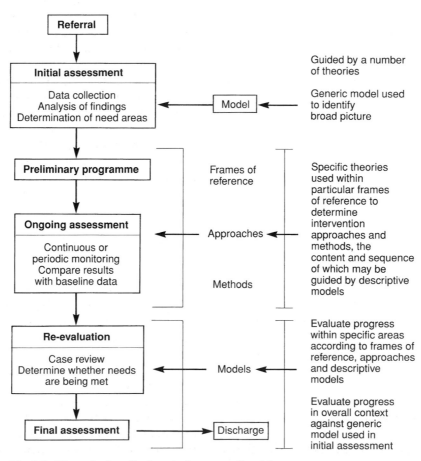

Fig. 2.2 Theoretical applications in the occupational therapy process.

LINKING TERMS

Frequently there is difficulty in linking the terms defined above, particularly when there is no consistent interpretation of the terms between texts.

In the context of the present volume, the *paradigm* of occupational therapy will be considered as the basis of the fundamental principles of the profession. It comprises the concepts that therapists hold in common concerning the ways in which people use and benefit from occupation, i.e. from involvement, interaction and activity in life. These concepts derive from and are supported by the profession's *philosophy* regarding the essential humanity of man and his participation with and in his environment.

Theories have developed from this paradigm (as well as from other areas of knowledge and learning) to reflect therapists' values and beliefs about the nature of occupation, the criteria for defining and achieving competence and the essence of humanism. These theories have further led to the development of a number of *frames of reference* with regard to how man learns, develops and performs within his environment. *Approaches* have been devised in order to apply the philosophies and theories within these frames of reference in clinical practice.

Within this hierarchy of professional thinking, *models* exist at two levels. Some models have been devised and drawn up to explain particular approaches in relation to frames of reference. Other models show the integration of frames of reference with theories. Thus some models, such as the behavioural model, may be confined to a particular aspect or area of practice, while others, such as the Model of Human Occupation, may be more broadly based, explaining the inter-relation of a number of frames of reference in a theoretical whole.

THEORY IN PRACTICE

The practice of occupational therapy is eclectic in that it draws selectively upon various schools of thought in addressing a wide variety of needs. This eclecticism has permitted the use of a number of frames of reference, each of which may be used to determine particular techniques and approaches in practice. Inevitably, these frames of reference overlap and to some degree may be integrated with one another, but each is significantly different in its underlying theories and beliefs. Humanistic, occupations/activities, and psychosocial theories support individual aspects of practice but also underpin wider frames of reference and are used concurrently to form the basis of many approaches to practice. In this way, *theories* and *frames of reference* complement one another. Within the occupational therapy process therapists focus on different aspects of theory at particular stages to guide their thinking and actions (Fig. 2.2). During the initial assessments, the therapist may use a broad theoretical base, to remain 'open minded' and unbiased towards the particular area of deficit. Frequently the individual may be referred for a particular item, but this may only be part of the problem. The therapist may therefore use one or more broad based 'generic' models to identify the overall situation, and gain a fuller picture of the problem in the context of the individual's unique circumstances. Following this the therapist may use one or more specific frames of reference to guide her thinking towards, and assessment of, individual aspects of deficit or need.

When making decisions regarding intervention, the overall 'generic' picture remains in focus, but particular frames of reference and individual theories guide the chosen specific approaches in order to meet the person's biomechanical, developmental or learning needs, or to compensate for dysfunction which cannot be overcome by other methods. The structure and sequences of these approaches and methods are more likely to be directed according to a 'descriptive' model, which defines the processes and procedures of the particular approach.

The progress made in a specific area will be analysed and assessed according to the descriptive model. However it will also be viewed in the overall context of the person's situation and needs, as identified in the generic model during the initial assessment.

THE USE OF THEORIES

The humanistic theory

This is based in phenomenology and existential psychology. Phenomenology focuses on subjective experiences — individuals' personal views of events in their own current environment — and believes that people are not acted on by external forces but are themselves 'actors capable of controlling their own destiny' (Atkinson et al 1985). Existentialists believe that knowledge differs for each individual, and is constantly changing as the result of personal experiences and the subsequent interpretations of these experiences. The person is seen as a whole being — a Gestalt — rather than a collection of parts.

Humanism perceives the person optimistically, believing that human nature is essentially 'good'. Such positive beliefs are reflected in the view that human beings have an innate drive to be creative, to love, to grow and to be productive. These views are demonstrated in the belief in 'the self' (as described by Rogers in 1984a) in the client-centred approach, which views the individual as a free and responsible agent capable of determining his own development. Maslow (1968) also reflected this positive view that man is motivated by a drive to satisfy needs. He described these needs in a hierarchy, the lower levels of this being devoted to satisfying needs for personal existence. When these have been largely met, the person is able to move on to strive to achieve higher needs for growth, self-esteem and aesthetic pleasure, and finally try to reach his full potential — self actualisation (see Ch. 32).

Humanistic theory in practice

In practice occupational therapists' use of phenomenological beliefs are widely applied through the humanistic ways by which the therapist respects people's autonomy and individuality throughout intervention. The therapist recognises the person's capacity for self-awareness, and his right and freedom to choose his own actions. This is the opposite of didactic authoritarianism, which dominated many professions' earlier practices — the 'professional knows best' syndrome — and is in line with current ideologies of patient autonomy, empowerment and patient-focused health care. When applying humanistic theory the therapist respects the individual as a partner in therapy. Partnership in assessment of needs and priorities, and in the negotiation of realistic, purposeful opportunities, is the basis on which the therapeutic relationship grows. The therapist's essential belief in individual self-determination is reflected in the ways in which she helps him to make informed choices from a range of suitable options without exerting control over his decisions.

Basic assumptions

- The person has the potential for awareness of personal needs, drives and goals and has the ability to change through opportunities and experiences
- The quality of intrapersonal and interpersonal relationships and rapport are important in the development of self-esteem
- The individual has the right to make choices and prioritise according to his personal perceptions of strengths and needs and the right to preserve or develop an internal locus of control
- The positive strengths and abilities of the individual to overcome difficulties, rather than his weaknesses, should be emphasised
- Merely 'being able to do' is not sufficient. Feelings of purposefulness, skill and achievement are vital components in self-actualisation and self-esteem.

Practices which reflect humanism

- Self-rating assessments
- Recognition of values, roles and beliefs
- Non-directive counselling
- Providing opportunities for expressive interactions

- Providing opportunities for informed prioritising
- Acceptance of opinions and choices.

The occupations/activities theory

This, the earliest theoretical base for occupational therapy, was founded on the belief that occupation and activity are instrumental in achieving and maintaining health. Theories regarding the value of occupation and activities developed from studies by Meyer (1922), Reilly (1962) and many others, but have their beginnings in the view of the relationship between activity and health as understood by the Romans and ancient Greeks (see Ch. 1).

The basis of the use of this theory in occupational therapy was summed up in Mary Reilly's (1962) well-known statement: 'Man through the use of his own hands, as they are energised by mind and will, can influence the state of his own health'.

In recent years many therapists have striven to explain the differences in meaning between 'occupation' and 'activity', in order to clarify the profession's philosophy. Occupation has been defined as:

- 'volitional goal directed behaviour aimed at the development of play, work and life skills for optimal time management' (Rogers 1984b)
- 'The dominant activity of human beings that includes serious productive pursuits, and playful, creative and festive behaviours' (Kielhofner 1983)
- 'Man's goal directed use of time, energy, interests and attention' (American Occupational Therapy Association 1976)
- 'Those activities and tasks which engage a person's time, energy and resources and are composed of skills and values' (Reed & Sanderson 1983)
- 'An active doing process of a person engaged in goal directed, intrinsically gratifying and culturally appropriate activity' (Evans 1987).

The majority of these definitions are American. The Concise Oxford Dictionary (1993) defines 'activity' as a 'task or action' or 'being active', and 'occupation' as 'profession or employment' and 'occupying or being occupied'. In order to clarify the meaning of terms Hagedorn, Creek, Turner and others met in 1993 to discuss definitions. The definitions suggested by this group are that 'activity is an action performed by an individual for a specific purpose on a particular occasion', whereas 'occupation defines and organises a sphere of action over a period of time and is perceived by the individual as part of his/her personal and social identity'. In summary, activity is *doing*, whereas occupation is a state of *being*, most frequently achieved through active participation in activity. Within the realm of occupational therapy, activity is said to be 'purposeful' when the value of its use is to 'achieve mastery and competence' in those activities which have significance to the person 'in terms of social, cultural and personal meanings that are describably real and symbolic' (Fidler & Fidler 1978).

While there has been some deviation from the occupations/activities theory, particularly when other ideas developed in the 1950s and 60s, the belief in the value of occupation has remained central to the profession. This may be seen through the direct use of purposeful activities in therapy, or through the use of problem-solving strategies to enhance the individual's ability in daily living tasks, thus achieving 'occupational' goals.

Recent analysis of occupations/activities theory (Kielhofner 1983, Cynkin & Robinson 1990) has led to a fuller appreciation of 'occupation' and a greater recognition of the value of activity in healthy living. This has been reflected in the modern 'generic' occupational therapy models, which have been organised to show factors and stages in the development of successful occupational performance. They have been able to integrate professional values concerning the belief in the individual, theories of achievement and motivation, and the implications of the individual's inter-relationship with the environment, to explain ways by which a broad range of activities may be used purposefully to achieve occupational goals and a balance in health.

Basic assumptions

- Occupations and activities are vital components of balanced healthy living
- Occupations and activities can be used in a variety of ways to overcome dysfunction, and promote health in body and mind
- The most positive outcomes are achieved through activities which are purposeful and goal directed, offering realistic challenges and achievable outcomes
- The greatest personal commitment is obtained when the activities chosen are relevant to the individual's life-style, roles, aspirations and needs within his environment, and relate realistically to his present level of function.

Generic models

Several conceptual models have been based on occupations/activities theory. Recent examples include:

- Cynkin & Robinson (1990) — Activities Health Model
- Kielhofner (1985) — Model of Human Occupation
- Reed & Sanderson (1992) — Personal Adaptation through Occupation Model.

Psychosocial theory

This theory concentrates on the attainment of interpersonal and intrapersonal skills in the environment. Initially it was considered particularly important for people with mental health problems, but many of its principles are equally important in areas of physical or cognitive dysfunction to achieve social integration and role performance. Psychosocial theory may have application for those who have to make adjustments to living as the result of trauma which affects cognitive function (for example following head injury), or for those who have disease or injury resulting in physical or perceptual dysfunction, or gross disfigurement. Additionally the initial acquisition of competent psychosocial performance may be limited or constrained through lack of opportunity or ability for those who suffer congenital impairment.

Many practitioners, recognising the psychological and social implications of impairment, have incorporated aspects of psychosocial theory into their frames of reference. These have been considered as factors to be included in planning holistic, humanistic intervention programmes, but have been combined with other aspects within the frame of reference rather than being considered as a theory per se.

Mosey's psychosocial theory

Use of psychosocial theory in occupational therapy was expounded by Mosey in the 1970s and 80s. Mosey based her views on psychoanalytical and developmental theories, together with earlier learning theories used in occupational therapy. These included limitations identified in early habit training as used by Slagle (1988), Fidler & Fidler's communication processes, and Ayres' neurobehavioural orientation theory, together with her own previous theories of adaptive skill responses, described in her *Recapitulation of Ontogenesis* (1966), a reflective summary of the stages of development of the individual.

Mosey's theory is based on the belief that individuals have an inherent need to explore the environment, which leads to a desire to be competent within that environment. The requirements to achieve competence are dependent on the nature of the society in which the individual wishes to function, and the social roles expected of and anticipated by him. The nature of the environment also has a significant effect on the process of learning.

According to Mosey (1986) the performance components which underpin psychosocial achievement are sensory integration, cognitive and psychological functioning, and social interactions.

Mosey (1986) defined sensory integration as 'processing of sensory information in such a way that the individual can act on the environment ... the central nervous system translates sensory impulses into meaningful information and organises that information so as to initiate an appropriate response'. This involves a process of filtering the many stimuli which are received from the different senses — sight, hearing, smell, and vestibular, proprioceptive and tactile sensations — and, by using cognitive functioning, perceiving and organising them to make the desired response.

Mosey identified these cognitive functions as attention, concentration, memory, orientation to the environment and thought processes which 'combine, re-combine and manipulate' associations of ideas through conceptualisation, intellect, known facts and problem-solving sequences, to plan and organise the most appropriate action.

Actions also depend on psychological functioning — individual's own perception of 'being'. This involves the person's values, needs, emotions, interests and motivation, his conscious and unconscious thought processes, and the psychodynamics of his behaviours, as well as his understanding or insight into his own and others' mental processes and actions. Psychological functioning also includes the self-concept — identity, sexual identity and body image, self-esteem and the awareness of one's own assets and limitations. Actions are also affected by object relations — 'the ways in which objects satisfy needs or interfere with satisfaction' — and the ways in which the individual 'seeks need-satisfying objects and attempts to eliminate objects that interfere with satisfaction'. This includes people's deliberate drives and courses of action, self-discipline, self-control and personal responsibilities, and the ways in which individuals deal with stress, failure and frustration. Besides their own perceptions of themselves, psychological functioning also includes individuals' concepts of others — how they view other people and how they come to these views.

Mosey identified the final element — social interaction — as the interpretation of people's perceptions and understanding of situations, their social skills in 'initiating, responding to, and sustaining interactions'. This includes communication, 'the ability to engage in meaningful interaction with another person — dyadic interaction' and group interaction skills in both structured and unstructured situations.

Basic assumptions

● The process of social integration occurs through psychosocial learning regarding roles and role needs.

● During illness the individual may lose skills, but these can be relearned and regained.

● Development of skills may be delayed by congenital impairment, but skills may be learned later through supported opportunities.

● Adaptation in each skill area occurs developmentally, and is dependent on and related to adaptation in other skill areas.

● Change (adaptation) occurs as a continuum from conscious learning and doing, through non-conscious action to the adoption of unconscious habit as mastery develops.

● Most adaptation occurs through practical interaction in a 'growth facilitating' environment which is realistic with regard to the area of need, and provides opportunity to explore the skill area and receive feedback from it.

Psychosocial theories have been important in models and frames of reference used by occupational therapists to underpin intervention to promote integration of the individual within the environment.

GENERIC MODELS

Generic models aim to provide a structure or format by which practitioners can integrate thinking to guide their intervention. Generic models can be applied across a number of areas of practice. While generic models may draw predominantly on one theory, most draw on a number of different theories, which reflects the eclectic nature of occupational therapy practice. They interlink a number of frames of reference with these theories to enable therapists to consider various different options for intervention according to the needs and situation of the individual and particular demands or preferences.

Model of Human Occupation (Fig. 2.3)

One of the most widely publicised current models is the Model of Human Occupation. This

for the activity to be considered from two perspectives:

- *the activity-centred elements* — the 'essential properties and characteristics that are intrinsic to the activity, always present, in spite of individual differences in the way the activity is performed' and the acquired characteristics which 'come from variations among individuals and groups in the ways they perceive, associate to, and carry out the activity'
- *the actor-centred perspective* — the 'degree to which the patient/client's activities performance adheres to sociocultural standards and norms, and individual's idiosyncratic approach to the activity, and the specific performance components that a particular actor uses to carry out the activity'.

The model identifies how activities may be used as a means to achieving activities health through learning of activities (client centred and developmentally) and through the various psychosocial, behavioural and developmental approaches.

The model also shows how an activities health approach can be used in the process of practice for clinical problem-solving through the stages of assessment, planning, implementation and evaluation.

Personal Adaptation through Occupation Model (Fig. 2.5)

This generic model outlined by Reed & Sanderson (1992) is also based on the assumption that 'a person adapts or adjusts through the use of various occupations'. It is based on a number of assumptions:

- By participating in occupations a person may adapt to the environment, and occupations

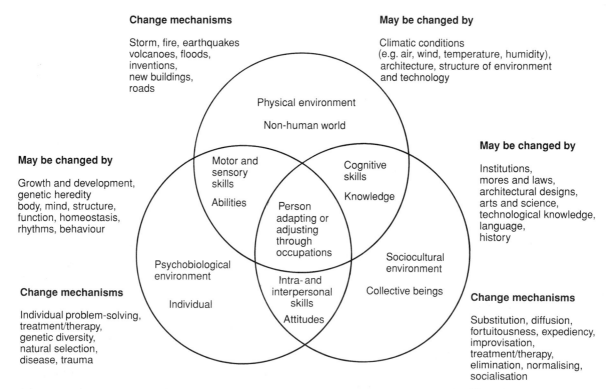

Fig. 2.5 Reed & Sanderson's conceptual model — Personal Adaptation through Occupation (from Reed K, Sanderson S 1992 Concepts of occupational therapy, 3rd edn, Williams & Wilkins, with permission).

may be a means of adapting the environment to the person.

• The degree of adaptation is determined by 'the occupations a person learns and is able to perform'.

• All occupations require knowledge, skills and attitudes in variable amounts.

• 'All occupations are determined by the environment'. They occur because of the need to maintain the physical environment for physical existence, because of sociocultural expectations, or because of the desire for particular pleasureable occupations.

• 'Change in occupation is affected by environmental change'. Change may occur at an individual level in terms of opportunities for skill acquisition and adaptation, or change may occur in the broader environment (medical, structural or geographical) which will impact on a number of people or whole populations. This may be positive change which enhances individuals' situations and opportunities, or negative change which restricts occupation. Occupational therapists can assist in the development of positive change in the environment, and in restricting the impact of negative change on the individual.

• Occupational therapists can have a positive effect on the extent and speed of an individual's abilities to adjust occupations through providing opportunities to relearn skills, to develop alternative skills, and to adapt the environment to facilitate occupation. 'Occupational therapy media and methods are designed to assist the individual toward maximum functional independence or adaptation to the least resistive environment that will meet the individual's needs' (Reed & Sanderson 1992).

• 'Functional independence and satisfaction can be achieved by promoting a balance of occupational performance in the areas of self maintenance, productivity and leisure' (Reed & Sanderson 1992).

• Occupational therapy aims to develop people's knowledge, skills and attitudes consistent with individual needs, to 'promote the maximum occupational performance to which the individual is capable'.

• Maintenance and development of skills is dependent on the occupations in which they are used, being 'relevant and useful to the individual in relation to the environment'.

The model is represented as three overlapping circles, at the centre of which is the person adapting or adjusting through occupation. Fanning out from the person are three skill areas which are used for adjustment and adaptation, namely motor and sensory skills (abilities), cognitive skills (knowledge) and intrapersonal and interpersonal skills (attitudes). The outer portion of each circle represents an area of the environment, and is surrounded by the elements which may cause change, and the change mechanisms which may alter the performance of skills or occupations. The physical environment or non-human world may be changed by gravity, temperature, altitude, humidity, soil, water, chemicals, air/wind, architecture and technology, and the change mechanisms which bring about these changes are cited as storms, fire, earthquakes, floods, volcanoes, new buildings, roads and inventions. The sociocultural environment made up of collective beings may be changed by institutions, mores and laws, architectural design, arts and science, technological knowledge, history and language. In this environment the change mechanisms are substitution, diffusion, fortuitousness, expediency, improvisation, therapy/treatment, elimination, normalisation and socialisation. The third aspect of the environment portrayed in the model is the 'psychobiological' environment — the organic features of the individual. These may be changed by growth and development, genetic heredity, mind, body, structure, function, homeostasis, rhythms and behaviour, through change mechanisms such as natural selection, disease, trauma, genetic diversity, individual problem-solving, and therapy or treatment.

Reed & Sanderson (1992) outline a number of concepts which are inherent in the model and the assumptions they make. These include detailed analysis of the different environments, exploration of change mechanisms, outlines of skill acquisition, maintenance and loss, and the definition and meaning of occupation. They also explore the ideas of need and satisfaction, the

ditions, has led to increased emphasis on the individual to develop people's coping strategies for managing their own situations. Use of cognitive problem-solving techniques, and transference and adaptation of skills, is crucial to successful functioning, particularly when impairments are likely to be permanent. Additionally, added recognition of the value of preventive as well as restorative care has increased the use of educative techniques to develop people's knowledge base, learning and understanding, in order that they may make informed judgements regarding their own health.

The frames of reference which will be described in this text as they may be applied to physical dysfunction are based on thinking regarding development, biomechanics, learning and compensation. Within the scope of the text it is not possible to address all the approaches which may be used within each frame, so the following will be given as illustrative examples of the application of the frame of reference:

- developmental frame of reference
  — neurodevelopmental approach: Bobath techniques
  — sensory integration approach: Ayres
- biomechanical frame of reference
  — biomechanical approach
- learning frame of reference
  — educational approach
  — behavioural approach
  — cognitive approach
- compensatory frame of reference
  — adaptive skills approach
  — compensatory approach.

Developmental

This has had a significant influence upon occupational therapy practice since the 1940s; many approaches have been based on the theories of physical development and human development described by Piaget (1950), Erikson (1950), Freud (1965) and others.

Development occurs because of continuous interactions between nature (heredity, genetic factors and maturation) and nurture (the effects of experiences and the environment upon the individual). The development process affects the sensorimotor, cognitive, perceptual, personal and social domains of life. It can be attributed to: natural maturation; conscious interactions with the environment and external stimuli; the processes of learning; analysis, evaluation and making choices; and uncontrolled occurrences which influence the individual.

Most frames of reference take into account some element of growth, progression and evolution but an understanding of human development is at the *core* of this frame of reference, dictating and guiding the stages of the approaches that derive from it.

Basic assumptions

- Dysfunction is due to incomplete, maladaptive or retarded behaviour. This may be the result of incomplete maturation, the inability to utilise input effectively or the paucity of stimuli and opportunity
- The person has the potential for development
- Development occurs sequentially, each stage building on the previous one. Approaches relate closely to the stages of normal chronological human development
- Development occurs in sequential stages from the person's present level of capability. Missing or jumping stages is usually counterproductive
- Active cooperation rather than passive participation on behalf of the person involved facilitates greater development in most cases.

Examples

Some examples of developmental frames of reference which have influenced approaches to physical dysfunction are:

- Ayres' (1973) sensory integration model
- Rood's (1954) sensorimotor approach
- Llorens' (1970) developmental model
- Bobath & Bobath's (1975) neurodevelopmental approach

- Brunnstrom's (1970) movement therapy
- Voss et al's (1985) proprioceptive neuromuscular facilitation approach
- Gilfoyle & Grady's (1990) spatiotemporal adaptation
- Mosey's (1986) sociodevelopmental approach.

Merits

- The developmental frame of reference uses developmental theory to good effect by incorporating the normal processes of physiological and psychological progression and maturation into intervention strategies
- The belief is one of optimism for each stage's completion, and there is a defined progression
- The commencement point for intervention is flexible, reflecting the person's present state, and there is no defined rate of progress. The programme is therefore adaptable to a variety of levels of need and rates of development.

Limitations

- Progress to functional performance may appear slower than in some approaches, as each stage should be successfully achieved before moving on to the next
- In the majority of situations the developmental frame of reference has limited application for people suffering with deteriorating conditions
- Most individual approaches within this frame of reference require high levels of expertise and tend to be labour intensive
- In order to attain maximum progress a coordinated, consistent approach is required from all members of the intervention team.

Approaches within the developmental frame of reference

The neurodevelopmental approach. A widely used approach which is developmentally based is the neurodevelopmental approach as proposed by Karel and Bertha Bobath in the 1940s and 50s in the treatment of children with cerebral palsy. In recent years this has been extended and modified for the treatment of some adult neurological disorders, particularly hemiplegia as the result of cerebrovascular accident (CVA) or head injury.

This approach makes use of positions which inhibit abnormal postures and patterns of movement, but facilitate normal equilibrium, balance and righting reactions and encourage normal movement patterns. Its basic principles are derived from the neurological learning theory and from theories of normal human development. The approach attempts to apply these principles to all aspects of activity throughout the day. It considers that the immature or damaged brain, because of the lack of opportunity to develop sophisticated balance control, or because of interruption or blocking of such patterns by trauma to pathways within the brain, gives rise to primitive or abnormal muscle tone and movement patterns. By inhibiting or suppressing these abnormal patterns, and then stimulating normal sensory, postural and motor patterns, the brain may be stimulated to develop normal patterns through alternative pathways. The neurodevelopmental approach is most successful if begun in very early life for the child with cerebral palsy, or as early as is practicable after a CVA or head injury.

The sequence of treatment follows the normal sequence of development of movement in children. Man is essentially symmetrical, and positioning and movement patterns aim to simulate and encourage bilaterality and symmetry while developing normal movement sequences. Alongside the development of motor patterns, stimulation of sensation and body awareness through touch and positioning is encouraged in order to assist the re-education of sensory pathways and to enhance the ability of the brain to interpret perceptual stimuli.

Integration of these principles within a programme of purposeful activities facilitates the development of sensorimotor control, which will then enable successful occupational performance.

Concern has been expressed by some occupational therapists that the exclusive use of neurodevelopmental approaches in occupational therapy neglects such aspects as volition, motivation or occupational needs. For use in the occupational therapy framework, 'it is necessary to expand knowledge of the logical continuity beyond inhibition–facilitation techniques to activity, and to ways in which sensori-motor treatment principles can be applied during the performance of purposeful activity' (Pedretti 1985, p. 5).

Examples of the use of neurodevelopmental techniques with hemiplegia are:

- games such as a posting box or bead-threading to promote bilaterality with the cerebral palsied child; these involve holding the container or thread with one hand while posting shaped objects or threading beads with the other
- positioning components (for example tools, ingredients or plants) on a table or bench in cooking or greenhouse gardening, which will necessitate the individual maintaining his sitting or standing balance and crossing the mid-line when making the cake or potting seedlings.

Sensory integration approach. This well-researched approach is based on the theories of neurosciences as expounded by Jean Ayres. Sensory integration is the process of organising sensory information in the brain to make an adaptive response (Ayres 1973). The approach focuses on information received by the brain from the auditory, visual, vestibular, proprioceptive and tactile systems, particular emphasis being placed on the latter three systems.

Basic assumptions of the approach which aim to explain the organisation of sensory stimuli in the central nervous system are:

- the plasticity of the central nervous system
- that normal human development occurs sequentially
- that the brain is innately organised to programme a person to seek out stimulation which is organising and beneficial in itself
- that input from one system has an effect on other systems and the whole organism
- that the central nervous system is

hierarchically organised — processing which occurs in the cortex depends on adequate organisation of stimuli received in the lower brain centres
- that stimuli must be registered meaningfully before the central nervous system is able to make a response, and permit higher level functioning to occur (Hinojosa & Kramer 1993).

Therapy aims to improve the ability to integrate sensory information by changing the organisation of the brain. Change occurs as the result of accumulated stimuli and brain maturation, which open up new neural pathways in order to allow sensory information to flow through appropriate channels and integrate with other sensory information. The approach stresses the importance of the control of sensory arousal and the use of functional support systems in order to stimulate and develop adaptive responses according to the person's developmental stage.

A number of assessments may be used to determine:

- tactile and vestibular proprioceptive sensory processing
- form and space perception and visual–motor coordination
- bilateral integration and sequencing
- coordination, dexterity and motor skills
- practice abilities and behaviours.

Activities are designed to include a variety of sensory stimuli, with the aim of facilitating appropriate physical and emotional responses, which can be transferred according to need to other situations. Through variation and variety in activities the person is able to build up a repertoire of responses to multiple stimuli. This usually commences with basic primitive responses and gradually builds up to more complex adaptive responses to multisensory stimuli according to the person's developmental level. These adaptive responses, or 'end-product abilities', aim to facilitate adaptation within the environment through independent emotional and motor control. The approach is particularly useful with children who are brain damaged or developmentally delayed for whom play activities may be used as the therapeutic medium, but it may also be used with adults who have suffered brain damage or have learning disabilities.

Activities such as press-button games or obstacle courses may be used to integrate actions with verbal or visual stimuli. Similarly activities which involve hammocks or swings enable the individual to experience changes of positioning, and make choices regarding whether to increase or diminish these by swinging with or counteracting the pendulum movement.

Biomechanical

This frame of reference has been the basis of many medical interventions throughout the century. It views the body as a functioning machine, made up of specific parts which may be damaged by disease or injury. This frame of reference is based in the desire to explain function anatomically and physiologically. Many of its basic premises formed the foundations on which exercise physiology, kinetics and dynamic orthoses developed within the medical model.

The body is seen as a combination of parts which work together to form a whole; however, the Gestalt (the sum of the whole being more than a combination of the parts) is not acknowledged. Treatment to overcome damage to a particular part results in return of function. Therapeutic exercise or activity improves functional performance; this in turn leads to a sense of well-being, which promotes recovery. There is the risk, however, that the exercise or movement becomes the main focus, at the expense of the activity medium.

Basic assumptions

- Successful human motor activity is based on physical mobility and strength
- Participation in activity involving repeated specific graded movements maintains and improves function
- Activity can be graded progressively to meet particular demands within an intervention programme.

Merits

- The biomechanical frame of reference makes good use of media and equipment to promote physical function
- It can be applied to a variety of creative and constructive activities
- It uses knowledge of activity analysis to good effect
- It utilises the increased knowledge of anatomical, physiological and kinaesthetic processes in man
- It has led to the development of specific techniques for measuring movement, strength and endurance.

Limitations

- The biomechanical frame of reference focuses on physical performance in the absence of volition, role duties or environmental influences. It is specifically based in physical activity with no reference to motivation or the psychological, emotional or social aspects of rehabilitation
- It does not address the need for balance in activity in daily life. It emphasises lower levels for survival — mobility and physical function — but does not follow through to the higher levels of self-esteem and self-actualisation
- It is not applicable to people whose central nervous system is impaired. The emphasis is on the promotion of physical mobility, therefore this frame of reference has limited application to people with chronic or deteriorating conditions which affect mobility
- There is the risk of didactic reductionism, the therapist controlling the programme and the person being the passive participant in an exercise regime which does not necessarily reflect personal interests or promote internal locus of control. The exercise may become the focus at the expense of the activity.

Current use of the biomechanical approach

Three slightly different biomechanical approaches have been developed:

- Baldwin's reconstruction approach

(presented in 1918, and one of the earliest documented 'physical' approaches) (Baldwin 1919)
- Taylor's (1934) orthopaedic approach
- Licht's (1957) kinetic approach.

While each of these approaches has a slightly different emphasis, all are based on the biomechanical frame of reference. They are used in physical rehabilitation in physiotherapy and occupational therapy to promote mobility, strength and activity tolerance (stamina). Their early popularity reflected the essentially scientific nature of medical development in the physical field in the 1960s, but they are less popular today, forming only a small part of the occupational therapist's treatment methods. The need to improve range of movement, muscle strength and endurance has also been reduced by modern medical and surgical techniques which no longer require long-term immobilisation.

The mechanistic compartmentalisation of functional performance into physical actions contradicts the holism and humanism of occupational therapy's philosophy. Overcoming specific biomechanical dysfunction is only part of the management of the individual's total needs, mobility being only one part of function. However, since mobility *is* an important aspect of life, the principles of the biomechanical approach may form a part, if not the whole, of the therapeutic programme.

The changing nature of occupational therapy practice (which can be seen in the shift from hospital- to community-based work, and in the increase in the proportion of people with complex, chronic disabilities and neurological conditions) further limits the use of this approach. Increased awareness of the merits of broadly based intervention as opposed to specialisation may further reduce the importance of this frame of reference in the total intervention programme.

Many occupational therapists have already abandoned the exclusive use of many biomechanical practices, although certain measurement techniques and activity analyses are useful in particular aspects of treatment. Some features of the biomechanical frame of reference combined with other, less reductionist, approaches retain importance in specific areas of practice, particularly orthopaedics, sports medicine and the treatment of physical damage resulting from trauma. Other professions, including physical medicine, nursing and physiotherapy are adopting more humanistic, holistic philosophies, which may further contribute to the decline in popularity of the biomechanical frame of reference.

Learning

This frame of reference is based on the work of educational and developmental psychologists, behaviourists and teachers. It is founded on the assumption that adaptation and change are based on the ability to learn. Learning may be cognitive, gained by insight from personal interpretations of subjective responses to sensory stimuli and cues based on studies by Beck (1976) and Piaget (1950). Learning may also occur through behavioural change based on predetermined objectives and reinforcement of good behaviours, as described by Thorndike (1932) and Bandura (1971). Formal teaching — the provision of information and guidance — also promotes learning for informed action and decision-making.

Therapists employ teaching skills in many aspects of intervention, but not all aim to promote learning. Similarly there may be an element of learning as a secondary gain with some interventions in other frames of reference, but theories of learning are central to the beliefs and aims in this frame of reference.

Basic assumptions

- The person has the capacity to learn through education and experiences
- The acquisition of knowledge, and insight into behaviour, will promote learning
- Learning occurs through different educational modes which may be cognitive, conditioned or educative
- Behaviours are learned. Poor or non-advantageous habits can be unlearned, and replaced by lasting, helpful, 'good' habits through positive experiences and practice.

This frame of reference is used to support some of the approaches within other frames of reference. It is a major influence in particular aspects of practice, for example:

- social skills training
- assertiveness training
- anxiety/stress management
- joint protection and time management education
- behaviour modification.

These techniques may be used in a number of ways in the management of physical dysfunction, not only with children to advance the stages of developmental learning, but also in facilitating the relearning processes following head injury, cerebrovascular accident or other changed circumstances resulting from trauma and physical dysfunction.

Approaches within the learning frame of reference

The educative approach. Occupational therapists aim to work in partnership with individuals and their family/carers, identifying a range of options for problem-solving and working with them to make the most appropriate choices of interventions.

In order that individuals and carers are able to make informed choices, it is essential that they have information concerning the importance of the issue at hand, the range of options available and the implications of choice of particular decisions.

An educative approach aims to provide the knowledge on which such choices may be made. Education may be provided through verbal discussion, but this depends on the recipient's memory and interpretation of what is heard. Many therapists now use visual educational means to support verbal guidance, in the form of booklets or leaflets which the individual may take away and study at leisure or discuss further with other people. These leaflets may provide information concerning the medical condition, the importance of particular aspects of health, and ways in which the individual may take some

responsibility for his future personal health care. Such leaflets may be used to inform people regarding the methods of joint protection in rheumatic disease, the importance of correct posture, exercise and suitable seating in the management of back pain, the care of the residual limb following amputation, and many other areas of self-care. In some instances this written information may also be supported by audio-visual means, such as tapes or instruction videos. Many such educative materials are provided in a number of languages and reflect the needs of people from a variety of cultural groups.

The therapist should discuss the information with the individual and be available to answer any queries concerning the content. The information may form the basis of decisions regarding intervention and the individual's future self-management. In many instances the provision of written or audio-visual information will be supported by other therapeutic approaches, usually involving practical and/or experiential techniques, to further the person's learning regarding a particular technique or issue.

The behavioural approach. This is based on the findings of behaviourists who believed that behaviours are learned in response to stimuli. Undesirable behaviours can be unlearned or modified through negative reinforcement of inappropriate behaviours and positive reinforcement of advantageous behaviours. A number of techniques may be used to change behaviour. Modelling may be used where the individual is able to model behaviour on good behaviour observed in others. Desensitisation, a gradual controlled build-up of exposure to a sensitive situation, may be used to change behaviour in relation to particular circumstances. Behaviour modification may be used to change inappropriate behaviours. This usually involves writing a contract with clearly defined predetermined objectives which the individual needs to achieve. Positive reinforcement or reward is given when such objectives are achieved, and this is gradually diminished as the new behaviours become established. However, at this stage care must be taken to ensure that the newly learned skills do not 'fade'.

Other modes of behavioural learning involve chaining — the gradual build up of actions towards completion of the task — and backward chaining. In backward chaining the individual is first responsible for completing the final stage of the task, and then gradually learns to do more towards the task in reverse sequence. Biofeedback is a behavioural technique which may be used in conjunction with other techniques, for example relaxation techniques, to develop individuals' abilities to learn how to cope with particular situations.

Behavioural techniques are rarely used in isolation by occupational therapists because of their reductionist nature. They are time-consuming to implement and monitor, and demand consistency of approach by all those involved with the individual if they are to succeed. However, they are useful in situations in which particular disadvantageous behaviours need to be unlearned, for example in cases of phobia following a particular incident, to develop appropriate social behaviours following head injury, or to change unsuitable practices in daily living or work settings.

The cognitive approach. This is based on the thought processes by which individuals link memories, perceptions, ideas and experiences within the context of their own environment, and use these to plan actions and problem-solve. Cognition is based on past experiences, and on past and present images and perceptions of oneself. If these are faulty or negative they will affect individuals' abilities rationally to address issues, process information and take a positive role in problem-solving. Analysis of the individual's reasoning processes forms the basis for the cognitive approach, which aims to re-focus thought processes to develop a more positive 'train of thought'.

A cognitive approach may be used to help individuals make informed adjustments to temporary or permanent changes in their circumstances. They aim to facilitate insight into the person's thought processes, to correct misinterpretations or distortions of ideas, and to promote a positive approach to future activities. By providing opportunities through information sharing, role play, reminiscence, reality orientation or exploration of stress management techniques, individuals are able to gain insight into their own and others' interpretations of the situation, and explore coping strategies for management of the situation in the future. Examples of how such techniques may be used with physical dysfunction may be seen in ways by which imagery or re-labelling may be used in the management of pain (see Ch. 28), or the development of assertiveness and stress management techniques to build self-confidence following disfigurement. Similarly, perceptual or memory training may be used to develop cognitive skills and awareness following cerebral vascular accident or head injury, or with people suffering memory problems.

In the learning frame of reference the prime focus is for the person to learn coping skills. While the three approaches have been outlined separately, they are frequently used in conjunction with each other, and with other approaches, to facilitate a broad-based approach to problem-solving, which employs theoretical, experiential and practical learning.

Compensatory

This frame of reference is based on the belief that man is a functional animal and that his ability to function — by whatever means — is essential to his well-being. It stresses the secondary benefit to be gained by improving performance in activity or occupation despite ongoing physical, cognitive, psychological or social dysfunction. A number of different compensatory methods may be used to perform an activity. The successful completion of the activity, rather than a specific change in anatomical, physiological or psychological attributes, is the primary goal, as this will enable the individual to survive in society.

Compensation may be used to facilitate performance in a variety of activities in daily life, through the use and adaptation of remaining abilities and strengths, by adapting the activities or by the provision of external compensatory means. These methods do not directly contribute to changing the person's biological, physiological or psychological deficits.

This is one of the oldest frames of reference for rehabilitation. It is not unique to occupational therapy and is also used by physiotherapists (for example in the provision of walking frames to compensate for lower limb weakness), by orthotists and prosthetists, and to some degree by speech and language therapists when alternative communication equipment or techniques are recommended.

Basic assumptions

- Completion of daily role activities is a basic human need; the disabled individual can benefit by learning alternative methods for carrying out these activities
- People suffer short- and long-term dysfunction which cannot be immediately or significantly improved by other therapeutic methods, so there is a need for compensation for lost or limited abilities
- Residual capabilities can be supplemented by external aids to promote problem-solving
- The individual's involvement in choosing appropriate methods can be advantageous in promoting some general aspects of 'well-being'.

Merits

- The compensatory frame of reference is a widely documented and widely used basis for therapy practice. Many therapists are familiar with it
- It is easy to explain and understand
- It makes good use of a problem-solving approach
- It can be used to meet immediate short-term needs or to compensate for long-term loss. It is therefore appropriate for acute needs, for example immediately following surgery, or for people with chronic or deteriorating disorders who are not likely to recover or improve
- A range of options is available, with considerable choice within them to meet a wide variety of needs
- There is no rigidly structured sequence of

progression, so there can be flexibility to meet the particular needs of the individual
- It is concrete and often visual. It is easy to understand and frequently brings speedy results.

Limitations

- Historically, this frame of reference has had a long association with the medical model, and so may be prone to reductionist or recipe-like thinking. The therapist may be tempted to 'prescribe' the 'best' method of compensating for a particular problem, rather than evaluate the range of options with the person concerned. A tendency, deriving from the medical model, to compartmentalise problems may fragment this potentially holistic approach into arbitrary divisions
- The recognition of permanence of loss of function as the basis for instigating this frame of reference may have negative connotations for the individual, who will then require considerable support
- In choosing solutions the therapist may be at risk of succumbing to external pressures concerning the quickest or cheapest way of compensating, thereby denying personal choice. Compensation per se may be seen as a solution in cases where the use of other approaches and frames of reference may in fact promote or facilitate physical or psychological recovery or improvement.

Approaches within the compensatory frame of reference

Adaptation of skills. An effective method of compensation for dysfunction is for the individual to adapt his existing skills to master problems and cope independently in particular situations. This method uses existing strengths to compensate for deficits. Techniques are based on:

- detailed knowledge of the present level of skill attributes
- clear identification of any previous techniques used for performing the activity

- exploration and identification of alternative techniques to perform activity using existing skills

Solutions may involve:

- modification of the techniques required to perform the activity
- development of new skills through exploration and practice
- transfer of existing skills to different activities
- the use of 'trick' movements to compensate for particular movement deficits
- adapting role or function to eliminate the need to perform the activity.

Techniques will obviously differ according to individual attributes and limitations. New techniques may be learned through exploration and development of skills, and practising using these skills in the task or situation. Such techniques as cognitive prompts may be used to aid memory, and individual movement skills may be transferred to perform activities in a particular manner, for example using manipulative hand skills in the non-affected hand to tie shoe-laces and dress one-handed, or using upper limb strength for non-standing transfers. Equally the addition or omission of a particular stage to a sequence of activity may facilitate independent performance. Regular practice develops familiarity and expertise in the adapted skills until they become automatic, and can be used with confidence.

The advantage of these methods of compensation over the provision of external support are:

- the enhancement of self-confidence and self-esteem through independent personal achievement — the methods are personalised and reflect individuals skills and attributes
- that they are flexible, adaptable and transportable — they may be used in a number of situations to a greater or lesser extent, depending on need, and are constantly available to the individual wherever he may be
- that, despite the time needed for the exploration of techniques, tuition and practice, they are usually cost-effective and their effect is long term

- that they reflect the basic philosophy of the profession regarding personal potential.

The compensatory approach. This approach is widely used to compensate for dysfunction in mobility, self-maintenance and domestic activities, and is also used to enable individuals to pursue work and leisure pursuits. It applies the basic beliefs of the compensatory frame of reference. Occupational therapists using this approach must recognise that the individual and carers need to be consulted and involved in the choice of the most appropriate form of compensation; this involvement will help to motivate users to accept and persevere with the chosen solution.

Methods of compensation may include:

- supply of adapted tools or equipment
- provision of prostheses or support orthoses
- modification of the environment
- provision of financial help
- organisation of manual / social assistance.

The therapist using this approach must acknowledge the need for flexibility and adaptability in responding to a person's individual circumstances. Support orthoses have the potential to solve a variety of problems in different locations, providing they are worn consistently and correctly. Adapted tools and equipment may have a wide application in some instances, but some equipment or tools may be specific to one particular task, and may not be easily transferable or transportable.

Environmental adaptations are often considered a more drastic measure, as they are more likely to overtly stigmatise the person with the problem and affect other members of the family; they are also more costly. An adaptation can usually be made to particular environments pertinent to the individual, e.g. home, work, school or vehicle, but their rehabilitative value is limited to these locations. The implications of restricted freedom in the wider environment will still have to be addressed.

Financial benefits may be used to purchase equipment or services to compensate for deficit; for example, a person who is unable to perform the full range of food preparation might buy an electric food mixer or microwave oven, or make arrangements for prepared food delivery. Such financial benefits may enable the person to pursue personal preferences, depending upon the range of options available and the funding provided, e.g. the Mobility Allowance or Care Allowance.

Arranging for helpers to assist with certain tasks will require the person to recognise his limitations and to decide that the tasks in question are essential to him, despite the loss of independence they entail. Increased dependence upon others may be viewed positively, by virtue of the social contact it brings. It also enables the person to conserve his energy for other personal priorities. Employing others to assist with particular activities also enables the individual to remain 'in charge', rather than being a grateful recipient of help.

Obviously, as there is such a wide variety of options available in the compensatory approach, detailed assessment of functional capabilities and life-style needs is essential. From these findings the priorities and options for problem-solving should be discussed so that optimum solutions are found. These will depend on personal preferences and volition, the level, nature and probable duration of the dysfunction, and the social environment. Additionally, the person's potential to learn new skills and use equipment or other resources should be considered.

It may sometimes be necessary to explore a number of different options before the optimal solution is found. For the person with a progressive condition it will be necessary to re-evaluate the choice of options as the condition progresses, but this should be minimised by forward thinking and proactive planning.

CONCLUSION

Without a theory base a profession has no foundation and no planned direction. Without a theory base the professional will be ill equipped to assess the situations she is faced with and to respond to them in a realistic and organised manner.

Understanding the theory base of occupational therapy is a complex task, given the eclectic nature of today's practice, the diversity of individuals' needs and the current emphasis upon humanistic principles in therapy. Appreciation of the individual needs and drives of her clientele and an understanding of theory will assist the therapist in her professional reasoning and reflection.

The therapist herself is an individual with personal values and beliefs which may influence her choice of frames of reference. Recognition of these within the context of other frames of reference and the broader pattern of theory will enable her to more fully understand her own professional approach and that of others.

No profession stands alone; a sound theory base is necessary to identify the strengths and boundaries of a profession in the context of multiprofessional health care provision.

No society stands still; theory is essential in guiding research and development in the profession, in order to meet the changing needs of individuals and ensure that the profession of occupational therapy remains up-to-date in its practices.

REFERENCES

American Occupational Therapy Association 1976 Occupational therapy: its definition and functions. American Journal of Occupational Therapy 20: 204

Atkinson R L, Atkinson C, Smith E T, Benn D J, Hilgard E R 1985 Introduction to psychology, 10th edn. Harcourt Brace Jovanovich, San Diego

Ayres A J 1973 Sensory integration and learning disorders. Western Psychological Service, Los Angeles

Baldwin B T 1919 Occupational therapy. American Journal for Care of Cripples 8: 447–451

Bandura A L 1971 Social learning theory. General Learning Press, New York

Barnitt R 1990 Knowledge, skills and attitudes: what happened to thinking? British Journal of Occupational Therapy 53(11): 450–456

Beck A T 1976 Cognitive therapy and emotional disorders. International University Press, New York

Black J A, Champion D J 1976 Methods and issues in social research. John Wiley, New York

Blom Cooper L 1989 Occupational therapy, an emerging profession in health care. Report of a Commission of Inquiry. British Association of Occupational Therapists, London

Bobath B, Bobath K 1975 Motor development in the different types of cerebral palsy. Heinemann Medical, London

British Association of Occupational Therapists 1995 Code of Ethics and Professional Conduct. British Association of Occupational Therapists, London

Brunnstrom S 1970 Movement therapy in hemiplegia. Harper & Row, New York

Clark F A, Parham D, Carlson M E et al 1991 Occupational science — academic innovation in the service of occupational therapy's future. American Journal of Occupational Therapy 45(4): 300–310

Creek J 1990 Occupational therapy and mental health. Principles, skills and practice. Churchill Livingstone, Edinburgh

Creek J, Feaver S 1993 Models for practice in occupational therapy. Part 1. Defining terms. British Journal of Occupational Therapy 56(1): 4–6

Cynkin S, Robinson A M 1990 Occupational therapy and activities health: toward health through activities. Little, Brown, Boston

Ellis M 1981 Why bother with research? British Journal of Occupational Therapy 44(4): 115–116

Erikson E 1950 Childhood and society. W W Norton, New York

Evans K A 1987 Definition of occupation as the core concept of occupational therapy. American Journal of Occupational Therapy 41(10): 627–628

Fidler G, Fidler J 1978 Doing and becoming: purposeful action and self actualisation. American Journal of Occupational Therapy 32(5): 305–310

Freud A 1965 Normality and pathology in childhood. Assessment and development. International Universities Press, New York

Gilfoyle E M, Grady A P 1990 Children adapt, 2nd edn. Slack, New Jersey

Hagedorn R 1992 Occupational therapy. Foundations for practice. Churchill Livingstone, Edinburgh

Hinojosa J, Kramer P 1993 Frames of reference for paediatric occupational therapy. Williams & Wilkins, Baltimore

Hopkins H L, Smith H D (eds) 1988 Willard and Spackman's occupational therapy. J B Lippincott, Philadelphia

Kielhofner G 1983 Health through occupation. Theory and practice in occupational therapy. F A Davis, Philadelphia

Kielhofner G 1985 The model of human occupation. Williams & Wilkins, Baltimore

Kielhofner G 1992 Conceptual foundations of occupational therapy. F A Davis, Philadelphia

Kielhofner G, Burke J P, Igi C H 1980 The model of human occupation, parts 1–4. American Journal of Occupational Therapy 34(9–12): 572–581, 663–675, 731–737, 777–788

Kuhn T 1970 The structure of scientific revolutions, 2nd edn. University of Chicago Press, Chicago

Licht S 1957 Kinetic occupational therapy. In: Dunton W R, Licht S (eds) Occupational therapy principles and practice. Thomas, Illinois

Llorens L A 1970 Facilitating growth and development. The promise of occupational therapy. American Journal of Occupational Therapy 24(1): 93–101

Lyons M 1985 Paradise lost! Paradise regained? Putting the promise of occupational therapy into practice. Australian Journal of Occupational Therapy 32(2): 45–53

Maslow A 1968 Toward a psychology of being. Van Nostrand, New York

Mattingley C, Fleming M H 1994 Clinical reasoning: forms of inquiry in practice. F A Davis, Philadelphia

Meyer A 1922 The philosophy of occupational therapy. Archives of Occupational Therapy 1: 1–10

Mosey A C 1966 Recapitulation of ontogenesis: a theory for practice of occupational therapy. American Journal of Occupational Therapy 22: 426–432

Mosey A C 1981 Configuration of a profession. Raven Press, New York

Mosey A C 1986 Psychosocial components of occupational therapy. Raven Press, New York

Parham D 1987 Toward professionalism: the reflective practitioner. American Journal of Occupational Therapy. 41(9): 555–560

Pedretti L W 1985 Occupational therapy: practice skills for physical dysfunction, 2nd edn. C V Mosby, St Louis

Piaget J 1950 Psychology of intelligence. Routledge & Kegan Paul, London

Reed K, Sanderson S 1983 Concepts of occupational therapy. Williams & Wilkins, Baltimore

Reed K, Sanderson S 1992 Concepts of occupational therapy, 3rd edn. Williams & Wilkins, Baltimore

Reilly M 1962 Occupational therapy can be one of the great ideas of 20th century medicine. American Journal of Occupational Therapy 16: 1

Rogers C 1984a Client centred therapy: its current practice, implications and theory. Houghton Mifflin, Boston

Rogers J C 1983 Eleanor Clark Slagle Lecture. Clinical reasoning: the ethics, science and art. American Journal of Occupational Therapy 37(9): 601–616

Rogers J C 1984b The foundation: why study human occupation? American Journal of Occupational Therapy 38: 47–49

Rood M S 1954 Neurophysiology reactions as a basis for physical therapy. Physical Therapy Review 34: 444–449

Slagle E C 1988 Historical perspectives of occupational therapy. In: Hopkins H L, Smith H D (eds) Willard and Spackman's occupational therapy. J B Lippincott, Philadelphia, pp 20–21

Taylor E, Mitchell M 1990 Research attitudes and activities of occupational therapy clinicians. American Journal of Occupational Therapy 44(4): 350–355

Taylor M 1934 The treatment of orthopaedic conditions. Canadian Journal of Occupational Therapy 2: 1–8

Thorndike E L 1932 The fundamentals of learning. Teachers College, Columbia University, New York

Voss D E, Ionta M K, Myers B J 1985 Proprioceptive neuromuscular facilitation: patterns and techniques, 3rd edn. Harper & Row, New York

Wallis M A 1987 'Profession' and 'professionalism' and the emerging profession of occupational therapy, part 1. British Journal of Occupational Therapy 50(8): 264–265

Yerxa E J 1979 The philosophical base of occupational therapy in 2001AD. American Occupational Therapy Association, Rockville, Maryland

Young M, Quinn E 1992 Theories and practice of occupational therapy. Churchill Livingstone, Edinburgh

FURTHER READING

Ackerman W B, Lohnes P R 1981 Research methods for nurses. McGraw Hill, New York

Alexander L, French G, Graham G, King L, Timewell E 1985 Who needs a theory of occupational therapy? Do you? Australian Occupational Therapy Journal 32(3): 104–108

Allport G 1940 The psychologist's frame of reference. Psychology Bulletin 37(24)

Argyle M 1978 Psychology of interpersonal behaviour. Penguin, Harmondsworth

Argyle M (ed.) 1981 Social skills and health. Methuen, London

Bandura A L, Walters R H 1963 Social learning and personality development. Holt, Rinehart & Winston, New York

Barris R, Kielhofner G, Watts H V 1983 Psychosocial occupational therapy. Ramsco, Maryland

Barton W E 1943 The challenge of occupational therapy. Occupational Therapy Rehabilitation 22: 262

Berger R M, Patchner M A 1988 Planning for research. A guide for the helping professions. Sage, California

Bobath B 1986 Adult hemiplegia. Evaluation and treatment, 2nd edn. Heinemann Medical, London

Bruce M A, Borg B 1987 Frames of reference in psychosocial occupational therapy. Slack, New Jersey

Calnan J 1984 Coping with research. Heinemann, London

Clark P N 1979 Human development through occupation: a philosophy and conceptual model for practice, part 2. American Journal of Occupational Therapy 33(9): 577–584

College of Occupational Therapists 1985 Research advice handbook for occupational therapists. COT, London

Conte J, Conte W 1977 The association: the use of conceptual models in occupational therapy. American Journal of Occupational Therapy 31(4): 262–264

Cracknell E 1984 Humanistic psychology. In: Willson M (ed.) Occupational therapy in short term psychiatry. Churchill Livingstone, Edinburgh, pp 73–88

Hilgard E R, Atkinson C A, Atkinson R L 1975 Introduction to psychology. Harcourt Brace Jovanovich, New York

Levins M 1986 The psychodynamics of activity. British Journal of Occupational Therapy 49(3): 87–89

Mocellin G 1988 A perspective of the principles and practice of occupational therapy. British Journal of Occupational Therapy 51(1): 4–7

Partridge C, Barnitt R 1986 Research guidelines. A handbook for therapists. Heinemann, London

Royeen C B (ed.) 1988 Research tradition in occupational therapy. Process, philosophy and status. Slack, New Jersey

Skinner B F 1938 The behaviour of organisms. Appleton-Century-Crofts, New York

Skinner B F 1968 The technology of teaching. Appleton-Century-Crofts, New York

Trombly C A 1989 Occupational therapy for physical dysfunction. Williams & Wilkins, Baltimore

Willson M 1987 Occupational therapy in long term psychiatry, 2nd edn. Churchill Livingstone, Edinburgh

Young M 1984 Models of practice for occupational therapy. British Journal of Occupational Therapy 47(12): 381–382

3

Life span development

Elizabeth Cracknell

INTRODUCTION

Human beings are bound by time. People can generally give the date of their birth, sometimes even their time of birth, and age is a measure of how long they have lived. Time provides a sense of continuity as well as an anchor of stability and security (Salmon 1985). Throughout life people encounter a variety of events which, through experience, become part of their personal history. These experiences are extremely influential as they colour people's perception of the world and thereby how they interact within it. Past experience also contributes to a present sense of identity, an awareness of being and personal aspirations. Current values, attitudes and ways of living prepare individuals for an unpredictable future of new relationships and unknown events, as the only certainty of the future is death. The annual cycle reminds us of the passing of time as another year is added to age, bringing gains, losses and change. As the writer of Ecclesiastes (3:1, 2) puts it:

To every thing there is a season, and a time to every purpose under the heaven: A time to be born, and a time to die; a time to plant and a time to pluck up that which is planted.

WHAT IS LIFE SPAN DEVELOPMENT?

Life span development is the period of the life span which creates the framework for life span psychological development. Unlike developmen-

61

tal psychology which tends to concentrate on the early periods of life development until adulthood, life span psychology focuses upon both change and stability throughout the whole of the life cycle. Life span psychology requires an understanding of both intrapsychic and interpersonal processes, and takes into account people's life experiences and phenomenology. It includes not only each person's individual history but also how that history was created, and thereby has particular relevance to the understanding of issues of health and illness.

Life span developmental psychology is broad in nature, encompassing the biological, cognitive, social, cultural and personality processes which are involved in change throughout a person's life. Experience arises from the activities of life which involve the whole person, although awareness of the impact of any one specific experience may not be very great.

Life span development assumes that:

- the potential for development is continuous throughout life
- development occurs in an ordered sequence
- each successive stage of development incorporates the previous stages
- each stage builds on the previous stage.

Any one person may be slow in development compared with his peer group, but he will nevertheless progress through the stages in the same order as his peers. A person cannot run before he can walk. Psychologists are not being original in their model of life as stages of development. In *As You Like It*, Shakespeare considered men and women to be actors on life's stage with exits and entrances. He wrote that human beings passed through seven ages, reaching the final one of old age 'sans teeth, sans eyes, sans taste, sans everything'. In contrast to Shakespeare's time, today's different living conditions, life-styles and good health means that a growing number of people in Western industrialised society are reaching old age hale and hearty, with all their faculties intact.

Attitudes towards life vary from person to person. Life can be regarded as a long journey with many hurdles to jump rather like a pilgrim-age, as described in *Pilgrim's Progress* by John Bunyan (Bunyan 1986), or it can be considered to be an exciting adventure into which one must pack as much as possible before death. Whatever the attitude a person has to life, events and situations are interpreted according to individual beliefs, values and experiences, i.e. through the person's own world view. It is the phenomenology of the person, his internal knowledge of the world, which is a powerful determinant of behaviour as a human being grows through life and deals with its affairs.

LIFE SPAN THEORIES

Life span theorists generally adopt one of two long-term approaches, either:

1. *maturational*, i.e. that development is basically biologically determined

or

2. *interactional*, i.e. that development is the result of the interaction of the biological and the experiential.

The second approach takes account of both human nature and the learning processes of nurture to which a person is exposed. Within the developmental perspective occupational therapists generally adopt a humanistic approach, arising from the philosophy of the profession (Ch. 1). Humanistic psychology assumes that human beings are unique organisms with their own particular values and attitudes, determined in part by perception. It is each person's own individual phenomenology, i.e. interpretation of the world, which is the springboard of behaviour.

The value of life span development

In common with all students of the medical and allied professions, occupational therapy students undertake case studies as part of their fieldwork experience. A personal history includes, among other things, people's past experiences, which contribute to the understanding of an individual's current state of being. A personal history explains so much. A qualified practitioner builds on previous learning when she assesses a person newly referred to her and asks questions in order to make case notes based upon his history. Similar procedures take place within the life span development framework, based upon the assumption that without such information a person cannot be really understood. If little understanding exists between an individual and his therapist it is very difficult for treatment to be effective. The therapist will take actions for the other person, based upon her objective assessment of his level of dysfunction, which may be out of keeping with the way in which the individual is experiencing the problems. Objective assessment also ignores the individual's anxieties, expectations, desires and plans for the future. It is as if treatment takes place in a vacuum.

Occupational therapists work with people who have suffered illness, trauma or disturbance of some kind. Their whole being has been disturbed by an event which was usually unplanned. The words *disease* and *dysfunction* reflect the limitations and reduced level of performance hampering people when they suffer and lose the ability to function in the way that they once did. Indeed dysfunction may be of such a degree that future life plans have to be revised. All events of life have the potential for transition and change, even those which are predictable (Neugarten 1977, Kimmel 1980), but unpredictable events can be traumatic and a source of great stress.

Illnesses, accidents and losses of function are unpredictable. Even a small accident such as cutting a finger in the kitchen can be a shock and be upsetting. Learning from this incident would lead to more care in future when using kitchen tools. However, not all illnesses are sudden. Some are gradual and may at first be hardly noticeable. Changes in accuracy of movement may be put down to clumsiness or failure of attention, and it may be some time before medical contact is made. Medical diagnosis can either be a relief or a shock; either way, if the person has a deteriorating neurological condition, there has to be a gradual adjustment to the loss of function, even though these changes call into question a person's sense of identity and social roles.

On the other hand an unpredictable event, such as a cerebral vascular accident which leaves a person with a hemiparesis, may well result in a serious crisis of being. Many occupational therapists work with people who have suffered some physical dysfunction, and the goal for both them and therapist is the development of maximum occupational performance to cope with future living. People vary in their experience of and response to disability depending upon personal disposition, but it has only comparatively recently been realised how much personal factors such as age and experience influence health and illness. An understanding of a person's personal life history, and thereby current disposition, puts the therapist in a more relevant and realistic position to assist the person reach his goals.

Many life events are routine, regular and managed with ease. Habituation has occurred, and little thought has to be given to actions required to achieve a goal. It is rather like learning to drive. The period of learning demands intense concentration, and can provoke anxiety and be very frustrating. However, with practice new skills are learned which gradually require less concentration as they become routine. The driving test is to demonstrate that the learned skills can be executed with a level of competence and ease. The satisfaction of passing results in joy and pleasure, and achievement levels increase as confidence grows. Other events, such as becoming a parent, mean taking on new responsibilities. However, other responsibilities may be lost if one has to leave or curtail employment, social and recreational contacts. A change of this magnitude demands fresh thinking which will create a variety of emotions and require great skill in management as one has to learn to adapt to the changing demands of the different roles. As a person reviews a year at its close it is easy to note the great events of that period which have led to personal change.

LIFE EVENTS

Any one life event comprises three components,

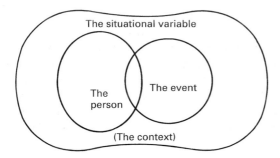

Fig. 3.1 The three components of a life event.

all of which interact with each other (Fig. 3.1). First, there are the people who participate in the encounter; then there is the event itself, which may or may not be expected; and third, there is the situation in which the event takes place — the situational variables. These three components are interdependent and influence the processes of personal change and the outcome. Each of these components will be looked at in turn, and then the process of adaptation and change will be considered.

THE HUMAN ORGANISM — PERSONAL FACTORS

Human beings are remarkable creatures. First, they are biological beings of matter, and their genetic inheritance lays down what they may become. Unless someone is one of identical twins, each person is unique, born with his or her own personal characteristics. However, people are not just biological creatures, and will only develop their potential if they are exposed to opportunities in the environment which allow them to develop their innate capacities. Human beings have a consciousness and a myriad of capacities which enable them to do wonderful things such as think, learn, create and imagine. They have a consciousness of self which appears not to exist in other creatures, and a host of cognitive processes by which sense is made of the world. Some psychologists believe that human beings have a spiritual dimension to their being, a part of them which transcends the human and material world as we know it and is in tune with

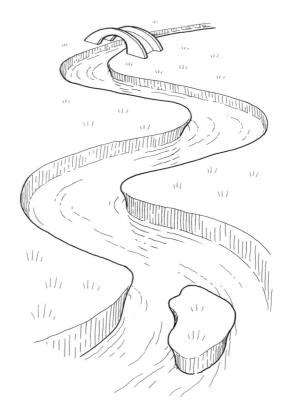

Fig. 3.2 Life is like a stream — it shapes and is shaped.

the Infinite. Whether or not this is so, a person who believes it has a very different perspective upon life from one who does not.

Emotions and feelings are experienced daily and can change dramatically within a short period, from joy to great sadness, from anxiety to calmness. In a society in which the emphasis is on what people think, rather than what they feel, many individuals find it difficult to say what their feelings are at any one moment. Human beings are never static, as all new experiences have the potential for learning and development. Living is like a stream which is both shaped by, and at the same time shapes, the banks between which it flows (Fig. 3.2).

The processes of change created by life events may enhance personal development and increase self-esteem and motivation, leading to further actions. The goal of growth in humanistic terms is the development of one's potential in order to become fully functioning or self-actualising.

Socialisation processes

The most formative years for a person are those of early childhood, and most babies are born into a ready-made family. In Western society it is more often a nuclear family than an extended one in which aunts, uncles and other kin are part of the community. It is through the interaction of the child and the family that the values, attitudes and behaviour patterns of that family are acquired by the child. The family itself represents to the child values of the community, class and race, and is permeated by the prevailing cultural and religious values. All these factors influence how a child construes and feels about the world.

Cultural influences (Fig. 3.3)

In a society such as that of the United Kingdom many people come from other cultural backgrounds. The majority of them are here as a result of British history, their parents and grandparents coming to find work when it did not exist in their own countries. Others have arrived more recently, and all have brought with them a whole new way of life from their native land. These people tend to live close to those from their own country and may not integrate with the host

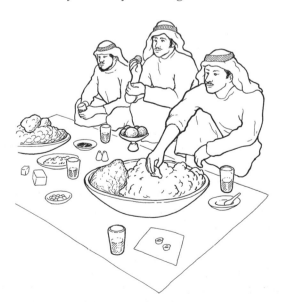

Fig. 3.3 Finger eating. Culture may determine the way in which daily activities are performed.

community. The international past of the United Kingdom means that, in reality, Britain is today a multicultural society. There are people of many faiths — Moslems, Hindus and Jews for example — many of whom have been here for generations. All these groups have differing values, attitudes, beliefs and ways of relating to each other which add to the richness of life in the United Kingdom as a whole.

In a multifaceted society such as ours it behoves all therapists to have a knowledge of cultures other than their own if a good working relationship is to be established with a colleague or other individual from a different ethnic background. Other religions are powerful determinants of certain values and ways of behaving which to Western eyes may be difficult to understand.

The 'social clock' (Fig. 3.4)

People who live in one society are bound by the legal requirements of that society, so in spite of differing cultural backgrounds they will experience certain common events. In the United Kingdom it is required that all children receive education; however, the types of school may be very different in their ethos, policies and procedures, leading to children having very differing school experiences.

The vast majority of human beings experience the arrival of a new family member and the loss of others, and will experience in their own lives the pressure of expectations laid upon them to follow the norms of the society in which they live. In the United Kingdom we are expected to leave school at 16 years of age and look for work, or continue into the sixth form and go to college. Whichever choice is made, human beings then become part of the adult world and, in response to biological and social demands, begin to look for a partner. The young woman in her early twenties is asked, 'Isn't it time you settled down now?', and the young married woman is asked whether she is thinking of starting a family. There is what has been referred to as a 'social clock' — times at which certain life events are expected to occur — and comment is often made if an individual does not follow the normal pattern.

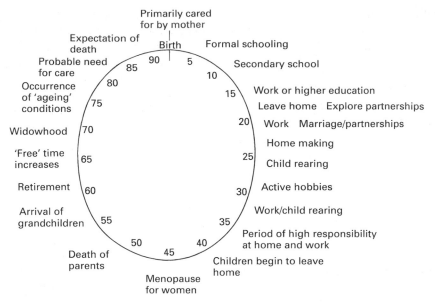

Fig. 3.4 The 'social clock'. Society has expectations of people's life patterns; in the United Kingdom a person's social clock may follow this pattern.

Childrearing takes a number of years and parents usually support their children through to independence. When children leave home parents find themselves with time they can spend together, something they have not been able to do for so long. For many this period may include coping with ageing parents and then their death, thereby losing one of the anchors to the past. Later years lead to a withdrawal from the economic market, a move into retirement and maybe the loss of a partner. Life is transient; it is but temporary and the last task is to prepare for one's own death.

Religious influences

The United Kingdom is nominally a Christian country, and although many Christian values permeate society few people go to worship in Church. It is not part of their experience even though they may believe in God. Other groups, however, do experience the equivalent of Church. The orthodox Jew worships on the Sabbath, Saturday; it is then that the scriptures are studied and the ritual of the synagogue is learned, whereas for many gentiles Saturday is the day on which families go shopping. Those of the

Moslem faith worship on Fridays and on other days pray five times. These beliefs and associated values strongly influence the family life patterns of daily living and the personal lives of each member. The broader dimension of all people who believe in God gives them common ground which enables them to communicate with each other with understanding. The same belief separates these people from those who do not believe: these people inhabit different worlds.

Contrasting life-styles

Other factors of socialisation will affect personal development. For example, a boy who is the third child in a family in which father is in the armed forces and moves every few years will have a very different life from the farmer's son who goes through the local schools with his peer group and eventually joins his father at work on the farm. Both styles of life have advantages and disadvantages. The farmer's son will have probably known stability and security, although his first-hand knowledge of the world may be very limited, whereas the soldier's son will have travelled and experienced a number of losses and new beginnings through moving house and school so many times, but at the same time he may have developed his capacity to adapt and make new friends quickly.

Physical handicap

The majority of babies in the United Kingdom are born biologically complete and with the potential to develop their capacities to the full, although a few are not so fortunate. Disability may be inherent due to some genetic fault or to failure to develop properly in the uterus, such as in those babies whose mothers smoked heavily or were HIV-positive. A baby may even develop perfectly to full term but be damaged during the birth process, and be left with residual functional limitations such as cerebral palsy. Development for these children will be partly determined by the residual handicap, which in turn will affect their perception and phenomenology. For example, the world of the blind child is very different from the world of the sighted, as the experiences of the blind child are filtered in perception through the fact of being blind.

Gender differences

Only comparatively recently, with the growth of feminist writings, has it been acknowledged how powerfully the biological differences superimposed by the gender differences of male and female influence perception and individual phenomenology. Men and women usually live in different realities because the interpretation of events and situation is shaped by the fact of being female or male. The experiences of the world for the two genders of the species differ radically, and influence thinking and conceptualisation. In a thorough analysis of how men and women use language and interpret ideas Tannen (1992) has shown that it is surprising that men and women communicate at all. Other issues associated with gender are explored by Beall & Sternberg (1993) in their stimulating and at times provocative text *The Psychology of Gender*.

The interactions of personality, the event and the situation are complex and multifaceted, and it is impossible to do justice to all aspects. Further information on the links between personality disposition and illness is to be found in Chapter 29, which discusses the work of Freidman & Rosenman (1974). Occupational therapists need to acknowledge that all people are different from others in inheritance and experience, so it cannot be assumed that other peoples' experiences are the same as ours or anyone else's.

THE EVENT ITSELF

Throughout life human beings are always involved in a variety of events with the family, at work, at college or at leisure with friends. Holidays are taken, birthdays celebrated and special events commemorated. Normal living comprises a succession of activities through which people are influenced and upon which they have an effect. Many of the activities of daily life are routine, requiring little thought or emotional response. Others may be very demanding, creating so much stress that a person may feel burdened.

Stress can vary in degree depending upon the person and the event. Some stress is good and essential to human healthy development: 'the spice of life' as Selye (1987) puts it. The psychological and physiological arousal created by stress leads to mental alertness and sound ways of managing events as they are met. From its close relationship with motivation we know that too little arousal leads to apathy, low energy level and lack of interest in anything, while too much arousal may lead to agitation and a feeling of being burdened. If these feelings are prolonged it may lead to physical and psychological ill-health. Moderately high stress was being experienced by one of my colleagues at a very busy time when she declared, 'Right, I have had enough, I'm going home'. She made an immediate withdrawal from a stressful situation.

Drawing on decades of physiological research Selye writes that stress is a word which everyone uses, yet few bother to find out what it really is. He defines stress as 'a nonspecific response of the body to any demand made upon it', and goes on to explain that, in general terms, it means 'the common results of exposure to any stimulus'.

Events are stimuli which are regarded by Selye as stressors, and it has already been noted that predictable events create less stress than unpredictable ones. Illness and accident, bereavement and loss, are all unpredictable events and may therefore be extremely disturbing in their effects. However, let us first take a look at common life events.

Life adjustment scale

One of the first studies which quantified life events and the degree of stress caused was by Holmes & Rahe (1967) who developed the Social Readjustment Rating Scale (SRRS). They argued that any life event that required the individual to adapt could be regarded as stressful. The investigators arrived at the life events scale after examining thousands of interviews and medical histories to identify the events of life which people found to be stressful. They found that marriage was a critical event for most people, so they placed it in the middle of the scale and gave it a value of 50. Then, by asking nearly 400 people, of differing marital status and from varying backgrounds, to rate the stress associated with a number of life events against that of marriage, they formulated the scale of 43 stressful events (Fig. 3.5).

As can be seen from Figure 3.5 the death of a spouse or child is rated as the most stressful life event and commands a value of 100, while minor breaches of the law gained a value of 11 points. Even Christmas, thought of fondly as a happy family time, was rated as a stressful period and rated at 12 point. Holmes & Rahe argued that people who collected a high number of points (200–300) over a period of two years were likely to develop serious illness in the following year.

Holmes & Rahe's Social Readjustment Rating Scale is a useful tool when trying to understand the relationship of stress and illness. It has, however, been seriously criticised, mainly because of the limitations of studying life events focusing on only one dimension, i.e. stress. It is possible to argue that the relationship events included in the scale go wrong because there are changes occurring in physical health, rather than the other way round. Cognitive processes are involved in any appraisal of a life happening, and these are not taken into account in this scale. Human beings differ in their perceptions of potential stressful events, and what one person views as stressful, another may not. For one person a minor breach of the law such as getting a parking ticket might be very stressful, whereas another person would take it quite calmly as an everyday occurrence. Culture and age may also affect perceptual differences, and people differ in their tolerance of stress. Some folk can work for long stressful periods without becoming ill, while others will become ill quite quickly. Finally, although the investigators established a significant correlation between the number of life events and physical illness, that does not mean that there is a causal relationship.

Since the work of Holmes & Rahe and Friedman & Rosenman (Ch. 29) many studies have established connections between life events and a spread of physical and psychological disturbance (McGrath & Burkhart 1983). Most research has focused upon the major events of life to which most are exposed, such as marriage, the birth of a baby and losing a close loved one through death. However, even minor events of daily living, such as rising prices or concern about personal weight, may create 'hassle' — a low level of stress (Kanner et al 1981).

Unexpected life events such as illness or a severe accident, unlike anything a person has previously experienced, can create overwhelming stress, producing trauma and great crisis. The experience of such events involving the total being may be a turning point which questions a person's sense of identity and social roles in a way previously unknown. It can lead to a loss of confidence and self-esteem, and a sense of failure and incompetence. To face the future, adaptation and personal change are essential, as new behaviours have to be learned to meet new circumstances, and where a person is feeling overwhelmed or fearful of the outcome of the change, he will need help in facilitating this adaptive behaviour. The event itself becomes a period of transition and one in which occupational therapists by the nature of their work may well be involved.

THE HOLMES AND RAHE SOCIAL READJUSTMENT RATING SCALE		
Life event		Mean value
1	Death of spouse/child	100
2	Divorce	73
3	Marital separation from mate	65
4	Detention in jail or other institution	63
5	Death of a close family member	63
6	Major personal injury or illness	53
7	Marriage	50
8	Being fired at work	47
9	Marital reconciliation with mate	45
10	Retirement from work	45
11	Major change in the health or behaviour of a family member	44
12	Pregnancy	40
13	Sexual difficulties	39
14	Gaining a new family member	39
15	Major business readjustment (e.g. merger, reorganisation, bankruptcy, etc.)	39
16	Major change in financial state	38
17	Death of a close friend	37
18	Changing to a different line of work	36
19	Major changes in the number of arguments with spouse	35
20	Taking on a mortgage greater than ...? (the maximum possible — author.)	31
21	Foreclosure on mortgage or loan	30
22	Major change in responsibilities at work	29
23	Son or daughter leaving home	29
24	In-law troubles	29
25	Outstanding personal achievement	28
26	Wife beginning or ceasing to work outside the home	26
27	Beginning or ceasing formal schooling	26
28	Major change in living conditions	25
29	Revision of personal habits	24
30	Trouble with the boss	23
31	Major change in working hours or conditions	23
32	Change in residence	20
33	Changing to a new school	20
34	Major change in type and/or amount of recreation	19
35	Major change in church activities	19
36	Major change in social activities	18
37	Making a large purchase, (e.g. TV, car, freezer etc.) or getting a small mortgage	17
38	Major change in sleeping habits (amount of time)	16
39	Change in number of family get-togethers	15
40	Change in eating habits	15
41	Vacation	13
42	Christmas	12
43	Minor violations of the law	11

Fig. 3.5 The Holmes and Rahe Social Readjustment Rating Scale. (Reproduced from Holmes & Rahe 1967 The Social Readjustment Rating Scale, Journal of Psychosomatic Research.)

THE SITUATIONAL VARIABLES

Factors surrounding any event make a difference to the response that is elicited in the people involved. An accident, such as a heavy fall at work, where there has been negligence in health and safety measures will create different responses from a similar accident where there has been

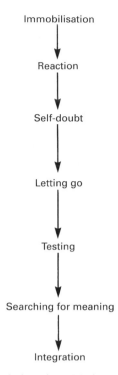

Immobilisation

↓

Reaction

↓

Self-doubt

↓

Letting go

↓

Testing

↓

Searching for meaning

↓

Integration

Fig. 3.7 Hopson's (1981) model of transition.

used to be, and upstairs is in chaos as all the drawers have been pulled out in a search for jewellery and money. Again think of being told that one has to have a serious operation when one has only been feeling a little under the weather, nothing really interfering with life. To such information there is a feeling of shocked disbelief, and one has to sit down to come to grips with what has happened.

2. Reaction — (i) mood swing, (ii) minimisation

Numbness gives way to elation or despair depending on what has happened. In the above incidents of theft and receiving bad news, despair may follow the events, but it is soon accompanied by an appraisal of the situation which, following a negative event, includes coping mechanisms, such as thoughts of how it could be much worse than it appears to be. In the case of positive events the appraisal includes thoughts of how things might be different in future.

3. Self-doubt

Even positive life events can lead to self-doubt. Marriage and becoming pregnant are events which normally are predictable and warmly anticipated. However, people become anxious as they question whether or not they will rise to the challenge of something which has been, to date, beyond their experience. The demands of the changes may give rise to not only anxiety but also even sadness, because as people move through life, change events often lead to losses as well as gains. Following negative events the self-doubt could well be associated with anger and despair, leading to depression.

4. Letting go

Up to this stage of transition a person may have been still attached to the past. Human beings find security in that which they know, and to leave the familiar takes courage as they step forward into the unknown. Tears may be shed and resentments felt at the demands of life, some of which may be felt to be unjust or unfair. If the clinging to the past continues for a long time there is little possibility of adaptation or preparation for the immediate future. To cast off is risky, yet it has to be done if the future is to be faced. It is the risk-taking in rising to a challenge and facing the unkown which may be a real turning point in personal development.

5. Testing

When the hold on the past has been released, the possibilities of action for the changed situation or stage of life can be considered. Options can be reviewed and tried. One might ask, 'What is appropriate for me in this place at this time'? It is an experimental period in which different identities may be tried and new bonds of affection established with varying degrees of success and failure, leading to rapid mood swings. From this low point of the transition cycle morale may begin to rise and self-esteem begin to emerge once again.

6. Search for meaning

At this stage of transition there is a tendency to look back and try to make sense of what has happened. It is here that one tries to learn from the event. One may ask, 'What is the learning issue in this?' It is a healthy period whereby the past is given meaning and thereby increases understanding of the changes and life experiences.

7. Integration

The transition period is completed with the incorporation of the event and associated crisis in a comfortable way into the life experience. The person who has had surgery, undergone trauma or is subject to a deteriorating condition has adapted to the limitations imposed upon him. Such a traumatic occurrence will have been extremely painful, driving him to question his concept of himself, but out of the questioning new understandings of self, others and life have been acquired. New insights, ways of coping and practical skills have been developed. Positive results may arise from painful, horrific events as the periods of transition are traversed. Growth takes place and the individual is strengthened so that future crises will be coped with more confidently.

MOOS & SCHAEFER'S MODEL OF TRANSITION

The model evolved by Moos & Schaefer (1986) (Fig. 3.8) covers both normal life transitions and crises, and differs from that of Hopson in a number of ways. In managing a life transition or crisis a person generally has five major sets of *adaptive tasks* to manage. The importance of each set of tasks varies depending upon the personality of the individual concerned, the nature of the crisis and the circumstances in which it occurs. Even so how these adaptive tasks are managed will first depend upon the cognitive appraisal that a person makes of all aspects of the event.

The processes of transition are complicated. Figure 3.8 is a representation of the overall processes involved in moving from the event to the outcome, but by its nature a model simplifies complex, intricate processes and can therefore only be regarded as a helpful tool to guide thinking.

1. First, the *significance* of the situation has to be understood. This does not happen immediately but may take time for the reality to be grasped. When a father has a heart attack, it takes time for the sufferer and his kin to realise the meaning and implications of all that has happened. Even though the situation is recognised at one level the effects of the trauma are not grasped.

2. The next set of tasks are those of *confronting the reality* of what has happened and dealing with what the situation demands. Some action is required. In severe illness affecting the breadwinner, moves to ensure financial security have to be made. The implications of the loss of one family member may lead to changes in roles and responsibilities of others. If children are involved preparations have to be made for living with one parent not fulfilling his occupational roles, while the other may become overloaded as she attempts to take on some of the roles herself,

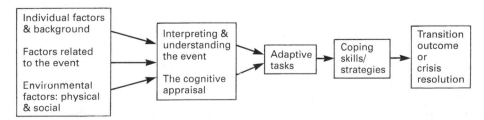

Fig. 3.8 A model of transition. All events take place within situational contexts which influence perceptions. (Adapted from Moos & Schaefer 1986.)

with the added burden of looking after her partner.

3. At the same time there is the task of *maintaining* relationships with family and friends who will provide support through the period of transition. Not everyone weighed down with the burden of a major life change is able to ask or accept support, yet it is at such times that it becomes essential, not just for emotional care, but also for the contacts and information they may give to ensure that the best decisions are made. Emotional distress may severely impede the processes of decision-making.

4. The fourth set of tasks is to maintain a *balanced* emotional life even though powerful emotions may be aroused by a life transition or crisis. Common reactions include self-blame, a sense of failure, tension and anxiety. Following traumatic illness, in which it is now known that self-care may play a part in recovery, all these feelings may prevail. Strong feelings may lead to the loss of hope and of the will to face the future. Hope is essential if the outcome is survival, and help may be needed to know that this is indeed a transitional period.

5. Moos & Schaefer believe that the fifth group of tasks are those concerned with the *preservation* of the self-image and maintaining competence. Transitions and crises can lead to a drop in self-confidence, particularly in relationships and the ability to live independently. Self-confidence may be so knocked that there is a crisis of identity, and confusion abounds as to who one is. Such a crisis requires a reassessment of values and attitudes, and a change in direction and purpose. A person who has had a cardiac arrest may have to redirect his life, change his life-style and develop a new sense of who he now is without some of his previous physical abilities and occupational roles.

Moos & Schaefer identify three groups of coping skills that are used to cope with the five groups of tasks associated with a crisis. These groups relate to a person's cognitive, behavioural and emotional domains of life, and together are holistic in approach. Within each group Moos & Schaefer define three types of coping skills, making in total a nine-item classification.

Cognitive coping skills

These skills are involved in the appraisal and understanding of the crisis. Appraisal occurs a number of times as the circumstances change following the event, and helps the person understand more fully the situation itself and the threat that it creates.

The three types of cognitive coping skill are:

1. skills of analysis and mental preparation
2. those skills involved in cognitive re-definition, which could be termed reframing
3. cognitive avoidance or denial, whereby the serious nature of the event may be denied.

Behavioural coping skills

These problem-focused skills by which the crisis is tackled practically with a view to easing the situation are:

1. skills to do with searching for information about the crisis and the possible lines of action
2. skills of taking action following a decision to deal with the crisis and its effects
3. skills involved in attempts to replace losses that have occurred due to the crisis, by changing patterns of living and finding new ways of meeting needs and gaining satisfaction.

Affective coping skills

These are emotion-focused skills whereby feelings aroused by the crisis are managed in an attempt to maintain an equilibrium:

1. the skills of controlling emotions and feelings when in a distressed state and holding on to hope
2. the skills of giving expression to feelings of despair, anger, and anxiety in whatever way the person chooses
3. the acceptance and coming to terms with the reality of the situation as it now is; this may vary from a resigned attitude of acceptance, believing that there is nothing more that can be done, to an avoidance of the situation.

Moos & Schaefer explore the factors which give rise to the variation of responses in people as they cope with crises, and what gives rise to successful outcomes.

These two models of transition provide structures and ideas which may assist occupational therapists when they are dealing with people who have recently encountered disturbing events of life. However, descriptions of processes of change do not do justice to the complicated nature of responses and adaptation to accommodate major life events. As already noted, some developmental psychologists differentiate between events for which a person may be prepared and those which are unexpected, but it is important for therapists to have a knowledge of tasks and coping skills, and be aware of the emotional reactions that people in crisis will experience. Occupational therapists who have a sound understanding of people can assist those who have suffered to adapt to a changing world. Through activity they can help people cope with their emotions at a time of transition and develop their coping abilities to the maximum, so that they can move towards independent living and functional autonomy.

THEORETICAL MODELS OF LIFE SPAN DEVELOPMENT

Many books entitled 'Developmental psychology' comprise models of development which focus mainly on childhood. It is as if there is an assumption that once a person has reached adulthood a state of stability is reached, and only minor changes occur from then on. Freud's (1901) proposition of psychosexual stages of development and Piaget's (1952) cognitive development stages structure are examples of childhood-focused models. Other developmental psychologists, such as Havighurst (1974) proposing role developmental stages, Levinson (1978) using task stages, Erikson (1965) considering psychosocial stages and Kohlberg (1969) focusing on stages of moral development, have observed that development continues all through life, and attempt to explain the pattern of changes which occur throughout the life span.

Some life span models emphasise the internal maturation processes while others focus upon the external social factors which trigger periods of transition. In spite of these differences in emphasis, each theorist offers some insights into how people change throughout life, and whereas they may have limitations, they provide particular perspectives arising from basic assumptions which may help occupational therapists better to understand their patients. Some theories seem to have particular relevance, as the ideas contained within them inform occupational therapy thinking. Two are outlined here, although it must be stressed that to understand them thoroughly it is important to read other texts.

Erikson's theory of life span development

Based upon clinical experience Erikson's developmental theory (1965, 1980) of psychosocial stages is an example of a model which encompasses the whole of life. In his thinking, the childhood development period is defined as having five stages, and that of adult development three. In this model each stage is a period of tension between opposing pulls which have to be negotiated by the individual. Successful development through each period leads to a positive outcome, such as the development of trust in the early years of life, while a failure to pass successfully through a stage may lead to the opposite state of uncertainty and failure to develop surely. In the early years failure results in mistrust. Positive outcomes to a stage of development result in surer foundations for future developments. These predispositions become part of the personality of the individual, and, as each stage builds upon previous stages, the developmental processes may take varying directions and result in different outcomes. As so much of occupational therapy is psychosocial in orientation Erikson's theory of psychosocial stages is a useful tool for occupational therapy practitioners, as Temple (1988) demonstrated when she discussed the use of art with patients suffering emotional disturbance at a particular stage of life.

Havighurst's developmental tasks

An older, but often overlooked, life span developmental theory which has relevance to occupational therapy is that of Robert Havighurst. Drawing on his educational experience and realising that learning is a life-long process, Havighurst proposed a theory of activity. In his 1974 text (p. 2) he wrote, 'Living is learning, and growing is learning' and although he recognised that learning intensity varied throughout life, depending upon a number of factors, he noted that there appeared to be particular developmental tasks associated with each period of growth. He defined a developmental task as:

one that arises at or about a certain period in the life of the individual, successful achievement of which leads to his happiness and to success in later tasks, while failure leads to unhappiness in the individual, disapproval by society and difficulty with later tasks.

Havighurst wrote that successfully completed tasks which are appropriate for that stage of life give a person a psychological boost (in today's parlance, a 'feel-good factor'), which strengthens him and enables him to face the next task with greater confidence and a likelihood of repeating the success. For example, a person who is having difficulty learning a new activity, such as pottery, will succeed if the whole task is broken down into small steps. As each step is successfully completed pleasure in achievement gives rise to improved self-esteem and confidence. The next step is then taken from a position of greater strength. In contrast failure to be competent and experience satisfaction may lead to a downward spiral of despondency and loss of motivation. The person develops a sense of incompetence, uselessness, low self-esteem and worthlessness. What could be a positive process of growth and development of individual functioning becomes one of reduced activity associated with feelings of defeat. Similar ideas about psychological processes leading to success or defeat are incorporated into Keilhofner's Model of Human Occupation, in the form of benign and maladaptive cycles of competence (see Ch. 2).

Both human and environmental factors contribute to the emergence of self and play a growing part in the development of the person. By acknowledging the part played by the processes of maturation, learning, the environment and the unique personality of the individual, Havighurst's concept of developmental tasks is an holistic one. He believes that successful involvement with the environment through the mastery of the developmental tasks of life constitutes healthy and satisfactory growth in society. Havighurst proposes that activity is an essential component of healthy living. Occupational therapists extend this thinking when they use activity in practice as a means of restoring health and occupational performance.

CONCLUSION

When a therapist works with a person with disability to assist him to regain his competencies, she is in a very powerful position, supported by all the authority of her profession and, usually, her employing authority. The goal is for the two people to enter a partnership from stances across a great divide, and bridges have to be built for the partnership to become an effective reality. For the two people involved in the interaction the point of meeting represents only a fraction of each person's being, yet important decisions will be made upon the knowledge gained in the encounter. To be truly 'holistic' one must consider not only the physical, psychological and social domains of the person, but also the developmental dimension past experiences, if the person with disability is to make the best decisions for himself.

The therapist is a facilitator in the processes of recovery. To work with another person towards restoration of holistic function she adopts a bio-psychosocial perspective to support her professional occupational therapy knowledge. To be effective she must not only assess objectively, but also understand the person's world as he experiences it. She is then in a position to direct her energies to help him work towards successful occupational performance. At first she may have to make decisions for the individual as his emotional state may preclude him from being able to make informed choices, but as recovery progresses and his equilibrium is restored, the therapist enables him to recover his dignity and be able to take more and more responsibility for his own life. The partnership is established and the two work together, each with responsibilities complementing those of the other (Fig. 3.9). The therapist can only do this wisely and sensitively if she is equally aware of her own motivations and sense of being. Her own needs are held in check so that they do not interfere with the process of meeting the needs of another.

The individual moves in a positive way from dependence towards greater functional performance. The transitions and adaptations which follow the period of pain and sorrow associated with a disturbing health event may in time lead

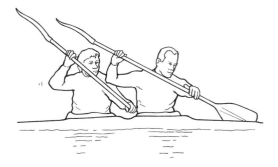

Fig 3.9 In partnership: the therapist ensures that both are pulling in the same direction.

to new insights about life and hope for the future. Development will then continue, albeit from a different baseline, so that life becomes worth while once again.

REFERENCES

Atkinson R L, Atkinson R C, Smith E E, Bem D J 1993 Introduction to psychology, 11th edn. Harcourt Brace Jovanovich, San Diego

Beall A, Sternberg R (eds) 1993 The psychology of gender. Guilford Press, New York

Bunyan J 1986 The pilgrim's progress. Penguin, London

Erikson E H (ed.) 1965 Childhood and society, 2nd edn. Penguin, London

Erikson E H 1980 Identity and the life cycle. W W Norton, New York

Freud S 1901 Cited in: Gross R D 1992 Psychology: the science of mind and behaviour. Hodder & Stoughton, London, p 591

Friedman M, Rosenman R H 1974 Type A behaviour. Knopf, New York

Havighurst R J 1974 Human development and education. Longman, London

Holmes T H, Rahe R H 1967 The Social Readjustment Rating Scale. Journal of Psychosomatic Research 11: 213–218

Hopson B 1981 Response to the papers by Schlossberg, Brammer & Abrego. Counseling Psychologist 9: 36–39

Kanner A D, Coyne J C, Schaeffer C, Lazerus R S 1981 Comparison of two modes of stress management, daily hassles and uplifts versus major life events. Journal of Behavioural Medicine 4: 1–39

Kimmel D C 1980 Adulthood and aging. John Wiley, New York

Kohlberg L 1969 Stages in the development of moral thought and action. Holt, Rinehart & Winston, New York

Levinson D J 1978 Cited in: Hayes N 1994 Foundations in psychology. Routledge, London, pp 791–793

McGrath R E V, Burkhart B R 1983 Measuring life stress: a comparison of different scoring systems for the social readjustment scale. Journal of Clinical Psychology 24: 83–110

Moos R H, Schaefer J (1986) Life transitions and crises: a conceptual overview. In: Moos R H (ed.) Coping with life crises: an integrated approach. Plenum Press, New York, pp 3–28

Neugarten B L 1977 Adaptation and the life cycle. In: Schlossberg N K, Entine A D (eds) Counselling adults. Brooks/Cole, California, p 44

Piaget J 1952 The origins of intelligence in children. International Universities Press, New York

Salmon P 1985 Living in time: a new look at personal development. Dent, London

Selye H 1987 Stress without distress. Corgi, London

Sugarman L 1986 Life-span development: concepts, theories and interventions. Methuen, London

Tannen D 1992 You just don't understand. Virago, London

Temple S 1988 Erikson's model of personality development related to clinical material. British Journal of Occupational Therapy 11: 399–402

FURTHER READING

Bee H L 1993 Lifespan development. HarperCollins, London

Donaldson M 1986 Children's minds. Penguin, London

Donaldson M 1992 Human minds. Penguin, London

Gilligan C 1982 In a different voice. Harvard University Press, Cambridge, Massachusetts

Gross R D 1992 Psychology: the science of mind and behaviour. Hodder & Stoughton, London

lem). These may be linked to the efficiency of the assessment process itself, the quality of the information gained, or to the degree of success of other interventions.

Impairment and disability

When determining the extent of the problem, the therapist should be aware of the sociological standing of the groups of which the person may be a part, as well as the immediate structure of the local society and living environment. Recognition of equal rights and acceptance of individual differences should form a part of the therapist's appreciation of the level of disability and the extent of the problem.

Conflict has arisen in recent years over the understanding of the terms 'impairment', 'disability' and 'handicap' between those who have worked to the World Health Organization (1980) definitions and those who prefer the social model definitions. The WHO defines the terms as follows:

- *impairment* — any loss or abnormality of psychological, physiological or anatomical structure or function
- *disability* — any restriction or lack of ability (resulting from impairment) to perform an activity in the manner or within the range considered normal for a human being
- *handicap* — a disadvantage for a given individual, resulting from an impairment or a disability, that limits or prevents the fulfilment of a role that is normal (depending on age, sex and social and cultural factors) for that individual.

In simple terms, impairment is seen as the loss or limitation of ability, disability is the effect that such loss or limitation has on functional performance and handicap is the restriction that these limitations place on the person's life-style.

Many people, particularly people who have impairments, no longer agree with these definitions. While the definition of impairment is generally accepted, the definitions of disability and handicap are contested because they take no account of the constraints imposed on the impaired person by society. The British Coalition of Disabled People (BCOPD) and the Union of the Physically Impaired Against Segregation (UPIAS) define disability as the 'disadvantage or restriction of activity caused by a contemporary social organisation which takes little or no account of people who have physical impairments and thus excludes them from the mainstream of social activities' (Oliver 1990).

Each person is a member of a number of different social groups, and it is the acceptance or restriction placed on the groups by society as a whole that causes the disability. Two people with the same levels of impairment may therefore have totally different disabilities, depending on the structure of their environment, the attitudes of people around them and the public view of their social groups. The support they receive may be less comprehensive because of their age or sex, rather than because of their level of impairment; this may, in turn, define the extent of their disability.

Locus of control

Studies of locus of control by Rotter may also assist the occupational therapist by providing another framework for understanding a person's problems (Rotter 1966, Rotter 1975, Lau 1982). People differ in their beliefs about how much control they can exert over their lives. The person who believes that control is located outside the self may feel that outcomes are dependent on fate, or may feel he is actively controlled by others. Such a person may show ready compliance with any suggestions made by the therapist because he perceives her as representing 'powerful others'; he may not even attempt to strive for success because 'his fate is already sealed'. Through increased understanding the person may be encouraged to exercise more control over his situation and the illness may then be positively affected by an active coping style. The therapist should therefore endeavour to educate him about his situation and involve him in making choices and initiating ideas at all stages of the programme.

Individuals who see control as lying within their own realm of responsibility are more likely to contribute their own ideas and to be more evaluative about others' suggestions. They are usually more motivated to overcome difficulties, provided that the goals are realistic in view of the person's perceived needs and wishes, and that emphasis is given to choice and personal responsibility.

Personal strengths

There is often a tendency for the occupational therapist to address the most obvious areas of deficit. The therapist's broad knowledge base and experience should ensure that associated areas of difficulty are not overlooked — in other words, that she approaches the difficulties from a wide perspective.

The basis of problem-solving is the identification of the individual's true problems. Frequently, therapists tend to focus on loss of function: impairment and dysfunction. However, it is equally if not more important to identify strengths and skills; these will be the foundations on which to build the future and base the programme. Particularly in the early intervention, when successful outcomes are important in maintaining the person's motivation to continue, the employment of these strengths and skills to achieve success, however small, will boost morale. They may be the means by which a problem is overcome or minimised in the long term. An example may be seen in the individual who is able to minimise problems, despite substantial impairments, by maintaining a willing support team to assist with daily needs by virtue of his strength of character and engaging personality.

Quality of information

Despite a wealth of information gained from case notes, interviews, observations and specific assessments, the true extent of a person's problems may not be clearly defined. This may be the result of the limited quality of the information gathered. The individual and his carers may, for whatever reason, not wish to reveal their real concerns. Language difficulties, limited understanding and other communication problems may restrict the exchange of information.

Identification of problems may rest with the therapist's appraisal of the quality of information gathered. She may be able to identify areas of difficulty which have not been addressed, or in some cases recognised, by the individual or his carers by utilising her understanding of the physical, psychological, social and clinical facets of the person's dysfunction and environment. A person who has difficulty rising from a chair is also likely to have problems getting up from the toilet, bath, bed or car seat. The therapist's understanding of movement from her learning in biological sciences, together with her awareness of living skills and environmental design, will enable her to identify those tasks which are likely to cause problems. Her clinical science base will assist her in planning the most appropriate approach to the problem in light of the pathology and prognosis of the person's impairment. Additionally, understanding of interpersonal dynamics and behavioural processes, together with astute observation, can help the therapist to identify whether the person is physically able to perform a given activity, or whether he is prevented from attempting to do so by, for example, an over-anxious or over-protective carer. The person may not be motivated to perform independently because of the secondary gains of disability (i.e. the attention provided by the carer may compensate for loneliness, when there is no real physical need for assistance) or because the activity is not perceived as personally valuable.

Outcomes of other treatments

Other intervention and treatment the person is receiving, or has received in the past, should also be considered when identifying the extent of his problems. The interrelation of other treatments with occupational therapy can be a significant factor in success. Both physiotherapy to improve mobility and speech therapy to increase communication will affect the occupational therapist's programme to reintegrate a person into school, work, the family and the social environment. Progress in other treatments will favourably influence the progress of the occupational therapy intervention; a lack of progress may indicate the depth and extent of the person's problems.

Prioritising (Fig. 4.3)

Once the therapist and the individual have jointly identified the problems that must be addressed, the next task is to establish their relative importance and urgency. Since it is unlikely that all problems can be dealt with simultaneously, it is important to prioritise them in this way before planning the treatment programme. Factors contributing to priority include:

- the wishes of the individual and his own perspective on his most vital needs
- the nature of the dysfunction
- the culture of the individual and the social climate in which he lives
- the complexity of the tasks which the person wishes to be able to perform.

The wishes of the individual

These are often referred to in American texts as 'personal causation' and 'volition' and are closely linked to aspirations and personal drives. Factors that determine a person's drives include:

- past individual life-style experiences
- locus of control
- life-style needs and social pressures.

The occupational therapist's belief in the autonomy, dignity and personal potential of the individual should lead her to take time to identify each person's desires and drives. She should not be tempted to interpret the range of a person's problems solely in terms of her *own* priorities and values. Similarly, care must be taken in the application of theoretical models to individual cases. Maslow's hierarchy of needs (1968), for example, identifies a structure of values which applies to many people — basic personal needs requiring satisfaction before higher, intellectual ones — and may help the therapist to understand human nature and personal preferences. However, like all models, it may not be directly applicable to every individual.

Every individual who is faced with a problem will bring to the situation his own personality and drives, his past experiences and his particular understanding of locus of control. Therapists have seen individuals who have overcome tremendous difficulties in order to succeed, and those who will not even attempt the first hurdle. These personality factors may contribute to the choice

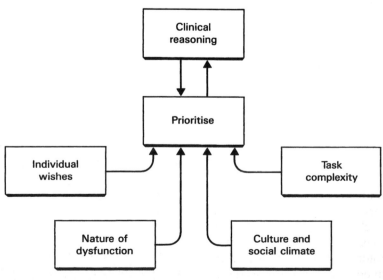

Fig. 4.3 Prioritising.

of priorities for activity. Those who appear to have a low level of drive, or a belief in an external locus of control, need to be actively involved in the choice of activity and to achieve success. Early intervention may involve the performance of small, simple tasks which are relatively unimportant in the total context of needs but whose successful outcome will foster self-respect and encourage the person to tackle more demanding or complex activities.

Identifying personal wishes may be relatively easy with some people. An individual with arthritis may be able to express a particular need in a daily living activity. However, where cognitive or communication skills are impaired — for example, following stroke or head injury — or where the person has no previous life experience on which to base judgements — as in the case of cerebral palsy in childhood — identification of personal drives may be more difficult. Observation of the individual's non-verbal responses to suggestions or levels of enthusiasm when participating in particular activities may give an indication of personal inclinations.

Many personal wishes are based on previous life experiences or life roles — parent, partner, breadwinner and independent being. Life-style needs and social pressures will almost certainly contribute to priorities. A person who lives alone may perceive mobility and safety in self-care activities as his most vital need. The breadwinner may rate gaining competence in work-related tasks in order to retain employment over achieving independence in all aspects of personal and domestic care.

The nature of the dysfunction

The therapist's knowledge of the clinical features of the disorder, together with an understanding of the anatomical, neurological and physiological processes of recovery, may help to determine her choice of approach and treatment plan. For example, when recovery or improvement is anticipated following motor neurone damage, priority will normally be given to achieving active mobility and strength in the proximal joints and to preventing secondary complications in distal joints until recovery commences.

Where dysfunction is likely to persist or deteriorate, priority will be given to maintaining skills and facilitating life-style adjustments. Many people are eager to find ways of retarding the deterioration and welcome advice on methods of maintaining function while recognising that they will not be able to return to previous levels of attainment. Education and practice in joint preservation techniques for the person with rheumatoid arthritis, and energy conservation programmes for people with multiple sclerosis are two examples of interventions appropriate to long-term dysfunction.

Where deterioration is inevitable a person may strive to maintain ability in one particular task, and assistance to achieve this aim may be the prime focus of intervention. This is often particularly evident when the illness causes severe impairment and achievement of a particular goal is the main priority. This goal may be as diverse as learning to play a musical instrument or to use a computer, or may involve completion of a task or plan already in hand. The person's energy and attention may be totally directed towards achieving success in the chosen task, while assistance is readily accepted in other areas of living.

If physical recovery is anticipated the occupational therapist's chosen approach will aim to promote such progress. However, where there is likely to be residual deficit, or deterioration, a compensatory approach may be more appropriate. Similarly, the psychosocial implications of the dysfunction may influence the therapist's choice of approach in order to address the person's needs for return to optimum participation in community life. For example, with the head injured person the therapist may use a combination of neurodevelopmental and behavioural or cognitive techniques to overcome the effects of hemiplegia together with behavioural or learning difficulties.

Culture and social climate

The therapist should make herself aware of the main beliefs and practices of the person's culture if she is not to risk offending him or his carers. In some cultures personal independence may not be highly valued because of the recognised duty of care within the extended family. Assisting a person to strive to perform self-care skills may in this context even be viewed as cruel.

Recognition of cultural or religious practices may be impeded by the therapist's lack of experience or knowledge and may be further complicated by language barriers. In some religions accepted hand dominance for personal activities (i.e. the right hand is the clean hand used for feeding and greeting others, and the left hand is for personal cleanliness) is vitally important and should be respected, if the person is not to be ostracised from his own community as unclean for using the right hand for all self-care activities. Personal cleansing may take priority over feeding or toileting because of its importance to religious practice. The therapist should inform herself about such cultural beliefs and respect them in planning intervention.

The social climate — the general attitudes or feelings of those with whom we come into contact — may also influence priorities. This may be related to social roles or may be determined by poverty or affluence.

The individual's social role in the family or local community may be an important personal driving factor. For example, cognitive, communicative and motor skills may assume prime importance for the person who is accustomed to the role of leader, organiser, extrovert or active participant.

Where poverty exists basic needs such as shelter, communication, food and toileting may take priority, along with financial concerns.

Complexity of the task

Some tasks are simple to perform, requiring only a relatively basic level of skills in limited areas of function. For example, switching on a light requires upper limb mobility, coordination and some dexterity in conjunction with visual and cognitive skills in locating and recognising the light switch. Putting on a round-necked jumper is a much more complex task, requiring a greater degree of upper limb motor skills and considerable ability in visual and cognitive functions to identify the correct parts of the garment — which is the front and which is the back — and to remember and follow the appropriate sequence for dressing.

The therapist's skills in activity analysis will enable her to identify the component parts of a task and to determine the particular skills required to perform each part in a successful sequence. By linking these requirements to the person's strengths and weaknesses she can judge the probable difficulty he will have in completing the task.

It is usual for the sequence of activities in a therapeutic programme to reflect this progression of activity complexity — commencing with activities which are less demanding and building up to those which require a particularly high level of skill in one or more areas of ability. Where there is a likelihood of deterioration the reverse procedure may be suitable, provided that the downgrading of the activity is managed sensitively.

However, when prioritising activities the therapist should bear in mind that for reasons of safety or particular need it may be preferable or even essential for the person to become competent in a relatively complex task early in the intervention programme. In such a case the task may be broken down into component parts, each part analysed in detail, and a range of options for successful completion of the task explored. After all the components of the activity have been analysed, a simple programme may be developed to reflect the person's present skill level. For example, a person living alone who needs to be independent in making a hot drink might be provided with an instruction chart to assist with cognitive sequencing and modified equipment which he can safely handle. Alternative methods, such as using a thermal jug, might be explored.

In conclusion, prioritising is itself a complex activity which is dependent on a number of factors. When determining the intervention sequence the occupational therapist may guide the discussions concerning the range of options but the wishes of the person and his carers should be respected when the final choice is made.

Clinical reasoning

The therapist's skills in clinical reasoning are vital to the sound analysis of information and to the planning and preparation of intervention.

Clinical reasoning (or clinical inquiry) is the thinking which guides the occupational therapist's analysis and helps her to work with the individual to come to a clinical judgement — an opinion or decision on the pertinent facts.

Rogers (1983, p. 601) sums this up in her statement that 'the goal of clinical reasoning is a treatment recommendation issued in the interests of a particular patient.' She describes clinical reasoning as a four-stage process involving:

- *deduction* — the formation of ideas about a possible range of problems from the pre-assessment information
- *induction* — modification of ideas from the person's specific details gained through assessment, which results in
- *dialectic reasoning* — logical interpretation and argument based on knowledge, observations, experience and reflection. Rogers (1983) states that, in this stage, the therapist 'argues or defends the interpretation of the data in much the same way as the lawyer pleads a case in court . . . the evidence supporting or opposing each alternative is weighed with the objective of rendering one explanation more cogent than another. Inferences that are compatible are retained and others are rejected or modified as contradictions appear. Through the dialectic process the model of the individual patient is polished and repolished. In this way, the therapist arrives at a cohesive conception of the patient, and, having grasped the whole, re-interprets the parts in light of this understanding'
- *ethical reasoning* — considering with the individual what ought to be done and the priorities for this.

In order to progress through this process successfully, Rogers (1983) identifies a sequence of questions that ought to be considered:

1. What is the person's status? What is his occupational role, what strengths does he have, what problems does he have and what is he prepared to try?

2. What are the available options? What can be done, what theoretical approaches can be used, what are the possible outcomes/results of each and how long are these likely to take to achieve?

3. What ought to be done? Which options concur with the person's wishes and values; has the person been informed of the consequences of each option; has the person been fully involved in the decision-making process?

Rogers maintains that clinical reasoning demands three basic attributes — science, ethics and artistry — and that 'without science clinical enquiry is not systematic; without ethics it is not responsible; without art it is not convincing'.

The scientific component of clinical reasoning is founded in the therapist's knowledge base. This includes knowledge she may have gained from theoretical learning and from previous experience and practice, as well as the knowledge acquired through the information gathering stage of the occupational therapy process.

The ethical component is based in the therapist's philosophy of valuing human dignity and is used in clinical reasoning to decide what option should be chosen from a range of possibilities. It is founded in the therapist's recognition of and respect for the person's own values and is reflected in the cooperative manner in which the determination of priorities and activities for therapy is made.

The artistry lies in the way in which the therapist uses her own personal skills to perfect her information gathering and analysis, and in her ability to impart values and guide decisions without imposing her opinions. Rogers (1983, p. 601) states that 'the artistry of clinical reasoning is exhibited in the craftsmanship with which the therapist executes the series of steps that culminates in a clinical decision.'

Clinical reasoning is therefore based on the therapist's understanding of the value and reliability of information, her knowledge of possible options and their merits and limitations, her posi-

commenced, a predominately rehabilitative compensatory approach will initially be appropriate in facilitating successful achievement in some essential activities. As recovery commences, other approaches may assume greater significance. For example, a neurodevelopmental approach may be used with someone who has experienced a cerebrovascular accident, and a biomechanical approach with someone who has suffered a hand injury. When maximum improvement is achieved any residual deficit may necessitate a return to the compensatory approach to overcome long-term problems.

In some instances the sequencing of activity will also be determined by the approach. When an educative approach is employed to teach or re-teach a skill, the activity will be graded according to the learning methods and the nature and complexity of the task itself. For example, when learning to prepare food it is usual to start with a simple drink and snack before embarking on the preparation of a full meal. In some approaches the progression will follow the process of expected recovery; for example, in the neurodevelopmental approach activities to improve sitting balance and posture will precede those which promote hand control and dexterity.

The therapist's abilities in identifying the person's interests, strengths and needs, and her skills in analysing and modifying activities will enable her to identify how a particular activity which the person values and enjoys may be used in a number of different approaches to meet the aims and goals specified.

Aims and goals

Having identified general aims, the therapist must plan her intervention in the context of achieving a particular goal. A range of options may be available and it is frequently necessary to implement a number of these to identify which is most helpful in achieving the desired goal. This may be illustrated by the different ways by which independence in toileting may be attained, i.e.: through the use of specific activity to improve strength and mobility in order to perform transfer techniques independently; by adapting clothing,

either in choice of design or modification of fastenings; through the use of assistive equipment such as seat raises, rails, frames or commodes; or through alterations to the environment to provide an accessible toilet. Through discussion of the merits and constraints of each option, the individual, his carers and the therapist can decide upon the solution most suitable for all concerned.

The individual and his carers

Choice of activity must be realistic in view of the life-style and needs of the individual, taking into account his personal, domestic, work and leisure experiences as well as his sociocultural environment. Activity should be chosen in light of the person's previous physical, cognitive and social competence, but should be graded according to his present strengths and deficits. This will be based on thorough baseline assessment and knowledge of activity analysis, application and grading.

Activities should be appropriate to the person's age, sex and culture, but care should be taken to ascertain suitability *in each case* and not to impose sexist, generational or cultural boundaries as a matter of course. Activities involving the use of modern technology, such as computing, may be more appropriate for the person wishing to return to paid employment, while cookery or creative craft activity may have more appeal to the elderly housewife. However, such assumptions should not be made without due consultation with the person concerned, as the elderly housewife may be an enthusiastic computer user from contact with her grandchildren. Such enthusiasm may motivate her to pursue computing and thereby gain cognitive skills or fine motor functions in excess of those acquired through cookery or other creative activity.

In many instances the needs of the carer will have equal consideration in the choice of activity. If a carer is willing to continue assistance with dressing, but is at risk of personal injury through helping with lifting or transfers, creative activity to strengthen the disabled person's limbs and develop balance for independent transfers may be more appropriate than daily dressing practice. Assistance with dressing, if given out of a genuine desire to help, may be the basis of secure friendship and trust, while the risk of personal injury through lifting may cause the carer anxiety and make him or her reluctant to continue in the caring role. Practice with mechanical hoists may overcome the carer's risks, but such equipment offers less flexibility than the acquisition of personal skill, and is expensive to provide.

While many technical factors may be considered in the choice of activity the therapist should not overlook the purely emotive aspect of personal interests. An activity chosen predominantly for pleasure and interest may be the driving force in motivating the person to pursue the treatment programme despite some discomfort and considerable effort. However, choice of an activity in which the person has had a previously moderate level of skill should be considered with care, as the negative effects of reduced capability because of impairment may only serve to reinforce a sense of loss.

The therapist's role and skills, and the options available

During the course of her duties an occupational therapist must, of necessity, adopt a very wide range of roles (Table 4.1). Commonly, she will enact the roles of assessor, information giver and receiver, educator, planner, interviewer and goal-setter. However, during specific interventions involving individuals or groups she may need to adopt still more diverse roles in order to assist people to overcome or come to terms with their difficulties. These roles may include advocate, counsellor, negotiator, mentor or carer.

An occupational therapist's key tool is her 'self', along with core skills, knowledge, attitudes and other attributes. It is often the approach and the role or roles adopted by the therapist which are the most significant factors in her intervention and an individual's progress. A therapist will continuously evaluate and modify her role(s) and adjust her expectations of the recipient of treatment. By increasing the degree of independence and autonomy offered, and by gradually reduc-

Table 4.1 Roles and the occupational therapist: a summary

Role	Function/purpose
Communicator/ interviewer	Giver/receiver of information Establishing working relationship Comprehension of individual and his perceived abilities/inabilities
Assessor	Identification of skills, problems, abilities Formation of baseline for intervention
Planner	Explorer of options in relation to needs Requires objectivity and realism
Negotiator	Influencing/exchanging ideas Mutual decision-making, agreeing on plans, resolving differences Motivating the individual
Advisor	Imparting information, knowledge, skills
Decision-maker	Selection/choice from range of options, increasing individual's ability to make own decisions
Role-model	Adopting roles to achieve empathy Modelling a desired set of behaviours
Problem-solver	Identification of problem, options and resources to aid solution, choice of solution
Educator	Transfer of skills, knowledge, abilities to individual/carers
Goal-setter	Establishing aim(s) and planning strategies for achievement
Advocate	Understanding individual's needs/ requirements and acting on his behalf
Counsellor	Listener, assistant, explorer of options/ values/needs/solutions
Mentor	Counsellor, with knowledge and skills to guide, usually in relation to specific topics
Carer	Concern for individual within programme of intervention, providing media/techniques to meet his needs

ing her support, she will pass responsibility to the individual.

Occupational therapists are recognised for their flexible approach to problem-solving. However, the therapist herself is an individual with particular skills which extend or limit her own capability and expertise. Individual differences between therapists may be the result of previous learning and experience, and of personal preferences with regard to areas of interest. Some therapists prefer to specialise in particular treatment approaches, activities, or areas of dysfunction and may develop in-depth knowledge and skill in these areas, often at the expense of other facets of practice.

The depth and range of the therapist's skills will be of vital importance in her choice of activities for an intervention. She may have specialist knowledge in the area of need and be the ideal person to assist the individual. She may have a number of skills available to her and she should use her clinical judgement, in consultation with the individual, in identifying the range of suitable options and making the most appropriate choices. On the other hand, she may have limited expertise in the area of need. In this situation she should consider the choices available. Is there someone else in the department or team who may be more appropriate and who is available to assist? Will other skills the therapist possesses be likely to achieve the same aims for the individual in the same time-scale? If the therapist feels that she lacks expertise in a given area it is important for her to recognise this, discuss options with the person and his carers, identify where such skills may be available and take steps to make the appropriate contacts and referrals.

The therapist should not see this as a shortcoming on her part, particularly where the person's needs are very specialised. Her knowledge of the expertise offered by a broad range of disciplines in the hospital and the community is a support in itself. The therapist's skills in recognising needs, and her communication and liaison with outside disciplines is a vital part of her role in facilitating the most appropriate solution.

Where the person has a long-term regular need for support, it is unlikely that this will be provided by the occupational therapist. Referral to others who are able to provide such support, for example the community nurse or a day centre, earlier rather than later in the therapy intervention, will enable this contact to be developed while the therapist is still involved and able to evaluate the adequacy of the provision for the person's needs.

Occasionally no one is available to help with a particular problem. This should be acknowledged with the individual and possible alternative coping strategies considered which, while not ideal, will minimise the disability in the short term in an acceptable way until such support becomes available. Take, for example, the case of a young woman with cerebral palsy who wishes to live independently and requires a modified living environment and considerable practice in domestic and life skills. The accommodation is not available at present and a place in a skills training programme will be available in three months' time. The therapist is not able to provide regular domestic or skills training but she may be able to assist the person and her carers in developing ways of gradually increasing her responsibilities and skills in the home and the community until such outside support becomes available. The therapist's contribution as facilitator and educator is thus no less important than the provision of direct treatment in the intervention process.

To summarise, choosing a solution is a complex task which depends upon many aspects of the individual's personal needs, experiences and drives, the environment in which he lives, the nature of the dysfunction and the services that are available. The therapist's skills in clinical reasoning will be vital in guiding selection.

Choice of activity should be realistic. That is, it should be geared to the person's requirements and wishes in accordance with the facilities and resources available. The activity should present a challenge which is valued and the goal should be perceived to be achievable. The part any activity plays in attaining a broader solution or aim should be clearly understood by all concerned.

IMPLEMENTING INTERVENTION

An intervention plan should set out *how* to meet short-term goals in the most appropriate way for a particular person. It will state the approaches and methods to be used and identify the therapeutic activity, chosen from the range of options that has been identified (Fig. 4.5).

Choices of *where* the activity should take place will be important. This may be the ward, the therapy department, the person's home, a day centre or some other suitable location. Obviously, if therapy is to occur away from the person's

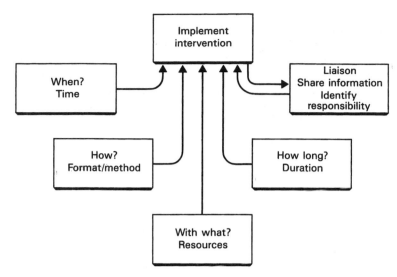

Fig. 4.5 Implementing intervention.

residence (whether home or hospital) the distance to travel and the method of transport should be anticipated, and the impact travel may have on the person's performance and gains should be considered.

Factors to consider

Time

The programme plan should also take into account the optimum length of time for each therapy session, and how frequently sessions should occur. This may be based on the dysfunction, its cause, course and prognosis, and the advantages gained by regular intervention, as well as on the contractual arrangement with the referring agent.

There may be particular times during the day when therapy is more advantageous. Activities to improve physical performance for the person with an arthritic disorder characterised by morning stiffness may be more successful in the afternoon. Similarly, in situations where the person has an increasing level of fatigue through the day, activities in the morning may be especially successful. However, it will be necessary for the therapist to observe some self-maintenance activities performed when the person is at the worst stage during the day, in order to consider

methods by which he can cope successfully in the daily routine. When the person has cognitive problems, particularly those affecting orientation in time or place, the timing and location of self-care and domestic activities should equate, as far as possible, with his 'normal' daily routine.

Format

The intervention should be carried out in the most suitable therapy format: on a one-to-one basis or in a group. The occupational therapist's basic philosophy of recognising individuality, together with the variations among different persons' goals, will demand that much of the intervention be on a one-to-one basis, particularly in the initial stages. Some goals, especially those related to the development of social and communicative skills, may be more readily achieved by participation in group activities. The format will also be affected by the choice of activity medium and the amount of direction or guidance required by the person to safely succeed in achieving the desired goal.

Resources

Having considered her plan for intervention in relation to the person's needs, the therapist should also consider whether the programme is realistic and achievable in practical terms. In an ideal world all things might be attempted. In reality, limitations of the therapist's knowledge and skill, together with constraints on practical resources such as staff, a suitable location, transport, tools, materials, equipment and finance may restrict the intervention programme. Demands made upon the therapist's time by her entire caseload and the unavailability of support may limit the frequency and duration of therapy. The therapist should weigh the ideal quantity or extent of her interventions against the need for quality assurance. She should also endeavour to ensure that the goals of those in greatest need are met. In many situations, excessive case overloads leading to the risk of unsatisfactory outcomes for all have led to the use of priority ratings for therapy intervention.

Duration

In some instances it may also be necessary to identify the anticipated total length of the intervention and the pattern of contact for purposes of contracting, caseload planning and clinical budgeting. For example, where the intervention aims to promote physical improvement, identification of an anticipated length of treatment may serve as a time framework for the evaluation of outcomes. This evaluation should be consistent with the aims and goals of the programme, and may provide a basis for consideration of the continuation or termination of therapy. It may be found that further goals remain to be achieved, or that discharge or referral to other sources is now indicated. While an estimate of programme duration is valuable for contracting, intervention planning and caseload and staff management, care should be taken to ensure that rigid time criteria are not applied at the expense of genuine benefit from further therapy.

Where major home adaptations are planned the occupational therapist's pattern of intervention may not be regular. It will often extend over a considerable period of time — from initial assessment of need, through planning and the monitoring of progress, to successful completion.

At some stages the person's needs will be urgent and particularly time-consuming for the therapist.

Liaison with the team

The personnel with whom the occupational therapist should liaise vary, depending on the nature of the problem, the choice of solutions and plan for intervention, and the setting of the therapy (Fig. 4.6).

In the hospital environment

The therapist may need to liaise with the medical and nursing staff and others in the rehabilitation team. She may also have to liaise with others outside the hospital, in addition to the family or carers, depending on the person's needs and the choice of activity. This may involve personnel in social services departments, the community occupational therapist, or other community resource personnel — for example, members of voluntary organisations, or staff from community health care, employment, education or leisure facilities.

Outside the hospital environment

Therapists may need to liaise with similar personnel in both the hospital and the community. They will be particularly involved with personnel outside the hospital environment in the majority of instances. Liaison with staff from local authority departments, particularly housing and social services, plays an important part in work in the community.

Why is liaison important?

Liaison is vital to successful teamwork. Professional communication is discussed in Chapter 11.

Membership of the intervention team should include the people who are most meaningful to the individual — family, friends, neighbours and/or carers. The contribution these people can make towards achieving the individual's wishes and meeting his needs is often vital to the success of the intervention process.

COMMUNITY SERVICES   **HOSPITAL SERVICES**

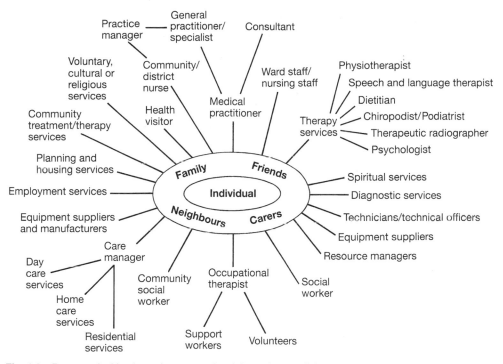

Fig. 4.6 Personnel with whom the occupational therapist may liaise.

Successful teamwork depends on:

- good communication between team members
- comprehensive identification of needs
- agreed aims and goals by all participating members
- agreed strategies and methods for how aims and goals may be achieved
- respect for, and effective use of, individuals' skills
- clear and agreed understanding of responsibilities
- efficient and effective sharing of information.

In particular, liaison is important:

- *To ensure that the programme of intervention is cohesive.* Liaison is a two-way process of giving and receiving information. The therapist should inform herself of other support or treatments the person is receiving and of the aims and goals of these. She should gain information on the frequency and timing of other activities, in addition to the details of the methods used. The therapist should also give information on her proposals. Any divergence or overlap should be discussed and outcomes negotiated to achieve optimum benefit for the person and the carers in the most appropriate format.

- *To identify responsibilities.* It is important to ensure that all members of the team clearly understand their duties and that attention to any area of need is not overlooked or duplicated. This promotes efficiency on the part of the team in terms of time and effort, and the best utilisation of individual skills. The clear delineation of responsibilities is likely to encourage a greater sense of duty and a desire for achievement, which in turn promotes quality of care.

When discussing the range of possible solutions with the individual, his own responsibilities should be negotiated with the therapist. When identifying the responsibilities of the provider — the therapist or carer — the demands these may make in terms of skills, knowledge and time should be discussed and agreed on.

Frequently, there is some role overlap among members of the multidisciplinary rehabilitation team. In some instances it may be more advantageous for one person to take the key worker role, thus preventing confusion and the duplication of effort. Conversely, in some situations which involve learning a particular skill, repetition by more than one person may promote or consolidate learning, provided the teaching is consistent.

When identifying needs and planning for intervention it will have been necessary to consider a wide range of factors. If these have been identified and fully explored with all concerned, the therapist, the individual and his carers should be well prepared for the programme of intervention.

In many cases intervention may proceed according to the chosen plan but there may be unforeseen factors, such as an alteration in the person's health or social situation, or in the facilities or resources available, which necessitate a change of course. The therapist should be prepared to modify her plans accordingly. This may be a total reappraisal of the intervention, or only a minor modification, or a delay or advancement of an activity already included in the programme.

The therapist needs to retain a flexible, positive approach to such changes to accommodate the needs of the individual and others in the team, in line with her duties of employment.

EVALUATING OUTCOMES

The aim of evaluation is to appraise and monitor the effectiveness of the intervention programme. This may be considered in terms of its success and limitations for the person concerned. Such information may also form part of an analysis of occupational therapy in the wider context of researching the value of specific strategies for a particular group in a given situation.

Evaluation may be carried out formally through specific tests, measurements and assessments or informally through observation and conversation with the person, his relatives, and others concerned in the intervention programme.

Why evaluate?

- *To measure progress* (or the lack of it) in order to determine whether the treatment should be continued or whether a change of activity or strategy is needed. This type of evaluation should occur at regular intervals throughout the programme and is usually made with reference to the specific goals identified when the intervention strategy was planned.

- *To plan for discharge or referral* to others for further intervention. This usually occurs at the end or in the later stages of the programme in order to measure the *extent* of the progress and identify any residual deficits which have not been overcome (Fig. 4.7). It is based on the aims

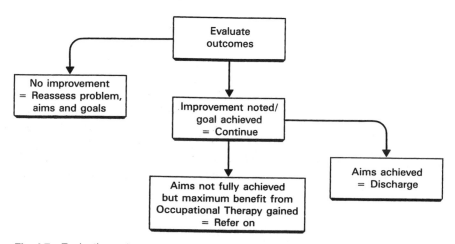

Fig. 4.7 Evaluating outcomes.

identified in the plan and is usually carried out through a formal assessment. Frequently this is a repetition of some or all of the initial assessments performed before planning the intervention.

A final evaluation carried out at the end of the programme provides a valuable record for future reference in the event of the person's re-referral to occupational therapy or another discipline at a later date. Information gained will also form part of the basis for the therapist's referral of the person to other sources to meet his residual needs.

• *To monitor or measure efficacy.* Information may be gained through evaluation of part or all of the intervention to identify the value of specific activities or the interrelation of a number of techniques in the total programme. Such information may be useful to the therapist in her justifications to others, such as management staff. It may also form a valuable resource for reflection on and analysis of practice and may lead to the development of new intervention strategies or therapeutic activities.

Evaluation is therefore a means for determining continuation or change — both for the individual and for the therapist. It confirms that intervention is progressing at the anticipated level and alerts the person and the therapist to any particular need for change. This illustrates the cyclical nature of the occupational therapy process: the earlier stage of analysis of information is returned to, in the reappraisal of priorities and the adjustment of preparation and planning. Gillette (1988, p. 211) writes:

Evaluation serves the purpose of keeping the therapist's work current, for it is a spiral building process. Each treatment session should be assessed, and each target area should be reviewed in order to determine the effectiveness of the activity process and to revise the objectives as they are mastered or found to be unreachable. Treatment should not persist in a straight line. It is the system of evaluation that is built into the treatment process that ultimately determines the effectiveness of treatment.

Evaluation is also one of the major bases on which research is founded, promoting wider change or development in professional practice. Evaluations of outcomes may provide evidence that helps to confirm or refute theories, ideas or beliefs about particular practices. Further investigation or analysis may identify the reasons behind the outcomes. Successful investigations in this area lead to an increased understanding which may be the basis for objective continuation or cessation of particular techniques, or may promote totally new thinking which enhances professional enquiry and development.

CONCLUSION

The practice of occupational therapy must follow a clearly identified process if the treatment it offers is to be organised, systematic and successful. As this process must aim to realistically and sensitively meet human needs in a wide variety of situations it will inevitably be somewhat complex.

The complexity of the process lies in the identification of needs, the recognition of individuality and the variety of options available for implementation. The greatest effort and detail are required in the investigative and preparatory stages. If these stages are managed correctly, the treatment programme based on their findings should be appropriate to the person's needs. Evaluation, ideally, will provide confirmation that all is well, and may give rise to new ideas for future development.

None the less, the therapist may find that a particular action has failed to meet a person's needs or to respond to changes in circumstance. In such a case, the ultimate success of her intervention will depend upon her objectivity, flexibility, 'artistry' and understanding of the individual and the situation as she finds alternative strategies to help him meet his evolving goals.

REFERENCES

Gillette N 1988 Occupational therapy and mental health. In: Hopkins H L, Smith H D (eds) Willard and Spackman's occupational therapy, 7th edn. J B Lippincott, Philadelphia

Kielhofner G 1985 The model of human occupation. Williams & Wilkins, Baltimore

Lau R R 1982 Origins of health locus of control beliefs. Journal of Personality and Social Psychology 42(2): 322–334

Macdonald E M 1960 Occupational therapy in rehabilitation. Baillière Tindall & Cox, London

Maslow A H 1968 Toward a psychology of being, 2nd edn. Van Nostrand Reinhold, New York

Oliver M 1990 The politics of disablement. Macmillan, Basingstoke

Rogers J C 1983 Clinical reasoning: the ethics, the science and art. American Journal of Occupational Therapy 37(9): 601

Rotter J B 1966 Generalised expectancies for internal versus external control of reinforcement. Psychological Monographs 80(1) No. 609. American Psychological Association

Rotter J B 1975 Some problems and misconceptions related to the construct of internal versus external control of reinforcement. Journal of Consulting and Clinical Psychology 43: 56–67

Wade D T, Langton-Hewer R, Skilbeck C E, David R M 1985 Stroke — a critical approach to diagnosis, treatment and management. Chapman & Hall, London

World Health Organization 1980 International classification of impairments, disabilities and handicaps. WHO, Geneva

Skills

The New Oxford English Dictionary (1993) defines skill as 'the ability to do something well, proficiency, expertness' that may be acquired through practice or learning.

Skills are combinations of inherited abilities and assets, which are developed and honed through learning and/or practical experience. According to the College of Occupational Therapists Position Statement (1994), core skills are 'the expert knowledge at the heart of the profession', which are 'related to the paradigm of occupational therapy'. The Position Statement cites the unique core skills of occupational therapy as the:

- use of purposeful activity and meaningful occupation as therapeutic tools in the promotion of health and well-being
- ability to enable people to explore, achieve and maintain balance in the daily living tasks and roles of personal and domestic care, leisure and productivity
- ability to assess the effect of, and then to manipulate, physical and psychosocial environments to maximise function and social integration
- ability to analyse, select and apply occupations as specific therapeutic media to treat people who are experiencing dysfunction in daily living tasks, interactions and occupational roles.

The Position Statement continues by identifying core skills for practice as the:

- enabling of people to maximise their physical, emotional, cognitive, social and functional potential
- anticipation and prevention of the effects of disability and dysfunction through education and therapeutic intervention in a functional context
- enabling of people to achieve a meaningful lifestyle by the preparation for or return to work, or the development of the quality use of time through leisure, education, training and opportunities for voluntary work
- provision of professional advocacy for people on access and equal opportunities matters
- provision of practical advice and support for the families and carers of people with disabilities
- ability to change, adapt and modify practices according to the needs of people with disabilities and their environment
- partnerships with others to facilitate development of services for people with disabilities
- ability to influence social policy and legislation relating to impairment, disability, handicap, and economic self sufficiency.

This section describes the ways in which occupational therapists analyse the component elements of activities and then use activities therapeutically in practice. The section continues by identifying the purpose and process of assessment, and outlines different methods for determining the need for intervention and measuring the success of same. Chapters 8, 9 and 10 explore the application of particular skills in different aspects of practice. These cover the development of life skills, different means of achieving mobility and the use of orthotics in practice. The final chapter describes the organisational and managerial components essential for maintaining efficient and effective professional practice.

These seven chapters identify the ways in which occupational therapists implement the profession's principles in their work, and are further expanded for particular areas of dysfunction in the practice section of the book.

College of Occupational Therapists 1994 Core skills and a conceptual framework for practice – a position statement. College of Occupational Therapists, London.

5

Activity analysis

Sybil E. Johnson

Absence of occupation is not rest,
A mind quite vacant is a mind distressed.
(Cowper 1731–1800)

INTRODUCTION

A glance at the philosophy and history of the use of occupation and activity in promoting health and alleviating ill health and dysfunction (see Ch. 1) will show that occupational therapy's underlying concepts have their origin in antiquity. Centuries later, it is still recognised that occupation is a 'key component in the maintenance of wellbeing' and it is therefore logical to use it as the 'medium through which to restore and acquire functional ability' (Meyer, quoted Ch. 1) and to recognise that, on a day-to-day basis, this involves people in activity.

A brief reflection on the words 'occupation' and 'activity' is of value here. Some may argue that occupation and activity are synonymous because there is a tendency to use them interchangeably, but evidence (and our subsequent understanding) shows that this is not so (Fig. 5.1). Occupation, according to Young & Quinn (1992) and Darnell & Heater (1994), is the concept and foundation of occupational therapy and the domain of concern of its registered practitioners. It is a 'descriptive and specific means of referring to human doing' (Darnell & Heater 1994) and the state of 'being', describing the purpose and manner of maintaining health throughout the life-span by balancing occupations relating to

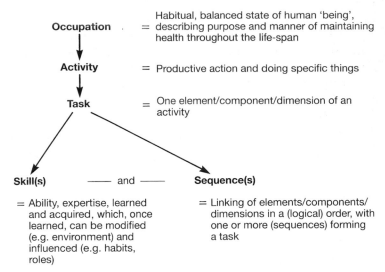

Fig. 5.1 Occupation — activity — task hierarchy. Readers are reminded that (a) this hierarchy and terminology represent the UK interpretation, and (b) hierarchy terminology within USA — therapist-derived models, in particular, often differs.

self-care, work / productivity, leisure, roles, habits, routines and sociocultural and environmental influences. Activity implies productive action, i.e. being active and doing particular things, for example making and then eating a toasted sandwich. Reed & Sanderson (1992) describe activity as a 'specific action, function or sphere of action', which involves 'learning or doing by direct experience'; Young & Quinn (1992) state that it is 'essential for maintenance and continuance of life'. So, we could summarise by saying that occupation gives us a framework of the broad life-sustaining elements to which we attach the day-to-day sequence of events (activities) whose nature changes as a person develops, ages and changes roles, for instance. It is these latter activities, their analysis and synthesis — the daily human doing and sequencing of tasks and skills — with which this chapter deals.

The use of activity is the basis, or core, of the profession. Activity encourages adaptive behaviour, meets specific objectives and fosters active involvement by the individual in addressing his specific problems and needs. In this context activity is taken to mean all the tasks which form the pattern of a person's life, and which are taken for granted until that individual suffers illness or trauma.

Activity used therapeutically may be drawn from the wide sphere of everyday life, including the arts, leisure pursuits, household and personal care tasks, work, education, sport, hobbies, family and social relationships. If an occupational therapist is to use some or all of these activities in her interventions she must do so in a manner which has meaning and purpose for the individual. Moreover, she must be able to optimise one of her core skills, i.e. her ability to analyse the component parts of an activity.

Activity analysis is a process used by occupational therapists to determine the characteristics of and the tasks involved in an activity with the potential for therapeutic use, and to translate that analysis into individual goal-specific intervention(s). In analysing an activity in detail the therapist must either physically participate in it or undertake specifically planned and detailed observation of it in order to understand its components and complexities. The therapist should, first, learn the 'how' of the activity and then concentrate on the 'why', 'what', 'where' and so on. These latter elements will lead to analysis of physical, cognitive, social, interpersonal, sensory, emotional and behavioural components. Once an analysis is complete the therapist must relate her findings to the individual's identified abilities and needs. Utilising the occupational therapy process (Ch. 4) she will reach the stage in an individual's programme where she has to select activities relevant to that person. Her skills of analysis, her use of imagination and creative thinking, her knowledge of activities and her problem-solving skills will enable her to discriminate between appropriate and inappropriate activities and to modify them according to individual needs.

Such analysis is used in conjunction with the assessment and treatment of function and dysfunction whereby the therapist determines the extent to which physical, behavioural and other abilities and skills affect an individual's ability to perform 'normally' and then plans, implements and evaluates appropriate intervention.

This chapter begins by reviewing the importance of activity to everyday life, including its contribution to the individual's roles, cultural and social status and life-style. The distinction between purposeful and non-purposeful activity is explained, with particular reference to the application of both kinds of activity to occupational therapy. In subsequent sections the definition and importance of activity analysis and synthesis is considered, along with the main features the therapist should look for when selecting activities to use in a rehabilitative programme.

The 'why' of activity analysis, that is, the kinds of information that analysis will yield, is then described, and types of models used in activity analysis are briefly outlined. The chapter then provides a detailed framework by which activities might be analysed and assessed. This includes general factors such as environment, safety, appropriateness and adaptability, and, more specifically, the potential physical, sensory, cognitive, perceptual, emotional and social demands that an activity will place upon the individual.

The next section of the chapter outlines methods by which activities can be graded, that is, how they can be adapted to the changing abilities and needs of the individual during the course of intervention. The final sections take three very different activities — making a cup of coffee; setting a line of type; and participating in a dis-

cussion group — and demonstrate in more concrete terms how the preceding frameworks for activity analysis and grading might be applied to each. Finally, the application of activity analysis to the therapist's overall therapeutic procedure is summarised.

THE RELATIONSHIP OF ACTIVITY TO EVERYDAY LIFE

Activity is necessary to man's survival. It occurs spontaneously in healthy people and, in addition to meeting his basic needs, activity may also give him pleasure (Fig. 5.2), ensure he is comfortable, solve his problems, enable him to express himself and to relate to others and allow him to earn a living in order to support himself and his family. Activity is characteristic of and essential to human existence (Cynkin 1979, Cynkin & Robinson 1990). It offers rewards and achievements as well as constraints and frustrations. Through activity a person not only develops skills, but also learns about his strengths and weaknesses.

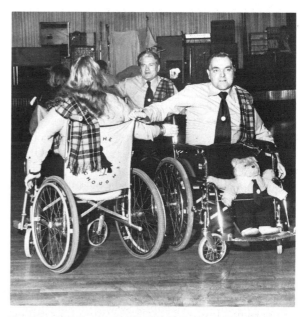

Fig. 5.2 Activity should offer pleasure, as well as physical, psychological and social well-being.

Activity and routine

Most of the activities an individual performs daily are so routine that he carries them out automatically. For example, a person's set pattern of rising from bed, going to the bathroom, washing, dressing, preparing and eating breakfast and leaving the house to catch a bus or start the car is part of an established routine involving a series of activities. If, however, that routine is disrupted for some reason it will disturb other routines and activities during the day; for example, oversleeping or tending a sick child may make the person late for work and a vital meeting and result in ill-humour, adversely affecting his usual objectivity and efficiency at work.

Activity and roles

Activity is very closely related to the roles an individual adopts each day. Roles comprise a combination of attitudes and strategies that are used to maintain an individual's status and self-esteem throughout his life cycle. They are modified and balanced according to his developmental stage and its associated roles, and their relevance to culture, family, beliefs, interests and productivity. The role of parent, breadwinner, teacher or therapist, for instance, is supported and defined by particular skills, functions and behaviours. Each role requires some activity on the individual's part. The parent role, for instance, involves effective communication, providing and caring for the family home, looking after and disciplining the children and setting an example. The individual may pursue some of these activities, such as playing with his children, with enthusiasm and anticipation while he finds others, such as spring cleaning, dissatisfying or boring, to be undertaken only as a matter of duty and social norm.

Activity, culture and social status

'In order to survive, humans must provide for their material, emotional and intellectual needs. These are satisfied by culture, a complex system that includes tools, language, arts and beliefs. Cultures vary because they must be compatible with their supporting environments. Thus different climates, terrains and sources of food evoke different cultural responses.'

(First People's Exhibit)

This description encapsulates the meaning of culture so succinctly for occupational therapists that it is impossible to resist its inclusion here. 'Humans must provide' implies 'doing', i.e. activity, which is significant as culture also influences social status, values and norms, which are also influenced by roles and environmental factors. In their 1991 work Christiansen & Baum discuss culture and its influences on performance, describing culture as a system of *learned* (as opposed to inherited) patterns of behaviour 'transmitted' to the young of a group by its older members. The influences can be significant geographically or in relation to the local community, one's family and oneself (Box 5.1). In reality each person strives to lead as satisfying a life as possible; therefore, he will endeavour to perform activities which are approved of by his social and/or cultural group, providing those activities also satisfy his personal needs and wants. There are, of course, exceptions and each individual will modify, to a greater or lesser extent, his activity

---

Box 5.1 Cultural influences on performance. (After Christiansen & Baum 1991)

Geographical	=	place of origin; its dialect, colloquialisms and/or main language; its climate, natural resources and staple diet
Community	=	its environmental strengths and weaknesses as an urban or rural area; its economy, social and health issues, including housing and the dominance of one kind of tenure over others; the population and its ethnicity
Family	=	structure, whether there is a set role structure and how strictly this is enforced; style of living and balance of productivity, leisure, self-care
Oneself	=	work ethic and use of time; sense and definition of personal space; coping mechanisms; ways of expressing emotions; role selection

within the parameters of his environment and what he believes is acceptable behaviourally. Envisage the person who enjoys work and leisure to a greater extent than caring for his home. He will work diligently and participate in his leisure interests and hobbies enthusiastically, excluding all but the most basic elements of self-catering and home care. However, if he were expecting relatives for the weekend his behaviours would change, influenced by social and cultural values and norms (which, for himself, he may have discarded). He would tidy, clean, shop and cook to meet the expected needs of his visitors. Therefore, his activity relates to the perceived expectations of his social/cultural group even if *personally* he has modified his own standards and activity levels.

Activity and time

The performance of activities also relates to time. The minutes or hours allocated to a particular activity on a specific day reflects the relative value attached to that task at that time. The value, or importance, of an activity may vary — the family breakfast will be a far more rushed affair on weekdays than at weekends, because family members are routinely preparing for school or work during the week. However, the time allotted to breakfast at weekends enters another time dimension altogether; even with events to attend, shopping to complete or visits to friends to make, the pressure to meet deadlines is relaxed.

Integration of activities

The integration of activities with roles, routines, time, social/cultural groups and the individual's environment will form quite distinctive activity groups relating to work, leisure, recreation, self-care and social interaction. They will also integrate each person's physical, psychological, cognitive and social functions; i.e. the performance of activity will unite the mind, body and will in the actual 'doing' of that task.

All activities which form the daily life pattern of a particular person are taken for granted until illness or accident and subsequent dysfunction intervene. Kielhofner (1985) (Fig. 5.3) describes man's daily functions in terms of a 'function/ dysfunction' continuum. That is, while man is well he performs at the functional level of exploration, competence and achievement, but when he is handicapped in some way he lapses to the dysfunction level in which he may display helplessness, incompetence or inefficiency in daily activities. Thus, moving from helplessness to achievement, the individual may, in succession, exhibit a complete deficit of skills, an inability to perform a particular skill routinely, a dissatisfaction with reduced ability, an investigation of skills in a secure environment, a striving to meet the demands of a skill, the development of new skills and, finally, a striving to maintain and enhance his performance.

Cynkin & Robinson (1990) summarise the importance and relevance of activity in daily life thus (Fig. 5.4):

- activity is concerned with the procedures of day-to-day living
- it involves the process of doing
- it is necessary to and characteristic of man's existence and survival

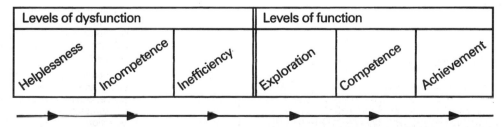

Fig. 5.3 An occupational dysfunction/function continuum. (Adapted from Keilhofner 1985.)

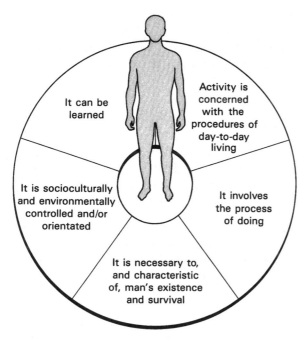

Fig. 5.4 The importance and relevance of activity in daily life.

- it is socioculturally and environmentally controlled and/or orientated
- it can be learned.

In the course of her intervention, utilising a very wide range of self-care, work, leisure and social activities, the occupational therapist must fully appreciate man's dependence upon activity if he is to function effectively and to maintain his general mental and physical health while meeting his sometimes complex needs and wants in a manner which suits his life-style and environment.

PURPOSEFUL AND NON-PURPOSEFUL ACTIVITY

Thus far, we have considered man's normal daily activities which have directed purpose. However, prior to detailed discussion of the analysis and synthesis it is important to reflect on both purposeful and non-purposeful activity. The latter is, one could argue, activity for its own sake rather than a (therapeutic) means to an end, for example, an individual playing solitaire for his own enjoyment rather than as a means of im-

proving his hand–eye coordination. It might also be understood as that which forms part of a recipe — that is, as activity undertaken because it is standard practice in the circumstances. For example a person with a fractured radius and ulna may use a prescribed range of activities in a certain manner at specific stages in his programme. Thus in the early stages he might participate in large remedial games and pottery, and as he improves he might be offered stool-seating or printing; finally he might be upgraded to heavy woodwork and wrought iron work. It may be argued that there is nothing adverse in this approach — nor, indeed, is there, *provided that* the activities used mean something to the individual, i.e. that he understands their purpose at that specific stage of his programme.

None the less, the occupational therapist should ensure that she does use specific (purposeful) activities, avoiding those which may be construed as merely exercise-orientated, especially if their purpose is unclear and unexplainable to both the individual and herself.

Purposeful activity is a concept central to occupational therapy theories, the implication being that activity (doing), when purposeful, leads to change. Henderson et al (1991) reinforced this in their multidimensional definition, stating that the purpose and meaning of activities are attributes of *people* rather than of the activities themselves. Furthermore, readers must understand that purposeful activity motivates a person to participate because it has meaning and is related to his goals, regardless of its actual or perceived unpleasantness, difficulty or pleasure. The therapist may argue that activity with some purpose relates as closely as possible to the recipient's daily life. However, she may also argue that at selected stages in an intervention programme she has to utilise activities that may not relate very closely to general daily life but do encourage, for instance, early reduction of oedema and the return of mid-range movement. The individual himself might also feel that any activity is 'purposeful' for him as long as it improves his function, whether or not it relates to his usual life roles and tasks. Without furthering the debate here, suffice it to say that the therapist *must* give serious thought to the ways she uses activity — to ensure it has purpose enables her to fulfil her functions and roles as an occupational therapist.

ACTIVITY ANALYSIS AND SYNTHESIS

DEFINITIONS

Occupational therapists' legitimate and essential tools are occupation and activity. Designed for intervention and evaluation they must be subjected to analysis and synthesis — analysis to ascertain its potential therapeutic value; synthesis to aid the matching process between person and activity.

Analysis provides the therapist with knowledge of how an activity can contribute to the balance between daily living skills, work and leisure and motivate the individual to organise routines and skills into behavioural patterns and roles. Analysis can be general in nature or related to a particular frame of reference or treatment approach and will reveal the complexities of an individual's function. It examines his mastery of or ability to learn skills; his possession of integrated concepts (such as size and weight); his neuromuscular control and coordination, sensation and joint stability; his problem-solving abilities and creativity; and his skill in making informed choices. It also requires cognisance of the individual's values, goals, roles, habits and interests to enable him to learn or relearn.

An activity is a step-by-step process involving a potentially large number of tasks in which sequencing is vital. Analysis allows the activity to be broken down into its simplest components, using the actual order or sequence of tasks.

Synthesis, also a process, combines 'component parts of human and non human environments . . . to design an activity suitable for evaluation or intervention' (Hopkins & Smith, 1993). This matching between individual and activity must develop within a frame of reference as this helps to define the choice of activity, those aspects of the activity that will promote goal achievement for the individual and those that will need emphasis for

and exploration with him. For instance, in the developmental frame of reference parallels may be drawn between levels of function expected or needed in particular activities and skill areas and (normal) developmental stages.

Features of activity

All activities utilised by occupational therapists are chosen for specific reasons, as summarised in Figure 5.5. In selecting activities, the therapist should bear the following points in mind:

- Each activity must have a purpose. It must be directed at a specific goal, such as enabling the individual to regain confidence and ensure safety when handling kitchen utensils while preparing a hot drink (Fig. 5.6).
- The task must be significant/relevant to the individual. Its level of significance may vary with his stage of treatment, but it must be seen, by him, to be of value and use even if its merits may only be fully realised at a later date. Hence, early workshop activity may make it possible for him to aim for a future goal, i.e. the motivation, coordination and neuromuscular control which will facilitate his readoption of one of his leisure roles.
- Any activity requires the individual's cooperation and consent to some degree. He must be involved in the actual performance of the activity, but he must also assist in the process of determining which activities are relevant. In this way he not only receives feedback about his physical and mental involvement with the activity but can redevelop and reaffirm his ability to plan, make decisions, initiate action, solve problems, transfer learning and take increasing responsibility as his programme progresses.
- In addition to maintaining and/or improving levels of function, activity should also aim to prevent any further dysfunction or disability (Fig. 5.7) and to improve a person's quality of life. The specific choice and type of activity used depends initially upon the individual's current functional level, including his ability to participate, but it must also facilitate his progress towards future goals.

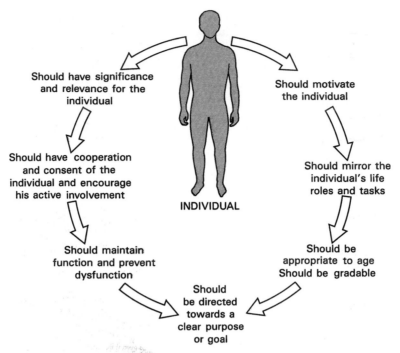

Fig. 5.5 Specific characteristics of activities appropriate for use in occupational therapy.

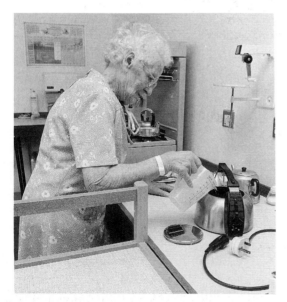

Fig. 5.6 Each activity must have a purpose and be directed at a specific goal.

● Most, if not all, activities in a programme should mirror an individual's life roles and tasks, enabling him to achieve or redevelop skills which are vital to him and which assist him to develop the required competence level. They should also encourage balance in his life-style, physical and psychological well-being and self-esteem, and recognise his worth and individuality.

● If the individual is to demonstrate and fulfil his commitment to his intervention he must be sufficiently motivated. Relating activity to his interests and involving him in the selection of tasks will help both him and the therapist to attain their objectives.

● In addition to the interest element, an activity must be age appropriate. As a person ages the nature of his 'doing' changes, influenced by role modification, different responsibilities and societal and cultural issues.

● It must also be gradable, i.e. adaptable, in complexity and time in terms of the minutes or hours he performs an activity which aims to increase his range of movement and improve his muscle strength or coordination.

● Activities are selected as potentially appropriate by the therapist based on her professional knowledge and judgement, thereby ensuring that

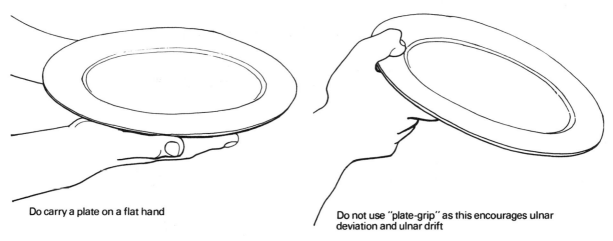

Do carry a plate on a flat hand

Do not use "plate-grip" as this encourages ulnar deviation and ulnar drift

Fig. 5.7 Preventing further dysfunction or disability may require a re-education programme, for example the 'do' and 'do not' of carrying a plate for the person with rheumatoid arthritis.

the activity meets the needs of the individual in a meaningful way.

THE PURPOSE OF ACTIVITY ANALYSIS

The therapist's skill in activity analysis and synthesis is essential if she is to utilise any activity with purpose and precision. The step-by-step analysis can be a lengthy and complex process but it can be vital in identifying and meeting treatment aims and objectives. The specific reasons for analysis are summarised in a 'Why?' checklist in Table 5.1 and can be described as follows:

• To observe and understand the numerous elements of an activity, i.e. the tasks which, when performed in the correct sequence, form the complete activity.

• To determine each activity's potential use as a treatment medium in relation to the people receiving occupational therapy, their perceived needs, their life-styles, and the frame of reference/ approaches being used.

• To determine whether an activity is viable in terms of:
— cost, including time and safety
— the space it requires
— whether it needs a particular environment because, for example, it is noisy and dirty
— the availability of materials, tools or equipment
— staff expertise and availability.

Table 5.1 The necessity for activity analysis: a 'Why?' checklist

Why?	In relation to . . .
To observe and understand	the numerous elements and sequences which form a complete activity
To determine an activity's potential use	treatment, individual's perceived needs and life-style frame of reference
To establish viability	cost, space, particular environment, materials, tools, equipment, staff expertise/ availability
To establish performance levels required	basic and essential skills required, e.g. coordination, standing tolerance
To identify potential for modification	adaptability and scope for grading
To break down into tasks	learning and teaching purposes, e.g. logical progression, tasks needing simplification
To identify more demanding components	facilitating change in behaviour

• To establish whether or not individuals can perform it. In order for an activity to meet a particular person's needs he must possess certain basic skills. If, for example, hand-press printing is used within his programme the skills he requires will include: sufficient coordination to handle the paper, adequate standing or sitting balance and tolerance to maintain his position, an adequate range of movement in his upper limbs to depress and raise the press handle, and motivation in order to complete the task set. However, if the intention is to increase his skill level then elements of the activity should be slightly beyond his current ability, thereby offering a further goal. In addition, the elements within the activity which are planned to be of specific use to the individual should form the greater proportion of the whole in order to make it worthwhile.

- To identify an activity's potential for modification, i.e. for grading and adaptation, thus ensuring that a selected sequence of tasks is a valued experience and applicable to the individual's ability and needs.

- To break down the activity into tasks for learning and teaching purposes. As the therapist undertakes this element of her analysis she can identify the tasks and consider whether they present a logical progression or stages which may need to be simplified or which can be eliminated, or whether the tasks themselves need further subdivision due to their complexity and subsequent required skill levels.

- In order to grade an activity appropriately. To facilitate change in an individual's behaviour the therapist must identify which components are more demanding and why. This will enable her to prepare the individual adequately for the activity and the challenges and problems it may present.

APPROACHES

There are many approaches in the analysis of activity, some quite straightforward, others more complex and lengthy. The form of analysis used by a therapist will usually be influenced by her treatment frames of reference and approaches. Models of analysis are described below, but initially the therapist must ask herself certain questions prior to the selection of an activity for therapeutic use:

- How is the activity performed? The therapist must know the basic components and processes involved in the activity and understand its po-

tential. She must undertake the activity herself, or undertake planned observation, in the same or similar circumstances expected or anticipated of the individual. She must be sufficiently competent to teach the person successfully, having considered the media to be used, positioning, movements, reactions, cognitive function required and so on.

- What activity is most appropriate to meet this individual's needs? With him she must select an activity which meets his needs, solves particular problems and relates to his interests and preferences.

- Why is a specific activity selected? The therapist must be able to establish a reason for the choice, which must be consistent with programme aims and objectives. It must be appropriate as well as meeting physical, psychological, cognitive, cultural and social demands.

- Where will the activity take place? Whatever the constraints concerning location, the therapist should endeavour to provide appropriate activity in its relevant environment, for example, personal care in the bedroom and bathroom, domestic skills in a kitchen, workshop activity in the therapy department, in the assigned area at home, or in the local community, utilising public services.

- When will the activity take place? Time, in this instance, may relate to time of day or week, season, or stage of a treatment programme. Timing may influence the activity chosen to meet a need, but whatever it is it must take place at its appropriate time or hour, thus confirming its credibility. Therefore, morning self-care will precede and/ or succeed breakfast, depending on the individual's normal routine; a seasonal activity such as making a Christmas cake will take place in the autumn.

- Who is involved in the activity? As well as the individual, carer and therapist, this may include other occupational therapy staff contributing to the programme and to whom the therapist has deployed particular elements. In this latter instance the therapist requires the ability and skill to involve support staff whose expertise in certain creative and practical tasks may far outweigh her own.

Within the question 'Who?', specific factors relating to the individual must be borne in mind. These include age, sex, past or present occupation, social and cultural background, his presenting problems, diagnosis and prognosis, his interests, approximate intellectual level and any disabilities other than the present one(s).

Assembling a 'pen-picture' of the person referred for intervention should precede analysis of potentially suitable activities and the planning of a programme appropriate to his functional and personal needs. Table 5.2 illustrates how the therapist may create such a picture for two individuals.

Table 5.2 Assembling a pen-picture prior to activity analysis and programme planning

Factor	Adult	Older person
Age	30	65
Sex	Female	Male
Past/present occupation	Teacher/mother with small child	Miner/retired
Social/cultural background	Settled in UK 20 years ago from Scandinavia. Lives with husband, no other family in area	From mining family, spent whole life in the town. Widower of 3 years, 2 children and grandchildren in same town
Diagnosis/ presenting problems	Depression following birth of child, early signs of rheumatoid arthritis?	Pneumoconiosis, CVA
Prognosis	Uncertain, due to non-confirmation of rheumatoid arthritis	Mediocre due to long-standing pneumoconiosis
Interests	Scandinavian folklore and crafts, wine making, travel abroad	Grandchildren, the local miners' club, gardening (allotment)
Intellectual level	University graduate	Left school at 14, well read
Other disabilities	None	Amputation distal phalanges little and ring fingers dominant hand

ACTIVITY ANALYSIS MODELS

An occupational therapist's skill in analysing activity is vital in order to establish valid use of the chosen tasks. She will select a method of analysis which is applicable to the frame(s) of reference, approaches and techniques she uses in treatment and one with which she feels most comfortable, i.e. which meets her needs and those of her clientele.

The following section describes two activity analysis models, of which one is quite simple, the other more detailed.

SIMPLE ANALYSIS METHOD

This entails answering the questions How? What? Why? Where? When? and Who? in the manner described above and summarised in Table 5.3. This technique has been used successfully by generations of therapists, often with additional questions in order to specify more accurately the potential benefits of an activity. For example:

- Does it provide a basic sensory skill?
- Does it need repeated use of the same skill?
- Can it be graded?
- Does it assist tolerance to noise?

Table 5.3 A simple activity analysis method

Question	'Answer(s)'
How is the activity performed?	Potential, basic components and processes involved; use of treatment media, positioning, movements, reactions, cognitive functions
What activity?	Appropriateness related to individual needs, problems, interests, preferences
Why is the activity selected?	Choice must be consistent with programme aims and objectives; must meet physical, psychological, cognitive, cultural and social demands
Where will it take place?	Whatever the constraints, choice of environment must be as relevant as possible
When will it take place?	At the appropriate time of day, week, season, year, in order to lend credibility
Who is involved?	Individual, therapist, other staff, carers

- Does it appeal to the individual?
- Does it have any vocational or educational value?

DETAILED ANALYSIS MODELS

These are described in many texts and vary only according to the preferences of the authors. These more complex frameworks itemise analyses in terms of the demands of a particular activity, that is, according to the physical, emotional, social, sensory, cognitive, perceptual and cultural demands of any task, its components and sequences.

Common factors

Factors common to all activities and their analysis include:

- The environment in which the activity does or could take place, including space and equipment, or the environment the activity creates, i.e. the relevance, value, emphasis, priority created by or given to the activity by an individual and his sociocultural group. The environment can also play a part in shaping and directing an activity, e.g. interaction with it, negotiation of it and orientation.
- The motivation an activity can evoke. How does it facilitate personal effectiveness and how does it relate to interests, roles, individual values?
- The appropriateness of any activity utilised in a therapy programme to the chronological age and developmental stage of the individual, regardless of his problems, to enable him to learn or relearn age- and role-appropriate skills and behaviours.
- The appropriateness of the activity to the sex of the individual. This will depend, of course, upon the sociocultural background of the person; for example, does his culture accept role-swapping or has it very stringent laws about the roles and behaviour of men and women?
- The adaptability of the activity. This is exceedingly important if optimum use is to be made of it. This is discussed in detail in Grading activity, below.
- The degree of vocational application of the

activity. The vocational element relates to the potential application of the skills within the activity to work (paid or unpaid), home care, leisure and social relationships.

- The cost implications of the activity. Intervention must be cost-effective and efficient in relation to staff time and departmental/service resources. Factors to consider include whether suitable equipment and materials are available, whether a completed article is to be produced, the time the individual has available and whether there are cost implications for the individual pursuing the activity elsewhere, for example at a sports club.
- The safety of the activity. While everyone lives with an element of risk, the person receiving occupational therapy has to be treated 'safely', i.e. the environment must be as hazard-free as possible, and intervention techniques must be safe for the individual and the therapist. However, the situation will vary according to the treatment venue. Compare, for instance, the individual's home environment with that of a local authority day centre, a sports club or a hospital department. Legislation and regulations will affect the safety precautions taken in specific environments.
- The time required to complete the whole activity. This may or may not have relevance, but the therapist must analyse the time factor, i.e. total time for the activity, time for particular elements or sub-tasks.
- The potential of the activity for individual and/group work. This knowledge is vital when planning individual programmes.

Specific factors

These factors should be applied to analysis as required, i.e. in respect of the individual and his discrete needs. Table 5.4 summarises them.

Prior to initiating her analysis the therapist must establish which frame of reference, i.e. developmental, biomechanical, learning or compensatory, and approach, e.g. neurodevelopmental, sensory integrative, cognitive or adaptive, she will use. Thus she can facilitate positive change related to a person's presenting functional abilities, problems and needs and utilise activity

Table 5.4 A summary of a detailed activity analysis model

Analysis area	Summary of demands	Analysis area	Summary of demands
Motor/physiological Position	• of individual and/or activity • does position of both/either change during the activity or not?	Problem-solving	• reasoning • abstract thinking and imagery • decision-making • planning
Movement	• joints involved • range of movement required • specific movements and ranges required • bilateral/unilateral • speed/rhythm	Logical thinking	• concrete/abstract thought • initiating action from thought processes
		Communication	• verbal • non-verbal • relevance of senses
Grading	• range of movement • strength and/or precision required • resistance • endurance • discomfort levels	Organisational ability	• in relation to cognition above
		Perceptual Agnosia	• non-recognition of familiar objects
Sensory Visual	• figure/ground discrimination • spatial awareness • appreciation of form, colour, tone	Apraxia	• loss of ability to perform previously learned task
Auditory	• language • cues • selective attention	Spatial relationship disorders	• relating to figure/ground, form constancy, depth/distance perception
Olfactory	• relevance in certain activities and environments • compensation for absence of other senses	Self-awareness disorders	• relating to body scheme, unilateral neglect
Gustatory	• relevance in certain activities • stimulus/pleasure/interest	*Emotional* Activity demands/offers	• e.g. inventiveness, gratification, expression of mood, exploration of feelings, impulse control, coping with feelings/emotion
Tactile/kinaesthetic	• temperature • texture discrimination • sensations of movement • body awareness	*Social* Activity demands/offers	• e.g. interaction, communication, cooperation/sharing, competition, role-play
Cognitive Motivation	• interest/fun • achievement potential • individual-directed activity	*Independence* Activity demands/offers	• opportunity to examine ability to plan, organise, use initiative, make decisions
Learning	• memory • information retention • transfer of learning • attention/concentration span • numeracy/literacy	*Cultural* Activity demands/offers	• cultural appropriateness in terms of values, roles, life-style

in different ways and for different reasons. An illustrative example is offered in Table 5.5.

Motor/physiological demands

These would be selected from the following aspects:

• position — of the activity and the individual. Does positioning remain unchanged throughout (Fig. 5.8) or are changes required at certain sub-stages?
• movement — which large and/or small joints are involved; degrees of range of movement required; specific movements entailed, for example flexion (Fig. 5.9) and extension; grips/grasps needed; muscle groups in action; type of muscle work necessary. What is the unilateral or bilateral involvement and

Table 5.5 Motor and sensory activity demands for a biomechanical and neurodevelopmental approach to intervention

Biomechanical	Neurodevelopmental
Deals with joint range, muscle strength and endurance. Full voluntary control of movement is usually present.	Used in relation to developmental and upper motor neurone disorders and other conditions with neurological deficit, e.g. CVA. Individual may no longer have full control of voluntary movement. Loss of voluntary movement may result from changed muscle tone and/or re-emergence of primitive reflexes. Equilibrium reactions and sensation may be impaired.
Prerequisite of activities used in this approach: movement needed must occur often enough to be therapeutic, and must facilitate grading to maintain pace with person's progress.	The nature of activity and the responses it elicits must be analysed in conjunction with the development sequence of learned movement at the appropriate level for the individual; for example, head control is necessary prior to undertaking activity in a sitting position.
Consider: Position of individual in relation to activity — position must be maintained to effect required treatment outcome. Which joints are used? Range of movement through which joints move. Which muscle groups are involved? Type of muscle work — eccentric, concentric, static? Degree of muscle strength involved/required Resistance offered Repetition and frequency of movement(s) Degree of coordination required Endurance/stamina required	*Consider:* Does activity encourage control of righting and equilibrium responses? Does it encourage normal/abnormal movement patterns? Does it provide stability/mobility at specified joints depending on the developmental sequence required? What sensory feedback does the activity provide (for example: proprioception, touch sensation), facilitating the learning/relearning of functional movement through sensory feedback?

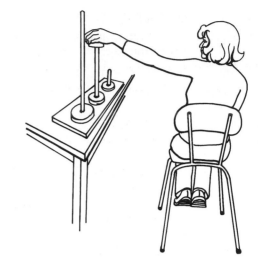

Fig. 5.8 Positioning should facilitate specific movements required, for example shoulder abduction.

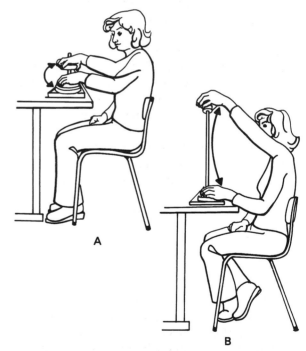

Fig. 5.9 Shoulder flexion. (A) Using a standard span game. (B) Increasing flexion with lengthened dowel rods.

is left and right comparison facilitated if appropriate? What fine or gross movement and coordination, rhythm and speed of movement are required?

- grading/adaptability — may include range of movement, strength and/or precision required, resistance offered, coordination necessary, endurance (for example, standing for extended periods of activity) and discomfort level.

Sensory demands

These relate to the sensory and perceptual qualities of an activity and should be considered in terms of sensorimotor integration and proprioception as well as the function of individual senses. All five senses should be considered:

- visual, for example appreciation of form, colour, tone
- auditory, including comprehension of language, use of auditory cues, use of selective attention
- olfactory — often overlooked but appropriate in home care, workshop and community activities and skills. In addition to offering pleasure, for example in cooking spicy foods, it may alert an individual to potential danger and it may become a well-developed sense in those with impaired vision
- gustatory/taste — also frequently overlooked but particularly important for people with severe disability and for whom mealtimes can be a source of pleasure as well as nourishment. As mentioned above, food can provide a much-needed stimulus and in this case the tasting of food in preparation as well as eating the completed dish can offer interest and pleasure to the cook and to others invited to participate
- tactile/kinaesthetic — includes temperature and texture differentiation, degrees of touch (light, firm), body awareness and sensations of movement.

Cognitive demands

These concern the level of function the activity requires in relation to:

- motivation — whether the activity promotes interest, fun, potential achievement, whether the individual perceives it as relevant; whether he is self-directed in performing the activity
- learning-level(s) required — use of memory (short-term, long-term or both); retention of information regarding procedures, stages and changes; transfer of learning; concentration and attention span; numeracy and literacy; motivation
- problem-solving — use of reasoning, abstract

thought and imagery; judgement and/or decision-making; planning versus trial and error

- logical thinking — concrete and abstract thought; use of imagery; initiation of action from thought processes
- communication — verbal (including written); non-verbal (simple and complex); relevance of hearing and vision
- perception — may be included in cognitive demands or dealt with separately. See Perceptual demands, below
- organisational ability in relation to all the elements enumerated above.

Perceptual demands

Difficulties with sensory integration can be grouped as follows (see also Chs 14, 15):

- agnosia — inability to recognise familiar objects; can be visual, auditory or tactile
- apraxia — the loss of ability to perform a previously learned task although the motor power, sensation, coordination and comprehension required are retained
- spatial relationship disorders — relating to perception of figure/ground, position in space, form constancy, depth/distance
- self-awareness disorders — leading to unilateral neglect, distorted perception of body scheme.

Proprioceptive and stereognostic functions may be included within perception, but some practitioners consider this incorrect. However, it could be argued that as poor proprioception involves a loss of postural or position sense it ought to be considered alongside other general sensory and specific perceptual deficits. Stereognosis describes a person's ability to recognise items by touch; this too is a sensory input, the perceptual element being described by subsequent sensory integration (followed in normal function by motor output).

Emotional demands

Does the activity demand or offer opportunities for: inventiveness and originality; destructiveness/

aggression; gratification; expression of a present mood, attitude, perception; exploration of feelings; structured or unstructured time; impulse control; independence or dependence; testing of reality; coping with feelings/emotions?

Social demands

What interaction is required? Is the activity undertaken alone, in a group, or both? What interaction with others is needed vis-à-vis: verbal communication, cooperation, dependence; sharing ideas, equipment, tools, materials; responsibility for others; consideration for needs and safety of co-workers; competition; testing reality; role-playing, e.g. leading, cooperating?

Independence

Does the activity offer the individual an opportunity to examine his ability to plan and organise, to use his initiative, to make decisions and to gradually relinquish dependence on others?

Cultural demands

The activity must be culturally appropriate in terms of values, roles and life circumstances. Some activities, for instance domestic tasks, may have underlying cultural assumptions rendering that activity unsuitable or inappropriate for some people.

Having analysed an activity in order to use it therapeutically the therapist must be an able teacher of the processes and procedures involved. If the individual is to benefit from the activity he must understand what he has to do, with minimum correction, and how and why he is doing it, particularly if he does not see its immediate relevance.

GRADING ACTIVITY

To what degree do the innate properties of any activity permit realistic adaptation relative to an individual's needs and personal style and to activity in the 'real world'?

While it is recognised that activity needs a sequence or routine for successful achievement, it must also possess a structure which facilitates the learning of skills beyond those currently possessed by the individual. An activity must stimulate and sustain eagerness and the will to learn. As well as being relevant and practical it must also be versatile, i.e. lend itself to a variety of processes, end products and environments, and be adaptable to individuals, their needs and environments.

Some activities have more potential for modification than others. The therapist must use her own judgement and ingenuity in deciding when and how it is necessary to change from one activity to another or when to grade or adapt an activity to meet individual needs. She must remember that all activities utilised need to be adjustable so that, with the individual's improvement or deterioration, they can be adapted to suit his maximum capability.

Grading methods

Whatever grading methods she uses, the therapist must adhere to the following rules:

- The activity must foster and maintain a good working posture and position
- The individual should know and understand why he is required to perform an activity in a way which may differ from the norm
- The therapist must ensure that adaptations secure a positive rather than a negative effect on the individual
- The therapist must consider the time required for modification and maintenance of adapted activities.

Additionally, the therapist should decide whether any grading method is activity-centred, in which case the task itself is graded to meet a particular need, or person-centred, in which case the individual's position, cognitive process and so on are 'graded'.

Adaptation

In this context adaptation concerns making an

adjustment to an activity, when necessary, to provide it in an alternative way so that it meets an individual's therapeutic needs. It may include adjustment to method, changing the components involved or modifying the environment in some way. Activity adaptation trends 'come and go' and depend upon a number of factors, such as the personal preference of the therapist, priorities in treatment, the types of problems an individual is experiencing, the therapy service itself and where it is based. Whether the adaptation of an activity relates to a specific skill or to the modification of the environment in which a task takes place, it must meet the specific needs of the individual. It must be simple, both for the individual to manage and for the therapist to implement (Fig. 5.10) and it must maintain the value of the activity for the person, i.e. focus on the activity rather than on the movements or processes involved.

Grading

Grading comprises the gradual increase or decrease in one or more of the measurable criteria of an activity, i.e. adjustments are made to meet the individual's changing needs in time and in particular circumstances. Activities are paced and modified to meet immediate needs — the individual's maximum current capacity. A variety of grading methods are used if the required movements, resistance, creativity and so on are not obtained when an activity is performed in its usual manner. For example, if injury to an individual's hand prevents him from gripping a saw, the saw handle may be enlarged so that he can grasp it sufficiently to perform the correct actions in safety. This enlargement will be decreased as his grip improves.

The following elements may be of importance in the grading of activity:

• *Resistance.* In order to strengthen affected muscles or muscle groups, assisted gravity may be decreased gradually; thus weights and spring resistance may be added to selected tasks so that the individual has to overcome the resistance in order to complete the activity. The person may use heavier equipment or tools, e.g. moving from a light plane to a surform. Textures of materials may be modified to offer greater resistance; for

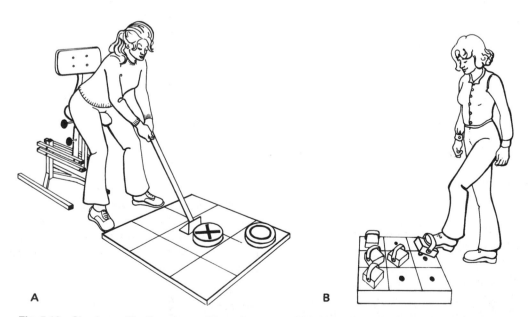

A   **B**

Fig. 5.10 Simple modifications to noughts and crosses which, in this example, enhance balance (A) in the early stages and (B) in the later stages.

example, the person may be given harder wood to work with, cutting with the grain initially and then against the grain.

● *Endurance/tolerance to activity.* This requires careful gradation. The therapist may use light work initially, grading the individual's programme until he can manage heavy work appropriate to his needs. The length of time spent on a particular activity can be increased, as can the number of sessions per week. These latter elements are of particular relevance for individuals whose work tolerance needs to be enhanced.

● *Organisation and integration of activities.* In terms of modifying and grading activity this includes:
— selection of appropriate activity based on needs, age, culture, environment and the individual's own goals
— structuring of activity in such a way as to render that activity therapeutic; the activity should include systematic learning stages, involve sequencing, and allow for modification, the monitoring of progress and the prioritising of goals
— timing of activities so that they are integrated into the individual's daily routine as soon as possible
— interaction between the therapist and individual, the therapist acting as a model of competence.

● *Techniques and tools.* The grading of these also relates to other elements. The 'how', or technique, of an activity must be integrated with the individual's physical and psychological needs; it must 'make sense' to him and interrelate with activities and situations in his environment. Tools encompass: equipment such as daily living aids, adjustable furniture, special crockery or orthoses; the environment, i.e. physical settings, people and objects of relevance to the individual. Tools and equipment, to a greater or lesser degree, will be important in the effective grading of activity for achievement and may be utilised temporarily, for example in the early stages of a programme, and then discarded as function improves.

● *Developmental grading.* This is relatively straightforward in that it adheres to the sequences of normal development; for example, the indi-

vidual must be able to sit before he can stand, and stand before he can walk. This is of vital importance for people with neurological deficit who may have to relearn normal movement patterns.

● *Positioning.* This is of great importance throughout therapy but can also be utilised to a large extent in grading. The relative positions of the individual, the activity and its accessories can be modified to meet specific requirements, for example by positioning paper for printing in such a way as to facilitate spinal rotation or extended reach. Positions will change as ranges of movement increase and joint function improves. Utilising vertical planes and horizontal positions for selected activity can add variety to a task; for example, placing a board game in the vertical plane may facilitate spinal side flexion, shoulder abduction and flexion and coordination.

● *Standing and walking tolerance.* These are vital elements of many individual programmes. The performance of many activities can offer: increases in the time spent standing; practice in transferring weight and balance; progression from static to mobile activity. The degree of physical support required can be decreased, e.g. by a gradual removal of trunk/pelvic supports and seats to facilitate a planned return to independent standing. The amount of walking in an activity can be increased, for example by encouraging free movement about the workshop to select tools and materials, or movement about the garden to select an activity.

● *Coordination and muscle control.* These are achieved primarily through increasing fine movements and decreasing gross ones. As a programme progresses the individual should undertake a large proportion of tasks requiring fine movement, control and coordination while gross movement decreases — even though it may not be eliminated from his schedule completely. If in his daily life the individual requires particular skills or unusual movement patterns, such as particular grasps used in handling large or awkward items, these should be introduced as soon as he can attempt them.

● *Dexterity.* Accompanied by *speed* when relevant, dexterity can also be upgraded. Timed activity related to particular objectives as well as tasks requiring greater manipulative skills will be utilised. Composing in printing, computer keyboard work and small table games provide the opportunity to practise fine movements, and speed and accuracy can be added dimensions which enhance potential to return to work. Where appropriate, skills can be transferred to other, more important tasks.

- *Complexity.* The very great variety of activities used in occupational therapy enables the individual and his therapist to select tasks requiring greater skill as his abilities increase. Activities with a large number of stages can be utilised. Printing, for example, involves a progression from a preliminary design to a finished article, thereby fulfilling not only physical needs, but providing opportunities for creativity, originality, achievement and feedback. If the individual has particular cognitive needs the complexity of activity must be developed to increase the demands on the individual. More demands can be made in a particular area of skill by adding more information to be remembered. Also, additional areas of cognitive function can be introduced, such as problem-solving and decision-making.

- *Social interaction.* The individual may begin by working alone, later sitting with one other person, and then with a small group. He might then begin to *work* with another person and, later, to participate in a small and then a larger group. To this type of grading can be added a number of additional functions, for example degrees of responsibility; expected interaction with one or more people; or initiation of a particular stage of the activity for the group.

Passive v. active participation

Passive involvement in activity requires no special effort by the individual, as in watching television or accepting a drink made by another person. Active participation, on the other hand, demands that he contribute. It significantly influences his health and well-being, and helps to prevent dependency that can arise from the inability to perform life skills. The individual's progress from passive to active involvement can be graded to meet developing needs, moving from straightforward and non-threatening activity which the individual wants to undertake to complex, challenging activity which he needs to be able to carry out in order to fulfil his chosen life-style and particular roles.

Creativity and spontaneity

Creativity and spontaneity are vital elements of the grading process and can be integrated with any of the other elements. The therapist should avoid stereotyped and structured activity when and where appropriate, stimulating the individual's creativity, self-expression, and originality and offering him the opportunity to plan, implement and review his selected actions.

Meaning and relevance

Finally, the meaning and relevance of activity and its grading or modification warrants particular attention. Any activity used in an individual's programme must be meaningful to him. It must relate to time and place and to his life-style. Activities must be acceptable to the individual and enable him to transfer his learning from one activity and environment to another. If activities have meaning then successful completion is more likely; in turn, success promotes the development of competence. The person's interest and involvement will be enhanced by feedback and once he is motivated by this process the therapist can facilitate further development and achievement. Additionally, the individual must be able to understand and interpret his improved function — for example, his greater range of movement or increased coordination; this is essential, as it leads him to perceive the psychological value of success and achievement.

Although the necessity for activity to be relevant or appropriate has been reiterated throughout this chapter, this requirement is so important that it warrants even further attention. Activity needs to be relevant for two key reasons:

1. In relation to personally determined attributes:
   — historical: past experience of activities and the attitudes, feelings and associations these offer
   — symbolic: the meaning of certain activities to the individual, including the process of completion and/or the end product
   — motivation and the variety of unconscious needs, drives and feelings the activity may satisfy
   — the new learning required and/or achieved
   — the retention of former skills or parts of those skills and their relevance now; for example, is it relevant that former skills be sequenced differently in order to achieve the required results?
   — the individual style of each person, his behaviour, his preferred ways, how he may have modified these in the past to suit his environment.
2. In relation to the socioculturally determined attributes of people, relationships, actions and objects which may be based on a person's age, sex, status (e.g. occupational, educational, socioeconomic), past roles, values and beliefs:
   — cultural background, including religious or ethnic elements and certain activities within this framework
   — the history of social trends and attitudes with regard to certain activities in the person's sociocultural environment
   — the relationship of activity or parts of activities to the person's current concepts of work, recreation and self-care
   — the relationship of the above to other daily living activity and its potential for integration in terms of learning achievement.

The application of all or part of these grading methods may seem potentially complex. However, with practice the therapist masters the elements which are most applicable to her frame of reference and approaches, work ethic, environment and speciality and refers to the less frequently used elements when necessary.

ANALYSIS OF THREE ACTIVITIES

The analyses below aim to clarify the essential elements of three areas of activity, i.e. a daily living skill, a creative or work activity and an interpersonal skill.

Daily living skill

Making a hot drink: the purposes of using this activity therapeutically may include assessment of previously learned skills and behaviours; safety in the kitchen; specific cognitive function; specific sensorimotor skills; ability to meet a particular need. Table 5.6 is intended to assist the reader in understanding and applying an analysis of this activity.

Creative or work activity

Composing type in printing: the therapist may use this particular element of the printing process to assess, enhance and reinforce cognitive function; specific sensorimotor function; use of tools/equipment; organisation; tolerance. Table 5.7 offers an analysis of this activity.

Interpersonal skill

Maintaining a relationship with a co-member of an educational group: physical dysfunction of all degrees of complexity and severity may have some effect on an individual's motivation, interests, roles, values, routines and practical skills. Therefore analysis of relationships and allied interpersonal skills is as important in predominantly 'physical dysfunction' practice as in any other speciality. The analysis in Table 5.8 demonstrates the value that such specific activity may offer.

Activity and treatment planning

The analysis and synthesis of any activity is a prerequisite to the therapist's plan to assist an individual to overcome or manage his dysfunction. The analyses illustrated above may be required before treating some people, but not all.

Table 5.6 Analysis: making a hot drink. *Task*: To make a mug of coffee, with milk, in the kitchen. The individual is ambulant, upper limb function and senses are intact and all equipment and materials are available

Component	Demands		Component	Demands	
General factors	Motivation —	thirst, wish for coffee rather than alternative beverage		Perceptual —	spatial awareness, visual/ tactile senses, figure/ ground discrimination, praxis, gnosis
	Relevance —	age appropriate, drinks coffee regularly, acceptable socioculturally, sex inapplicable in this instance, role as provider to self acceptable	3. Filling the kettle, i.e. unplugging kettle, removing lid, moving kettle to sink, placing under tap, turning on tap, filling kettle, turning off tap, returning kettle to work-top, replacing lid, plugging in, switching on	Motor —	as above and moving in small area; upper limb movements: flexion and extension of joints, shoulder ab/adduction and rotation, forearm pronation/supination, various grips
	Time —	routine, habit		Sensory —	coordination, particularly hand/eye; proprioception; tactile sense: degrees of touch, temperature and pressure, body awareness, sensation of movement; auditory sense
	Risk —	aware of potential risk factors			
	Emotional —	gratification			
	Social —	coffee for two			
	Cultural —	coffee for visitor			
Stages				Cognitive —	appreciation of safety, sequencing, memory, concentration, organisation
1. Enter kitchen	Motor —	walk independently; coordination; balance; weight transference; lower limb, pelvic and trunk joints and muscles enable mobility, balance and maintenance of upright posture		Perceptual —	spatial awareness, figure/ ground form constancy; visual sense: praxis and gnosis, figure/ground discrimination, spatial awareness, appreciation of form, colour
	Sensory —	proprioceptive awareness; coordination; visual sense to aid mobility	4. Putting coffee and milk into mug	As above plus:	
	Cognitive —	motivation (thirst); social; knowledge of activity and where it occurs; decision-making		Motor —	grips: prehensile, spherical, tripod
				Cognitive —	judgement/decision re quantities
				Perceptual —	stereognosis
2. Assemble equipment and materials, i.e. kettle, mug, spoon, coffee, milk from cupboard(s), fridge, drawer, shelf	Motor —	walking, standing, balance, weight transfer, bending, reaching/ stretching; lower and upper limbs involved in gross movements; upper limbs required to produce finer, skilled movements and grips, for example, lateral, spherical, cylindrical, hook, prehensile	5. Making drink once kettle has boiled	As above plus:	
				Sensory —	olfactory
				Perceptual —	tactile/temperature
			6. Drinking coffee	Motor —	mobility, coordination, sip and swallow
	Sensory —	coordination and proprioception, visual/ tactile senses used in unison and independently		Sensory —	thirst satisfied; olfactory, gustatory and tactile senses
	Cognitive —	memory and knowledge, logical and sequential thought, organisational skills		Emotional —	gratification
				Social —	communication, interaction and social skills

For instance, the more complex a person's needs the more likely the requirement for attention to detail in activities in order to enhance abilities and to begin to address difficulties. If the therapist is working with an individual who has motor, cognitive, social and sensory deficits as the result of a head injury she may need to divide tasks into component parts, whereas an indi-

CONCLUSION

The opening paragraphs of this chapter refer to the philosophy and history of the use of occupation and activity, founded on the belief that the performance of activity promotes and enhances physical and mental health. Occupational therapists believe that dysfunction can be modified, changed and reversed through activity. Such activity enables an individual to direct his time, energy, attention and interest productively and in such a way as to offer him opportunities for learning, development and satisfaction.

There is no universal method for analysing activity — a therapist's approach often depends on her area of speciality and expertise, her frames of reference and her personal preferences. Her analysis and synthesis of activity contributes to the productivity and satisfaction of the individual and offers the therapist scope to identify how activity may motivate him, assist him in organising skills, behaviours and routines and make a contribution to role and task balance. Analysis also indicates the flexibility, simplicity / complexity and relevance of a task, and enables the therapist to design effective intervention which, building on a person's existing abilities, helps him to achieve the desired results.

The occupational therapist's knowledge and application of the therapeutic use of activity (see Ch. 6) is enhanced through activity analysis and synthesis. Any activity used in an individual's programme must have certain qualities to enable him to learn, explore, experiment and achieve. These qualities are discovered through thorough analysis of activities which have a wide range of potential as therapeutic media.

REFERENCES

Christiansen C, Baum C (eds) 1991 Occupational therapy: overcoming human performance deficits. Slack Inc, Thorofare, NJ

Cowper W 1731–1800 Retirement. In: Cohen J M (ed) 1974 The Penguin dictionary of quotations. Penguin, Harmondsworth

Cynkin S 1979 Occupational therapy: toward health through activities. Little, Brown, Boston

Cynkin S, Robinson A M 1990 Occupational therapy and activities health: toward health through activities. Little, Brown, Boston

Darnell J L, Heater S L 1994 Occupational therapist or activity therapist — which do you choose to be? American Journal of Occupational Therapy 48(5): 467–468

First People's Exhibit (undated) Royal British Columbia Museum, Victoria, BC

Henderson A, Cermak S, Coster W, Murray E, Trombly C, Tickle-Degnen L 1991 The issue is: occupational science is multidimensional. American Journal of Occupational Therapy 45: 370–372

Hopkins H L, Smith H D 1993 Willard and Spackman's occupational therapy, 8th edn. J B Lippincott, Philadelphia, PA

Kielhofner G 1985 The model of human occupation. Williams & Wilkins, Baltimore

Reed K L, Sanderson S R 1992 Concepts of occupational therapy, 3rd edn. Williams & Wilkins, Baltimore

Young M E, Quinn E 1992 Theories and principles of occupational therapy. Churchill Livingstone, Edinburgh

FURTHER READING

Bee H L, Mitchell S K 1984 The developing person — a lifespan approach, 2nd edn. Harper & Row, New York

Earhart C A, Allen C K 1988 Cognitive disabilities: expanded activity analysis, Colchester, CT: S & S Worldwide

Finlay L 1993 Groupwork in occupational therapy. Chapman & Hall, London

Kielhofner G 1983 Health through occupation — theory and practice in occupational therapy. F A Davis, Philadelphia

Lamport N K, Coffey M S, Hersch G I 1989 Activity analysis handbook. Slack Inc, Thorofare, NJ

Mosey A C 1986 Psychosocial components of occupational therapy. Raven Press, New York

Nelson D L 1988 Occupation: form and performance. American Journal of Occupational Therapy 42: 633–641

Punwar A J 1988 Occupational therapy principles and practice. Williams & Wilkins, Baltimore

6

The therapeutic use of activity

Ann Turner   Charlotte MacCaul

INTRODUCTION

Occupational therapy philosophy (Ch. 1) tells us that activity is fundamental to well-being and occupational performance. Where this has been interrupted a person can use or modify activity in order to facilitate its return. We assume that, in order to have maintained appropriate occupational performance throughout evolution, people have adapted to changes that occur naturally in the environment and society, and that healthy people respond positively to change by adapting their activities to meet changing needs. The human need for occupation and adaptation is therefore grounded in evolution, and it is this need to use activity to acquire adaptation that forms the core feature of intervention by the occupational therapist. We engage in occupations in order to solve problems related to adaptation, and this engagement continues to be necessary for developing and maintaining well-being throughout life. To be a healthy and productive member of society a person must be seen to be, and see himself as, contributing to it at some level, and must feel effective and efficient in order to remain purposeful. Without a sense of purpose, productivity, the sense of self and ultimately health are at risk. John Dewy, an early 20th century American philosopher, saw evidence of learning through doing and felt that 'Activity is the human endeavour that feeds people's souls and meets their needs' (Brienes 1995, p. 17).

Success in performance leads to self-confidence and a willingness to continue. When an inability

125

using a cash machine or video) and social interactions assume high priority for many. This causes a dilemma for the therapist endeavouring to enhance performance through purposeful activity when society's skill base has changed radically and rapidly and may not 'fit' with the skills and facilities with which she is equipped.

USING ACTIVITY THERAPEUTICALLY

The occupational therapist's ability to use activity must be based on an assessment of the skills the individual possesses and applied through the use of appropriate media. Traditional craft-based activities may be appropriate for some, but for the majority they are not. Many therapists have, however, had difficulty replacing them with a cluster of media which are appropriate for the skills possessed and required by the people they treat. As this occurs the invasion of technique-based processes, exercise regimes or assessment schedules undertaken for their own sake will advance to fill the gaps left by inappropriate or dated activities. Such actions only emphasise occupational therapy's slowness in shifting its media base to reflect the skills and needs of the people being treated.

The ways in which occupational therapists use activity must reflect the fundamental philosophy of the profession. Equally, in order to consider the choice of activity, it is important to distinguish between media and technique as they are used to improve occupational performance. Theoretically, media, the means by which the activity is applied, are of infinite variety. Gardening, cookery, photography, vehicle maintenance, brick-laying and puppetry are all media which have been employed by occupational therapists, and while their scope is theoretically endless their choice is generally constrained by the skills of the therapist and the facilities and finances available to her.

In contrast, technique is the manner in which an activity is carried out and the way in which the therapeutic medium is harnessed. Setting up table tennis in a way that encourages maximum trunk balance for a person in a wheelchair, learning specific sequences and methods for getting dressed, or weight-bearing through an upper limb while buttering toast all show the application of technique to an activity.

To decide which media have therapeutic potential requires accurate activity analysis (see Ch. 5). However, in order to be successful the medium must fulfil certain universal criteria (Box 6.2). Additionally, when evaluating a medium to see whether it should be continued, adopted or discarded, the factors described by Reed (1986) form a useful basis (Box 6.3).

Occupational therapists, however, not only improve function through the use of a chosen medium. They also work creasingly with people for whom increase in physical capacity is no

---

Box 6.2 Determining the success of a medium for use within occupational therapy

To be successful a medium must be:

- **Flexible** — able to be used in a variety of ways, for long and short periods of time, and to offer a wide variety of therapeutic components

- **Adaptable** — able to be used within and outside its normal domain

- **Relevant** — to the therapeutic needs and cultural, age and gender requirements of the people who use it

- **Rich in therapeutic components** — so that it offers sufficient of these to be relevant to the user group. The therapeutic components should not be outweighed by the non-therapeutic elements

- **Usable by a wide variety of staff** — and not dependent on the skills or whim of one or two people with specialist training, but be objectively analysed and costed

- **Therapeutically and professionally justifiable** — while many outcomes are measurable, can the therapist justify activities whose outcomes she considers non-quantifiable? Can the activity be justified within professional boundaries? Does it fit within the ethos of departmental practice?

- **Usable within existing resources** — including staff, time, environment and cost. Is the activity cost-effective? Is there an outlet for any tangible output?

- **Robust and replaceable** — and conform to any Health and Safety regulations, or other local or national policies. Storage, availability and maintenance of equipment and materials must be viable

- **Aesthetically, culturally, gender and age appropriate** — to those who will use it

---

Box 6.3 Factors influencing the choice or abandonment of media by occupational therapists. (Based on Reed 1986.)

- **Cultural** — whether the activity fits within the culture of the individual being treated
- **Social** — social acceptance of an activity is influenced by marketing and changing values which lead to fads and fashions
- **Economic** — changing relative cost and availability of equipment and materials. For example, woodwork has become a relatively expensive medium while the cost of using computers has greatly reduced. A far wider variety of programs is available and, universally, therapists' skills are increasing
- **Political** — shifts in practice brought about by legislation
- **Technological** — the introduction of new materials has changed orthotic techniques, while the development of computer printing has reduced the appeal of handpress printing
- **Theoretical** — some techniques have evolved as direct result of an increase in theoretical knowledge. Therapists must evaluate the status of the technique against the need for increased functional activity
- **Historical** — activity continues if materials, facilities, personnel, etc. remain available. However, it must be regularly evaluated therapeutically — activity may disappear because of a perceived change in status
- **Research** — increased knowledge in fields of neurology, grief reaction and ergonomics, for example, have increased attention on these areas

longer possible or appropriate. For those who have undergone a full programme of rehabilitation, or whose capacity continues to fail for whatever reason, other means of facilitating occupational performance must be used. In these circumstances the therapist uses her knowledge of adaptation in order that the method, environment, equipment for or role performance of the activity is adjusted instead of the person's ability to perform it.

Five discrete ways in which occupational therapists use activity in order to enhance or facilitate occupational performance are described in Figure 6.1. The five methods relate directly to the statement within the philosophy that describes the facilitation of occupational performance.

Developing the adaptive skills required to restore, maintain or acquire function

1. Using activity as a direct intervention to reduce dysfunction

This is perhaps the most traditional way in which occupational therapists use activity. The process of identifying through assessment the dysfunction and needs of the individual, and then selecting via analysis an activity medium which directly addresses this shortfall, is a method well studied and practised by therapists. When used well such a process has infinite scope, limited only by the resources and skills of the therapist. The process and completion of the activity brings its own rewards.

This relies, however, on the therapist ensuring that the individual has sufficient input into the whole activity, and that the outcome is relevant and acceptable to him, otherwise the activity will not be sufficiently therapeutically valuable. A person who, for example, only chops apples for chutney which will then be made by another group the following day is unlikely to feel sufficiently motivated to work conscientiously. Similarly if the production of a slab pot or jam tarts to increase upper limb function is replaced by the rolling of therapeutic putty, the full potential of the activity is not being utilised. Further difficulty may arise when a frequently encountered diagnosis leads to a prescriptive, pre-arranged series of activities which does not allow flexibility to meet individual need. Such a situation can be seen on occasions when the treatment of some people with hand injuries or post hip replacement follows a fixed regime based on the diagnosis, rather than being a response to the person's need.

2. Improving functional activity following a shortfall in the existing level of competence

This way of using activity relates directly to the person's need to perform specific tasks. It relates the shortfall in his performance level to his need to fulfil certain role duties. It is used in cases in which a non-specific pathological deficit

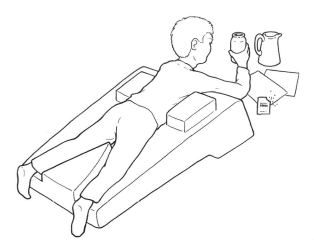

Fig. 6.3 Applying a therapeutic technique (prone lying on a wedge to enhance head and upper limb control) through the medium of an activity.

making leaf or seed pictures on a surface in front of the plinth, may be appropriate (Fig. 6.3).

Modifying activity in order to facilitate occupational performance

4. Adapting normal activity to enhance functional ability

For a person who enjoys gardening as a hobby a permanent loss of function may at first appear to put the hobby out of reach. Throughout life individuals develop and employ adaptive skills to meet the demands of a particular situation. Thus if a person has reached his maximum potential in terms of physical skills, the therapist can help to increase functional ability by adapting the way activity is carried out. This may involve teaching him how to use adapted tools and equipment which are manufactured for particular areas of difficulty. It is not just equipment, however, that may require adaptation. With careful planning and imagination the environment and the method can also be reorganised to enable the person to continue to enjoy gardening.

Tools and equipment. For people whose upper limb function is poor, lightweight tools are available. The lightest tools will have plastic, aluminium or carbon fibre handles. Long-handled tools extend reach for people who have difficulty

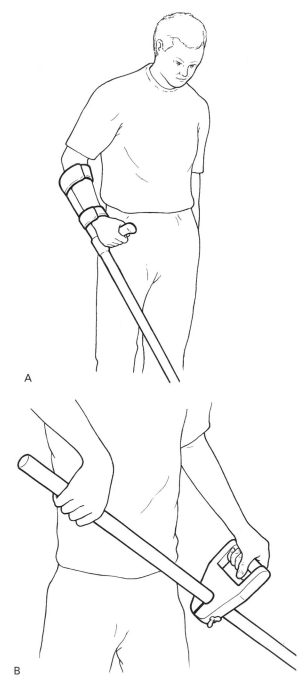

Fig. 6.4 (A) and (B) Adapting equipment to enhance functional activity.

bending and additional adaptations may be made to these for those with weak grip. (Fig. 6.4). For indoor gardeners the same principles can be applied to modify tools. Handles can be enlarged to assist weak grip, and loops may be attached to handles so that minimal grip is required.

The environment. One of the more well-known methods of adapting the environment for a disabled gardener is to build a raised garden or use a raised tub for planting flowers or vegetables. This is ideal for a person who spends the majority of his time in a wheelchair, such as a person with paraplegia, but is not always possible owing to limitations of space and finance. Planting and weeding of ground-level beds is easier from a wheelchair where the beds are small, to enable the person to reach the centre. If beds are to be reduced in width it may be appropriate, at the same time, to incorporate a slab or concrete border to facilitate access in a wheelchair. Wider pathways will also aid wheelchair access.

A sloping garden can create great difficulties for the disabled gardener. For the real enthusiast levelling, terracing or re-landscaping may be the long-term answer.

Where bending, stretching and stooping are a problem, planning a garden which requires little maintenance at ground level, or above shoulder height, can be considered. Eliminating heavy weeding by using gravel, paving, woodchips or ground-cover plants will help those who cannot stoop or kneel. Growing plants that require maintenance without bending or stretching, such as flowering shrubs, standard roses or dwarf fruit trees, enables the gardener to maintain his hobby without physical strain. ·

For the person who does most of his gardening indoors and whose mobility is limited, the installation of a gardening table will prove invaluable for potting up, sowing seeds or pricking out (Fig. 6.5). Space on the side to store tools while not in use leaves more room on the work top.

5. Adapting the content of occupational performance following or during the demise of existing skills

There are circumstances in which it is not possible, owing to safety problems or the continuing diminution of functional ability, to adapt either the tools or the gardening environment to suit

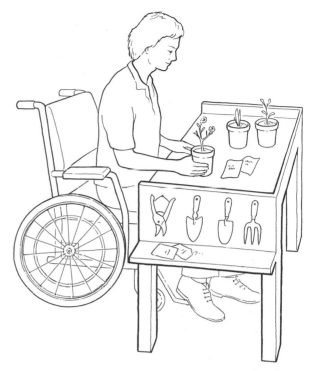

Fig. 6.5 Adapting the environment to enhance functional ability by providing a gardening table.

the gardener's remaining abilities. However, it is important that the individual retains at least part of his gardening role for as long as possible if this is important to him. The occupational therapist can help to adapt the content of the activity, and thus maintain associated roles, despite the inability to perform the gardening functions or tasks related to it. A person who can no longer tend a garden due to the severity of his dysfunction may turn his attention to indoor gardening. Growing pot herbs for cooking, tending house plants or window boxes, creating a terrarium or a mini-desert of cacti and succulents, or developing skills in fresh or dried flower arranging may capture his imagination. Skills may be used to create an environment in which to keep tropical fish, lizards or tree frogs.

Interest and responsibility in gardening can be retained through planning what should be grown and where. In a vegetable plot the organisation of crop rotation, what should be grown and when it should be planted and harvested, enables the person to maintain an important role. The gardener's experience and knowledge can still be used and respected, even if the physical process of ground preparation, planting, tending and harvesting is devolved to someone else.

A gardener can also maintain responsibility through visits to garden centres or exhibitions to choose varieties of seed and colours of annuals, and to select the most suitable and healthy specimens from those available. Advice or knowledge may be given to others — talks may be offered to local groups. Where dysfunction or energy preclude even these activities interest and knowledge can still be maintained by listening to media broadcasts, reading catalogues and magazines or watching the changing seasons. Outings to parks, formal gardens and country areas with suitable access for those with limited mobility will help the person to maintain contact with nature and provide a valuable source of interest and conversation.

Where the severity of dysfunction has caused a person to lose his role as provider or breadwinner he may find that gardening, particularly growing produce, will not only reduce costs but will help him to maintain an image of himself as a contributor to the household.

CONCLUSION

There is clearly enormous scope for the use of gardening as a treatment medium. It can help a person to regain specific areas of lost function, can provide purposeful use of leisure time, increase stamina to enable daily tasks to be accomplished, and help to maintain a person's sense of self in the presence of severe dysfunction. In order to achieve this the therapist must have a good knowledge of the activity, an ability to think both concretely and creatively, and the skill to analyse an activity and solve its related problems.

THE USE OF COMPUTERS AS A THERAPEUTIC MEDIUM

INTRODUCTION

Today the microcomputer is used in the home,

workplace and school. It is not surprising therefore that it is increasingly part of the occupational therapist's tool-kit. A decade has passed since the Department of Trade and Industry's (DTI) Project supplied over 40 microcomputers to various occupational therapy departments in the United Kingdom. This jump-started their use within the profession. But just how well has the microcomputer been incorporated into the profession's repertoire?

Talk of CD-ROMs, modem links, CAD, ergonomic analysis and computer access assessment may so overwhelm the occupational therapist as to make it difficult for her to keep therapeutic objectives in view (Okoye 1993). However, occupational therapists have a long tradition of incorporating technology into practice to improve or maintain the functional performance of the people they treat (American Occupational Therapy Association 1992). Such technology ranges from simple mechanical aids like tap turners to everyday equipment such as microwave ovens in assessment kitchens. When dealing with more 'high-tech' solutions, such as the microcomputer, it is necessary to apply the same principles, using a functional perspective focusing on the individual person's needs for such technology. On occasion high and low technology may be combined, by for example using a mouthstick or keyguard with the computer.

However, the computer is not just a tool for direct therapeutic intervention, but also a tool for accessing information. We live in an information age, and the ability to access and use technology has become a survival skill in our society. This provides another reason for incorporating the computer into our professional practice and perceiving it as part of meaningful activity and human occupation (Hammel & Smith 1993).

This section examines present-day computer use, both in terms of restoring, maintaining or acquiring function, and modifying it to facilitate occupational function.

Associated issues of training and research will also be considered, and since the computer is used for administration and documentation, this will also be briefly touched on.

COMPUTERS, COMPETENCE AND CLINICAL APPLICATIONS

Toffler (1971) maintains that the three critical skills for a super-industrial society are learning, relating and choosing. Applying these skills to computer use in occupational therapy raises some interesting points.

Competence

What do occupational therapists need to learn or be able to do to use computers safely and appropriately? Training is obviously of paramount importance, not only at pre-registration but also in post-graduate continuing education programmes. Such training should be part of a module or package which addresses technologies per se.

Hammel & Smith (1993) detail the technology competencies for American occupational therapists at a foundation and specialist I level. Competencies for a specialist II level are in hand. These levels are based on a taxonomy of awareness, knowledge, utilisation (emphasising skill development) and proficiency (skill application). These levels equate to basic grade or staff unfamiliar with computers/technology, Senior II and Senior I.

Lecturers and trainers need to enable their students and staff to take on responsibility for their own learning and to adopt a strategy of learning, unlearning and relearning. In terms of computers and technology this means that the therapist should:

- keep up to date
- decide what should be kept or discarded
- look at problems from a new perspective.

Keeping up to date can be achieved by accessing information via membership of groups (such as the National Occupational Therapy Special Interest Group in Microcomputers and the Disability Section of the British Computer Society), databases, periodicals, exhibitions, visits and liaison with other colleagues.

Adopting a person focused approach will enable the therapist to decide whether old or new technology is most appropriate. Merely supplying new technology because it is more advanced may not answer the person's particular needs (Easton & Millar, undated).

Problem-solving skills, professional judgement and an openness to new ideas and different ways of working are needed to explore alternative or improved methods of computer application to attain a person–technology fit.

The learning needs of the disabled person must also be taken into account. These needs are twofold: first, to learn how to operate the system, and second, how to make the most effective use of it. Discontinuing treatment once the system is installed may negate the latter objective (Vanderheiden 1987).

Relationships and teamwork

Matching technology to individuals' needs requires teamwork. Such a team involves the 'inventors' — the engineers, computer scientists and programmers — the 'appliers' — the clinical team (occupational therapists, speech therapists, physiotherapists, psychologists) — and the 'users' — the individual and his carers.

Computer technology has also been harnessed to improve communications via networking and 'electronic mail' (Email) systems. Bulletin board systems and computer conferencing systems are examples of this type of networking. Global academic electronic networks include INTERNET and JANET (Joint Academic Network) (Colbourn 1991). These networks allow people to share information and ideas via computers.

In terms of enabling people to relate to each other, one of the most worthwhile developments has been the use of computer technology to assist those with severe speech impairments. Here technology is being used to extend the range and capabilities of alternative and augmentative communication technology, including the mode of operation (input), method of representing the message (symbol set) and method of conveying the message (output) (Easton & Millar, undated). With spoken output, the non-speaking person gains a voice. As research into computer technology continues, research into virtual reality is

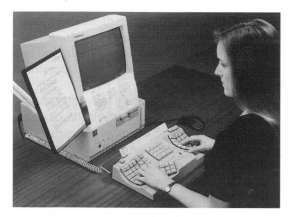

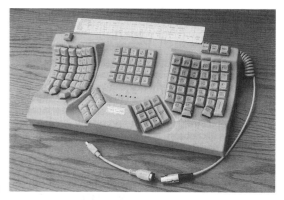

A   B

Fig. 6.9 The Maltron keyboard. (A) In use with a mouse. (B) Detail of the keyboard. (Reproduced by kind permission of PCD Maltron Ltd.)

to motor, sensory and cognitive dysfunction, and the part they have to play in life skills (self-care, work/education, leisure).

Developing the adaptive skills required to restore, maintain or acquire function

1. Using activity as a direct intervention to reduce dysfunction

Motor. *Improving function in upper limb.* While the standard keyboard can be used to improve function of the hand, the MULE Exerciser (Microprocessor Controlled Upper Limb Exerciser) (Fig. 6.10) has been specially designed to assess and improve range of movement, increase strength or maintain function in the wrist and hand (extension and flexion in the metacarpophalangeal, proximal interphalangeal and distal interphalangeal joints of the hand). With the spade handle and the elbow stabilised, pronation and supination can also be improved. The Exerciser comes with its own set of games programs and assessment options.

Biofeedback and the computer. In the treatment of people with a physical disability, biofeedback is a valuable adjunct to rehabilitation. It is often difficult for a person to evaluate his own performance without an objective monitor; for example the therapist may tell him to 'try harder' but he may not know how much better he is

performing without constant feedback (Crofts 1995).

Box 6.5 gives examples of biofeedback devices, while Box 6.6 gives a case study.

Sensory. While the computer can be used with a concept keyboard or touch screen to desensitise finger or thumb stumps, or a 'feely board' (textured overlay on a concept keyboard) to resensitise them, its main use in this area is in vision training (Okoye 1993). Okoye maintains that training of smooth scanning patterns, simultaneous visual attention to multiple stimuli, and integration of peripheral with central vision is more effectively achieved with computer applications.

These functions, together with postural head control and visual–motor skills, are critical for success in daily living skills. Occupational therapists should play a key role in such training and take a proactive approach in developing software in this area (Seale 1995).

Cognitive rehabilitation. While remediation of physical dysfunction is reliant on special inputs and supporting software, in cognitive rehabilitation it is the software which is of critical importance, input usually being adequately gained via a joystick or mouse. Box 6.7 outlines the areas in which computer programs are being used to assess, remediate and maintain cognitive function. Identification of cognitive deficits and involved systems will enable retraining to target the more basic functions first. Difficulty with sustaining visual attention for all tasks may be

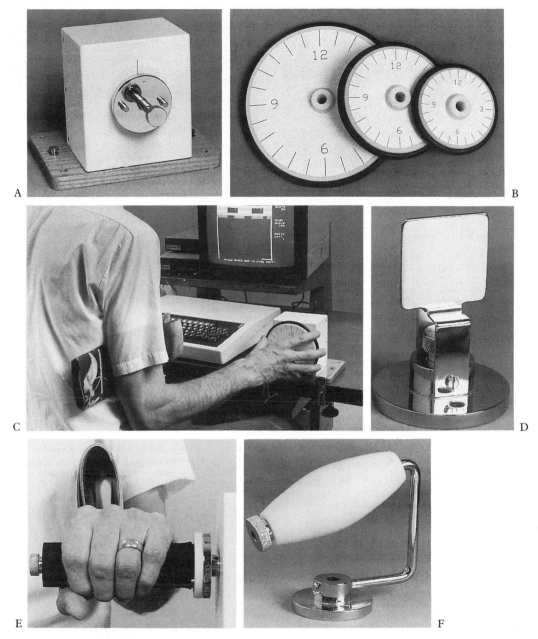

Fig. 6.10 The MULE Exerciser and attachments. (A) Device without handle. (B) 3″, 4″ and 6″ span handles. (C) Mule Exerciser with 5″ span handle. Markings on span handle guide hand positioning. Compensatory movements are avoided by holding magazine close to the ribs. (D) Key handle. (E) Cylinder handle (padded). Unpadded handles can also be used. (F) Spade handle. (Reproduced by kind permission of Southern General Hospital, Glasgow.)

initially addressed, for example, by just looking for a few seconds at a single picture being built up on the screen (Fairbairn 1990).

The complexity of visual or spatial information to be processed can be gradually upgraded. As far as possible the computer task should parallel the real-life situation (Skilbeck 1991).

Computerised games may be used to assess

Box 6.5 Examples of computerised biofeedback devices

1. The *Myolink* (Fig. 6.11, Box 6.6) uses electromyography to provide feedback about muscle tension to the client

2. *Pressure Pads* (see Fig. 6.6B) for weight-bearing exercises by walking on the spot and increasing speed of movement. The client steps on the pressure pads to activate or respond to actions on the screen

3. *Goniometer*: the client can see the increase/decrease of the angle of the joint concerned. With the MICE (Movement Incentive Coordination Exercise) system multi-axis sensors are attached to the user's joints. In this way the range of movement at the hip, knee, ankle, elbow and wrist can be assessed and exercised (Crofts 1995)

4. *The Compex Board* is designed to allow children to gain practice at balance and weight shifting. Software which accompanies the board provides biofeedback to inform the user of his centre of pressure during standing, sitting, kneeling or arm support (Seale 1995)

The above devices can be obtained through Nottingham Rehab but there are many 'one-off' accessories which have been developed for particular purposes (Crofts 1995).

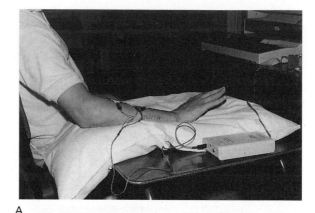

A

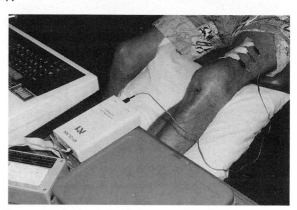

B

Fig. 6.11 Myolink. (A) Working for wrist extension following surgery. (B) Maintenance of the quadriceps muscle group while non-weight-bearing. (Reproduced by kind permission of Felicity Crofts, Cedars Rehabilitation Unit, Nottingham.)

or improve cognitive skills. Birnboim (1995) describes 'Bagles' — a computer version of a well-known game of guessing a number — to improve reasoning skills, which are then applied to simulated and real-life events.

While research still needs to be done to evaluate the effectiveness of computer use in cognitive rehabilitation, evidence is accruing of its usefulness in improving attention and information processing abilities and transfer of these skills. Memory dysfunction is also considerably improved (Skilbeck 1991). Box 6.8 gives three case studies to demonstrate computer use in this area.

2. Improving functional activity following a shortfall in the existing level of competence

Pre-work skills. The therapist can assess and develop skills in computer use, customising the system to the person's needs. She should assess

accuracy as well as speed before progressing to work skills. Box 6.9 gives two case studies illustrating computer use in this area.

Computerised work simulators are also available which can measure and record progress (strength and endurance) using static/isometric and dynamic/isotonic tests (Fig. 6.12).

For people who will return to their previous jobs graded sessions on the computer can be instigated. For example, a secretary who suffered a Colles fracture was able to use the computer to regain typing speed and accuracy following removal of her plaster.

Social skills. The computer can be used to practise social skills affected by disability. Playing chess and other board games with another

---

Box 6.6 Case study: biofeedback using Myolink

A man aged 50, working in a supervisory position for a large organisation, had a cerebral tumour excised. He was subsequently referred for rehabilitation for residual left hemiplegia. On initial interview his left arm was flaccid, with a mere flicker of voluntary contraction in the finger muscles with the limb supported. He was able to walk with a stick and compensated for his left foot drop by abducting the hip. Speech was slightly affected owing to paralysis of his left facial musculature. The man was very depressed by his physical limitations, particularly with regard to his left arm which he described as 'dead'.

To show this man that there was some potential for return of function in the left upper limb, the Myolink was used. With the surface electrodes over the wrist extensors and the threshold set for minimum performance, he was instructed to waggle his fingers. The contraction of the extensors produced an upward movement of the cursor on the monitor, which enabled him to play simple games. The therapist was able to point out that the arm could not be 'dead' as voluntary contraction could be demonstrated. This motivated him and regular sessions were undertaken.

Although he was only able to regain minimal function in his left upper limb, it was sufficient to enable him to put his hand in his pocket. This gave him control of the limb and was more comfortable when walking than having the weight of the arm pulling on his shoulder. It also helped him psychologically, showing that his own effort, although weak, could be developed.

In view of the severe weakness of his left arm, it would have been difficult without the Myolink to find any other activity which this client could have done to encourage voluntary movement.

Box 6.7 Cognitive rehabilitation (Skilbeck 1991)

- Attention/concentration: immediate, sustained and speed of cognition
- Perceptual–spatial abilities: colour, shape, size and form differentiation and recognition, figure ground discrimination, directional and spatial skills
- Sensori–integrative (perceptual–motor) abilities: hand–eye coordination
- Numeracy and literacy and other educational subjects
- Problem-solving: information processing, decision-making, forward planning
- Memory: immediate/delayed recall, mnemonic strategies
- Psycholinguistic abilities, e.g. training tasks for reading deficits for clients with aphasia (Katz & Nagly 1984)

---

person, or doing quizzes or problem-solving games in a small group can all assist.

Activities of daily living. Programs which deal with money management, home finance, shopping and budgeting can be used to reinforce skills in self-care.

3. Applying therapeutic techniques through the medium of activity

Placing equipment and positioning the user are ways in which, for example, developmental techniques can be incorporated into computer use, the computer being used to motivate and encourage the person to persist with the activity. Using the Bobath neurodevelopmental approach sitting and standing balance can be practised by reaching forward with the hands clasped together to reach and touch the screen or concept keyboard. The user is positioned further and further away from the input device so that his bottom gradually comes off the stool. Weight-bearing through the affected arm or elbow in order to improve muscle tone can be obtained by operating the concept keyboard positioned for maximum reach.

Modifying activity in order to facilitate occupational performance

4. Adapting normal activity to enhance functional ability

Matching input and output devices to a person's needs enables access to the computer for work, leisure and education. Whether people suffer from orthopaedic conditions, neurological problems or sensory impairments, there are many devices available which can compensate for their limitations. Indeed with nearly 500 access devices available it can be a daunting task selecting the most appropriate. Anson (1992) has devised a RoadMap to Computer Access Technology to enable therapists to match the person's requirements following the occupational therapy assessment. By following the directions on the RoadMap and answering a series of yes/no questions the therapist is led to a small group of devices which should answer the person's access needs.

Box 6.8 Case studies: cognitive rehabilitation

Case study 1: Use of computers to assist in electric wheelchair assessment

A man aged 30, suffering from cerebral palsy with epilepsy, was referred to occupational therapy. He had considerable brain damage and personality difficulties, spastic rigidity in his left arm but some useful movement in his right arm and right thumb. He had been provided with a wheelchair, to which he was transferred once a week, although he needed constant attention because he was found to be a danger to both himself and others.

He used the computer twice a week with a four-way joystick and software that involved directional use of the joystick. This was used to:

- assess his directional/spatial awareness
- find out his physical ability to use a joystick (similar to his wheelchair control)
- to assess, in conjunction with his weekly episodes in his wheelchair, the best functional position of the joystick, and to adapt his wheelchair accordingly.

Using the computer program and joystick he was able to have more practice at directional activities. He was also given more opportunity to see whether or not it was possible for him to improve. It was also easier to assess whether his problems of bumping into people were due to personality or perceptual difficulties.

Case study 2: Assessing perceptual and cognitive function in people with dysphasia, and grading programmes according to their ability

A man aged 35 suffered a left cerebrovascular accident (CVA) that left him with a right hemiplegia and dysphasia. Initial assessment showed that he had no useful speech except repetitive sounds. He lacked confidence but was highly motivated to improve.

After an initial assessment it was found that he had an understanding of some written words. His expressive abilities (i.e. speech and his ability to press the correct key on the keyboard) were poor. The following programs were used in conjunction with some simple maths programs.

1. The first program he used required him to read a short sentence and type in one of two words to complete the sentence, e.g. 'The man . . . on his coat' (choosing either 'put' or 'push')
This program required minimal keyboard skills, but he was able to gain confidence by reading the sentence and knowing that he had understood the meaning. He did not have to remember how to spell the word as the correct word was on the screen and he only had to copy it.

2. When he found that the first program was becoming easier he was upgraded to a program that involved sentence ordering. Four sentences were on the screen and they had to be put in the correct sequence, e.g.:
She poured the boiling water over the tea in the pot
She boiled the kettle of water
She put the tea in the pot
She filled the kettle with water
This program required more complex cognitive skills such as reading and sequencing but only required limited use of the keyboard (space bar and return key).

3. Memory game — this is a graded program. A choice can be made of between two and six words. The words are displayed on the screen, with a number alongside, for as long as the person requires. The words disappear and a number is displayed. The word relating to the number must be typed.
The words are short. The program involves short-term memory to remember and spell the words. The program can be gradually upgraded by increasing the number of words selected. He found this program difficult but slowly progressed to six words.

4. Word ordering — this was an upgrade of the first and second programs. A short sentence appeared on the screen with the words in the wrong order. Each individual letter had to be typed, e.g. 'He in the drive a for car went'.
This involved far more keyboard skills as he had to type in each individual letter. However, the words were still on the screen for him to copy.

5. Word processing — writing his own sentences.
This required him to remember the word, to spell it correctly and to order the sentence. He is now spending most of his computer time improving these skills. His increase in confidence and self-esteem cannot be measured but are obvious from his expression and enthusiasm.

While doing the programs and in conjunction with speech therapy he was encouraged to speak the letters and later words that were on the screen.

Three years after the CVA he is continuing to recover speech and is now writing and speaking sentences. He has been motivated to buy his own computer so that he can work on his own at home.

N.B. With clients after a CVA or similar disability it has been found that, by carrying out a program on their own with the computer, their confidence and ability (both written and spoken) have increased long after the initial rehabilitation has ceased.

Box 6.8 (Cont'd)

Case study 3: Assessing and improving intellectual and educational ability in a partially sighted person classified for educational purposes as learning disabled

A man aged 25 with a left hemiparesis, registered blind and having spent his education in schools for children with learning disabilities, was referred to occupational therapy. In the initial assessment he recognised a few letters but was not able to read Braille or text, and he only knew the names of a few letters.

Assessment was carried out using an enlarged text program on an IBM-compatible computer. He was encouraged to learn the keyboard and also the names of the letters by using the enlarged text program along with a screen reader. He later transferred to a talking wordprocessor that could also enlarge the text. It appeared he was keen on computers, and showed that he was both motivated and able to learn.

In conjunction with the remedial teacher a program was set up to help him learn to read both text and Braille. This is a slow process, but with special software the computer is used to practise the words and letters that he is learning with the teacher.

Another person has written a small program in BASIC which, together with a 'speech' program, speaks the words to be typed, speaks the letters that are typed, and then says whether the words have been typed in correctly.

After a year of attending twice a week he is now managing to read and type short sentences, and is tackling maths- and puzzle-based speech output programs to help him educationally. There is also a program that assists with mobility in making him aware of relationships between streets in a town.

N.B. This client has increased in confidence, motivation, independence and the ability to learn since he started learning to read.

Box 6.9 Case studies: prevocational assessment

Case study 1

A 40-year-old man was referred following a cervical disc lesion resulting in a right brachial neuralgia. He had not worked for two years and had a period of hospitalisation for alcohol-related problems. His previous occupation had been clerical, organising specialist holidays.

He used the computer to learn to type, and also to learn the basics of wordprocessing, spreadsheets and databases. He was well motivated towards this kind of work and went on to be accepted on a part-time course for Business Administration (NVQ level 5) at his local college of further education.

Case study 2

A 30-year-old landscape gardener had a sudden onset of rheumatoid arthritis. He responded well to medication, and eight months after the diagnosis was referred to an assessment unit. He was advised not to return to heavy work but was keen to keep an interest in horticulture and perhaps teach adults. He held a National Diploma in Nursery Practices and was studying for an A level in environmental science at evening classes. His biggest problem was adjusting to the limitations imposed by his illness.

Following discussion it was felt appropriate for him to work on the computers in order to learn to type and to learn basic programming skills. He discovered a leaning towards computers, and with the help of the Disability Employment Advisor (DEA) secured a training place with work experience in Information Technology (NVQ level 3).

In any assessment for such devices, be they low or high technology, account must be taken of not only the person's capabilities but also his preferences. The four students (two with spinal cord injury and two with muscular dystrophy) in Lau & O'Leary's (1993) study, for example, produced the highest input with the mouthstick, but rated it the least attractive when compared with the TongueTouch Keypad and HeadMaster (similar to Headstart shown in Figure 6.6). The mouthstick was not only the least expensive device, but also, with its own 'docking station' clamped to the work surface, did not require any assistance to fit it, unlike the other two devices. All the subjects in this study preferred the TongueTouch Keypad, although this gave the slowest input and was the most difficult to learn to use.

However, there is a still further input to consider. With voice recognition systems non-speaking, severely physically disabled people, such as those with spinal cord injury, are able to enter data and process information fast enough to compete with and even rival those without disabilities. Assistants may still, however, be required for support tasks and self-care activities.

With the advent of robotics, however, it is possible to design voice-controlled robotic work-

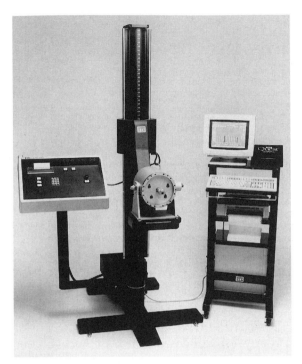

Fig. 6.12 Computerised work simulator. The BTE Work Simulator consists of two components mounted on a pedestal base and Quest, the system's software. The exercise head (centre) can be raised or lowered and/or angled from vertical to horizontal. It has over 20 attachments which can be used to simulate many different work tasks, e.g. crank handles, screwdrivers, pliers, various knobs, D-handle, steering wheel, lifting tool, etc. As well as providing immediate feedback to user and therapist and a standardised assessment, the software also includes tests, daily treatment and progress charts, which can all be printed out to provide a permanent record. (Reproduced by kind permission of Baltimore Therapeutic Equipment Co., Hanover, Maryland, USA.)

stations to reduce such dependence with a robotic arm, replacing or supplementing a person's manipulation skills. The desktop vocational assistant robot described by Taylor et al (1993) gives vocational support and assistance with activities of daily living and environmental control. The tasks the pilot robot was programmed to carry out included selecting, loading and returning floppy discs; selecting and dispensing medication (throat lozenges); retrieving and returning a phone receiver; and scratching an itch on the user's face.

Environmental control units (ECUs) first be-came available with the POSSUM, developed in the 1950s. They can be operated by a number of devices, such as a special input like the Headstart, an electronic communication aid or, as mentioned before, voice recognition. These devices can be used to switch on and off various household appliances such as a lamp, TV, radio or fan; make and receive telephone calls; release door locks; and open and shut curtains (Dickey & Shealey 1987). Sophisticated systems can operate over 200 infrared functions, including running a com-puter and controlling all the features on a remote control television (Curtin 1994).

Spoken output, enlarged text on the screen or printouts, and Braille embossers are particularly useful for people with poor vision.

Where input and output devices enable the disabled employee to hold down a job they may be obtained via the Employment Service's 'Access to Work' scheme.

Computerised 'filofaxes', like the Psion Series 3 personal organiser, can be used to compensate for memory deficits (Giles & Shore 1989, Barrett & Herriotts 1994).

5. Adapting the content of occupational performance following or during the demise of existing skills

Severely disabled people may wish to learn com-puter skills for application in future work, to con-tinue their education, or to expand their leisure interests. The computer can be used to maintain valued activities and roles — for example a dis-abled housewife producing a shopping list for her carer to do the shopping; a non-speaking per-son writing poetry or books; or enjoying leisure pursuits such as chess, music and letter writing — when disability prevents a return to previous roles (Box 6.10).

Batt & Lounsbury (1990) devised a flowchart to teach a particular person with left hemiplegia to use the computer for leisure. He had impaired memory, concentration and constructional skills, but using the flowchart allowed him to bypass the menu (which he had difficulty in under-standing) and access the computer. The flowchart used coloured symbols and a limited number

Box 6.10 Case study: using the computer for leisure

A 48-year-old man had a left CVA resulting in a right hemiplegia, with a very slight speech problem, no active movement in the arm and a rather 'spastic' gait. Six months after the onset of his disability he was discharged from the hospital and referred for work assessment.

Prior to his CVA he had worked for a large electrical firm as a shop technician in their model shop. He now expressed a keen desire to use computers, in the hope that this might lead to a future career. It was found that when under any pressure muscle tone increased in his right arm and leg. He was recommended not to attempt to return to employment and was medically retired.

Fortunately he was able to afford his own computer at home, and he has built up his system to include colour printers and flat-bed scanners. He has gone from strength to strength, and computing is now a substantial hobby. To quote from a letter received from him shortly after his medical retirement:

'But the computer which is helping me with this letter gives me the most pleasure. I am now looking forward to my future not with any bitterness but with my new found interests; I now know that what I have done in the past is not possible and it is no good looking back. For my immediate plans I want to try to develop the ideas that I have inside my head onto paper. These are the ideas I have thought about when I have been trying to cope with my disability. This is where my new found interest in my computer will help. I find the standard drawing package very limiting, so I hope to get a computer-aided design package which will allow me to put my ideas into drawings.'

of words, and compensated for his impaired memory as he did not have to remember the previous instruction or the instruction to come. Eight months later he was using the computer for letter writing to friends, politicians and government officials.

In education the National Federation of AC-CESS Centres seeks to support and empower students with physical disabilities. The Computer Centre for People with Disabilities (CCPD), University of Westminster, London, is part of this national network.

For those with speech impairment the computer can be used as a tool for communication, various augmentative communication systems now being available (Detheridge 1993).

Psychological considerations

The therapist should introduce the user sensitively to the computer and allay his fears.

The computer gives strong motivational rewards. Feedback is consistent and non-judgemental. User-friendly software is important not only in this respect, but also in reducing frustration and anxiety. The therapist should look for programs which allow more than one attempt to get the right answer, have different levels of difficulty, give appropriate rewards, etc.

Computer technology enables disabled people to achieve tasks for themselves, thus increasing their self-esteem and sense of achievement. Self-expression and creativity are increased with the use of the wordprocessor, desktop publishing, graphics and music packages.

RECORDS, REPORTS AND STATISTICS

Computerised records, reports and statistics enable staff not only to meet demands for increased accountability and accurate data, but also to do so efficiently within a standard framework. Computer systems may be used for:

- *administration* — patient records/activity, staff workload, service level agreements
- *clinical support* — referral, assessment and treatment records and reports, plans for home adaptations (using computer-aided design packages)
- *education* — student progress records, timetabling, student training programmes, post-registration programmes
- *research* — projects including statistics

(Maslin 1991, Korah 1994, Joyce 1995)

Wordprocessing, spreadsheet and database software can now be purchased in a single package. Joyce (1995) describes such a package and its implementation.

Virtual reality — whereby a person interacts with a three-dimensional imitation of the world — may soon find its way into occupational therapy clinics. Already architects are using it to explore design problems before building commences. In America a wheelchair simulator is available which enables different environments and buildings to be tested for accessibility by disabled people (Fyson 1995).

FUTURE POSSIBILITIES

This section has examined computer technology and applications based on Toffler's three critical skills of learning, relating and choosing. However, there remains yet another consideration — his 'strategy of futureness', which is described as an ability to look ahead, to anticipate the future. Toffler sees this future-orientation as the basis for successful adaptation. We need not only enable the people we treat to take a look at the future, but also to do so ourselves.

If the profession is not to be overtaken by events it needs to increase research now into when and how technological advances should be applied to occupational therapy practice, and to keep up this commitment. Bearing in mind our philosophical base in meaningful activity and our skills in activity analysis will answer the 'when' and the 'how'. We need to ask ourselves just what part CD-ROMs, multimedia, interactive videos and virtual reality should play in the professional curriculum and in assessment and treatment. We should be prepared to debate the challenges and ethical dilemmas that may be posed. Will technology alienate and depersonalise people, for example in the development of robotics? Can 'virtual reality' be considered a meaningful activity?

As Seale (1995) points out, we need to be proactive and seek funding to undertake the research that will take the profession into the 21st century and beyond. It is beginning to happen. Korah (1995) describes a study using virtual reality in the treatment of unilateral neglect. However, research is a responsibility that lies with every member of the profession and should be part of every therapist's practice.

ACKNOWLEDGEMENTS

The authors gratefully acknowledge the help of students and colleagues who have assisted in the preparation of this chapter. These include a group of willing volunteers of second-year occupational therapy students at St Andrew's School of Occupational Therapy, Nene College, Northampton, for their most constructive criticism of the first section of the chapter; Anne Goodrick-Meech, Head of Department of Occupational Therapy, Christ Church College, Canterbury, for her contribution to the gardening section; Felicity Crofts, Cedars Rehabilitation Unit, Nottingham, for supplying information, photographs and case studies for the computer section, and for the software evaluation in Figure 6.7; and Val Wall, Flightways Resource Centre, Barnet Community Services, and Roberta Perrin, St Leonards Hospital, Ringwood, also for supplying case studies for the computer section.

USEFUL ADDRESSES

ACE (Aids to Communication in Education) Centre
Ormerod School
Waynflete Road
Headington
Oxford OX3 8DD

Apple Special Needs Alliance (ASNA)
Dane Centre
Melbourne Road
Ilford
Essex IG1 4HT

Baltimore Therapeutic Equipment Co.
7455-L New Ridge Road
Hanover, Maryland 21076–3105
USA

Bristol SEMERC (Special Education MicroElectronics Resource Centre)
Bristol Polytechnic
Faculty of Education
Redland Hill
Bristol BS6 6U2

British Computer Society — Disabled Specialist Group
Tom Mangan, c/o The Computability Centre
PO Box 94
Warwick
Warwickshire CV34 5WS

Compaid Trust
Pembury Hospital
Tunbridge Wells
Kent TN2 4OJ

Computability Centre
PO Box 94
Warwick
Warwickshire CV34 5WS

Computer Centre for People with Disabilities (CCPD)
University of Westminster
72 Great Portland Street
London W1N 5AL

Disabled Living Foundation
380–384 Harrow Road
London W9 2HU

National ACCESS Centre
Hereward College of FE
Bramston Crescent
Tile Hill Lane
Coventry
West Midlands CV4 9SW

National Occupational Therapy Special Interest Group in
Microcomputers
c/o Mrs C. V. MacCaul
Swale Day Hospital
Keycol Hospital
Sittingbourne
Kent ME9 8NG

NCET (National Council for Educational Technology)
Science Park
University of Warwick
Coventry CV4 7EZ

Northwest SEMERC
Fitton Hill Curriculum Centre
Rosary Road
Oldham OL8 2QE

Nottingham Rehab
Ludlow Hill Road
West Bridgford
Nottingham NG2 6HD

P.C.D. Maltron Ltd
15 Orchard Lane
East Molesey
Surrey KT8 0BN

RCEVH (Research Centre for the Education of the Visually
Handicapped)
Birmingham University
Selly Wick House
59 Selly Wick Lane
Birmingham B29 7JE

SNRU (Special Needs Research Unit)
The Polytechnic
1 Coach Lane
Coach Lane Campus
Newcastle NE7 7TW

REFERENCES

ACE Centre 19 Switches and interfaces, 2nd edn. ACE Centre, Oxford

American Occupational Therapy Association 1992 Use of adjunctive modalities in occupational therapy. American Journal of Occupational Therapy (46)12: 1075–1081

Anson D 1992 Finding your way in the maze of computer access technology. American Journal of Occupational Therapy (48)2: 121–129

Anson D 1993 The effect of word prediction on typing speed. American Journal of Occupational Therapy (47)11: 1039–1042

Barrett J, Herriotts P 1994 Employment and the workplace. The Disability Information Trust, Oxford, pp 108–142

Batt R C, Lounsbury P A 1990 Teaching the patient with cognitive deficits to use a computer. American Journal of Occupational Therapy 44(4): 364–367

Birnboim S 1995 A metacognitive approach to cognitive rehabilitation. British Journal of Occupational Therapy 58(2): 61–64

Breines E B 1995 Occupational therapy activites from clay to computers. F A Davis, Philadelphia

Clark E N (ed.) 1986 Microcomputer: clinical applications. Slack, New Jersey, pp 7, 20

Colbourn C J 1991 Issues in the selection and support of a microcomputer system. In: Ager A (ed.) Microcomputers and clinical psychology. John Wiley, Chichester, pp 21–45

Colven D, Detheridge T 1990 A common terminology for switch-controlled software. ACE Centre, Oxford

Creighton C 1985 Three frames of reference in work-related occupational therapy programs. American Journal of Occupational Therapy 39(5): 331–334

Crofts F 1995 Personal communication

Cromwell F S 1986 Computer applications in occupational therapy. Haworth Press, New York

Curtin M 1994 Technology for people with tetraplegia. Part 2. Environmental control units. British Journal of Occupational Therapy 57(11): 419–424

Data Protection Act 1984 HMSO, London

Detheridge M 1993 The contribution of I.T. to working with symbols. In: Symbols in practice. Aspects of the use of symbols in learning. NCET, Coventry, pp 13–14

Dickey R, Shealey S H 1987 Using technology to control the environment. American Journal of Occupational Therapy (41)11: 717–721

Easton J, Millar S (undated) High technology communication aids. In: TAAC. Technology & Alternative and Augmentative Communication. ACE Centre, Oxford

Eliason M L, Gohl-Giese A 1979 A question of professional boundaries. American Journal of Occupational Therapy 33(3): 175–179

Everson J M, Goodwyn R 1987 A comparison of the use of adaptive microswitches by students with cerebral palsy. American Journal of Occupational Therapy (41)11: 739–744

Fairbairn J 1990 Computers in the treatment of brain injured patients at the Wolfson Medical Rehabilitation Centre. Headway, Spring, pp 10–11

Fyson N 1995 Almost real. Therapy Weekly (16 March): 7

Giles G M, Shore M 1989 The effectiveness of an electronic memory aid for a memory-impaired adult of normal intelligence. American Journal of Occupational Therapy 43(6): 409–411

Hammel J M, Smith R O 1993 The development of technology competencies and training guidelines for occupational therapists. American Journal of Occupational Therapy 47(11): 970–979

Health & Safety Executive 1994 Working with VDUs. HSE Books, Sudbury

Hobday S W 1994 Computer related upper limb disorder. A keyboard to eliminate the stress and the pain. Paper presented at the 19th Annual Congress of IMART, 4 May, London

Hope M H 1987 Micros for children with special needs. Souvenir Press, London

Joyce J 1995 Department statistics and activity monitoring the easy way (a departmental management system for occupational therapy staff by occupational therapy staff). OT Micronews (February): 32

Kaldor C, Kinsey C, Millar S, Head P, Poon P (undated) Evaluation and design of software. In: TAAC. Technology & Alternative and Augmentative Communication. ACE Centre, Oxford

Katz R, Nagly V T 1984 Cats: Computerised Aphasia Treatment System. In: Ager A (ed.) Microcomputers and clinical psychology. John Wiley, Chichester, p 101

Korah M 1994 A study to investigate the use of computers in occupational therapy for administration and management. OT Micronews (May): 13–21

Korah M 1995 First Experiments into the application of virtual reality as a tool in the treatment of unilateral neglect. OT Micronews (February): 17–26

Lau C, O'Leary S 1993 Comparison of computer interface

devices for persons with severe physical disabilities. American Journal of Occupational Therapy (47)11: 1022–1030

Maslin Z B 1991 Management in occupational therapy. Chapman & Hall, London

Millar S V, Nisbet P D 1993 Accelerated writing for people with disabilities. CALL Centre, Edinburgh

National Council for Educational Technology 1993 CD-ROM — a matter of access. NCET, Coventry

Newell A F 1985 Developing appropriate software. British Journal of Occupational Therapy (August): 242–243

Okoye R 1989 Computer technology in occupational therapy. In: Hopkins H L, Smith H D (eds) Willard and Spackman's occupational therapy, 7th edn. J B Lippincott, Philadelphia

Okoye R 1993 Computer applications in occupational therapy. In: Hopkins H L, Smith H D (eds) Willard and Spackman's occupational therapy, 8th edn. J B Lippincott, Philadelphia, pp 341–353

Reed K L 1986 Tools of practice: heritage or baggage. American Journal of Occupational Therapy 40(9): 597–605

Reed K L, Sanderson S R 1992 Concepts of occupational therapy, 3rd edn. Williams & Wilkins, Baltimore

Rogers J C 1982 The spirit of independence: the evolution of a philosophy. American Journal of Occupational Therapy 36(11): 157–160

Ross M 1987 Using microcomputers: a guide for occupational therapists. Paradigm Press, Perth

Seale J 1995 Information technology for adults with learning difficulties. OT Micronews (February): 14–16

Sietsema J M et al 1993 The use of a game to promote arm reach in persons with traumatic brain injury. American Journal of Occupational Therapy 47(1): 19–24

Skilbeck C 1991 Microcomputer-based cognitive rehabilitation. In: Ager A (ed.) Microcomputers and clinical psychology. John Wiley, Chichester, pp 96–118

Smith R O 1991 Technological approaches to performance enhancement. In: Christiansen C, Baum C (eds) Occupational therapy. Overcoming human performance deficits. Slack, New Jersey, pp 748–786

Taylor B, Cupo M E, Sheredos S J 1993 Workstation robotics: a pilot study of a desktop vocational assistant robot. American Journal of Occupational Therapy 47(11): 1009–1013

Toffler A 1971 Future shock. Pan, London, pp 374–386

Vanderheiden G C 1987 Service delivery mechanisms in rehabilitation technology. American Journal of Occupational Therapy 41(11): 703–710

Van Denson Fox J 1983 Selected measures of patients motivation and creativity and their relationship to occupational therapy outcome. Occupational Therapy Journal of Research 3(2): 121–122

Williams R, Westmorland M 1994 Occupational cumulative trauma disorders of the upper extremity. American Journal of Occupational Therapy 48(5): 411–419

FURTHER READING

General

Barris R et al 1988 Occupational therapy in psychosocial practice. Slack, New Jersey

Cynkin S, Robinson A M 1990 Occupational activities and activities health — toward health through activity. Little, Brown, Boston

Kielhofner G 1992 Conceptual foundations of occupational therapy. F A Davis, Philadelphia

Keilhofner G 1983 Health through occupation — theory and practice in occupational therapy. F A Davis, Philadelphia

King L J 1978 Towards a science of adaptive responses. American Journal of Occupational Therapy 32(7): 429–437

Sabonis-Chafee B 1989 Occupational therapy, introductory concepts. C V Mosby, St Louis

Taylor E, Manguno J 1991 Use of treatment activities in occupational therapy. American Journal of Occupational Therapy 45(4): 317–322

Wood W 1993 Occupation and the relevance of primatology to occupational therapy. American Journal of Occupational Therapy 47(6): 515–522

Gardening

Fleet K 1991 Gardening without sight. Royal National Institute for the Blind. Peterborough

Hagedorn R 1987 Therapeutic gardening. Winslow Press, Bicester, Oxon

Hollinrake D 1991 Gardening with arthritis. ARC Cards Ltd, Notts

Hollinrake D 1992 Gardening equipment for disabled people. Disability Information Trust, Oxford

Llewellyn R, Davies A 1993 Grow it yourself (gardening with a physical disability). Cedar Reed, London

Computers

ACE Centre 1993 Aids to communication. Where do I go?, 3rd edn. ACE Centre, Oxford

ACE Centre 1994 Basics to back technology. An introductory guide to non-electrical access equipment for computers and writing. ACE Centre, Oxford

Gray C 1988 The importance of correct seating. ACE Centre, Oxford

From other medical personnel

In the community the therapist frequently receives referrals from other members of the team. They may be from the person's general practitioner, the health visitor, community nurse, home help or social worker to name but a few, and the level of information received will therefore vary considerably according to that person's knowledge of and involvement with the individual and occupational therapist.

In hospital the therapist may similarly receive referrals from a variety of personnel. Other members of the paramedical team, e.g. the physiotherapist, speech therapist or social worker, may identify a need for occupational therapy. In some instances, especially in wards where the majority of residents would benefit from occupational therapy, a 'blanket referral' system may operate. In this instance the occupational therapist has permission to commence treatment with any of the residents when she feels it necessary without having to notify the doctor and gain his permission in each individual case.

The British Association of Occupational Therapists (1995) Code of Ethics and Professional Conduct states: 'Occupational therapists shall accept referrals which they deem to be appropriate and for which they have the resources. It is the duty of occupational therapists to obtain sufficient information to enable them to determine the appropriateness of the referral. Subject to any legal requirements to provide a minumum service, if the basic standards of treatment or intervention cannot be met at any time, for whatever reason, occupational therapists should decline to accept a referral or to initiate treatment.'

From the general public

In the community the occupational therapist may receive the referral from a member of the public. Requests may be made by the individual himself, or by the family, carers, neighbours or friends. In most instances the referral is with the approval and knowledge of the person concerned but this is not always the case.

From clinics

In hospital it is common for referrals to be received from outpatient clinics, particularly those concerned with rheumatology, neurology, physical medicine or orthopaedic disorders. These referrals may not necessarily be on the directions of the doctor or consultant. In some instances the occupational therapist may attend the clinic to receive direct information on the person referred. If this is not possible it is important to ensure that those in charge in the clinic have a clear understanding of the role of the therapist and the facilities available. Although proportionately fewer referrals in the community are received from clinics, some may be initiated from chiropody, speech therapy or possibly such sources as 'Age Well' clinics.

In both the hospital and community, referrals may be received from members of the primary health care team, usually via the general practitioner.

From case conferences

In many places case conferences have replaced the rigid formal ward rounds because they give the opportunity for fuller discussion in a less threatening environment for the person concerned. Medical and paramedical staff may attend the conference and it is not uncommon for the person concerned and his relatives or carers to be present and contribute equally. These conferences may take place in the hospital setting or in the community and are a common aspect of the social services procedure in many areas. For those with special needs, educational or employment case conferences form part of the programme planning process and the occupational therapist may contribute to such conferences or receive referrals from them.

From ward rounds

Ward rounds are most frequently conducted by the consultant, the team of doctors and the ward sister/charge nurse responsible for the ward. Other paramedical personnel involved with the ward residents may attend. During attendance at such rounds it is possible to gain information about people to be referred and to report on those whom the therapist has already seen. If the therapist is not present at the ward round, she may still receive referrals from this source, if those conducting the round are familiar with the occupational therapist's role.

The method of referral

Occupational therapists may receive either written or verbal referrals, but when there is no formal written referral it is important that formal documentation is completed for the records. This may not necessarily be completed by the person making the referral.

In many departments there are specifically designed occupational therapy referral forms. These vary considerably in design and the amount of information requested. Such forms may be available in the wards, clinics or departments in the hospital, or in the health clinics or general practice centres in the community.

When a written referral is received by other means, for example a letter from a doctor, or a relative, or an entry in a person's case notes, the occupational therapist will usually complete the referral form herself, attaching a letter of referral to it.

If a verbal referral is received, it is also usual to complete a written form, either at the time of the verbal referral, which may be by telephone, or at the initial interview. In some instances, particularly in social services, the referral may not initially be received by the occupational therapist, but may be passed to the intake/duty officer for the day, who may be a therapist or a social worker, for later redirection.

However, by whatever means the referral is received, certain information is essential. This information will include:

- The person's full name, both surname and forenames
- The full address *where the person may be seen.* Confusion may arise if the home address is given and the person is staying with relatives. If he is resident in hospital, the

ward and the hospital record number should be given. The latter will enable the therapist to accurately locate the case notes
- The date of birth
- The consultant/doctor responsible for the person referred
- The date of the referral
- The diagnosis and/or presenting problems and any secondary complications or diagnoses. This is the ideal. However, particularly in a lay person's referral in the community, the diagnosis may not be known and the therapist has then to ascertain this information from any other persons involved, for example the general practitioner, and the initial visit
- The name of the person initiating the referral.

Other useful information will include:

- The persons' religion
- The person's marital status
- The person's next of kin
- A specific reason for referral. This may give some indication of the specific expectations of the therapist but may not in itself be definitive; for example a request may be received for a person who is having difficulty standing up from his easy chair. While this may be so, there may also be many other related mobility problems concerning stepping in and out of the bed or the bath, or going up and downstairs or getting in and out of a car
- The person's occupation. This may be appropriate if the person is of employable age and wishes to return to work. It will also give the therapist an indication of previous functional levels
- School age/pre-school age . . . school attended.

Making contact

It is essential that a good working relationship is established between the person and the therapist if the contact is to be successful. This does not always occur immediately but the first meeting is vitally important as initial impressions tend to colour opinions, and too formal or too casual an approach can hinder the development of a thera-peutic relationship. A good relationship will lead to mutual trust so that all parties can feel at ease in future contacts. In some cases it may be ad-visable to see the person only briefly prior to the first full assessment because:

- the person's situation is not appropriate to carry out the initial assessment. He may be awaiting a meal, a visitor, transport or another treatment — or he may be too unwell — or the venue of the initial contact may not be appropriate, for example a busy clinic or day room
- the therapist may not be prepared — she may not have the relevant information or be in the middle of a treatment session when she first meets the person. However, in this instance the therapist should introduce herself clearly and explain the purpose of the proposed interview and how she hopes to help, especially as occupational therapy is a frequently misunderstood label. The therapist should explain the format of the interview and a further appointment should be made. A written explanation of the interview and the date, together with a contact point for the therapist, should be given to the person as a reminder, or to assist him to explain to others. He may also use this to contact the therapist in the event of illness, transport problems or unanticipated inconvenience of the date/time proposed.

The initial interview preparation

The purpose of this interview is threefold. To be successful both the therapist and the interviewee will be required to:

- give information
- receive information
- establish a rapport.

In order to facilitate this, various factors need to considered.

The venue of the interview

The therapist should remember that most people feel more relaxed and secure if approached on their 'own ground'. If this is not possible, the familiar surroundings of the bedside or a quiet corner of the day centre and day room will usually be better than a strange department or office. The venue should be as quiet and private as possible so that both parties feel free to ask and answer questions.

Positioning

The therapist should ensure that the person is secure and comfortable and does not feel hemmed in, by respecting 'personal space' and not sitting so close that the interviewee feels threatened. The interviewee should be at the same level as the therapist so either person can take the initiative to make or break eye contact. The therapist should not dominate the interview by standing over him, neither should she lurk behind a large untidy desk with books and telephones creating a barrier to free exchange of information (Fig. 7.1).

Understanding the purpose of the interview

It is vital that both parties clearly understand the reason for the interview. The therapist must know what information she aims to gain from the interview to help her plan further action, and she should ask the appropriate questions to gain this knowledge. The interviewee should understand the reason for referral and the role of the thera-pist. This may need frequent reiteration by the therapist as interviewees are often confused about the many and varied roles of the host of members of the multidisciplinary team involved with one person. Equally, opportunity should be given for the interviewee to express anticipa-tions or anxieties regarding the outcome of the interview to ensure that they are realistic and not threatening; for example he may envisage com-plete recovery from a deteriorating condition, or fear admission to a home or the provision of an unwanted wheelchair or home care aid. Such hidden agendas can inhibit free exchange of information and lead to future misinterpretation or mistrust.

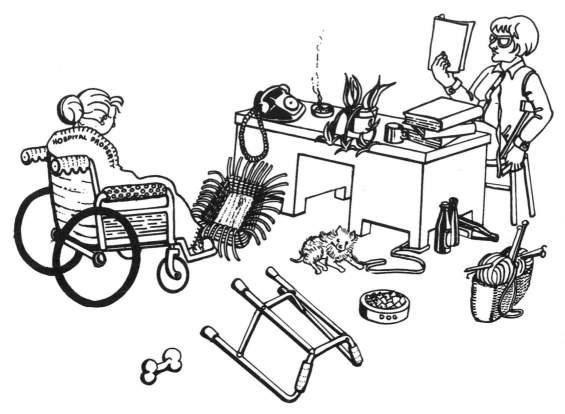

Fig. 7.1 Lurks behind an untidy desk. . . .

The therapist's presentation

The therapist should be neat, tidy, well prepared and unhurried. She should have read any relevant notes and organised the interview at an appropriate time in the person's daily routine. The therapist should be aware of any communication problems such as deafness or language barriers, and take the necessary steps to overcome them. She should also be familiar with the clinical features of the diagnosis and any other routine treatments. She should be able to address the person by name, have any information about the referral to hand, have any assessment equipment prepared and be prompt. The therapist should show empathy, i.e. understanding without over-involvement. This may be shown through:

- her listening and observation skills
- her questioning skills
- her recording method
- her social skills.

Listening and observation skills consist of allowing the interviewee time to express himself and maintaining a positive regard for him. Observation of non-verbal communication is especially important as this may more accurately reflect true responses than the spoken reply. When relatives or carers are present the therapist may have to maintain a balance diplomatically, between respecting their responses and ensuring the interviewee's true wishes or views are noted. She should observe the interviewee's non-verbal cues to the carers' responses. If there is a conflict, she should clarify this by asking the interviewee if there is agreement with the carer and listening carefully to his verbal response while observing the non-verbal cues.

Questioning skills. Using language and terminology which the interviewee understands and asking pertinent questions relevant to the situation are an indication of the therapist's awareness of potential problems and her sound professional knowledge base. Care should be taken to ascertain the interviewee's understanding of his situation and his attitude to it. The therapist should never assume the interviewee is aware of his diagnosis; so such shocked responses as 'Well, the doctor didn't tell me I had multiple sclerosis' or 'Do you mean Billy is a spastic?' are avoided. The therapist should offer the interviewee (and the carer if appropriate) the opportunity to reveal his knowledge of and attitude to his condition by asking, for example, 'How long have you had difficulty walking?' This may disclose an open 'Well the doctor told me last month I have multiple sclerosis but I'd had my suspicions for a year or so' or 'It's been awkward for a month or two, but it's getting better and I'll soon be fully recovered.'

Questions should be clear and concise and free of ambiguity. They should be delivered in a natural tone which is neither demanding nor patronising. Where possible, open questions should be used which encourage the interviewee to explain or elaborate, as these will yield more information than those requiring a 'yes' or 'no' answer.

Recording method. Most therapists prefer to make notes during the interview, but there should be a balance between writing and paying visual attention to the interviewee. A clear explanation of the need for notes to ensure that the record is accurate should be given to the interviewee. The opportunity for him to either read the notes or agree them verbally with the therapist allays any anxiety concerning their content. Accurate notes and records will enable the interviewee and therapist to plan the outcome of the interview, and will provide a sound baseline from which to measure progress.

Social skills. In most situations the therapist is the interviewee's 'guest'. Whether she is interrupting the interviewee's conversation with a person in the next chair or bed when visiting him on the ward or making a home visit as a guest, she should observe the normal social graces of introducing herself, asking permission to handle an injured limb or measure a toilet height, and thanking the interviewee at the end of the contact.

METHODS OF ASSESSMENT

The following methods of assessment are described in detail:

- interview
- observation
- specific tests
- physical measurement
- self-evaluation.

The interview

Much has already been said regarding the venue of the interview, the understanding of its purpose by both parties and the presentation skills of the therapist. This method of assessment has the advantage of sufficient possible flexibility of content to be appropriate in the majority of situations and enables the therapist to give information, receive information and begin to establish a rapport. In order for the interview to be successful the therapist should respect normal interview progression — the opening of the interview, its development and the method of closing or terminating the interview.

In the opening, following introductions, the therapist should define the reason for the interview, the type of information to be discussed, the time it is likely to take and the use to which the information will be put.

As the interview develops, the nature of the content will depend on the initial purpose. This may be a need to investigate a particular area of difficulty which will be explored in detail, or the interview may aim to cover a range of topics to compile a total picture of the individual's circumstances. The therapist should be aware that the first interview may be an emotional experience for the interviewee as this may be the first occasion he has been asked to face the facts of his situation, let alone share them with the therapist. She must be prepared for emotional outbursts such as crying or aggression which may result from the frustration of adjustment to a residual disability or limitation, or anger at himself or towards the professionals with whose help he expected to achieve a complete recovery. Interviewees may respond unrealistically to some questions, either because they are too embarrassed to acknowledge the problem which they consider to be of a particularly private nature, or because they overrate their skills and are genuinely unwilling to accept the situation. The therapist should endeavour to use her knowledge, her awareness of non-verbal communication and her observation skills to identify such discrepancies, and either raise the topic again at a later time when the interviewee appears more relaxed or check the verbal assurance of ability with an appropriate functional assessment.

The therapist should recognise signs of distress and respect these by (a) allowing the interviewee to share concerns, or, if he does not wish to do so at this time, by (b) giving him the opportunity to continue the interview and discussing another topic, or by (c) terminating the interview. It may be necessary to terminate an interview early if the interviewee is showing signs of fatigue. Over-running the pre-arranged time should be avoided, especially in the initial interview.

The therapist or interviewee may bring the interview to a close. Summarising the topics which have been covered is an accepted way of concluding it. This acts as a check on the information shared during the interview and indicates that both parties have understood the points made. Unless there is a particularly urgent item which has not been addressed, new information should not be introduced at this stage, but a further interview date should be arranged. The interview should be concluded by the participants making shared decisions regarding priorities from the topics already discussed, and identifying the date and format of a further appointment. Occasionally it may be possible to make firm decisions and recommendations from the initial interview, but it is more usual for a number of options to be considered by both parties; or a further form of assessment may be necessary to ensure that the aims and goals are accurate, appropriate and achievable.

Observation

Observation in the formal interview has already been considered. The skills of successful observa-

tion are based on the therapist's ability to listen well and to identify relevant observations from the surrounding information. Observation may be an appropriate part of assessment in structured situations, such as the performance of a particular functional task, or in less formal situations, such as having a meal on the ward or talking with a member of the family in the home.

Verbal responses

People communicate in different ways in different situations. Short, terse comments or over-wordy responses may both be signs of anxiety. Only through observation of other non-verbal cues can these verbal responses be categorised as normal for the individual, or indicative of the tension of the situation. The tone of the response may also indicate the emotions or attitudes of the speaker. Similarly, the choice of words may be an indication of the level of cognitive ability, emotion or culture.

Non-verbal cues

Observation of body language and non-verbal responses is equally important. Frequently these embellish the verbal or written responses, but when they contradict each other it is frequently the non-verbal cues which give a more reliable picture of the true response. Non-verbal cues may also indicate mood, cognition or behavioural patterns which may influence the subsequent success of the therapeutic relationship and activity programme.

When observing performance the therapist should consider both the process and the product. In addition to noting the person's physical capabilities in terms of function, the therapist may observe the attitudinal and behavioural factors through the way the task is approached. Facial expression and posture may indicate pain or discomfort, while attention to detail and the standard of performance may demonstrate the individual's values. The willingness or hesitancy to participate may be a measure of interest in the activity, personal volition or level of confidence in performance.

Interpretation of observations

Objectivity in observation is based on the therapist's knowledge of the biological and clinical features of the impairment, awareness of the demands of the activity or task and appreciation of the personal or interpersonal dynamics of the situation. A child with cerebral palsy may knock over a cup, which could be misinterpreted as naughtiness rather than lack of muscle control by the uninformed observer. An understanding of the behavioural sciences will help a therapist interpret her observations, not only when analysing non-verbal responses, but also in acknowledging the influence of personality, culture and life roles on performance. Recognition by the therapist of her own interpersonal skills and ways of communicating will enable her to more fully understand her observations of others.

It is vital to consider the observations in the context of the situation and the environment. These external circumstances may alter the person's usual behaviour, both in practical performance and in the tone of the responses. Past experiences in similar environments may also influence responses. This frequently occurs in formal clinical situations where the normally relaxed outgoing person may become anxious and hesitant. Environmental influences may also affect the therapist. Her familiarity with the situation and the routine of the assessment may lead her to anticipate the response in the light of previous assessment experience. She may be at risk of overlooking minor details of the person's performance in favour of the more obvious anticipated information. Assessment interpretation is rarely truly objective, but the therapist should endeavour to minimise her own perspectives by checking her observations through other assessments, specific tests or measurements. In this way risk of personal bias in observation can be minimised.

Specific tests

A large number of specific tests are used by occupational therapists to assess function. Some tests have been devised by therapists but many have been designed by others and are used by the occupational therapist to measure a specific function. Many visual perception tests were originally created by psychologists or neurologists, but may now be used by occupational therapists to assess visual perceptual skills following stroke or head injury, or with children affected by cerebral palsy.

Occupational therapists may test motor, sensory, cognitive and perceptual skills and their use in areas of self-maintenance, role duties and leisure activities. Assessment of the environment, the cultural and social situation, and the carers' needs and quality of care may also be part of the occupational therapist's role. In addition, attitudes, volition and motivation, and behavioural and social skills may be assessed. With such a breadth and diversity of areas of assessment it is inevitable that a wide variety of specific tests may be used. Vital factors in determining the value and success of any test are the therapist's skills in:

- identifying the need for the test
- identifying the most appropriate test for the situation
- administering the test accurately and sensitively
- interpreting the results correctly.

Specific tests may be considered in three main groups — standardised tests, non-standardised tests and checklists.

Standardised tests

Some tests used by occupational therapists have been standardised, but unfortunately many have not. Standardisation provides two main advantages to the measurement:

1. It provides a valid and reliable standard or 'norm' against which to measure individual performance
2. It sets out the content of the test and explains how it is to be carried out to achieve maximum validity and reliability.

In order to appreciate the value of standardisation it is important to understand its process and the ways in which validity and reliability may be achieved.

Standardisation involves the establishment of a 'norm' or standard, both for carrying out the test and as a basis against which to measure individual results. This is achieved by using the test with a large sample group which reflects the group for which the test is intended. A standard set of assessment tools and instructions is formulated to ensure the same procedure is carried out under similar conditions each time. Analysis of the results of the sample group will determine the range of variation. The 'norm' or standard will be the result or small band of results which contains the majority of the group. The extent of this may vary according to the sensitivity of the test, the accuracy of control and the nature of the skill being measured. Acceptable variations to each side of the 'norm' are usually referred to as standard deviations.

Validity is the extent to which the test *truly* measures what it is intended to measure. Consideration should have been given to the face validity, construct, content and criterion-related validity of the test.

Face validity is how far the test appears to do what it is supposed to do. This is a lower form of validity as it cannot easily be tested. It is, however, important for the individual participating in the test as he may be less motivated to perform to his optimum if the test procedures do not clearly reflect the skills to be tested. The therapist's own perceptions of face validity may influence her opinion of the test.

The circumstances of the dysfunction and their effect on the test procedure may affect face validity. An example may be seen when testing perceptual function with a person with receptive dysphasia. It may be difficult to determine how far the results truly reflect perceptual performance or how far they have been influenced by the person's difficulty in understanding the instructions. Similarly, the distraction of pain may influence performance; so while the test appears to be measuring a specific function, the results may be biased by other unseen impinging factors.

Interpreting results of tests which have only face validity may involve considerable personal opinion on the part of the therapist. She should confirm them, wherever possible, by carrying out other tests which have greater validity before making clinical judgements.

Construct validity considers the components which act together in the construction of the activity. These may be defined through task analysis to ensure all contributory skills are identified. This may seem a relatively simple logical process for occupational therapists who are skilled in such analysis. However, the true complexity of this task may be realised when they attempt to define the constructs of visual perception, memory, intellect or self-maintenance — all areas familiar to many occupational therapists and included in many therapy tests.

Content validity considers whether the contents of the test adequately measure the areas of the construct and are sufficiently exact to identify variables in performance. Content validity cannot exist without the construct.

Criterion-related validity is how far the findings from one test can be used to make particular inferences. It is derived from the belief that comparison of the results against some other measurements or criteria can be used to interpret particular test findings.

Criterion-related validity has two subdivisions:

1. *Concurrent validity* says something about what *is* at the time of the test. We can say that something is now because this criterion exists now.
2. *Predictive validity*. Because some criteria exist now, predictions can be made about the future.

Rothstein (1985) states that 'criterion-related validity is lacking in many physical tests and measurements'. This may be because of the difficulty in obtaining accurate initial criteria against which to make comparisons. Measurement of a specific factor, for example sensation, may be more easily criterion-related than performance in a functional task such as feeding. Human task performance is frequently difficult to define accurately in criterion-related terms, as successful performance will involve a combination of physical, cognitive and psychological factors as well as social, cultural and environmental influences. Criteria for concurrent or predictive validity would need to accommodate these factors and would therefore result in a vast range of criteria interpretation data against which to make comparisons.

However, attention to the development of criterion-related validity would add to the accuracy of the interpretation of the person's test results, both in the recognition of the present levels of function and in identifying possible future outcomes.

Reliability is the consistency of the measurement when all conditions are thought to be held constant. The same results should therefore be obtained when the test is repeated under the same conditions.

Kerlinger (1973) stated that 'high reliability is not a guarantee of good scientific results, but there can be no good scientific results without reliability.'

Various forms of reliability have been tested in the process of standardisation.

1. *Intratester reliability* is the consistency of the test over time when the same person measures the same thing on different occasions.

2. *Intertester reliability* is the consistency of the test between testers when different testers measure the same thing.

To ensure that both the above forms of reliability are achieved the actual procedure for performing the test must be *constant*. The test tools and materials must be the same on each occasion, and the test instructions must be described in detail and adhered to. This attention to detail is sometimes viewed as being unnecessarily complex, but is essential to ensure reliability.

Specific tests are frequently used to measure progress, so it is vitally important that the procedure is intratester reliable if the results are to be accurate. Intertester reliability will enable different therapists, or other personnel, to use the same test with an individual to obtain accurate results. This is a useful asset when the person may be seen in different environments during the rehabilitation process.

Intertester and intratester reliability are also necessary when making comparisons between individuals, either for the purpose of a more objective measure of the standard of each person's results, or for comparative research.

3. *Parallel reliability and internal consistency*. In some situations it may not be possible for exactly the same assessment tools and materials to be used with an individual. Where this is so, and more than one assessment tool is used, it will be necessary to consider parallel forms of reliability. These determine how far one method is consistent with the other. An example of this is measurement of grip strength which may be carried out using a vigorimeter, dynamometer or sphygmomanometer (see Physical measurement). Parallel reliability is the level to which all these tools yield the same measurement.

In some tests involving a number of procedures, different parts of the test may be designed to assess the same skill. Internal consistency is the level to which each of these different parts yields the same result. Significant variations in internal consistency may bring into question the sensitivity or validity of the procedure. Consistency within the test will confirm or consolidate a skill measurement about which the therapist may be unsure if it is only measured on one occasion.

4. *Population-specific reliability*. This is the degree of reliability the test has for the specific person being measured. Many tests have been standardised with particular age, sex and disability groups, and nationality and cultural factors may have been considered.

When using and interpreting tests, occupational therapists wish to consider individual performance as accurately as possible. Standardised tests describe the population group or groups with which they were standardised. Obviously not all factors related to the particular person will have been represented in these groups.

The therapist should therefore consider the clinical relevance of the test, i.e. how far the particular person equates to the group or groups for which the test has been standardised. Using her theoretical and clinical knowledge she should consider the reliability of particular findings in light of the person's individual differences from the standardisation groups.

Objectivity and accuracy. It is virtually impossible to achieve total objectivity and accuracy in any assessment involving human performance.

There is usually some subjectivity by the assessor and the person completing the test. The assessor has usually chosen the particular test and will often be responsible for interpreting the results, which may be affected by her relationship with the individual and her view of the actual test.

The individual's volition and motivation when participating in the test will affect the outcome. Intratester reliability is rarely 100%, as most people will experience some change over time. Merely having completed the test on a previous occasion may alter anxiety levels which in turn will affect performance.

Accuracy in intertester and intratester reliability is difficult to achieve in tests involving significant levels of visual observation, or complex test procedures. However, if the need for making some allowance for human subjectivity and individual differences is recognised, validity and reliability are valuable components for achieving optimum accuracy and objectivity when obtaining and interpreting the results of a test performance.

Interpretation of results. Comparison of results against a predetermined 'norm' to enable the individual and the therapist to make a judgement and identify an outcome or need, should not contradict the therapist's basic philosophy of valuing individuality. Deciding actions from the outcomes of tests should be a shared activity, and the person should have the right to accept or reject any suggestions made by the therapist. The person may be content to recognise his lack of ability to perform the task in the normal way and he should not be expected to adjust accordingly (provided the outcome is satisfactory to him). However, by alerting him to his performance he may be able to make an informed, as opposed to an uninformed, choice. The test may have provided an accurate measure against which to evaluate individual performance, but the 'norm' should not be used too rigidly to dictate aims or objectives.

Non-standardised tests

These have been devised to test skills and measure performance but have not been standardised to determine the 'norm'. They may or may not have valid or reliable procedures.

Many occupational therapists devise tests to meet the needs of particular groups or situations. While these may have been developed and refined to improve reliability within a given environment, many lack the detailed preparatory analysis to determine the validity of the construct. Similarly, the precise description of the use of the assessment tools and materials frequently lacks definition, which risks producing discrepancies in both intertester and intratester reliability.

Therapists should not be dissuaded from developing such tests as they may form pilot studies for further developments which may later be standardised. However, the therapist should not 'reinvent the wheel' by duplicating standardised assessments which are already available, but may require more experience in analysing the results to reflect her client group. This adjustment should not take place in the actual test procedure as this will render the results invalid.

A non-standardised test may be an indicator of functional level at a specific time in a particular setting if it is valid and reliable. However, it cannot be used to measure this performance against the population 'norm'. Non-standardised tests may therefore have very restricted use because they are limited to a particular environmental or client situation. Similarly they have limited use in comparative research. Keith (1984) reflects this concern in his article 'Functional assessment in medical rehabilitation' which states: 'Many organisations still prefer to construct measures to fit their particular situations. Since these *ad hoc* methods have not been well developed, many assessment instruments have uncertain validity for clinical, research or programme evaluation.'

Scoring. This is an important aspect of any form of assessment and many different methods are used. Most tests involve the completion of some form of record sheet. This may include a grading structure which indicates outcomes simply in terms of able/not able, or has interim categories. Some record sheets may show times taken to complete the action and have a grading of time acceptability.

Grading scales also have different ranges. Some have 3-, 4- or 5-point scale; others are more dependent on the variations available, for example they grade ability with the variables, not able, able with manual assistance, able with support equipment, able with verbal prompts, able with extra time, fully able. Many such gradings are based on observations which risk the bias of subjectivity on the part of the assessor unless strict scoring criteria are defined.

Weighting. Some test scores are allotted weighting. This is often in number form. When all tasks are given the same numerical range they are all measured as equally important, and any differences between the value of the tasks or their complexity are lost. Equal weighting of activities therefore indicates equal 'disability value'. Therapists recognise that identification of the perceived level of dysfunction for particular tasks is very individual and varies considerably from person to person and such variations are lost in equal weighting.

Where unequal weighting or categorisation of tasks does occur, it is not always clear how such differences have been devised. Some tests seem to group the essential or most important tasks in one section, and organise subsequent sections in order of perceived importance, with greater numerical scores allotted to those in the first section, or at the top of each subgroup. Other tests accord different weightings to particular tasks, and it is not always clear whether these reflect the complexity of the demands of the task or its perceived importance in the activity as a whole. Frequently this does not relate to the individual's perceptions of the task's importance for himself.

Dangers may occur when such scores are totalled to identify levels of function or predict outcomes. Individual strengths and needs will inevitably be masked in the total score. A person may score highly in many aspects of the test, but may be totally unable to perform in one crucial area. Unless this area is very heavily weighted the final score is likely to be high, despite the person's inability in a vital area of personal need.

Score totalling may be a useful part of analysis of data in quantitative research. However it has limited application in enhancing the occupational therapist's information for individual problem analysis, or for measuring progress in particular performance skills. Score totals are equally unreliable in predicting outcomes, as much progress is dependent on individual volition and the levels of support provided.

Checklists

These are frequently used by occupational therapists and are sometimes referred to as 'performance checks'. A checklist aims to ensure all areas are addressed and particular aspects are not overlooked.

Most checklists are comprehensive lists of activities or factors to be noted in a particular area. Checklists may be general, i.e. covering a variety of areas or skills, or they may be specific to one particular aspect, for example a home visit or communication checklist.

While it is useful to ensure all areas are addressed, a checklist cannot be considered as an assessment because it does not include tools or procedures for measurement, and it is not tested for validity or reliability. However, it may be used to identify a particular area of concern which requires a more detailed assessment.

Conclusions

When analysing specific tests, consideration should be given to variations in 'normal' human performance. When making clinical judgements there are a number of advantages of tests which have been standardised over those which have not and over checklists. Standardised tests are likely to be more reliable and valid. They may be used by a number of professionals in different situations and the results can be compared against a standard or 'norm'. However, interpretation of results of some standardised tests may require a particular skill level which is confined to one group of professionals or those who have had specific education and training in this area.

Physical measurement

Specific physical measurement may be the most appropriate method of ascertaining the level of function in particular areas. In order to ensure any measurement process is efficient, and as comfortable as possible for the individual, the therapist should make certain preparations:

- All necessary equipment should be to hand and in working order. The therapist should be familiar with the equipment and able to use it accurately and confidently. Accessories such as record cards, or a comfortable stool or chair on which the person can sit while measurements are taken, should also be available.
- Measurement should be carried out in a well-lit warm environment where there is adequate space for both the therapist and the individual to move freely. Privacy is important to avoid embarrassment, particularly in the first measurement session when the required actions are being explained and the individual may be particularly apprehensive.
- The therapist should explain the procedure and the reason for measurement. A simple short explanation of the method and importance of the measurements will put the person at ease and make the procedure quicker and easier.
- The therapist should know the particular measurements required and the methods of achieving them. She should handle and move the person's limbs with care and confidence, thus causing minimal discomfort. If she wishes the person to perform an action independently, a simple demonstration may clarify the task.
- Any support or tight clothing which may restrict the movements to be measured should be loosened or removed unless contraindicated.
- Whenever possible, measurement of one person should be carried out by the same therapist, as familiarity will increase confidence and minimise the possibility of any minor discrepancy in measurement technique.
- Where possible, measurements should be taken at the same time of day and at the same time relative to any treatment. The importance of this may be illustrated by differences in the levels of hand function in individuals with rheumatoid arthritis between early morning, when stiffness may limit function, and later in the day. Similarly, the movement of a joint is likely to change from the beginning to the end of a treatment session, so measurements should be taken consistently either before or after treatment, but not at random.
- Measurements should be taken regularly and recorded clearly and accurately for further reference.

Areas of measurement

- Muscle power
- Range of movement
- Swelling
- Muscle bulk.

Measuring muscle power. Reduction in power may result from muscle wasting following a period of inactivity, reduced or absent nerve innervation, or a mechanical disturbance such as damage to the tendon or muscle body. In such circumstances it may not be possible to measure muscle power against gravity, but some measurement is necessary to determine the existing level of strength and chart recovery of power. Ultimately, as improvement occurs, the therapist may assess power through comparison with the unaffected limb.

A method of manually estimating muscle power around a particular joint, known as the Oxford Rating Scale, has been developed for this purpose. The person is asked to move the particular joint as far as possible in a given plane, so muscle power around the joint can be noted. The power is graded on a scale from 0 to 5 in the following way (an example is given for the elbow joint in brackets).

0. *Zero.* No muscular contraction or joint movement is evident. (With the arm supported to compensate the effects of gravity, no muscle contraction or elbow movement is felt or seen.)
1. *Flicker.* A flicker of muscle contraction is seen or felt, but no joint movement is evident. (With the arm supported as above, a muscle

flicker or twitch can be seen or felt, but no elbow movement occurs.)

2. *Poor.* Movement is only possible with compensation for gravity and no other resistance. (The elbow joint is only able to move in a horizontal plane when both the upper arm and forearm are supported.)

3. *Fair.* Movement is possible against gravity but no other resistance. (The elbow can be flexed in a vertical plane without support.)

4. *Good.* A full range of joint movement is possible with some resistance. (The elbow can be flexed in the vertical plane with an object held in the hand, or against the counterforce of pressure on the volar aspect of the forearm.)

5. *Normal.* A full range of movement is possible against gravity and resistance in comparison with the unaffected limb. If both limbs have been affected, measurements should be compared to that person's previous level of performance. (The elbow can be fully flexed when holding a weight in the hand or against volar counter pressure, consistent with the unaffected limb.)

Grip strength. Occupational therapists are frequently required to assess specific aspects of muscle power, especially grip strength in the hand. A number of pieces of equipment are specifically designed for this purpose.

1. *The vigorimeter or dynamometer.* The bulb-type vigorimeter consists of a pressure gauge to which one of three bulbs of different sizes may be attached. When assessing cylinder or whole hand grip it is usual to choose the bulb which the person can hold comfortably in the palm of the hand. The smallest bulb is usually used to measure pincer or tripod grip. Both needles on the gauge are set to zero and the person is asked to squeeze the bulb securely and then relax. The coloured needle will remain static on the dial at the maximum point reached, from which the reading may be taken. The dial is then reset to zero. Usually the measurement is performed three times and the average of the three attempts

is recorded. Vigorimeters produced by different manufacturers have variations in gauge scoring so there is no uniform system of recording. It is therefore important to accurately record the gauge readings in case of equipment changes between assessments.

2. *A spring vigorimeter or sphygmomanometer* may also be used to measure grip strength. The spring vigorimeter consists of a metal rectangle, or two metal bars, which are spring loaded together and attached to a gauge or dial. By squeezing the bars together the dial or gauge records the pressure applied to the springs. This equipment offers more resistance than the bulb vigorimeter and is therefore more commonly used to measure stronger grip strength. However, the thumb is involved less in the grip action.

The sphygmomanometer records small pressure changes on a column of mercury and is therefore more suitable for detecting minor changes in the hand which is particularly weak. The equipment consists of a small hand-held bag which is attached to a column of mercury. The bag is inflated to a basic pressure (for example 20 mm mercury) and the column of mercury will rise to detect any pressure change when the bag is squeezed. Pressure should be released on the mercury column when the equipment is not in use.

It is usual to take the average of three readings with both these pieces of equipment in the same way as with the bulb vigorimeter.

Measuring range of movement. Joint range of movement may be measured in a variety of ways. The therapist should check both active and passive range within the joint for each action. When moving a joint through a passive range the therapist should always support the limb above and below the joint. Passive joint movement enables the therapist to demonstrate the movement she wishes the person to perform actively, and she may be able to identify some possible causes for limitation of active joint range of movement. For example, a joint which moves freely through a passive range of movement, but is limited when moved actively, will indicate that muscle weakness is inhibiting the range despite freedom to move in the joint articulation. A joint which is limited in both active and passive range may indicate other limiting factors, such as contractures, oedema, soft tissue or bone damage.

However, the therapist must also be aware that a discrepancy between expected active joint movement, based on its passive range and muscle strength, and actual active movement, may have other causes. These may include a misunderstanding by the person regarding the movement required, pain, or fear of pain on active movement. It may also be due to conscious or unconscious inhibition of joint movement by the individual for further gain — often referred to as compensationitis'. This may occur when a person is involved in a formal claim for compensation following trauma when the level of impairment may be a basis for insurance payment. It may be a less obvious desire for attention by the family or carer, or be a means of avoiding a particular situation or responsibility.

When measuring joint range of movement the therapist should never force the joint to move beyond the range which can be easily achieved passively. Apart from causing considerable pain to and loss of trust by the individual, by forcing a joint to move beyond this range the therapist may cause myositis ossificans which will further delay or inhibit joint movement.

Principles of measuring joint range of movement.

- Starting position. The most widely used method of recording joint movement is one in which all joints are measured from a specifically defined starting position which is taken as zero (0°). In the majority of joints this zero starting position is the anatomical position of the joint. For example, at the elbow the starting position is extension (Fig. 7.2(i)).
- Measuring joint movement. The joint movement is measured in degrees from the starting position (0°) to the furthest point of travel. For example, for the elbow joint the measurement is taken from 0 to the point of greatest flexion (Fig. 7.2(ii)).
- Measuring limited range of movement. If the joint cannot be placed in the anatomical starting position (0°), measurement should be taken

from the angle nearest to this which the person can achieve. For example, in Figure 7.2(iii) the measurement of flexion at the elbow joint would be taken from (a) to (b).

- Measuring a joint which hyperextends. Should the joint fall into hyperextension then this extra movement can be recorded as a 'minus' reading. In Figure 7.2(iv), for example, the measurement at the elbow joint would be taken from

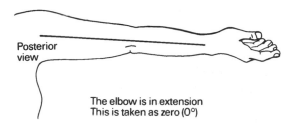

The elbow is in extension
This is taken as zero (0°)

Fig. 7.2(i) Starting position for elbow measurement.

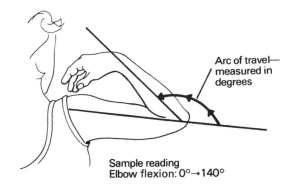

Arc of travel—measured in degrees

Sample reading
Elbow flexion: 0°→140°

Fig. 7.2(ii) Measuring joint movement at the elbow.

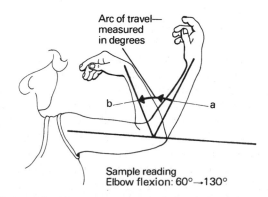

Arc of travel—measured in degrees

b   a

Sample reading
Elbow flexion: 60°→130°

Fig. 7.2(iii) Measuring a joint which is unable to reach the normal starting position.

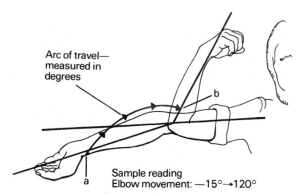

Arc of travel—
measured in
degrees

b

a

Sample reading
Elbow movement: —15°→120°

Fig. 7.2(iv) Measuring hyperextension.

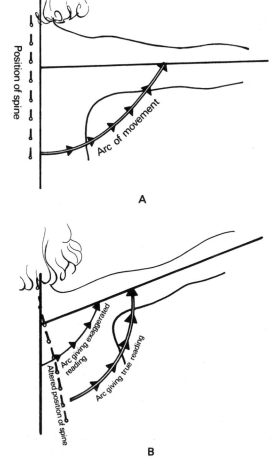

Position of spine

Arc of movement

A

Arc giving exaggerated reading

Arc giving true reading

Altered position of spine

B

Fig. 7.2(v) Allowing for compensatory movement around a joint. (A) Correct movement. (B) Compensatory movement of the spine exaggerating shoulder movement. (*Note*. The fixed arm of the goniometer must remain parallel to the spine to give a true reading)

the furthest point of hyperextension (a) through to the furthest point of flexion (b).

● Measuring a unilateral disorder. When measuring someone with a unilateral disorder, measurements of the unaffected side should always be taken as a guide to the expected level of recovery. Where both sides are affected the average range of movement of the joint should be used as a guide (see Table 7.1.) The therapist should remember, however, that this can only give a rough guide to the expected level of recovery, as this will depend on the age, physical build, race and occupation of the individual.

● Handling the person. Moving an affected joint is often painful and, therefore, all measurements should be made as quickly as possible.

● Compensatory movements. It is important to identify whether a person is making compensatory movements when asked to perform a certain joint motion. This may be conscious or unconscious and usually takes the form of an apparent exaggeration in the movement performed which is the result of a sympathetic movement of a joint close to the one being examined. For example, when the person is asked to abduct the arm he does so in conjunction with side flexion of the spine, thus exaggerating the shoulder movement (Fig. 7.2(v)).

This compensatory movement can be overcome by:

— telling the person he is doing it (frequently he will be quite unaware of this) and correcting the movements he is making
— asking him to perform shoulder movements bilaterally, so that the spine remains static
— supporting the part which is not required to move, either manually or by resting it on a firm surface so that it remains still
— asking him to perform the action in front of a mirror so that he can check his own compensatory movements.

If these methods are not successful the therapist should make allowances for the additional movement when she is measuring the joint.

Joint measurement using the goniometer. The goniometer is the most commonly used instrument for measuring the exact range of joint

Table 7.1 Points of reference for joint measurement

Joint	Starting position	Fixed line	Axis	Mobile line	Average range of movement
Shoulder	Anatomical position	Line parallel to the spine	Acromion process	Shaft of the humerus	Elevation through flexion 0°–158°. Elevation through abduction 0°–170° Extension 0°–53°
Elbow	Anatomical position (with the shoulder flexed for ease of measurement)	Shaft of the humerus	Lateral (or medial) epicondyle of humerus	Shaft of radius (or ulna)	0°–146°
Wrist	Anatomical position (with elbow flexed) for flexion. Forearm in pronation (and elbow flexed) for extension	Shaft of ulna	Ulnar styloid	Shaft of fifth metacarpal	Extension 0°–71° Flexion 0°–73°
Metacarpophalangeal joints of fingers	Anatomical position	Shaft of metacarpal	Over dorsum of MCP joint	Shaft of proximal phalanx	0°–90°
Proximal interphalangeal joints of fingers	Anatomical position	Shaft of proximal phalanx	Over dorsum of PIP joint	Shaft of middle phalanx	0°–100°
Distal interphalangeal joints of fingers	Anatomical position	Shaft of middle phalanx	Over dorsum of DIP joint	Shaft of distal phalanx	0°–80°
Carpometacarpal joint of thumb	Anatomical position	Parallel to metacarpal of middle (3rd) phalanx	Base of 'Anatomical snuffbox', that is over base of 1st MCP	Shaft of 1st metacarpal	Extension 15°–45° Abduction 0°–58°
Metacarpophalangeal joint of thumb	CMC joint of thumb in abduction	Shaft of 1st metacarpal	Over dorsum of joint	Shaft of 1st proximal phalanx	0°–53°
Interphalangeal joint of thumb	CMC and MCP joints of thumb in extension	Shaft of 1st proximal phalanx	Over dorsum of joint	Shaft of 1st distal phalanx	0°–81°
Knee	Anatomical position, that is extension (patient seated on plinth with knee at the edge of the plinth)	Shaft of femur (or in line with the greater trochanter)	Lateral condyle of femur	Shaft of fibula (or in line with the lateral malleolus)	0°–134°
Ankle	Anatomical position (patient seated on table with knee bent over edge)	shaft of fibula (or in line with head of fibula)	Lateral malleolus (or the indentation just below it)	Shaft of the fifth metacarpal	Dorsiflexion 0°–18° Plantarflexion 0°–48°

Note. The reader will notice that several joints/movements are not mentioned in the above table. This is because, in the experience of the author, they are not usually measured with a goniometer by the occupational therapist. The measurement of these joints/movements is discussed later. Those which do not appear at all, for example the movement of the toes, are rarely measured by the occupational therapist.

movement. Several different designs are available but the standard goniometer consists of:

• the central protractor marked in degrees
• a fixed arm
• a mobile arm.

Figure 7.3 shows a standard large goniometer for general use (B), a standard smaller instrument specifically designed for measuring the joints of the hand (C) and a more modern model capable of measuring most joint movement (A). To use the standard goniometer the therapist

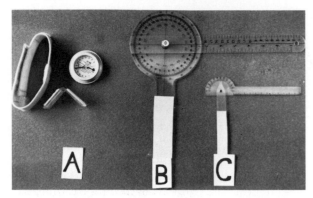

Fig. 7.3 Goniometers for measuring joint movement. (A) Swedish OB goniometer 'Myrin'. (B) Standard-size goniometer for measuring large joints. (C) Small goniometer for measuring joints in the hand.

must first find three points related to the joint to be measured:

1. The axis (or fulcrum). This is the point on the body surface which most closely corresponds to that around which the joint movement occurs.
2. A fixed line. This is the line close to the joint which acts as a reference point from which movement occurs.
3. A mobile line. This is the line close to the joint which acts as a reference point to show the arc of movement of the joint.

For example, at the wrist joint the axis can be the ulnar styloid, the fixed line can be the shaft of the ulna and the mobile line can be the fifth metacarpal. With the joint held in the starting position (see Table 7.1) the goniometer is lined up with the relevant reference points (Fig. 7.4A).

The person is then asked to perform the required movement while the therapist, ensuring the fixed arm of the goniometer remains parallel to the fixed line on the body surface, moves the mobile arm to lie along (or level with) the mobile line when the movement is completed (Fig. 7.4B). The central screw (if there is one) on the protractor is tightened to secure the reading and the person is allowed to relax while the therapist reads and records the movement obtained. Table 7.1 shows the starting position, fixed line, axis, mobile line and average range of movement of

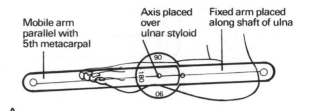

A

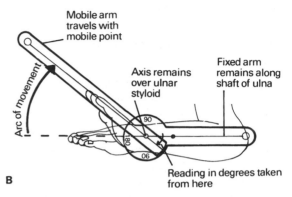

B

Fig. 7.4 Using the goniometer. (A) Starting position. (B) Position to read movement.

those joints most commonly measured with the goniometer by the occupational therapist.

Joint measurement using a tape measure or ruler. In some cases it is difficult or inappropriate to measure the range of movement of a joint or series of joints in degrees, so a tape measure or ruler may be used. An example is the span of the hand which is a combination of abduction of the fingers and extension of the thumb. This is frequently measured as the maximum distance between the tips of the little finger and the thumb (Fig. 7.5).

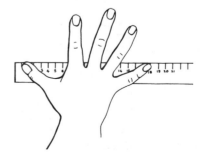

Fig. 7.5 Measuring span of the hand with a ruler.

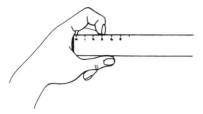

Fig. 7.6 Measuring composite movements of the finger with a ruler.

Other joints which can be measured in this way include:

- Joints in the hand. Composite movement of finger flexion can be measured as the distance between the palm and the finger tip (Fig. 7.6)
- Joints of the spine. Composite movement of joints involved in forward flexion can be measured by recording the distance between the spinous processes of C7 and S1, first with the person standing erect and then when he is bending forward in flexion.

Visual assessment of joint movement. The person is asked to perform a specific movement while the therapist makes a visual assessment of the range of movement at the joint. Under these circumstances, the movement cannot be recorded in specific units of measurement such as degrees or centimetres; it is therefore often expressed as a percentage or fraction of the person's normal range of movement (in comparison with that of the unaffected side). The recording may, for instance, show that a joint can move through 50% (or one half) of the expected range.

Visual assessment is often used to estimate movements which are particularly difficult to measure using the goniometer. These movements include medial and lateral deviation and internal and external rotation at a joint. The joints where visual assessments are used most frequently are the spine, the shoulders and hips, the forearm and thumb, and occasionally radial and ulnar deviation at the wrist (Figs. 7.7(i)–(iv)). While visual assessment is a recognised form of measurement, it is very subjective and the results are prone to variable accuracy.

Joint measurement using a joint outline. The range of movement at a joint may be measured either by drawing around the outline of the joint or by tracing the joint outline with a soft thin wire (this latter method is used less frequently).

For the former method the therapist must locate the fixed point, axis and the mobile point near the joint which is to be measured. The fixed point and axis are then placed over the area marked on a prepared piece of card, and the person is asked to move the joint through its maximum range while the therapist marks the furthest point reached (Fig. 7.8).

This method is usually used for measuring the finger joints where a composite reading is required. The visual record enables the person to see changes in range of movement over a series of measurements.

Measuring swelling. It is often necessary to

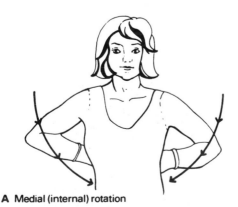

A Medial (internal) rotation

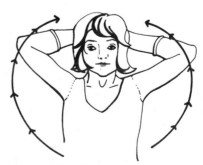

B Lateral (external) rotation

Fig. 7.7(i) Estimating movement at the shoulder. Method 1.

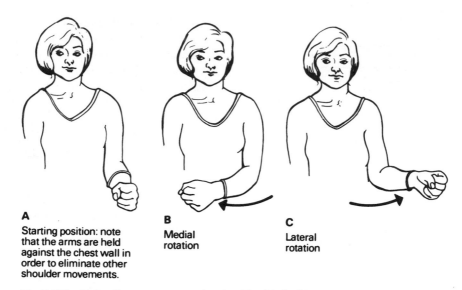

A

Starting position: note
that the arms are held
against the chest wall in
order to eliminate other
shoulder movements.

B

Medial
rotation

C

Lateral
rotation

Fig. 7.7(ii) Estimating movement at the shoulder. Method 2.

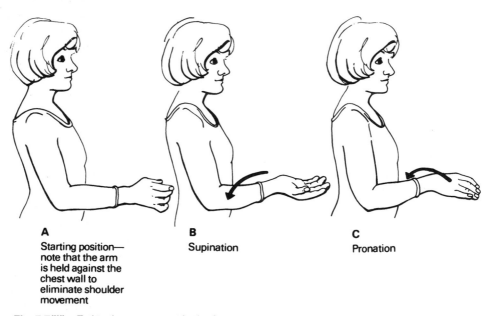

A

Starting position—
note that the arm
is held against the
chest wall to
eliminate shoulder
movement

B

Supination

C

Pronation

Fig. 7.7(iii) Estimating movement in the forearm.

measure swelling around a joint. The therapist should note whether any reduction is occurring during treatment and the healing process, as persistent swelling is likely to inhibit joint mobility.

Measuring swelling with a tape measure. The simplest method of assessing swelling is by measuring the circumference of the swollen area with a tape measure. The tape must always be placed around the same point of the limb for accuracy. If swelling is present in the hand, this may be measured by placing the tape around the palm, just proximal to the metacarpophalangeal joints.

Measuring swelling by immersion in water. It is possible, though less common, to estimate the

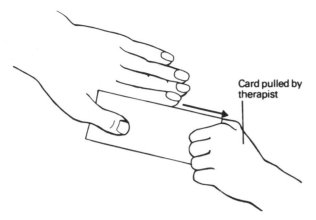

Fig. 7.7(iv)   Estimating adduction of the thumb.

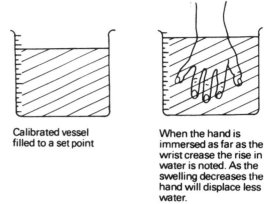

Calibrated vessel
filled to a set point

When the hand is
immersed as far as the
wrist crease the rise in
water is noted. As the
swelling decreases the
hand will displace less
water.

Fig. 7.9   Measuring swelling in the hand by immersion in water.

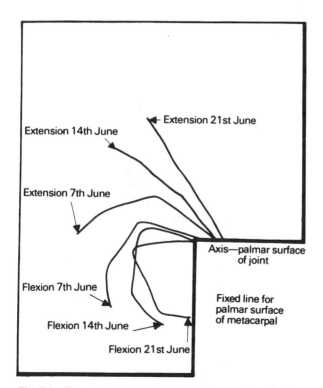

Fig. 7.8   Estimating joint movement with an outline chart.

amount of swelling in the whole hand (rather than around the level of the palm) by measuring the amount of water displaced when the hand is immersed up to the wrist crease (Fig. 7.9).

Measuring muscle bulk. The muscles most commonly measured in this way are the quadriceps group. These muscles waste very quickly during a period of inactivity and their rate of recovery can be checked by measuring the muscle bulk. The measurement is usually made with a tape measure and the circumference around the thigh is taken at a set point each time (for example 150 cm (6 in) above the proximal border of the patella). Other muscle groups may be measured in this way.

Self-rating

This is sometimes referred to as self-evaluation and usually takes the form of a written questionnaire or a rating scale which requires the respondent to answer statements or prioritise them. The individual completes the questionnaire independently of the therapist who then uses the response to identify the individual's personal perceptions of his achievements and his levels of expectation, or his rating of priority skills or needs. In so doing the individual is actively involved in the identification of his own level of function, which may improve his motivation to prioritise needs. Such an assessment may also indicate an over-optimistic or a pessimistic attitude.

Self-evaluation or self-rating tests are difficult to design to ensure the questions or statements elicit the information accurately and are free from bias. Many such tests lack clarity in the questions and are ambiguous, thereby producing confused responses. Familiarity with the assessment may affect subsequent responses, particularly in the assessment of cognitive or perceptual performance.

Hidden agendas about the purpose of self-evaluation tests may skew the responses. The individual may complete the form in a way which he believes will please the therapist. For example he may indicate an improvement in ability following treatment when this is not so. Alternatively the respondent may deny a problem area if this is likely to necessitate further treatment or delay returning home.

However, despite these difficulties this form of assessment does have considerable merit. When used in conjunction with other assessments the therapist is able to identify the individual's personal perspectives in relation to observed or measured performance in more formal assessments. This insight adds to the total picture and will increase the extent of information on which to plan and prioritise intervention. The opportunity for the individual to be actively involved as the assessor as well as the recipient may raise his view of the value of assessment and improve his volition on the possible outcomes.

CONCLUSION

Assessment is a process in which the occupational therapist identifies the individual's requirements for restoration and enables him to make an audit of his own needs. Once agreement has been reached, they can move together towards their goal.

(see p. 786)

A wide variety of methods of assessment are available to the occupational therapist. No one measure will provide all the necessary information. Care should be taken to ensure the most appropriate types and methods of assessment are used to yield the most useful information, and the individual is not subjected to unnecessary, inappropriate tests or measurements.

No assessment involving human performance can be totally objective, and the very nature of the tests, where results are judged against a defined standard or 'norm', frequently conflicts with the occupational therapist's philosophy of valuing individuality. However, without some form of reliable comparative measurement it may not be possible to ascertain individual needs or to identify progress. The therapist should involve the individual with the findings to facilitate a shared understanding of the data so that it can form a basis on which to plan priority needs and therapy intervention. Having acquired such information it should be accurately and concisely recorded for further reference and interpretation.

As the therapist becomes proficient with different facets of assessment she will be able to identify particular strengths and limitations of individual methods. It is important for such expertise to be developed in order to more fully evaluate the use of particular methods in specialist situations, and to improve the quality of assessment and measurement in all areas of practice. Campbell's (1981) comment on research education in measurement and technical skills outlines this well in the statement:

If therapists want to claim efficacy for their practice they are totally dependent on the quality of the measurement used to show change in patients. As more and more therapists have adopted the role of assessors and treatment planners, as well as that of treatment givers, it is ironic that they have not been more concerned with the measurements that justify this role.

The importance of the quality of assessment cannot be underestimated in the total therapy process.

Successful completion of an assessment should not be an end in itself. It is merely a part of the occupational therapy process and should be used to plan, implement, evaluate and change intervention as necessary.

While respecting confidentiality, the findings may be used as a basis for liaison within the multidisciplinary team. They should therefore be clear, concise and accurate, and expressed in communicable terms without risk of ambiguity.

REFERENCES

British Association of Occupational Therapists 1995 Code of Ethics and Professional Conduct. British Association of Occupational Therapists, London

Campbell S K 1981 Measurement and technical skills — neglected aspects of research education. Physical Therapy 61: 523

Keith R A 1984 Functional assessment measures in medical rehabilitation: current status. Archives of Physical Medicine and Rehabilitation 65(2): 74–78

Kerlinger F N 1973 Foundations of behavioural research, 2nd edn. Holt, Rinehart and Winston, New York

Rothstein J M 1985 Measurement in physical rehabilitation. Churchill Livingstone, New York, pp 23–24

Rowntree D 1987 Assessing students. How shall we know them? 2nd edn. Harper & Row, London

FURTHER READING

Eakin P 1989 Assessment of activities of daily living: a critical review. British Journal of Occupational Therapy 52: 11–15, 50–54

Granger C V, Gresham G E 1984 Functional assessment in rehabilitation medicine. Williams & Wilkins, Baltimore

Hopkins H L, Smith H D 1988 Willard and Spackman's occupational therapy, 7th edn. J B Lippincott, Philadelphia

Kane R A, Kane R L 1984 Assessing the elderly: a practical guide to measurement, 4th edn. Lexington Books, Massachusetts

Kanfert J M 1983 Functional ability indices: measurement problems in assessing validity. Archives of Physical Medicine and Rehabilitation 64(6): 260–267

Maczka K 1990 Assessing physically disabled people at home. Chapman & Hall, London

Open University 1981 Research methods in education and social sciences. Open University, Milton Keynes

Pedretti L W 1985 Occupational therapy: practice skills for physical dysfunction, 2nd edn. C V Mosby, St Louis

Trombly C A 1989 Occupational therapy for physical dysfunction, 3rd edn. Williams & Wilkins, Baltimore

Wade D T, Langton Hewer R et al 1985 Stroke: a critical approach to diagnosis, treatment and management. Chapman & Hall, London

8

Life skills

Margaret Foster

INTRODUCTION

Life skills constitute a vast subject for study which has implications for all areas of occupational therapy practice. It is impossible in one chapter to provide detailed information on the entire range of life skills and on all the possible rehabilitative options for dysfunction. Whole books have been written on particular areas of living and there is a wealth of reference texts on the assessment and management of particular dysfunctions related to life skills.

This chapter, therefore, aims to present an overview of life skills. It identifies requirements for success in individual areas of function and illustrates ways in which the occupational therapist may be involved in assisting individuals to address problem areas. Specific techniques and items of equipment are offered only as illustrative examples; the references given at the end of the chapter will provide the reader with more detailed information in specific areas.

The present chapter begins by defining what is meant by 'life skills' and describes their classification into three overlapping categories: self-maintenance, role duties and leisure. The general development of life skills is described, together with the implications for the individual of any disruption in his ability to perform everyday tasks. Next, the role of the occupational therapist in helping the individual to recover his competence in life skills is outlined.

The chapter then discusses each of the three categories of life skills in turn, describing what types of functional ability each entails, the kinds of assessment appropriate to each area, and ways in which the therapist can help the individual to optimise performance and meet his own priorities for activity. The discussion of self-maintenance activities includes sections on mobility, processing skills, feeding, toileting, dressing, personal cleansing and grooming, communication, sexuality, and manipulative hand skills.

The discussion of role duties first examines the responsibilities and skills associated with the homemaking role. Next, the role of carer is discussed, with particular attention to the needs of those who provide support to disabled people and to the statutory and other assistance available to them. The special needs of disabled carers are described, as well as the needs of parents of disabled children. Following this, the worker role is considered. This discussion explores the value of work in maintaining the individual's self-esteem and the occupational therapist's role in assessing the disabled individual for resettlement in his former job or in alternative employment. In addition, the various kinds of support available to disabled workers and trainees are outlined. Finally, two roles related to the worker role — that of student and of volunteer — are briefly considered.

The final section of the chapter examines the importance of leisure pursuits in helping the disabled individual to achieve a healthy balance of interests and activities, especially where the worker role can no longer be fulfilled. Leisure activities provide an avenue for socialisation, relaxation and mental stimulation and can form a vital component of the rehabilitative programme. Options for leisure activities are described, along with ways in which the therapist can help the individual regain the confidence necessary to take up new interests and make social contacts beyond his family circle.

Throughout the chapter, a problem-solving, compensatory approach, by which the individual can find ways of compensating for loss of function, predominates. It must be stressed, however, that the therapist's approach must be determined by the particular needs of the individual and his carers, and that her treatment plan must, above

all, reflect the aspirations and priorities of her client. Other therapeutic approaches may be used to improve performance and overcome rather than compensate for impairment.

WHAT ARE LIFE SKILLS?

Life skills are the abilities individuals acquire and develop in order to perform everyday tasks successfully. As well as varying from person to person, these may change throughout the life span. Evolving roles and responsibilities will influence the individual's balance of activity, his perception of the relative importance of various activities, and the very nature of the activities in which he is engaged (Fig. 8.1). The emphasis given to particular skills in an occupational therapy intervention should reflect the individual's own priorities, taking into account his desires and aspirations and the demands placed upon him by his various roles.

The acquisition or recovery of a life skill depends not only upon the level of its complexity in relation to the individual's dysfunction, but also upon the person's motivation and accustomed life-style and roles. The therapist needs to understand the relevance and importance of people's roles in their particular family, culture and environment. Illness, dysfunction or other disruption to a person's routine life pattern will disrupt roles he accepts as normal. Individuals' priorities will vary; for some individuals, independence in self-maintenance activities will be the prime concern. Others may prefer to accept ongoing assistance with self-care tasks in order to conserve energy for other pursuits. For others, the acquisition of skills that will allow them to return to paid employment will be the prime objective.

The occupational therapist must also consider the nature of the skills which she proposes to address in her treatment programme. She will need to analyse each in terms of its physical, sensory, cognitive, perceptual and social components, and consider to what degree these components may be transferable from one area of living to another. Her primary concern will be with how the individual's skills *interrelate* in the perform-

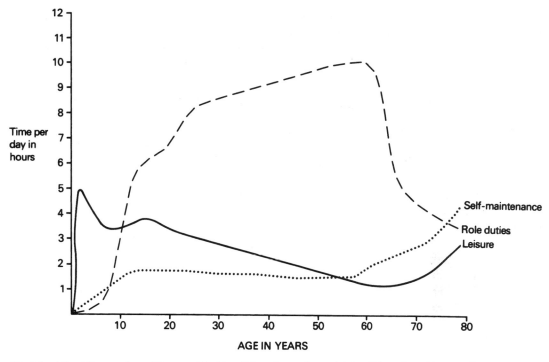

Fig. 8.1   Life skills map for a 77-year-old widow living alone who maintained the roles of housewife, parent and part-time employee until 60 years and nursed her disabled husband until his death when she was 63 years old.

ance of activity. Therefore, while she may make frequent use of the specialised measurements taken by other professionals in order to locate specific areas of functional weakness, her particular contribution will lie in her ability to take a holistic view of the performance of functional tasks and perceive their relative importance in the wider context of the individual's life pattern.

Categorisation of activities

Life skills may be grouped into various categories, such as 'domestic activities', 'work activities' and 'activities of daily living' (ADL). Such categories, although useful, often overlap; money-handling skills, for example, may be related to work or to domestic activity. While bearing this fluidity of categories in mind, this chapter considers activities under three main headings: personal self-maintenance, role duties, and leisure (Fig. 8.2).

● *Self-maintenance.* Skills related to self-mainte-

nance include personal care activities such as feeding, toileting, dressing, personal hygiene and grooming, mobility skills, communicative skills, sexuality, fine manual skills and processing skills.

● *Role duties.* Duties which are demanded by the individual's roles and which are not (primarily) related to self-maintenance or leisure may be termed role duties. These may include the domestic duties of the homemaker, the academic duties of the student, the work duties of the employer/employee, and the duties of the carer.

● *Leisure activities* are those tasks in which the individual participates in order to socialise, relax, or pursue interests and hobbies.

Again, the activities included in each of the above categories will vary from one context to another. A lucrative hobby, for instance, may be classified as work or as a leisure pursuit. Eating a meal may be a matter of self-maintenance, but a business lunch may be seen as a role duty and dinner with friends as a leisure activity. Moreover, role duties may be perceived differently

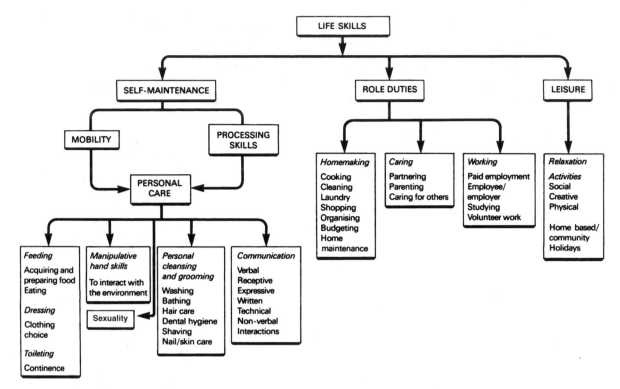

Fig. 8.2 Categorisation of activities.

from one culture to another. A more extensive exploration of such difficulties of classification may be found in *Occupational Therapy and Activities Health* by Cynkin & Robinson (1990).

However problematic, the categorisation of activities can provide the therapist with a starting-point for assessment, and help to ensure that the full range of an individual's activities is given consideration. It is instructive to ascertain not only the individual's level of performance of a given activity, but how he perceives and categorises that activity, as this will provide some insight into his attitudes and priorities. In a study of time-use by adults with spinal cord injuries, Yerxa & Locker (1990) identify differences in the perception and classification of activities between the study group, a parallel non-disabled group, and occupational therapists. Their study suggests that the increased value accorded to some activities by the disabled group may be linked to the loss of the work role and reflect a desire to find alternative occupational competency.

To sum up, although the therapist will need some kind of structure through which she can isolate and assess the various activities which constitute life skills, she should not apply any categorisation rigidly, but should take time to identify the significance that each activity has for the individual concerned.

THE DEVELOPMENT OF LIFE SKILLS

Skills in self-maintenance are acquired gradually throughout childhood. They improve with practice and are finally taken for granted. Consider the process of getting up each morning and preparing to go to work or school. On waking one automatically stretches, gets out of bed and walks to the bathroom and toilet. One washes, dresses and prepares breakfast, all without much thought. But imagine the thinking and preparation required for those who rely on a wheelchair or prosthesis for mobility, or are only able to use one hand, or have difficulty with balance and reach.

These simple tasks which are taken for granted by the able-bodied person take on vastly different proportions for the person with a disability.

For some people, the impairment may be short term and advice regarding ways of overcoming temporary dysfunctions in certain aspects of living may be all that is required. For the person with long-term problems the learning, relearning or modification of techniques may be necessary, and entail considerable practice. The therapist who guides such learning must be able to analyse tasks and adapt their performance to individual needs and capabilities.

When assessing each individual's condition, abilities and limitations, the therapist should consider that the ultimate success of intervention lies in the person's willingness to maintain a programme of strenuous practice and exercise to strengthen weakened muscles, improve coordination and agility, and consolidate skills. Periods of frustration, anxiety and depression may affect motivation and drive. Much will depend upon the encouragement and support that the individual receives. It is also important that *realistic* goals be set. The number and nature of the activities which a person can manage independently will depend on his level of ability, his own standards and those of his family, and the resources available to him.

Consideration should be given to the priorities determined by the individual. If work is a high priority it is pointless to strive for complete independence in a morning self-maintenance routine if this leaves the individual too fatigued to meet the demands of his job. In such a case it might be preferable for the person to accept help. Similarly, for the person living alone, eating breakfast in night clothes may be more acceptable than getting dressed in day clothes only to become too fatigued to prepare breakfast. The person who is independent only in the self-maintenance activities which are important to him may be better able to fulfil his role duties and to enjoy leisure pursuits than the person who is totally independent in self-care. The desire for independence should be weighed against the benefits of a good balance between the physical, psychological and social aspects of life.

Box 8.1 Developmental stages and associated roles: a summary	
Developmental stage	**Associated roles**
1. Infant	Total dependence — player, learner Family member role commences
2. Small child (pre-school)	Family member role increases Player role expands — experimentation with roles observed in others Friend role commences
3. Child (junior school age)	Increase in roles and experimentation Schoolchild Family member role continues to increase Friend role increasingly important Begins to perceive certain roles
4. Adolescent	Student Family member role subject to change over time Role experimentation — adulthood Friend role important — both sexes Worker — assumes equal importance with friend role Player — greater diversity
5. Adult	Partner, parent, homemaker Worker/breadwinner Leisure and friendship roles Social, organisational, cultural roles
6. Older person	Role continuity/gains — family, friends, work (paid or unpaid), leisure, education Role loss: bereavement, retirement, moving house

Skills in role duties develop through education and practice, as experiences change in line with chronological age and life roles (Box 8.1). The schoolchild learns about role expectations in the classroom and playground environment, but he can be prepared for some of these demands before entering school. Similarly, skills learned in the school environment relating to socialisation, adherence to rules, structure and organisation, as well as many of the performance skills related to mobility, communication, reasoning and creative activities prepare the child for adult role duties. Provided that adequate resources are available to enable a disabled child to integrate practically and socially, experience of the normal education system will give him the opportunity to prepare for the rigorous demands of adult living. Additional post-school training schemes may continue this preparation after formal schooling is completed.

Those whose activities as employee or homemaker have been interrupted by illness or disability may need support in regaining the skills and confidence to resume their former role. Similarly, those whose disability has had a significant impact upon performance in their usual role may need help to make the necessary readjustments. Practice in domestic skills in the therapy department, in a training flat or (with support) at home may prepare the disabled person for a return to homemaking. Activities which simulate the working situation may be used to assess or build levels of competence for return to employment. Further training schemes or additional education may also be necessary.

A child learns leisure activities naturally through play. As he develops, his interests expand, in accordance with the opportunities available. Such developments often form the basis of life-long leisure interests. For example, the person who enjoys music at school is likely to pursue it in later life, either actively or as a listener, and the child who is keen on active games or sports may have similar interests in adulthood. Those who enjoy precise or individual activities such as model-building, reading or sewing are more likely to pursue individual rather than team leisure pursuits. For this reason, introduction to play experiences and activities is vital for the disabled child if he is to mature in leisure skills. Frequently, such opportunities are denied because of the limitations imposed by the impairment or because the demands of daily care leave little time or support for play. Family support and introduction to community resources for leisure activities are of great importance for the disabled child's future development.

Dysfunctions in adult life may lead the person to devise new ways of pursuing favourite activities or to take up new interests altogether. The therapist should encourage the person's involve-

ment in leisure activities by providing information about the resources available in the local community for both disabled and able-bodied participants.

THE ROLE OF THE OCCUPATIONAL THERAPIST

Habilitation or rehabilitation in life skills involves the individual and his family or carers as well as medical, paramedical, employment and community services personnel. Success will depend upon the ability of team members to work together, understanding and supporting one another's roles, on the drive of the individual, and on the resources available.

The role of the occupational therapist will vary in accordance with her clients' circumstances and needs. As well as providing direct treatment, she may act as facilitator, planner, educator, resource person, advisor and liaison officer. She should know and understand the roles of her colleagues in the medical, educational and employment fields, be familiar with community provision for support in self-maintenance and domestic tasks, and be aware of local facilities and support for leisure pursuits. She should be familiar with legislative provision for disabled people and with the financial support available to them and their carers. She should appreciate the importance of independence in specific skills for each individual and should also be sensitive to the demands of caring that have been placed upon those close to the disabled person.

The therapist's intervention must begin with a thorough assessment of the person's strengths, weaknesses, needs and wishes. In identifying areas of difficulty and selecting goals for treatment, she must also be able to analyse daily tasks and recognise the specific skills or attributes necessary for their successful performance. In almost all cases, her intervention will be based in a problem-solving approach. However, she will need to be conversant with specific treatments to overcome particular difficulties and improve bodily function. Biomechanical, neurodevelopmental, cognitive and behavioural techniques might all be used to overcome impairment and promote independence in life skills. However, for many people with permanent dysfunction, a compensatory rehabilitative approach may be the most appropriate. This will involve the modification of techniques and the development of strategies to compensate for functional limitation.

SELF-MAINTENANCE

Self-maintenance activities are usually the primary focus of the occupational therapist's intervention, since for most people these are the basic essentials for independence and dignity. Assessment in self-maintenance activities aims to identify which activities the person wishes to perform, those he can and cannot do, how far activities can be improved and the most appropriate methods by which problems can be overcome. 'Baseline', 'progress' and 'final' assessments will be necessary to identify needs and monitor progress.

Assessments may take place in a number of different places, some of which are more appropriate than others. The hospital ward may provide a setting with which the person is familiar and the opportunity to evaluate such activities as dressing at a realistic time of day. However, ward assessments are often unrealistic in the style of furniture they provide and in their lack of privacy for intimate personal activities.

The occupational therapy department or assessment flat may afford a more realistic environment along with many special facilities for testing, but will be unfamiliar to the person being assessed and may therefore raise levels of anxiety or embarrassment.

The home environment is the most familiar setting; here, the assessment can take place using personal equipment and facilities in the presence of relatives and carers. However, for hospitalised clients this may only be possible through a short home visit after considerable practice in basic self-care skills has taken place in the ward.

MOBILITY

Some form of mobility is essential for inde-

pendence in almost all areas of self-maintenance and for most role duties and leisure activities. The ability to control specific limb movements, to transfer from place to place and to interface with equipment and the environment are vital to success in the wide range of tasks necessary for independence.

The occupational therapist should assess the person's mobility skills in relation to his environment and consider whether he will be able to improve his physical abilities in order to overcome problems or whether it will be necessary to use a compensatory rehabilitative approach to facilitate independent function. The ability to negotiate stairs, for example, may be gained through specific treatment to improve balance and lower limb strength and range of movement. This will usually have greater urgency for the person who is living in a two-storey house than for someone who is living in a bungalow. Where disability is likely to cause long-term difficulties in negotiating steps and stairs, consideration should be given to choosing a more suitable residence or adapting the existing home, either by the addition of downstairs facilities or by the provision of a stair raise or lift.

Additionally, the occupational therapist should consider outdoor mobility — in the garden, in the neighbourhood, at the shops, on the way to work or school — in accordance with the individual's life-style. Chapter 9 describes mobility needs, techniques, equipment and facilities in detail and should be considered in conjunction with the present discussion.

PROCESSING SKILLS

The ability to be independent extends beyond physical capabilities for performing tasks to include the cognitive and intellectual skills necessary for problem-solving and decision-making.

It is impossible to predict and rehearse all of the situations which a person might have to cope with in the community, at home, at work or in a recreational setting. A wheelchair or other piece of essential equipment may break down; a helper may fail to arrive; an unexpected social, educational or business opportunity may arise. It is therefore important to facilitate the development of the independent processing skills that will enable each individual to deal with situations as objectively, positively and autonomously as possible.

For the disabled person who has had previous life experience, the development of processing skills may involve re-education and/or an adjustment of attitudes to take account of the changed situation. Where disability has occurred early in life, opportunity to practise processing skills may have been limited; such skills may have to be learned and developed from a theoretical base rather than from previous experience.

Processing skills enable the person to interpret information and make the most appropriate response in a given situation. They involve the receptive abilities to take in and absorb information; knowledge; understanding; analytical and discriminatory skills to interpret the facts; imaginative, judgemental and evaluative skills to consider possible implications and outcomes; expressive skills to deliver a response; and practical skills to pursue a solution. Processing skills may be developed gradually; the person may progress from simple choices, such as which items of clothing to wear, to more complex decisions in such areas as budgeting or home modification. In each situation, the basic facts should be identified and the pros and cons of the available options explored. The individual should then decide upon and pursue the option he prefers, provided that all the possibilities have been addressed and that there are no major negative factors or health and safety hazards. In some instances, the individual's choice may not be in line with the judgement of the therapist or others, but provided it does not entail unacceptable risk, unnecessary expenditure or an unreasonable burden upon others, the decision should be respected. Where the outcome turns out not to be as the person had anticipated, the therapist can help him to analyse the possible reasons why.

The therapist's objective is to enable the individual to perform such actions practically and independently in his own environment. However, where there are major difficulties with thought processes, such as those which may occur following a stroke or head injury, or where experience is limited and important decisions are involved, it may be safer for learning to occur through theoretical exercises before practical action is attempted. Games, problem-solving exercises using case situations or audio-visual materials, individual counselling, and group discussions may be used to promote learning. The therapist may take a guiding or facilitating role in such activities, depending on the needs and skills of the individual or the group.

SPECIFIC SELF-MAINTENANCE ACTIVITIES

Feeding

The consumption of nourishment is the most basic voluntary activity for sustaining life. While those who are unconscious or severely ill may be fed by artificial means through tubes or drips, the usual way of gaining nourishment is through taking meals. This involves acquiring and preparing food as well as eating and drinking. The hierarchical scale of independent function defined by Katz et al (1963) recognises feeding as the first activity to be regained (and probably the last to be lost) following impairment. Difficulties in eating and drinking may relate to the acquisition and preparation of food, the structure of the environment in conjunction with the mechanics of feeding, and problems with mouth control, chewing and swallowing.

Acquiring and preparing food

The general level of a person's mobility, the accessibility of shops, and the availability of transport need to be considered here. Large supermarkets with wide aisles and parking space close to the entrance enable the wheelchair user to take an active part in shopping, although the height of shelves and freezer cabinets may make total independence difficult. Some ambulant disabled people cope well in this environment, using the shopping trolley as a substitute walking aid, but many find the hustle and bustle of the busy supermarket frightening and prefer to use a small local shop where personal service compensates for difficulties in reaching and handling foods.

For those who are unable to use supermarkets or small shops themselves, home delivery may be arranged; alternatively, a member of the family, neighbour, friend or home help may be able to shop from a prepared list. It is important for the individual to retain some control over the shopping, even if only by deciding which items should be bought.

Food preparation may involve a wide range of skills, depending on the type of meal to be made, the ingredients necessary and the equipment available in the home. Successful practice in the preparation of simple meals will help to build the confidence to tackle more ambitious menus. Frozen or partly pre-prepared meals will reduce the task demands, as will the use of a microwave. In all situations safety is of paramount importance.

A large variety of small domestic equipment is available for the disabled cook. Many everyday labour-saving items designed for the general user will also be of assistance. Kitchen layout and equipment design should be assessed; modifications may be required to improve manoeuvrability for the wheelchair user or to increase accessibility for the person with limited reach or poor manipulative skills. Impairments of vision, motor control or bilaterality may also restrict the use of some kitchen equipment, but with ingenuity and minor modifications many problems can be safely overcome.

The environment and mechanics of feeding

When assessing feeding difficulties the therapist must consider the accessibility of the family dining area, the choice of tableware and furniture, the positioning of the person's head, arm and hand in relation to the food and the need for any protective clothing.

When considering the dining area and furniture the therapist needs to ascertain whether the disabled person will sit at the table on a dining chair (or in his wheelchair or other chair) or whether he will use a tray attached to his wheelchair. Any of these situations may enable the disabled person to dine in the same room with the family, but for some people this may not be possible and meals will be taken in bed with a stable over-bed table of a suitable height.

The suitability of existing tables and chairs for the disabled person requires consideration, particularly regarding aspects of balance and stability. A chair with arms will provide more support than one without. A slightly higher table and chair may be required for the person with stiff lower limbs. The wheelchair user requires clearance under the table apron and the table must be stable enough to withstand any inadvertent knocks from the wheelchair. Domestic armrests on the wheelchair will facilitate closer positioning at the table. If the person cannot use the dining table he may be able to use a cantilever table or detachable tray.

A winged headrest on the wheelchair may assist the person with limited control of head and neck movements while eating, but if tremors or spasms are severe independent feeding may be unfeasible. Where weakness of the upper arm and forearm are the primary cause of difficulty, stabilising the wrist with a lightweight orthosis and using ultra-light cutlery may help. The technique of pivoting the forearm of the feeding hand on the clenched fist of the other hand, resting on the table, will facilitate greater hand mobility without upper arm movement.

Finger feeding is much easier than using cutlery but is contrary to etiquette in many Western cultures. However, in many Eastern cultures finger feeding is the norm and should be respected. Equipment for feeding should be as similar as possible to that used by a non-disabled person; special equipment which draws attention to the individual's problem should be avoided as far as possible.

Western cutlery is held like a small tool, with the handle pressed into the palm and stabilised by thumb pressure against the middle finger. It is stabilised and guided from above by the index finger and additional downward pressure for picking up or cutting food is exerted by flexion of the wrist joint. If any of these abilities is limited or absent, as in median nerve lesion, rheumatoid arthritis or tetraplegia, efficiency is considerably reduced. The therapist must identify the deficit and either suggest alternative methods of holding cutlery or recommend substitutes or equipment, such as clip-on cutlery, cutlery with padded handles, or small orthoses to hold the fingers in the normal grip position.

If cutlery handles are thin and slippery and the person has poor grip, is in pain, or has generalised muscle weakness, one of the many types of lightweight cutlery with or without enlarged or modified handgrips may be used. People who can use only one hand may become very dextrous when using an upturned fork or a spoon, but may need assistance when cutting food. Independence in cutting can be achieved by using a Nelson knife, Dynafork, 'Spork' or 'Splayd', or a sharp, curved cheese knife. Cutlery such as this has a sharp cutting edge incorporated with a fork and the therapist must ensure that the individual and his family are aware of the potential danger of cutting the side of the lips if it is used for taking food to the mouth. Many people with strong Islamic beliefs may prefer to be fed rather than use the 'unclean' hand for one-handed feeding.

For people with limited range of movement and restricted reach in the upper limbs, angled and lengthened cutlery may prove to be a suitable solution. This must be adjusted to meet individual needs. Swivel cutlery is also available for people with limited wrist and elbow movement or slight loss of motor control.

Suitable crockery may enable the person to become independent and retain dignity when eating. Deep, rimmed plates are available to match some ranges of crockery but these are often expensive and quite heavy. Their weight may make them unsuitable for those living alone who have to do their own washing-up. Some specifically designed tableware, such as the Manoy range, includes dishes which incorporate a shaped rim to assist in pushing the food onto the spoon or fork. Plate guards fitted to a dinner or breakfast plate may be used in the same way but these are more obtrusive.

The type of food may affect the success of independent feeding. Such foods as tough meat, spaghetti, peas or meringues cause difficulties for everyone and the disabled person is no exception. Foods which require slicing and cutting may pose problems. While the person should not be restricted to a diet of minced meat, mashed potatoes and yoghurt, particularly difficult foods may be best avoided, especially when eating out.

Drinking difficulties may be overcome by only partly filling a cup, mug or glass and by using a lightweight beaker, flexistraws or a small piece of narrow plastic tubing clipped to the side of the cup or glass. Bottle carriers of the type used by cyclists can be adapted for the severely disabled wheel-chair user. (The carrier and bottle are attached to the side of the chair and fitted with a longer piece of plastic tubing.) For people who have severe problems with motor control, non-spill beakers may be used. Insulated beakers help prevent cooling of hot drinks for those who are slow to drink and afford protection to the hands for those with sensitivity problems. Modern thermal containers with dispensers may be used to make hot drinks available throughout the day for those who are unable to manage a conventional kettle or pan safely.

Crockery can be stabilised with a varnished cork table mat or PVC-coated cloth or mat. These are easy to clean, pleasant to look at and do not draw attention to the person's problem. Other forms of stabilising material include Dycem sheeting or mats and pimple rubber. Even a damp cloth will serve to steady a plate. For people with severe coordination problems a rimmed tray with a non-slip surface may be necessary.

Difficulties with mouth control, chewing and swallowing

Children may readily accept bright towelling or plastic bibs to protect clothes during meals. However, these are very demeaning for most adults. A fabric napkin tucked into the neck of a shirt or, in the case of ladies, a large, detachable floppy bow clipped to the front of the garment will absorb drips in a less obvious manner. A plastic-backed fabric bib that matches the person's clothing is less obvious than one made from white towelling.

Choice and presentation of food may obviate

some of the difficulties with eating. Severe temporomandibular joint involvement in rheumatoid arthritis may cause pain and difficulty in opening the mouth. Similarly, the person with facial burns may have limited mouth opening, and foods cut into small pieces and which require little chewing will be easier to manage.

For people with oral spasticity, eating can be very difficult. Spasms may occur when anything touches the teeth or gums, so food should be sucked from a fork or spoon with the lips. Others may have tongue-thrust problems. Placing food to the side or back of the tongue will reduce food loss. People who have difficulty controlling head movements should eat from a central forward position. Under no circumstances should the head be tipped back to retain food in the mouth, as this adds to difficulties with swallowing and may cause choking.

Problems with the fitting of dentures should also be addressed, particularly following a cerebrovascular accident (CVA) which has affected the facial muscles.

Obviously, the choice of food consistency and texture will be important. Foods may be minced, shredded or liquidised, but where a number of different foods are treated in this way they should be prepared individually to retain their separate flavours and colours. Small, regular snacks may be easier and quicker to prepare and eat. The diet should be nutritious and appealing and include adequate fibre and vitamins, protein and carbohydrates. Difficulties with mouth control and diet may be discussed with the speech therapist and dietitian to find the most appropriate solution for all concerned.

In conclusion, feeding is a complex task vital to human survival. Emphasis has been placed on the essential tasks necessary to obtain adequate nourishment. These should be given priority, but it should also be remembered that eating is frequently a social activity with accepted norms of behaviour. Inability to perform such behaviours may cause embarrassment and anxiety for the disabled person, his relatives and carers. The individual may become reluctant to join others at mealtimes or to eat away from home. The therapist has an important contribution to make in identifying the precise nature of the individual's problems, which may be as diverse as an inability to respond to a waiter's questions or a loss of inhibitions in drinking and chewing food, and devising ways in which they can be alleviated or overcome.

Toileting

Toileting is the area where most disabled people first wish to regain or maintain independence. For those with severe impairment it is one of the most difficult areas of self-maintenance and one which is crucial to retaining dignity and remaining independent in one's own home. Difficulties in toileting may be divided into those which are caused by difficulties in coping with the environment and manipulating clothing, and those which are due to medical conditions causing continence problems. Frequently the two aspects are interlinked — the person with problems resulting in urgency may be incontinent because of additional difficulties with mobility which prevent him from reaching the toilet in time.

Environmental problems

The toilet is usually the smallest and most inaccessible room in the home. Generally, the more disabled the person is the more space he will require for manoeuvring. Even when the toilet is separate from the bathroom there is not always adequate or suitable space. Access to the toilet is often hindered by steps and stairs, narrow doorways, corridors and awkward corners. These will often necessitate major structural alterations, particularly for the wheelchair user. Where the toilet and bathroom are separate, the removal of the dividing wall to integrate the two rooms may provide more space for manoeuvring. Access may be improved in some cases by widening the doorway and providing good lighting, a gentle ramp or shallow step, and handrails. Installing a sliding door or rehanging a door to open the opposite way may add space and facilitate mobility.

The positioning of equipment in the room is

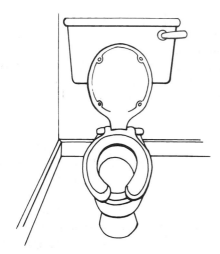

Fig. 8.3 A horseshoe-shaped toilet seat.

also important. Wheelchair users often find that sideways transfer is easier if the toilet pedestal is set further forward from the wall than is usual. The majority of less able people prefer a pedestal seat which is higher than usual. A variety of raised toilet seats are available, some of which clip to the toilet bowl and others which incorporate handrails in their design. The type of seat may make a difference to comfort and ability; for example, the horseshoe shape (Fig. 8.3.) makes perineal cleansing easier, but may be less stable for some people. Ideally, there should be a washbasin close enough to the toilet to save additional movement and exertion.

The size and positioning of handrails is a matter of individual need and preference. Horizontal and vertical rails usually offer more assistance and stability than those which are inclined, although some people find inclined rails of great assistance when rising from the toilet because they support the forearm as well as providing a firm hand grip. A matt finish, either ridged or rubberised, is safer than a chrome finish and a rail 3.75–5.00 cm in diameter is more serviceable than a slimmer one. Texts such as *Designing for the Disabled* (Goldsmith 1984), *Coping with Disability* (Jay 1984), *Designing Bathrooms for Disabled People* (Kings Fund 1985) and *Cracking Housing Problems. A Practical Guide to Problem Solving for Disabled People, Occupational Therapists and Carers* (Walbrook

Housing Association 1992) are useful sources of reference.

Transfers

Transfer techniques to and from the toilet should be considered, particularly for people who are wheelchair users.

Some people may be able to stand up, take one or two steps, turn around and sit down. The continued use of such abilities should be encouraged, as this will enable the person to be more independent in toileting both at home and elsewhere.

For permanent wheelchair users the most suitable technique will, ideally, be one that requires the minimum of environmental adaptation. Consideration of transfers should be included in the choice of a wheelchair. If the individual is unable to manage a direct sideways transfer, a portable sliding board may enable him to transfer independently by using the mobility and strength of his upper limbs, shoulder girdle and trunk. Detachable wheelchair armrests, chassis design which permits close approach and, occasionally, folding or removable backrests may all facilitate independent transfer. Some people, most commonly those who have double above-knee amputations, will transfer forwards on to the toilet and function sitting back to front.

Sanichairs are available for people who cannot transfer from the wheelchair to the toilet. These can either be propelled by the occupant or wheeled by a helper and positioned over the toilet pedestal.

Management of clothing

Undressing, cleansing, washing and dressing must all be assessed in conjunction with actual use of the toilet. These activities are usually undertaken in a confined space, thereby adding to some people's difficulties. Alteration to clothing, especially underwear, and instruction in alternative methods can enable some people to become independent.

If the person is no longer able to stand and balance, he may be taught to slide forward on the toilet seat and wipe himself from the back, or to slide back on the seat and clean himself with his legs apart. Simple cleansing aids such as paper tongs, Maddak toilet aid tongs or the Sunflower bottom wiper may assist people with limited reach or poor manual dexterity. For the severely disabled person the use of a bidet or electrically operated toilet such as the Clos-o-mat or Medic loo, which dispense warm water followed by warm air, may solve cleansing difficulties.

Menstruation can cause discomfort, embarrassment and sometimes depression. Periods are often painful, with a heavy loss of blood, and the person may seek medical advice to suppress or regulate menstruation. Therapists should assist women to manage as easily as possible and may be able to offer advice, particularly to younger women, about the most suitable and easily managed forms of protection, such as self-adhesive pads which adhere to the inside of the pants. The need for perineal hygiene to prevent odour and secondary skin problems should be emphasised.

Assessment in toileting skills should consider the person's need to use a conventional toilet. Some people may find that using a bottle or commode or chemical toilet is preferable to making major alterations to the home or expending the energy necessary for them to use an ordinary toilet.

Assessment should include both day- and night-time needs. For night-time it may be necessary to make arrangements different from those used during the day, taking account of relatives' and helpers' needs. Carers who are heavily committed to supporting the person during the day will need an uninterrupted night's sleep if they are to continue in this role. Urinals, commodes and chemical toilets may provide safe and convenient alternatives for night-time toileting. Whatever method is suggested and followed, safety is of paramount importance.

Continence problems

Incontinence is symptomatic of various conditions and may be a major contributory cause for admission to care. Some elderly people, those with neurological disorders such as multiple sclerosis, CVA, peripheral neuropathy or para-

plegia, and some people with cognitive and emotional disorders may require help with the management of continence problems. An understanding approach is necessary for all involved, for incontinence of urine and/or faeces causes the individual acute embarrassment, misery and discomfort. A number of ways of overcoming difficulties can be devised by the occupational therapist, nurse, continence advisor and carers. If a regime has already been formulated, all members of the treatment team should be aware of it and adhere to it.

Training in a particular regime is important, whether the person is wearing an appliance which needs emptying at regular intervals or whether urgency or frequency of micturition is the problem. Worrying only makes the situation worse, and so people need help and reassurance in timing visits to the toilet. This is a very individual matter. Some people may need to empty the bladder every hour by manual expression, while others may have to go to the toilet following meals, and during the mid-morning and mid-afternoon. Curtailing fluid intake throughout the day is not usually advised because of secondary risks to the urinary tract, but some people may be advised to restrict intake in the latter part of the day to avoid nocturnal incontinence. Medical advice must be sought in this regard.

A variety of appliances are available for coping with urinary incontinence. Men are often able to manage problems more readily because their anatomy makes the wearing of condom-style appliances easier. Most women prefer to wear some form of absorbent one-way pad inside protective pants. Several types of pad are available, together with a range of pants which may be pulled up in the usual way, or which have drop front panels or side openings.

Clothing for the lower half of the body should be kept to a comfortable minimum, and made from easy-care fabrics which are not likely to cause secondary friction or sweating problems. Wide openings and concealed zips in trousers will facilitate undressing. Separate upper and lower garments are usually easier to manage and a short upper garment is less likely to be soiled than a longer one. Skin care and odour control are also important for comfort and self-respect. Regular hygiene and skin care, together with the use of products to disguise odour, promotes confidence and reduces the risk of skin breakdown.

It is common for psychological stress to affect urinary habits and control. Discussion, counselling and reassurance regarding any emotional difficulties and anxieties can help to relieve stress. Continence problems may also be associated with confusion, disorientation or loss of memory following neurological damage, with ageing, or with chemotherapy. Identification of the cause of the individual's incontinence, together with the introduction of a regular regime, will help to alleviate his difficulties.

When using a compensatory approach to overcome toileting problems, modifications to the home environment or the provision of major items of equipment should be considered only if they are absolutely essential, since their value will be limited to facilitating ability within the home. Modification of techniques or clothing, introduction of a timing regime, and the provision of advice or small transportable items of equipment may be more helpful overall.

It should be remembered that there are many different habits concerning toileting in various cultures and religions, particularly Islam; these should be identified and respected.

The therapist should be able to advise the individual and his carers about the range of help available locally and the advantages and disadvantages of particular equipment and techniques. Detailed information can be gained from the Disabled Living Foundation information service, Equipment for the Disabled booklet *Incontinence and Stoma Care*, and texts such as *Coping with Disability* (Jay 1984) and *Incontinence and its Management* (Mandelstam 1986). (The reader is referred to Useful addresses, p. 223 and References, p. 224.) In addition, information on local services may be obtained through the social services community nursing service.

Dressing and undressing

Both able-bodied and disabled people express their personality and sexuality in their choice of clothing. Anyone may draw attention to himself by virtue of his dress and appearance and the disabled person is no exception. Clothing may exaggerate deformity or may disguise it, depending upon the wishes of the individual. Careful selection or adaptation of clothing may help to conceal deformities and to compensate for difficulties with dressing activities.

The ability to undress, dress and make one's appearance presentable and pleasing to oneself and others requires balance and coordination, joint mobility to facilitate reach, dexterity and muscle strength, insight into the task to be undertaken, sensation, and a degree of spatial awareness.

General principles

Everyone should be encouraged to change into day clothes rather than spend every day in night clothes and slippers. This is a primary move to boost morale and initiate the psychological move back to 'normal' living away from the 'sick role'. Full independence in dressing should not be rigidly pursued if such activity is likely to fatigue the person unduly. Practical assessment of undressing and dressing abilities should be undertaken and expectations for rehabilitation should be realistic. Practical assessment will identify those areas in which the individual is independent and those which require practice, teaching of alternative techniques or assistance from others.

Undressing is easier than dressing. It is less tiring and should be tackled before dressing in the treatment programme. It is usually carried out at a time of day which is comparatively relaxed, i.e. in the evening. This may contribute to success, but cumulative fatigue from the activities of the day may counteract this.

Garments on the upper half of the body should be removed first, followed by those on the lower half and, finally, the shoes. Footwear is usually left until last in case the person has to stand, when he will be much safer in shoes than in socks or stockings, but with tight trousers footwear may need to be removed before taking the trousers off.

When undressing the individual should be

encouraged to think ahead in preparation for dressing. Clothes to be worn again should be left with the right side out, and in the order in which they will be put on.

In most cases, dressing will occur in the bedroom. Clothing should be stored to hand and both the bed and a bedside chair may be used for dressing practice. The chair should be firm and stable, with arms if the person's balance is affected. The seat should be of a suitable height to enable the individual to place his feet flat on the floor. A good level of balance is required to reach up to pull clothes over the head, to lean forward and twist the trunk when managing the lower half of the body, and to reach back fastenings. For some people, sitting or lying on the bed may be easier for dressing the lower half of the body.

The room should be warm, comfortable, and as private as possible, remembering that some degree of privacy may have to be given up in the interest of safety. When planning techniques for dressing and undressing, consideration should be given to the person's level of ability, his choice and style of dress and any habitual techniques which he has retained. It is useful to respect the differences between men's and women's habits in removing jumpers, sweaters or other upper-half garments. Men tend to grasp the upper back of the garment to pull it over the head, while women will more frequently pull it up over the arms and head from the waistband. Such strongly automatic techniques may be retained despite perceptual problems or confusion. Special garments, adaptations or equipment to assist dressing should be used only as a last resort, when alternative manual techniques have been fully explored and found to be inadequate.

The dressing sequence should be considered carefully. Pants and trousers should be put on before transferring to a wheelchair. Prostheses and shoes must be put on before the person stands.

Timing is also important. As far as possible, the person's dressing schedule should fit into the family routine, particularly if he requires help. The therapist should try to fit into the person's normal routine when conducting dressing practice, as this will give her a realistic picture

of his level of capabilities at the relevant time of day, and will facilitate normalisation for those who are confused or disorientated. Ample time should be allowed for dressing practice, but the person should not be permitted to become cold or too fatigued. The therapist should decide at what stage help should be suggested, considering the person's pain, stiffness, slowness and weakness. This help may only be required temporarily, as specific difficulties may be overcome with practice.

The person should practise dressing first his upper half and then his lower half, with the therapist observing, advising and assisting when necessary. He should be encouraged to persevere in trying to attain standards which are personally acceptable. Particular methods of dressing or undressing must be suited to the individual's needs; those which have been worked out by the person himself are usually best for him and most likely to be continued without supervision.

Clothing

Where possible, it is best to select clothing which is currently available in high-street shops. It is almost always possible to find ready-made garments which meet the person's taste, are suitable for his age and capabilities, and conceal deformities, appliances and wasted muscles. Each person's needs, circumstances and disability must be considered in the choice of garments. Particular attention should be paid to comfort, as some disabled people have to spend many hours in the same position. Any specially made clothing should be skilfully designed to disguise the problem and should be produced in contemporary materials, styles and colours.

Shopping for clothes is often difficult and frustrating. Many people find that the larger stores are more accessible, have larger fitting rooms and offer a wider choice. If shopping locally is not possible, reputable mail-order firms may provide a solution, as clothes can be tried on at home and returned if unsuitable.

Ideally, garments should be simple and loose fitting, with a minimum of fastenings and with ample openings and gussets. Elasticated waists, cuffs and shoulder straps are easy to manage if they are not too tight. In cool conditions many people with limited mobility need warmer clothing than those who are able to maintain body temperature through physical activity. They should be advised to choose warm fabrics rather than to wear many layers of clothing which will require considerable effort in dressing and undressing.

Personal cleansing and grooming

Personal cleansing comprises the generalised activities involved in washing all or part of the body. Grooming includes such activities as hair care, dental hygiene, shaving, nail care and make-up. Some of these activities are essential to the maintenance of good hygiene and the prevention of infection, but personal cleansing and grooming also affect general well-being, morale, and confidence in social settings.

Habits vary considerably from person to person. Some people wash the whole body daily while others wash only certain parts daily and bathe the whole body weekly. Hair care and methods of washing may be determined by religious practices and cultural norms, or by familial habits.

Washing and bathing are areas of self-care where most people have a desire to be independent for reasons of privacy and dignity, whereas grooming activities are generally less private in nature.

Washing

Most people are able to wash the hands and face, provided they have access to hot water, soap, a flannel and a towel. If the bathroom wash-basin is inaccessible it may be possible to use a bowl of water on a stable over-bed table. Tap turners, flannel mittens or soap holders may make manipulative tasks easier.

The whole body may be washed in a bath, under a shower, by means of a 'strip' wash or, for those who are unable to attend the bathroom, in bed.

Bathing is a difficult task for many people with a disability. Considerable strength, agility and balance (including the ability to stand on one leg) are required to step in and out of the bath safely in the conventional manner. The provision of suitably placed fixtures and equipment, such as rails, boards, seats, non-slip mats, stools and hoists, may make the task easier and safer. The use of this equipment is described in Chapter 9.

It should be remembered that sitting on a board or seat over the water can be cold if the room is not adequately heated. Deeper water which enables the person to be immersed will be soothing and relaxing for those with painful muscles or joints.

Taps and other fittings should be of a design and in a position that facilitates their use. People should be discouraged from using taps, inset soap dishes and the wash-basin as additional grab rails, for the stability of these fittings may not be adequate to take extra weight. For those who are unable to operate conventional taps, lever taps or a tap turner may be of assistance. Soap, flannels, sponges, nail brushes and other accoutrements should be within easy reach; suitably positioned bath bars, trays and shelves will assist.

It may not be possible for the person with upper limb dysfunction to reach all parts of the body without assistance. Long-handled sponges, brushes or loofahs may extend reach. Trick methods are often helpful — for example, using one foot to put soap onto the other.

For many people, a well designed and positioned shower provides a more suitable and safer method of washing than a bath. Showering may be easier to manage, more hygienic and more economical, but it can be an uncomfortable task if the room is cold. The person's capabilities should be carefully considered before a shower installation is recommended. Shower sprays attached to taps may be easy to manage but thermostatically controlled showers are generally safer for elderly and disabled people.

The position of the shower rose is important; those fixed overhead are generally unsuitable for the disabled person, who is likely to have difficulty balancing in either a standing or a sitting position when bombarded with water over the face and head. The rose should be at chest height, and it should be moveable to allow all-over washing from a seated position.

In the case of an independent shower unit, the choice of tray is important. Those who are ambulant may be able to use a lipped shower tray, but a fixed handrail may assist when stepping over the rim into and out of the shower. A shower tray flush with the floor and with sloping drainage will facilitate the use of a wheeled shower chair, on which the individual can move into the cubicle.

Shower stools or chairs should have rubber ferrules, similar to those attached to walking aids, to prevent the seat slipping or damaging the shower tray. Some cubicles have built-in seats and others may have seats attached to the wall. These should be positioned at a height and depth to suit the person's needs for transferring and sitting comfortably. Some seats may be hinged so that they can be hooked back against the wall when other members of the family are using the shower.

If it is not possible to install a separate shower cubicle, a shower spray attached to the bath taps may suffice. Care must be taken to control the temperature of the water. Sitting on a bath board or seat, the individual may be able to use the shower to wash himself, with or without the bath filled with water.

Drying the body requires grip and coordination to control the towel, to reach the extremities and to apply sufficient pressure to dry the skin. A warm room and facilities on which to warm a towel or bathrobe are most useful. The person who is wrapped or wraps himself in a warm robe or bath towel will dry with a minimum of effort. A length of towel with handles or tape loops at each end facilitates drying of the back or legs (Fig. 8.4), and thick, soft, towelling mittens may be used by people with severely impaired grip.

In all instances safety is of paramount importance. Heat, condensation and steam may make surfaces slippery and may cause light-headedness and fatigue. Floors should have a non-slip surface and any unnecessary mats or clutter should be removed. Care should be taken when making transfers, and where appropriate the individual

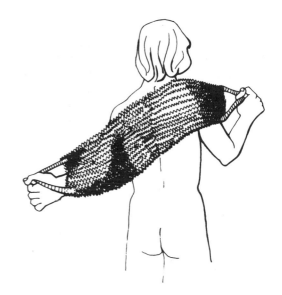

Fig. 8.4 A towel with tape loops.

should be advised not to lock the door, and to bathe only when someone else is in the house, in case he should need assistance. If bathing is required for health reasons the community nursing service may provide assistance for people who live alone or whose relatives are unable to help.

Some people may prefer to have a strip wash seated or standing at the wash-basin for reasons of safety or because of difficulties with transfers to the bath or shower. Problems in reaching the lower parts of the body or the back may be overcome with a long-handled sponge or brush. The room should be warm, as this method of washing can be very cold.

Washing the body is a very important ritualised activity in some religions. Every effort should be made to ensure that cultural norms are understood and that the wishes of the person and his family, particularly regarding privacy and techniques, are respected.

Hair care

If it is not possible to wash the hair independently at the hand-basin, it may be possible to wash it when bathing by using a shower attachment. For people who are unable to attend a local hairdresser, a mobile service can usually be engaged to attend the person at home. If the disabled person is confined to bed, a hair-rinsing tray may be used.

Hair washing, setting and drying is often difficult. Short, simple, minimum-care styles which do not require regular pinning, setting or plaiting are easiest for the disabled person to manage independently. A more complicated style may be managed with the cooperation of a willing carer if the person is not able to cope alone.

Dental hygiene

This is important for everyone but is particularly difficult for people who have problems with mouth or upper limb muscle control. A regular mouth wash may help to maintain oral hygiene. Tooth-brush handles can be enlarged to assist people with weak grip. Handles may be lengthened and/or angled to assist people with impaired upper limb mobility in reaching the mouth. An electrically operated tooth-brush may be essential for the person who wishes to maintain independence in oral hygiene despite serious impairment in hand function.

Shaving

While women may be able to use a depilatory cream to remove underarm or leg hair, this method is not acceptable for removing men's facial hair. Wet shaving with a hand razor is a hazardous business which can only be performed satisfactorily with a steady hand. A battery-operated or electric razor is safer. If the disabled person is unable to hold the razor it may be fitted into a holding bracket angled at the required height or may be attached to the hand with an elastic or leather strap.

Shaving may be particularly problematical for the person who has suffered facial burns. The skin may be sensitive and uneven; great care should be taken when shaving. Growing a beard might not be a suitable solution as many hair follicles may have been destroyed, resulting in uneven growth.

Nail care

Proper care of finger- and toe-nails is essential for reasons of hygiene and appearance, and the care of toe-nails is closely linked with mobility. Nail-files and clippers may be attached to small boards to assist stability and grip when cutting fingernails. Toe-nails often present insurmountable problems and it is advisable to obtain help from the family, the community nursing service or a chiropodist, particularly if the feet and toe-nails need professional attention, for example for the person with diabetes.

When cleaning the finger-nails the person with weak grip may find a curve-handled nail-brush which clips around the fingers easier to manage. Suction pads which attach the nail-brush to the side of the basin may be helpful for those who are only able to use one hand.

Make-up and skin care

A person may have had previous experience of skin care and the use of cosmetics, but due to the present dysfunction the former regime may be difficult or impossible. Alternatively, changes in the condition of the skin may necessitate a change in skin care.

Provision of adequate lighting and easily managed containers for beauty preparations may ease the problem for people with limited hand function. A suitably placed mirror (which may have a magnifying facility for the person with poor vision) may be of assistance. Extended handles for powder pads, make-up brushes or lipsticks will enable the person with limited reach to apply make-up.

People who have suffered skin damage may benefit from the advice of a trained beauty therapist on types of cosmetic preparations and their application. Some baby products or non-allergenic skin preparations can be recommended. Camouflage make-up may be used to boost the confidence of those who are particularly conscious of facial or hand disfigurement. Those who have had skin damage should be particularly careful in bright sunlight, as their skin may be more sensitive than prior to the injury.

Personal cleansing and grooming are essential parts of everyone's daily routine. It is important to encourage the person to take a pride in his appearance, for the sake of morale and hygiene and in order to be socially acceptable to carers, friends and workmates.

COMMUNICATION

Communication may be defined simply as the 'passing of information, ideas and attitudes from person to person' (Williams 1968). Communication is an extremely important life skill. We may need to move, to eat and to toilet in order to survive, but we also need to communicate from birth to death in order to gain assistance with any of these activities, and to become accepted members of society. The baby or young child laughs or cries to express feelings, the adult modifies and refines communication skills according to his environment and personal wishes, and the elderly rely on communication to maintain contact with others in the face of many losses. Whatever our age, our success in communicating with others determines a large measure of our quality of life.

What is communication?

The range of communication methods is vast. Communication may be direct or indirect: it may take place face to face or via an intermediary, in verbal, written or expressive form, or through the use of technical appliances. Messages may be conveyed by a smile or frown across a room, or by a fax transmission across thousands of miles. Whatever its form, communication consists of the same creative and receptive processes: a message or idea is initiated, formulated and presented, to be received, decoded and understood. This process becomes circular as messages are transmitted and responses given (Fig. 8.5). Problems may occur at any of these stages; some difficulties will be directly attributable to impairment, others to factors related to learning, culture or social

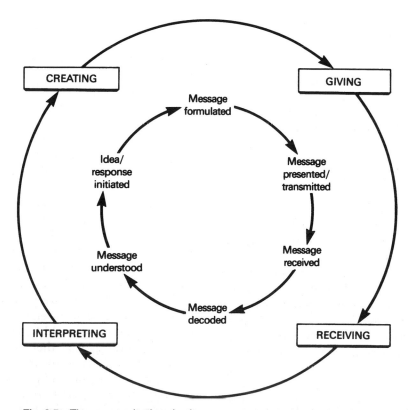

Fig. 8.5 The communication circuit.

context. The interpretation of messages is not always straightforward. A smile, for example, may be a sign of friendship or welcome or a signal of ridicule or disrespect. The receiver's interpretation may depend on his previous contact with the sender, on the formality of the situation, or on his self-image and self-esteem.

Communication problems related to impairment may occur in both the receptive and expressive domains; these are discussed below.

Receptive problems

These are usually caused by sensory or perceptual impairments, but may also reflect a limitation of intellectual capability resulting from, for example, head injury or some types of cerebral palsy. Receptive problems may also be the result of lack of experience, orientation or cultural understanding.

Sensory impairments affecting communication are predominantly those associated with limited hearing or vision. Visuo-perceptual problems and receptive dysphasia also affect communication. Limited cognition may impede learning and understanding of the verbal and written language, as well as the interpretation of non-verbal communications.

Hearing difficulties may be overcome in a number of ways. A hearing aid or voice amplifier, for example, can improve reception of sounds and various forms of apparatus can be used to compensate for a lack of hearing. The latter may include flashing lights on door bells or alarms, and such equipment as a vibrator pad placed under the pillow to act as an alarm clock. In all cases, instruction in the maintenance and use of such equipment must be given. Alternative communication techniques such as sign languages and lip-reading require considerable education and practice and are frequently acquired more successfully by those who developed their hearing impairment early in life. The Royal National Institute for the Deaf, speech therapists, audiologists, social workers for the hearing impaired and equipment suppliers such as British Telecom may provide assessment of needs and specialist support.

Some visual impairments may be overcome through the use of optical aids such as magnifiers or large-print books. Where these are not adequate, more specialist means of communication such as braille texts, sensory maps and taped books or scripts may be of assistance. The Royal National Institute for the Blind and social workers for the visually impaired are the experts in this field.

Perceptual deficits should be identified by the occupational therapist through specific assessments. Once the problems have been identified, her role is to inform the person and his carers of the deficit, to help the person practise techniques to overcome particular difficulties, and to find alternative ways through which he can communicate.

Problems with reception or understanding may be due to purely linguistic barriers, that is, difficulties in translation, differences in dialect, or even a lack of familiarity with technical jargon. The therapist should be aware of language or dialect difficulties and every effort should be made to facilitate interpretation by spoken or written means. Professionals tend to use jargon; this should be avoided when discussing issues with the disabled person or his carers because, besides limiting understanding, it further accentuates any perceived disadvantaged role.

Expressive problems

A number of expressive communication problems occur as the direct result of impairment. These problems may be with verbal or non-verbal expression or with the practical management of communication equipment.

Verbal problems may be the result of damage to the speech centres of the brain resulting in difficulties with remembering and formulating speech. Problems may be due to damage to the mechanisms for articulating speech, e.g. the muscles of the mouth, the tongue, the larynx or the trachea. This can occur with neurological disorders such as multiple sclerosis, cerebral palsy or motor neurone disease, or may be the result of surgery (for example, laryngectomy). The occupational therapist should liaise with the speech therapist to identify the specific problem and the most appropriate ways of overcoming it. Rehabilitation may include practice in speech sounds or words in conjunction with visual stimuli, the introduction of equipment such as letter or word boards through which the individual can indicate a request or response, or instruction in the use of more sophisticated means of communication such as voice synthesisers or electronic communicators.

Non-verbal expression may be limited by impairments which affect the control of the muscles of the face or upper limbs. Limited mobility of the facial muscles, such as that which occurs with Parkinson's disease, affects the ability to show emotions or responses facially. Where hyper mobility of the facial muscles occurs, as in some people with athetoid cerebral palsy, the control of a facial response may be difficult. Speech may also be impaired in both situations, further adding to communication difficulties. The listener or 'receiver' should be attentive to any response and check its validity. (In this the 'sender' should, where possible, employ an alternative method of communication, for example head-nodding, pointing or a written response.)

Uncontrolled movements of the upper limbs also hinder non-verbal communication. A hand or arm may be used to point, gesticulate, initiate contact by beckoning or emphasise a point. A sudden spasm of an upper limb may be misinterpreted as an invitation or a rejection. It is important for the therapist to explain such problems to the relatives and carers and to encourage them to verify the meaning of the person's non-verbal cues with him, thus ensuring understanding.

Written communication may be affected by limitations in hand function or by visual impairment. Various modifications may be made to pens to assist with grip and control. For those who are not able to write, alternative means of communication by word such as an electric typewriter with modified keyboard, a word processor or the possum system (Patient-Operated Selector Mechanism) may be considered. The use of a tape recorder to transmit the spoken rather than written word may be more appropriate for people with visual impairments who are unable to use a keyboard. Impairments of hand function may also affect the use of other pieces of communication equipment such as the telephone. A number of modifications are available from British Telecom.

Communication problems may also occur because of difficulties with language, or as the result of limited mobility or social experience. These difficulties may affect anyone, but often are an additional handicap for the disabled person.

People with mobility problems have difficulty keeping in touch, even with other members of the family in different rooms in the house. A simple intercom system may facilitate room-to-room communication. Where there is a need to make contact outside the home, either for pleasure or in the case of an emergency, a portable telephone or alarm system may be used to alert neighbours, family or friends. A large number of systems are available and careful choice should be made, bearing in mind the needs of all parties involved.

Limited social experience can impede the development of communication skills. This may lead to anxiety in social situations because of uncertainty regarding the most appropriate type of behaviour. In some instances inappropriate behaviour may lead to embarrassment and further handicap the individual. Appropriate instruction and support should be provided to enable the disabled person to develop skills and confidence in social communication in a secure environment. Following this, opportunity should be made for him gradually to integrate in a number of social settings, with support as necessary.

SEXUALITY

Human sexuality has been defined as a:

complete attribute of every person, involving deep needs for identity, relationships, love and immorality. It is more than biologic, gender, physiologic processes, or modes of behaviour; it involves one's self-concept and self-esteem. Sexuality includes masculine and feminine self-image, expression of emotional states of being, and communication of feelings for others and encompasses everything that the individual is, thinks, feels or does during the entire lifespan. Sexual behaviour, more than any other behaviour, is intimately related to emotional and social well-being.

(Kuczynski 1980).

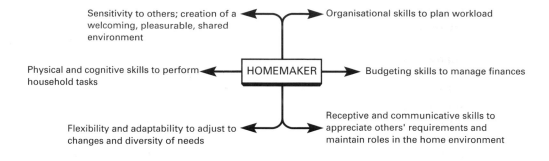

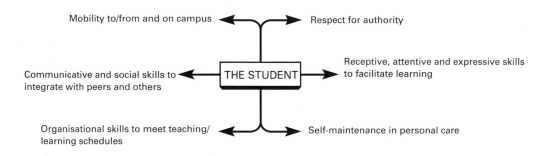

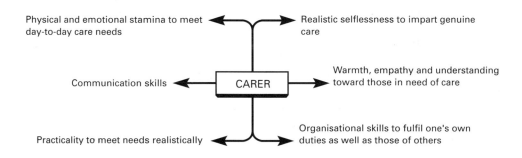

Fig. 8.6 Some aspects of role duties.

maintain a home environment physically and emotionally suited to the needs and wishes of all the occupants. This will vary, depending on the other occupants and their roles in the home-making process. Sharing responsibilities for the planning and execution of activities may ease the burden of homemaking for each individual, whereas responsibility for young children, dis-abled or elderly relatives or members of the family who take no part in domestic tasks will add to the demands placed on the homemaker. Many homemakers also have a worker role and must manage the essential demands of employ-ment alongside their domestic tasks.

Assessment and training or retraining of the disabled homemaker is an area in which the occupational therapist can make an important contribution. Assessment should include details of the type, design and organisation of the person's home, of how many there are in the family, of what help is available from the family and/or other agencies and of whether the appropriate re-organisation of any of these will make the person more independent or the homemaking role less demanding. When selecting specific areas for intervention the therapist should take account of the person's level of disability, his personal wishes and priorities and other roles he is pursuing.

Intervention must be realistic and practical. The therapist can assist the person who has been in hospital for some time to regain confidence and re-establish a routine. She may help in organising tasks so that each family member has his own duties, for example bed-making, cleaning his own bedroom, shopping, or preparing vegetables for a meal. For the disabled person, training in specific areas may be necessary, such as balancing on a kitchen stool, safe mobility in the home, optimum working positions or lifting techniques. The therapist can help the person to build up physical stamina and to improve physical and organisational skills, and can recommend appropriate and safe labour-saving techniques.

If the disabled person is not able to perform homemaking tasks other avenues should be explored. Trombley (1989) states that the 'severely disabled homemaker may be an effective home manager, directing the efforts of other family members or paid household help. She can manage the finances and oversee the shopping.' Trombley states that the experienced householder may manage this with little training but the 'inexperienced homemaker may need practice in hypothetical financial management and in directing others effectively by words alone'. Others may prefer to retain a more active role in home management through modification of methods or techniques or changes to equipment or the domestic environment, only accepting manual assistance in a small number of activities. Whichever role is pursued, careful planning is important to ensure that the workload is evenly distributed and needs are met appropriately.

Forward planning of the week's activities and organisation of tasks, labour and equipment are essential prerequisites to successful completion of activities. Where the person is an active participant, it is important to plan the day so that necessary tasks can be completed comfortably, allowing for rest periods and leisure time with family members or friends.

A compensatory approach may be used where previous methods are no longer possible. New techniques may be tried and the most appropriate ones adopted. Practice in these new techniques will be necessary in most cases. Reorganisation of the home layout to minimise difficulties and facilitate mobility, modification to storage, selection of major items of equipment such as cookers, cleaners and washing machines, and the provision of suitably sited power sources and small items of specialist domestic equipment may all assist the disabled person in many household tasks.

When tasks cannot be completed independently or with the assistance of family members, other sources of help may be sought. Local authority home-help provision varies from area to area in the duties the helpers are permitted to carry out. Some may only provide assistance with shopping, food preparation, cooking and serving meals, while others will do laundry and cleaning. The local Meals on Wheels service can meet the needs of the disabled person who has difficulty shopping and preparing food, but this is usually not available every day of the week. Various voluntary organisations in many localities also provide assistance with domestic tasks in the person's home. Specific individual requirements for the disabled person and his family may be financed in some instances by the Social Fund, a community care grant or the Family Fund. In many areas, local privately organised services exist to help with domestic care. These may be engaged through the use of benefits such as the Independent Living (1993) Fund or Disability Living Allowance. The therapist should be aware of local facilities and services and should advise the disabled person and his family on how to make applications and gain the most benefit from such services.

CARING

In many instances the occupational therapist is involved in assessing the disabled person for community living. This may be with a view to an individual's return to the community following hospitalisation. It may also be undertaken to find the most appropriate environment in which the home-based disabled person can continue in community living. It is therefore vitally important that the therapist be conversant with the needs, demands and resources for successful community care for both the disabled person and his carers.

Emphasis is often placed on the needs of the disabled person in the assumption that a partner or member of the family will take an active part in his care. Such assumptions infringe upon the rights as individuals of those concerned. Open, informed discussions should take place to identify the resources and options available; each person's wishes should be considered before decisions are made regarding future care. In many situations the outcome may have to be a compromise by both parties in light of the limitations of available resources. However, where compromise decisions are made they should be considered as sensitively and positively as possible to limit any feelings of anger and bitterness which may mar personal relationships between the carer and the disabled person. Information should be provided on services and personnel available to cope with unexpected pressures or crises in caring and, where possible, regular appraisal or reviews to monitor the situation and any changes in needs should be carried out.

The carer

Care may include help with any aspect of life skills. It may be given in the form of advice, guidance and stimulation to support the disabled person in learning how to safely perform a given activity himself, or it may extend to practical assistance to compensate for the person's inability to do the task independently. Each of these forms of care has its own particular strains. The former requires genuine respect and unflagging patience in promoting the person's achievement according to his own wishes and without the imposition of the carer's own standards. The latter type of care may be physically demanding, for example in terms of lifting and moving the disabled person, and may impose impossible or unrealistic physical strain on the carer. In either case, care is time-consuming, either in terms of the total number of hours devoted to the care of an individual or by virtue of an ongoing commitment to a daily or weekly schedule.

The Disabled Persons Services, Consultation and Representation Act 1986 extended the provision of the Chronically Sick and Disabled Persons Act 1970. Section 8 of the 1986 Act recognised the rights of carers to request an assessment of needs for the disabled person for whom they are caring which takes account of their ability to continue to provide care. For the purposes of the Act, carers are those who provide a substantial amount of care without remuneration on a regular basis for a disabled person who is living at home. The NHS and Community Care Act 1990 introduced the principle of care management, in which a designated care manager is responsible for assessing and monitoring an individual's needs and the use of support services.

Many carers are themselves elderly or disabled and the burden of caring for a loved one who is also disabled, over and above managing their own problems, can cause considerable physical, mental, social and financial strain. Successful caring requires a partnership in which each party recognises and respects the wishes and needs of the other. This should be viewed not just in terms of the demands each places on the other when they are together, but should also be considered in terms of the need for personal space, privacy and periods of freedom from the patient or carer role. Much will depend, therefore, on provision of and access to resources for support to permit respite periods to occur on a regular basis, without feelings of guilt or bitterness and without any sacrifice of safety.

Where the carer has a close relationship with the disabled person, changes in this relationship precipitated by disability may place heavy demands on both partners in their emotional and/or sexual interactions. Sensitive discussion of each other's feelings and needs may enable each partner to come to terms with his own and the other person's wishes and roles, and to find ways of modifying and continuing the close relationship.

Caring also includes child care and parenting. The stresses of looking after a disabled child may affect the entire family physically, emotionally, financially and socially. In addition to the pressures on parents, those imposed upon siblings must be considered. Siblings may feel jealous of the attention given to their disabled brother or sister, angry at the limitations imposed on the family or burdened by their extra duties toward the disabled child. These feelings should be shared and discussed and the family should be encouraged and supported in finding ways to achieve an acceptable balance of attention and activity for all its members.

Where a parent, particularly the mother, is disabled, practical difficulties may arise in caring for the children, especially when they are very young. Specialist equipment and practical assistance with caring duties may enable the disabled person to fulfil the parenting role safely. Where possible, such assistance should be home based; this will enable the children to develop in their own environment and permit the parent to retain maximum contact with them. Day nurseries should be considered only when home care is not possible, or where it seems to be necessary for the social development of the older child, as early separation of the child from the parent may affect emotional bonding. As children grow older they should be encouraged to take responsibility for their own personal care but should not be over-burdened with unrealistic domestic duties over and above those normally expected of children their age.

On a more positive note, it should be emphasised that caring can be a pleasure. It can provide friendship and companionship for both parties. Maintenance of abilities and small achievements can be a source of pleasure and pride to the disabled person and to the carer, adding to a fuller appreciation of life and living.

Needs for caring

The support required by carers in order to successfully fulfil their role includes:

- Information about the services available, how to make an application, how decisions are made and how to make an appeal against unfavourable or unsuitable decisions. This information should be given in easily understood terms in the languages of the local community.
- Separate assessment of needs for the disabled person and the carer. Both parties are entitled to this service and the legitimate interests of both parties should be considered equally.
- Consultation: this should occur at all levels *before* care plans are formulated. This should extend beyond the disabled person and the carer to include appropriate external agencies, for example voluntary organisations, social services or housing agencies, before decisions are made for future care.
- Practical help, which may include assistance with self-maintenance or domestic activities, mobility, employment or home adaptations. Practical help may also include financial provision in the form of benefits, or emotional support through counselling, befriending or self-help groups.
- Relief from care for both parties. Both short and long spells of relief should be considered, ranging from the occasional social or shopping trip to holiday periods. The type of relief should be compatible with each person's needs. However short the relief may be, a regular, predictable service is usually valued most.

Sources of information

These include the National Council for Voluntary Organisations, which provides a directory of voluntary agencies and their roles; DIAL UK, Disability Alliance and the Citizens' Advice Bureau, all of which provide information on rights and services; the Equal Opportunities Commission; the Department of Social Security and the appropriate acts of Parliament, which provide information on statutory provision; the Association of Carers and the Association of Crossroads Care

Attendant Schemes, which consider specific care provision; and many other agencies which provide information and assistance for specific groups of disabled people and their carers.

WORKING

Work may be defined as the purposeful application of effort. Over the century work and work patterns have changed considerably. Whereas in previous decades many people spent long hours in heavy manual labour, employment in less physically demanding tasks and more flexible, shorter working periods are now becoming the norm. Advances in technology have enabled tasks to be completed by push-button control, which in some instances has led to a need for fewer employees to meet production demands and higher levels of unemployment.

Gains from working

Independence

Work may provide the means to be self-sufficient. Many people work to earn sufficient income to sustain independence in daily living for themselves and their dependents. It is important to consider that those in low-paid employment may not benefit financially from work. Equally, statutory benefits do not usually provide sufficient funding for holidays, outings or other luxuries.

Additionally, many illnesses carry added expense; special dietary requirements, extra heating and transportation costs, and expenses for personal care and home cleaning can add to the strain for those on a low income.

Self-esteem/status

It is interesting to note that social class may be determined by occupation (Box 8.2). Some jobs have a status image attached to them which affects the ways in which the individual is perceived by society. The work people do may determine the type of house in which they live, the area in which they live, the people they meet, the items they can afford to buy and, in some instances, the opinions they hold.

Box 8.2 Work and social class
(Registrar General, Somerset House, National Records Office)

Category	Occupation
Social class I	Professional occupations
Social class II	Intermediate occupations
Social class III (N)	Skilled occupations: non-manual
Social class III (M)	Skilled occupations: manual
Social class IV	Partly skilled occupations
Social class V	Unskilled occupations

Work carries with it a sense of purpose and worth, a role in life, and a responsibility to or for others. Unemployment, by contrast, is still commonly associated with an image of laziness. Many people who cannot work feel a 'burden on society'. Some lose their self-respect and feel they cannot contribute to the society in which they live. Some still think of themselves as living on charity when receiving benefits or other services to which they are entitled and for this reason (as well as others) they may not apply for the help available to them.

Group membership

Man is a naturally gregarious animal and his need to be part of a group and to have a defined role in society is a constant pull. People can gain support and social contact from those with whom they work. For many people, the primary focus of work is not financial gain, but the benefits of meeting others, getting out of the house and being a useful member of society or part of a social and employment circle.

Structure

Everyone enjoys the freedom to do what he wants to do, when he wants to do it, for a limited period, but for many people this freedom may lose its attraction after a time, as they lapse into apathy because of a lack of variety or purpose to the day. Work, on the other hand, can provide structure to the day, week, month and year. It may determine the individual's allocation of time, type of dress and social behaviours. In so doing it may add to his appreciation of non-work time — in the evening, at weekends, or during holidays — because of the change and freedom it brings.

The role of the occupational therapist

In some instances assessment for work may be part of an individual's comprehensive programme of treatment; thus the occupational therapist will be familiar with the person's skills and limitations. In other instances the individual will be referred to the therapist specifically for work assessment or work preparation, and thus may have had no previous contact with her. In either case both parties should be clear of the purpose of assessment or work preparation, and be able to discuss anxieties, difficulties and options openly.

The demands of the worker

In order to sustain employment the worker must be able to meet the demands of the job adequately. These may be many and varied, depending upon the type of employment and the work situation.

Physically, employment demands extra effort and, in some cases, a sustained level of strenuous physical activity throughout the working day. In addition to fulfilling the demands of the actual work tasks, considerable effort may be required by the disabled person in order to travel to and from work. Some work, such as computing or fine assembly tasks, demands a high degree of coordination and dexterity. For some people these demands may prove too great if such skills are unpractised, or if illness has resulted in significant dysfunction.

Psychologically, any work demands a degree of concentration and adherence to routine. Certain rules and regulations must be followed; acceptable dress, language, social habits, time-keeping and personal hygiene must be displayed. Skills of communication and organisation are required to perform adequately in many situations. Social skills necessary to relate appropriately to em-ployers and workmates, and independence in all activities of self-maintenance, enhance the possibility of successful work resettlement. Awareness of current trends and societal opinions may assist the individual to gain acceptance by workmates in both work and social contexts.

Skills in budgeting, in adjusting personal life around the work routine, or in using public transport, work canteens or specialist equipment may be necessary for successful integration into the workforce.

Work assessment

The work assessment should aim to ascertain whether the person will be able to return to his former occupation or, where this is not considered feasible, to discover his ability to undertake a new job, and the training it may demand. The activities performed in a work assessment may vary, depending on the nature of the employment and the level of dysfunction. Certain skills will be required to greater or lesser extent, depending on the nature of the job. For example, it may be necessary to note the ability of a clerk to sit for long periods, use a typewriter or computer, and write legibly. Lifting, climbing and carrying skills may need in-depth assessment for a bricklayer. However, according to Jacobs (1991) skills will fall into four main groups:

1. Work behaviours (sometimes known as 'pre-vocational readiness' skills [Jacobs 1991]). These include ADL, intellectual and social skills such as personal grooming, social conduct, interpersonal skills, self-control, punctuality and time management, attention span, ability to follow instructions, ability to start and finish an activity, problem-solving, independent coping skills and adherence to regulations.

2. Aptitudes and abilities. Jacobs (1991) says that these include 'intelligence; verbal, numerical and spatial ability; form perception; clerical perception; motor co-ordination; finger dexterity; manual dexterity; eye-hand-foot co-ordination; and colour discrimination.'

3. Work skills and attainments. These are the skills that the person has previously achieved:

through formal employment, in daily living, and through previous academic and practical education.

4. Physical capabilities. These include gross motor skills, such as bending, kneeling, crouching, walking, climbing, lifting, carrying, pushing and pulling, strength and stamina; upper limb skills such as feeling, reaching, handling, grasping, holding and manipulating; and sensory skills such as smelling, hearing and seeing.

When assessing a person's ability to return to work the therapist should ensure that she is conversant with the skills demanded by the job; this will entail making an ergonomic job analysis. This can usually be done by asking the person himself what the job involves, but where this is not possible, the therapist should ensure she receives accurate information by contacting the person's employer or another reliable source.

Additionally, through questioning, observation of non-verbal behaviours, exploration of previous work patterns and discussion of future options, the therapist should aim to identify the person's motivation and attitude to work, and his priorities for future employment. These may also give insight into the realism the person has regarding his attributes and skills, and the situation of the labour market.

Work preparation

The intervention to prepare the person for work will vary, depending on the nature and type of work, the level of dysfunction, the setting of the intervention and the resources available. The therapist should aim to develop work skills and tolerances, guide the individual in developing realistic aspirations and refer him to appropriate sources for further assistance. This may include any or all of the following:

● Teaching coping strategies in self-maintenance activities. Where personal independence is limited the therapist aims to minimise dysfunction by suitable means. If the person is severely impaired, and needs to attend a work assessment or training centre, it will be necessary for him to have adequate skills or support for coping with

self-maintenance before embarking on such a scheme.

● Teaching or improving basic skills. Where confidence or abilities are limited the therapist will be concerned with improving the person's level of function. This may include practising using public transport, handling money or developing appropriate social skills. Driving a car may require specialist assessment and practice, which may be available through a disabled driving centre or a driving school such as the British School of Motoring.

● Improving psychological and communication skills. If concentration, perception, or other mental processes have been affected, the therapist may devise activities to improve these skills. Similarly if verbal or written communication is impaired, advice and support from the speech and language therapist and practice with various forms of written communication may develop skills and confidences.

● Improving physical ability. As part of the overall intervention process the occupational therapist will be aiming to help the person to regain or optimise physical function when this has been impaired or is limited. The interventions may include activities to improve range of movement, muscle strength, dexterity, coordination and balance. Liaison with the physiotherapist may be advantageous in some instances to coordinate activities to improve specific functions.

● Building or improving work tolerance and work behaviours. Following illness or a long period away from work, many people have difficulty regaining the work habit or sufficient stamina to cope with a full day's work. Impairments, either congenital or acquired, may further affect work tolerances and behaviours. In such situations the occupational therapist can begin to build up the person's work tolerance through his performance of tasks similar to those required by the job in a simulated work station. Time periods and output demands should be gradually increased to equate, as far as practicable, to the real work situation. Effort and concentration may be improved through changes in the demands of the activity in terms of muscle strength or complexity of the task. It may also be necessary, when designing the work station, to consider developing tolerances for specific environmental conditions, for example, heat, cold, noise, dust, heights, outdoor work or fixed bench work, where these will form part of the real job. The person may need practise to acquire the confidence to work unsupervised, or to attain the necessary levels of stamina and work behaviour suitable for open employment.

• Improving intellectual skills. Assessment enables the therapist to identify the person's level of intellectual performance. Deficits may be the result of injury and impairment, or may have occurred through lack of opportunity to develop specific skills. Standardised assessment or specific tests may be carried out by the therapist, or in conjunction with the psychologist. Following the results of the test the therapist may provide specific activities to meet or overcome particular areas of deficit, or make recommendations for referral to an appropriate educational agency.

It is often difficult for the therapist to simulate the demands imposed by a full day's work in industry or commerce but, where work behaviours and tolerances are limited, improvement in this area can be initiated while the person is regularly attending the hospital or rehabilitation centre. Practice in simulated work tasks builds up skills and confidences before returning to open employment or making an application for alternative training. Employment regulations and health and safety legislation have restricted opportunities to practise work-related tasks in other areas of the hospital or community, but the employment services work training and Job Introduction Schemes (p. 217) provide opportunities to further work preparation.

Advances in technology, in the form of computers, faxes and electronic links to employers, enable people who have difficulties with mobility, self-maintenance activities or verbal communication to work from a home base. In this situation the psychological demands for concentration and adherence to routine are particularly important to maintain the work pattern in the domestic environment. In the past, home-based employment has frequently been in poorly paid assembly or packing tasks, but advances in information technology have raised job status and the level of remuneration for some people who work from a home base.

Following comprehensive work assessment and/or work preparation the occupational therapist may recommend return to previous employment. Where this is not possible, the therapist should complete a report for the Disability Employment Advisor, to assist with advising the individual on the employment opportunites available through the Employment Services. The therapist may also be required to present a report to the consultant, general practitioner or other personnel concerned with the person's future or with his compensation claim.

Giving information and guidance

Frequently, people whose employment prospects are doubtful have little idea of the type of help available to them either for building up fitness for return to work or for retraining for alternative employment. It is often a source of great concern to the person that his future employment prospects seem poor. The occupational therapist should be able to supply accurate and appropriate information on the sources of help available (Fig. 8.7) and on what benefits the person may receive. The therapist may be a member of the team which assesses the person's capabilities and makes direct referral to the Disability Employment Advisor (DEA) or other appropriate agency.

Ordinary further education courses provide pathways for some disabled people to gain experience and qualifications at an academic and social level which may enhance employment opportunities.

The resettlement clinic

In some hospitals or specialist rehabilitation centres a resettlement clinic may be held regularly to determine the future work prospects of individuals undergoing treatment. Such clinics are usually run by the doctor in charge of the unit or the consultant responsible for rehabilitation services. They are usually attended by the occu-

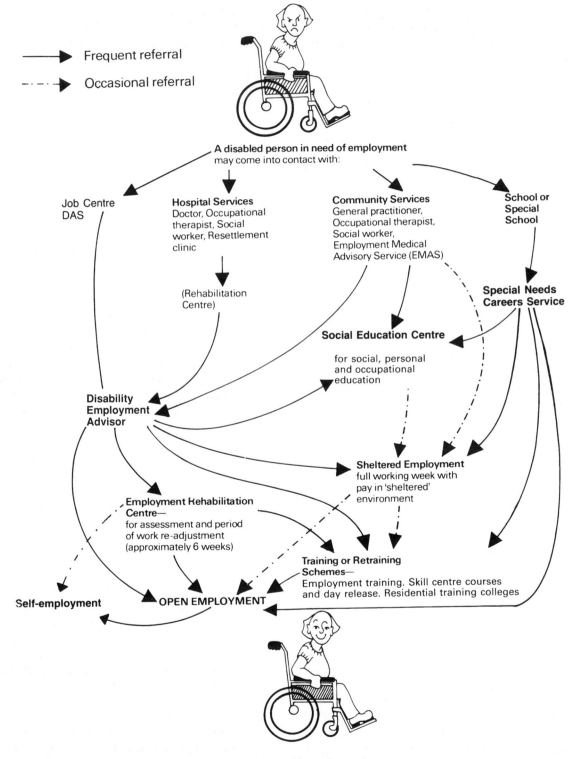

Fig. 8.7 Services available to help the disabled person with employment.

pational therapist, physiotherapist, social worker, a senior nurse attached to the unit (where appropriate) and the DEA. Occasionally, the psychologist or the person's relatives may also attend. The person's case is presented, his progress charted and his future prospects and options discussed. Where further intensive medical treatment is considered advisable, he may be referred to a medical rehabilitation centre. Alternatively, it may be considered that he has reached his maximum potential and that referral to employment training or support services would be more suitable.

Medical rehabilitation centres

These provide an intensive programme of rehabilitation following serious illness or injury. Individuals may be referred to such centres following initial assessment and treatment in hospital. Such centres have the facilities to build up a higher degree of physical fitness and work tolerance than is possible in most hospital departments. Treatment is provided under medical supervision by a team comprising physiotherapists (who may conduct hydrotherapy and gymnasium work), occupational therapists, speech therapists and social workers. The centres offer a non-hospital atmosphere. Some centres are residential on a weekday basis; residents are encouraged to be personally independent and make their own arrangements for transportation and entertainment during their stay.

Sources of assistance for the disabled worker

The Disablement Advisory Service (DAS)

This is part of the Employment Service Agency and is usually based at the Employment Service area office or Job Centre. The DAS exists to assist both employers and people who are already in employment or are seeking work. It can provide advice on developing and implementing a sound company policy on the employment of people with disabilities, as outlined in their *Code of Good Practice on the Employment of Disabled People*. Specific advice may be given regarding the

recruitment, career development and retention of workers with disabilities. A number of special schemes exist to overcome particular difficulties. These include the Job Introduction Scheme, the Special Aids to Employment Scheme, the Adaptations to Premises and Equipment Scheme, the Personal Reader Service for the visually impaired and the Working at Home with Technology Scheme.

Placing, Assessment and Counselling Team (PACT)

These teams, based in Job Centres and consisting of Disability Employment Advisors and Occupational Psychologists, aim to provide coordinated services to help people with disability into employment, to promote the value of people with disabilities to employers, and to help employers recruit and retain people with disabilities.

They provide advice and guidance regarding employment opportunities, counselling and assessment for work, contact with organisations providing work preparation and training, practical help for employment, work placements and continued support for employers and disabled employees.

Training and work preparation programmes usually extend for a period of six weeks in an environment as similar as possible to the 'real' work situation. Here the person is closely monitored and supported to help establish or re-establish a work routine. Alternatively the PACT team may advise on educational opportunities in specialist colleges or in mainstream educational establishments with adequate student support.

Practical help may involve the provision of equipment to minimise the effects of the impairment when working, funding for adapting work premises, or help with costs for funding a support worker for a person with a severe impairment, or for additional expenses incurred by the disabled person when travelling to work.

Work placement aims to place the worker in the most appropriate work environment. This may be in open employment with the necessary support, or may be in sheltered or supported employment, with organisations such as Remploy,

Scope or the Shaw Trust. The DEA acts as a source of information for both the employer and prospective employee. The Job Introduction Scheme provided financial incentives to employers to provide a trial period in a particular job for prospective disabled employees.

The DEA also acts as an advocate for employment of people with disabilities by working with people with disabilities and employers 'to help more employers employ more disabled people more effectively'. The use of the Disability Symbol promotes this. The commitments of employers using the disability symbol are:

- to interview all applicants with a disability who meet the minimum criteria for a job vacancy and to consider them on their abilities
- to ask disabled employees, at least once every year, what can be done to ensure they can use and develop their abilities at work
- to make every effort when employees become disabled, to make sure they stay in employment
- to take action to ensure that key employees develop the necessary awareness of disability to make the commitments work
- to revise the commitments each year by reviewing what has been achieved, planning ways to improve these achievements, and informing all employees of progress and future plans.

DEAs may provide practical information about ways of putting the commitments into practice, where to access expert guidance if an employee becomes disabled, and advice on ways of developing disability awareness. They may also aim to give a speedy response to help recruit someone with a disability where a suitable vacancy exists, and provide advice and individual help to access specialist support to facilitate successful employment of a person with a disability.

Employment Rehabilitation Centres (ERCs)

These centres provide opportunities for people who have not been employed for some time following illness or injury and who need a chance to adapt themselves gradually to normal working conditions. The ERCs also assess people's employment capabilities. Courses vary according to individual needs and the facilities offered aim to simulate working conditions and a realistic work atmosphere.

During the stay at the centre individuals are paid a tax-free maintenance allowance which is at a higher rate than basic unemployment and sickness benefit. Each person's programme is regularly discussed and reviewed at a case conference.

Employment training

A number of employment training schemes are available for the disabled person on a residential or daily basis. Residential colleges provide training courses for disabled people in a range of commercial and vocational skills. Trainees receive an allowance while on the course. Applications should be made through the local DEA. Local employment training initiatives vary from area to area and information is available through the DEA at local employment training or skill centres. Some further education establishments provide day release courses and other employment training courses suitable for disabled people.

Sheltered work

Where the disabled person is unable to work in open employment sheltered work provides an opportunity for him to offer a productive day's work under realistic conditions. Sheltered employment, established under the Disabled Persons (Employment) Act 1944, can be provided through Remploy Ltd, local authority workshops or schemes organised by voluntary organisations. Remploy provides jobs for severely disabled people under sheltered yet realistic commercial conditions. Products include furniture, leather goods, textiles and equipment for disabled people. Employees are paid a wage for their work. Local authority workshops and those run by voluntary organisations such as the Royal British Legion and Scope also provide work, usually under contract to local firms. In most workshops people must be capable of putting in a standard working week even though their output is low.

Social education centre

For those who are unable to cope with either open or sheltered employment, social education centres run by the local authority offer social and occupational education. As well as simple work tasks performed in a realistic work atmosphere (again, usually under contract to local firms), these centres provide education in life skills such as self-maintenance, homemaking and social interaction. Trainees receive standard state benefits while attending the centre and a small remuneration for the work they produce. Some people may progress to further courses after a period at the centre.

Other initiatives

A variety of local community programmes are available to help the less disabled person who has not worked for some time to regain confidence. These differ from region to region and rely largely on local initiatives.

Some specialist training courses are offered for people with particular impairments; for example, training schemes for visually impaired people are offered by the Royal National Institute for the Blind.

The Rehabilitation Engineering Movement Advisory Panels (REMAP) will also design and provide special items of equipment to assist the disabled person to overcome a particular problem at work.

Self-employment

Able-bodied and disabled people alike may wish to become self-employed, using their skills in a creative or consultative capacity. Starting one's own business can seem very attractive but there are many factors to consider before embarking on such a venture. Realistic, reliable advice regarding available resources and potential pitfalls is of vital importance. Consideration should be given to the viability of the skill or product in

question, and to financing the venture in terms of materials, premises, marketing and production costs. The physical, psychological and social demands of such a project should be assessed realistically in light of the person's impairment, and the stress that self-employment is likely to cause to the individual and his carers should be considered. The DEA may be able to advise the disabled person regarding the opportunities and schemes available to him, and advice from banking and business agencies will be invaluable.

The disabled employer

Many people are able to maintain their role as employers despite substantial levels of physical disability. Much will depend on the type of work involved. Cognitive and communication skills are usually the disabled employer's most important personal assets. Modern technology and good support staff have enabled people with limited mobility and very restricted physical skills to continue in the managerial role, using their knowledge and experience to organise and negotiate effectively, and retaining their pride, dignity and the respect of employees and customers.

The Employment Service Agency may provide advice concerning specialist equipment or other resources available to the disabled employer.

THE STUDENT

Studying is included here under the work role because many of the skills necessary for successful schooling are similar to those needed in employment. Both roles require adherence to the rules or regime of the establishment, social skills to communicate with those in authority and with one's peers, practical skills to meet the demands of set tasks, and mobility skills to travel to, from and within the school or campus.

The occupational therapist's role is also similar in both situations. She may be involved in assessing and developing skills in relation to the demands of the role, reporting to others about individual needs, and providing advice, guidance and liaison between the individual and the establishment to facilitate successful integration.

The 1981 Education Act encouraged increased placement of disabled children in mainstream schools. The occupational therapist may be involved in detailed assessment of the child's abilities for the Statement of Special Needs. Areas evaluated may include independence in personal care tasks, fine and gross motor skills, and perceptual, cognitive and social skills. The Statement aims to ensure that the necessary provision is available for the child at school. The therapist may be involved in the development of these skills in readiness for school and she may also be required to provide advice to parents and teachers. This may include recommendations on site modifications, handling techniques, and special equipment to promote mobility or facilitate teaching and learning.

For the older student, the therapist may assist with the assessment and development of skills for future study, employment and community living.

Many adult and elderly disabled people who are unemployed or retired may consider study as a means of purposefully filling the day without the direct objective of attaining gainful employment.

THE VOLUNTEER

Some disabled people who are not in paid employment use their knowledge and skills in a voluntary capacity to assist others. The range of voluntary activities is extensive and provides assistance to all age groups. People who have skilled knowledge and experience in managerial activities may be valued members of voluntary groups, while others who have particular physical skills or communicative abilities may be able to use these in teaching or assisting others. Personal experience of problems often promotes greater understanding of the difficulties others may be facing. Some people with disabilities become active members of disability organisations or pressure groups which aim to improve recognition and facilities for disabled people in general.

Many people who do not wish to join the paid workforce find that their volunteer 'work' provides structure, satisfaction, pride in their abilities and recognition. In some instances, volunteer work has led to paid work in open employment or to educational or managerial roles in charitable organisations.

In conclusion, purposeful occupation — whether as homemaker, carer, worker, employer, student or volunteer — is a vital component of the disabled person's quality of life. Many disabled people are able to fulfil some if not all of the duties associated with their roles, and the occupational therapist may assist them in recognising, maximising, and utilising their skills and in identifying techniques, equipment and resources that will help them to overcome particular areas of difficulty.

LEISURE

Leisure-time pursuits are an important part of any person's daily life. These may include hobbies, sports, exercise, entertainment, holidays, relaxation, and play. For the disabled or elderly person who is not able to work, leisure plays an even more important part in living. Leisure activities and involvement in local organisations are a substitute for work and provide opportunities for participation in creative activities and for maintaining or increasing social contacts. They may introduce the person to broader areas of interest and compensate him for the lack of status associated with unemployment.

Initially, leisure activities may help the more severely impaired or elderly person to adjust to a new life-style, but later these activities may become more than a time-filler. They may encourage the individual to strive for more knowledge and skills than he had time for previously.

Individual needs differ considerably, depending on the temperament, personality, interests and level of intelligence of the person, as well as on the impairments he may have. The therapist must be aware of such factors before she can guide the person towards fulfilling his needs. She needs to take into account previous interests, for these may still be pursued to advantage by some people; however, for others who have a significant level of impairment, returning to previous activities may cause frustration and accentuate functional losses. Much will depend on the person's desires and the facilities and resources available locally to meet his requirements.

EXPLORING LEISURE OPTIONS

The most important task is to identify what the disabled person would like to gain from leisure pursuits. For some people socialisation may be the prime objective, while others may see creativity as the most important aspect. Socialisation may involve active participation with others in a social setting or group; alternatively, the individual may be a passive receiver in a social environment such as the cinema, theatre or at a football match. The range of possible creative activities is immense. Some people may wish to join others in classes or groups, while others may prefer to be creative in their home environment if the facilities and materials are available. Others may wish to expand their education and knowledge through adult classes or independent learning methods.

Leisure pursuits may be explored individually, giving an opportunity for the development of relationships away from the carer or family. Such wishes should be clearly identified and discussed to avoid any feelings of rejection on the part of the family or carers. Alternatively, the disabled person and the family may wish to identify activities that all members can participate in together. This may be particularly important for holidays.

Issues such as travel, transport, cost of materials or activities and any special equipment should be explored. Some financial assistance may be available either through reduced attendance fees or through grants or loans from charitable organisations such as the British Sports Association for the Disabled or the Royal National Institute for the Blind. Jay (1984) suggests that many disabled people do not participate in the wide range of leisure opportunities available to them because of:

- lack of confidence in their ability to

participate, which reduces motivation to explore options
- lack of knowledge of how or where to find information about leisure activities.

Confidence

Some people do not wish to join activities specifically for disabled people. They would prefer to participate in activities with people who are not disabled, but are concerned about others' attitudes to them and whether they will be able to participate equally. Unfortunately, many may have suffered rejection or over-protection by their non-disabled peers because of their impairment.

The therapist can help such individuals to discuss their anxieties and societal attitudes and can provide opportunities for assertiveness training and confidence building. Where he lacks confidence in his practical abilities to pursue the activity, the disabled person may be able to explore the activity in a day centre before joining a local group or club. Many centres provide a wide range of social and leisure activities with help and guidance from centre staff or peers. Books and reference texts may be obtained from the local library to assist learning.

If communication skills are impaired they may be improved through regular practice in communication techniques in a safe environment in one-to-one and group activities. Social skills training may occur in discussion groups, role play, video exercises and organised excursions. Cognitive skills may be developed through reality orientation, problem-solving games and simple quizzes or through activities or exercises that involve following verbal or written instructions.

A one-to-one introduction may assist both the organisers and the disabled person to share concerns and discuss any special arrangements which may ease anxieties about participation in a club, class or group. In some instances a relative or carer may be able to accompany the disabled person; this may reassure him, particularly on the first visit. However, if he is happy with his choice of activity he may not wish the relative or carer to continue attending, as this may impede his social integration. It is possible in some instances for the occupational therapist to fulfil this introductory role.

Sources of information and range of options

Nationally, information may be obtained from a number of sources. Many charities provide information on the range of activities available to their members. Additionally, the Disabled Living Foundation information leaflets, the Equipment for the Disabled booklet *Leisure and Gardening* and the *Directory of Sports and Leisure for the Disabled*, as well as many other leaflets and books, provide a wide range of information on organisations and equipment specifically for disabled people (see Further reading on p. 224). On a local basis, information can usually be obtained from the Citizens' Advice Bureau, leisure or education services departments of the local council and from the social services department. Access information and details of facilities available in particular areas can be obtained from city information and access guides, and organisations such as the National Trust provide their own information booklets.

Information about travel can be obtained from the Department of Transport *Door to Door* booklet, RADAR publications on holidays and travel, and from RAC and AA publications. A number of holiday organisations have details of access and mobility facilities in holiday accommodation in resorts in Britain and abroad. Some organisations provide holidays specifically for disabled people and their families.

The range of leisure options available to a disabled individual may include:

- practical pastimes such as model-making, gardening, photography, cookery and needlework
- intellectual pursuits, including further or higher education, adult education classes, study and appreciation of music, art, literature, computing and many other areas of interest which may be used for intellectual stimulation or pleasurable appreciation
- active participation in sports or games, ranging from card or board games to more active pursuits such as archery, swimming, riding or skiing
- specific interest collections such as stamps, coins, books, records and many other collectable items
- interests requiring little or no active participation, such as theatre, cinema, television and radio, music or spectator sports
- social clubs which organise particular social activities or outings, either specifically for disabled people or as a broader facility for all.

In conclusion, a wide range of opportunities are available for the disabled person to pursue leisure activities at home or in the community. The occupational therapist may introduce leisure interests through therapeutic social activities or may provide information on where to obtain details of services or equipment. She may stimulate the disabled person to explore old skills or interests or encourage him to consider new leisure pursuits. For those who are not able to obtain paid employment, leisure activities provide structure to the day and enhance self-esteem.

Satisfaction, pleasure or achievement in recreational activities can add quality to the day or week and promote a sense of purpose and well-being for the disabled person, and may ease some of the emotional burden on relatives and carers.

CONCLUSION

This chapter has attempted to outline the life skills necessary for successful community living. Of necessity, the coverage of each particular area has been superficial. The chapter has addressed the main aspects of self-maintenance, role duties and leisure, but the reader will need to explore particular areas in more detail to meet the specific needs for a given individual. The practice chapters in this volume will identify some of the problems resulting from specific diagnoses, but other texts which provide detailed information on equipment, techniques or particular life skills should be explored.

Many of the techniques used by the occupational therapist in helping the disabled individual to develop life skills are based on the rehabilitative approach, and thus explore ways of compensating for loss of function. However, these techniques should not be used in isolation as many problems may be minimised or overcome by the use of other therapeutic approaches to enhance physical, intellectual or social performance, and thereby improve function.

Realistic consideration of the individual's personal wishes in the context of his present physical, social, psychological and environmental situation is the crucial factor in devising a strategy which will meet his needs and those of his relatives and carers in developing life skills.

USEFUL ADDRESSES

Association of Carers
29 Chilworth Mews
London W2 3RG

Association of Crossroads Care
Attendant Schemes Ltd
10 Regent Place
Rugby
Warwickshire
CV21 2PN

Association to Aid the Sexual and Personal Relationships of People with a Disability (SPOD)
286 Camden Road
London N7 0BJ

Banstead Place Mobility Centre
Park Road
Banstead
Surrey SM7 3EE

British Sports Association for the Disabled
34 Osmaburgh Street
London NW1 3ND

Centre on Environment of the Handicapped
35 Great Smith Street
London SW1P 3BJ

DIAL UK
Dial House
117 High Street
Clay Cross
Chesterfield
Derbyshire
S45 9DZ

Disabled Living Centres Council
c/o Disabled Living Foundation
380–384 Harrow Road
London W9 2HU

Disabled Living Foundation
380–384 Harrow Road
London W9 2HU

Disability Alliance
25 Denmark Street
London WC2 8NJ

Equal Opportunities Commission
Overseas House
Quay Street
Manchester M3 3HN

Equipment for the Disabled
Mary Marlborough Lodge
Nuffield Orthopaedic Centre
Headington
Oxford OX3 7LD

Kings Fund Centre
126 Albert Street
London NW1 7NF

Mobility Advice and Vehicle Information Service
Department of Transport TRRL
Crowthorne
Berkshire RG11 6AU

National Council for Voluntary Organisations
26 Bedford Square
London WC1B 3HU

Rehabilitation Engineering Movement
Advisory Panel (REMAP)
25 Mortimer Street
London W1N 8AB

Royal Association for Disability
and Rehabilitation (RADAR)
25 Mortimer Street
London WIN 8AB

Royal National Institute for the Blind
224 Great Portland Street
London W1N 6AA

Royal National Institute for the Deaf
105 Gower Street
London WC1E 6AH

REFERENCES

British Telecom 1989 Action for disabled customers. British Telecommunications, London

Bullard D G, Knight S E 1981 Sexuality and physical disability — personal perspectives. C V Mosby, St Louis

Chronically Sick and Disabled Persons Act 1970. HMSO, London

Comfort A 1978 Sexual consequences of disability. Stickley, London

Cynkin S, Robinson A M 1990 Occupational therapy and activities health: toward health through activities. Little, Brown, Boston

Department of Transport 1989 Door to door. A guide to transport for disabled people. Department of Transport, London

Disabled Persons (Employment) Act 1994. HMSO, London

Disabled Persons Services, Consultation and Representation Act 1986. HMSO, London

Education Act 1981. HMSO, London

Goldsmith S 1984 Designing for the disabled, 4th edn. Royal Institute of British Architects, London

Jacobs K 1991 Occupational therapy: work-related programs and assessments, 2nd edn. Little, Brown, Boston

Jay P 1984 Coping with disability. Disabled Living Foundation, London

Katz S, Ford A B, Moskowitz R W, Jackson B, Jaffe M W 1963 Studies of illness in the aged. The index of ADL: a standardised measure of biological and psychosocial function. Journal of the American Medical Association 185(12): 914–919

Kings Fund 1985 Designing bathrooms for disabled people. Kings Fund, London

Kuczynski J H 1980 Nursing and medical students' sexual attitudes and knowledge. Journal of Obstetric, Gynecological and Neonatal Nursing, Nov–Dec: 339–342

Mandelstam D 1986 Incontinence and its management. Croom Helm, London

Trombly C A 1989 Occupational therapy for physical dysfunction, 3rd edn. Williams & Wilkins, Baltimore

Walbrook Housing Association 1992 Cracking housing problems. A practical guide to problem solving for disabled people, occupational therapists and carers. Walbrook Housing Association Ltd, Derby

Williams R 1968 Communications. Penguin, London

Yerxa E J, Locker S B 1990 Quality of time use by adults with spinal cord injuries. American Journal of Occupational Therapy 44(4): 318–326

FURTHER READING

British Association of Occupational Therapists. Occupational Therapists Reference Book. Parke Sutton, Norwich in association with BAOT, London (Published biennially)

Charities Aid Foundation. Directory of grant making trusts. Charities Aid Foundation, London (Published annually)

Cochrane G M (ed.) 1990 Equipment for disabled people. Series of information booklets. Disability Information Trust, Oxford

Disability Alliance and Educational Research Association. Disability Rights Handbook (Published annually), Anderson Fraser, London

Disabled Living Foundation Hamilton Index 1994 DLF, London

Disabled Living Foundation 1993 Handling people — equipment, advice and information. DLF, London

Fenton M, Hughes P 1989 Passivity to empowerment. A living skills curriculum for people with disabilities. RADAR, London

HMSO. Department of Health Disability Equipment Assessment Programme Reports. Series of reports on specialist equipment. DOH Publications, Heywood, Lancashire

Honey S, Meager N, Williams M 1993 Employers attitudes towards people with disabilities. Institute of Manpower Studies, University of Sussex & College Press Ltd, Brighton

Maczka K 1990 Assessing physically disabled people at home. Chapman & Hall, London

Mandelstam M 1993 How to get equipment for disability, 3rd edn. DLF, London

Oliver M, Zarb G 1993 Ageing with disability. What do they expect after all these years? University of Greenwich, London

Roper N, Logan W W, Tierney A J 1990 The elements of nursing: a model of nursing based on a model of living. Churchill Livingstone, Edinburgh

Smith P, Porall M, Floyd M 1991 Managing disability at work. Improving practice in organisations. Jessica Kingsley, London

Swain J, Finkelstein V, French S, Oliver M 1993 Disabling barriers, enabling environments. Sage, London

Skills for caring 1992 A series of teaching/learning handbooks for carers and care workers. Churchill Livingstone, Edinburgh

9

Mobility skills

Ann Turner

INTRODUCTION

Independent mobility is a skill which develops throughout normal infancy and childhood into adult life. From the baby's first attempts at lifting, moving and controlling his head to the adult's proficiency at dancing, cycling, running and climbing, many forms of independent mobility are practised, improved upon and mastered.

Alongside this increasing ability to move and control our bodies we develop our cognitive and social abilities. Together, all these abilities allow us to explore, control and adapt to our environment and to create and maintain our personal, social and working lives. Our ability to move, therefore, becomes an integral part of our lives, and something we take for granted. Not until it becomes affected in some way do we realise the wide-reaching consequences that the loss of independent mobility may have on all aspects of our lives. Stepping on a nail, for instance, may cause a relatively minor injury, but can temporarily render someone unable to walk without the assistance of sticks or crutches, climb up stairs, get into a bath with ease, drive to or at work, dig the garden or play with the children. Not only may the person's activities be limited, but any activity he does perform may take twice the time and energy that it did before. In the short term this interruption to daily activity may be viewed as an enforced 'holiday', an opportunity to rest, sit back and let others take on the work and responsibility for a while. However, should such a state of restricted mobility continue for

with caution. The weight of the user determines the amount of spring assistance built into the chair. Different types of controls are also available to suit individual needs.

Chair to chair

Types of independent transfers from one chair to another are:

- Corner transfer (Fig. 9.2)
- Side transfer (Fig. 9.3)
- Transfer using a sliding board (Fig. 9.4)
- Front transfer (Fig. 9.5).

Bed transfers

Transfers onto or off a bed can be made easier if the following points are borne in mind.

- *The bed frame.* For many disabled people a standard divan bed is too low to allow easy transfer. Where possible the height of the bed, i.e. the distance from the floor to the top of the mattress *when compressed,* should be as near as possible to the height of the seat of the chair onto which the person will transfer. For a standing transfer onto or up from a bed the compressed mattress should be at the optimum height to allow easy transfer. The height of the bed can be altered by

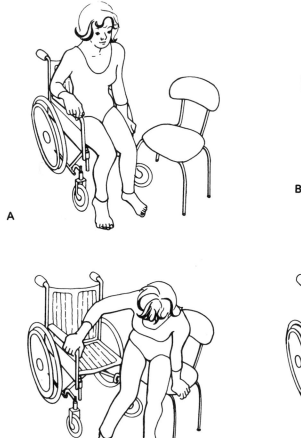
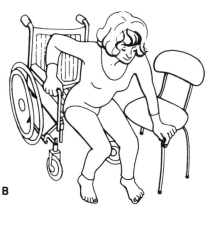
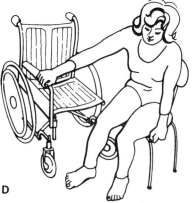

Fig. 9.2 Corner transfer.

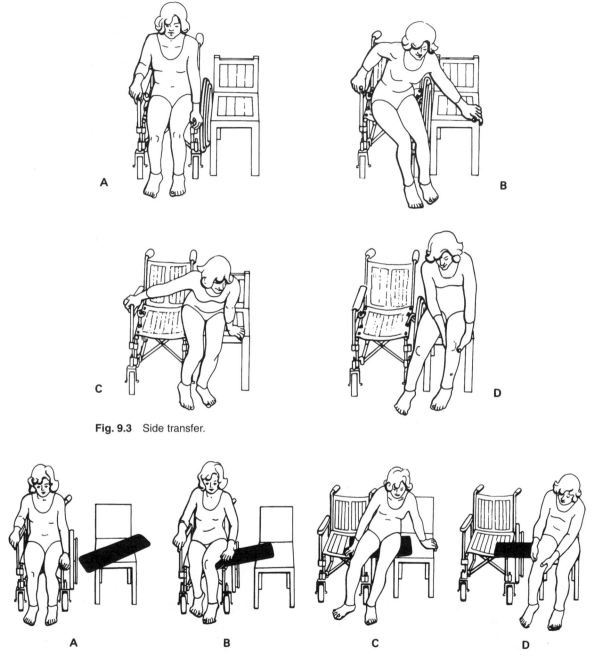

Fig. 9.3 Side transfer.

Fig. 9.4 Transfer using a sliding board.

lengthening or shortening the bed legs or by the use of *secure* bed blocks. In some cases it may be advantageous to remove the castors from the bed legs, as these may cause the bed to move during transfer.

• *The mattress.* This should be the same width as the bed frame. A firm-edged mattress is easier to rise from. If the mattress edge is soft, boards can be placed between the mattress and the bed frame to provide a firm base for transfers. Ideally,

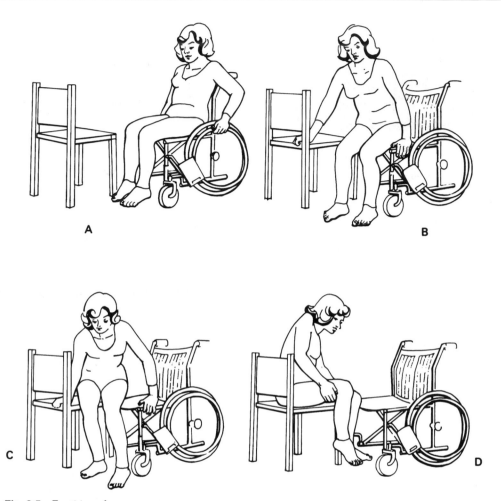

Fig. 9.5 Front transfer.

the boards should cover the whole width of a single bed and at least half the width of a double bed so that the individual does not have the additional problem of negotiating a ridge in the mattress.

● *Positioning*. When the person needs to transfer to a chair or walking aid there must be sufficient space at the side of the bed for these manoeuvres.

Sitting up in bed

See Figure 9.6.

Sitting over the edge of the bed

See Figure 9.7.

Getting up from the bed

The same principles apply here as for getting up from a chair. If additional support is needed a bed aid, head or foot board, or *stable* piece of furniture, such as a chest of drawers placed permanently by the bed, can be used for the person to push up on.

Sitting down on a bed

The same principles apply here as for sitting down on a chair.

Lifting legs onto the bed

This can often cause a problem if legs are weak

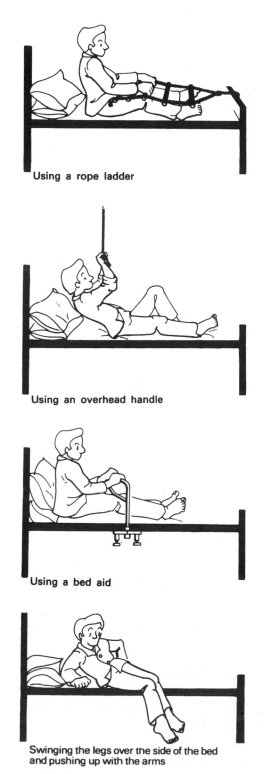

Using a rope ladder

Using an overhead handle

Using a bed aid

Swinging the legs over the side of the bed and pushing up with the arms

Fig. 9.6 Sitting up in bed.

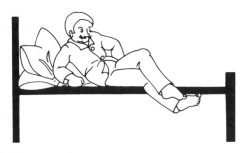

Hooking the weak leg over the strong leg

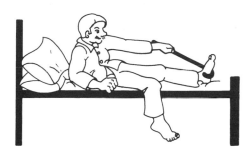

Lifting the weak leg with the aid of a stick handle

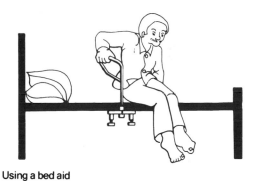

Using a bed aid

Fig. 9.7 Sitting over the edge of the bed.

and/or oedematous. It may be possible to hook one leg over the other or to use a walking stick handle (see Fig. 9.7). Alternatively, a stool or a low chair may be used as a 'half-way house'. Leg ladders and other commercial equipment are also available and may be tried to see if they help an individual where the above methods do not.

Bed to chair, chair to bed

The transfer used depends on the person's ability

and the space available around the bed. Consequently, a standing, corner, side or sliding board transfer, as already described, may be used. If none of these is appropriate a forward transfer (Fig. 9.8) may be tried.

Toilet transfers

When transferring to and from a toilet several points should be borne in mind:

• Many toilets, especially modern ones, are quite low and the seat may, therefore, need raising to allow easy transfers. Various designs of seat raise are available and the therapist must ensure that a raise fits *securely* before issuing it. Ejector and sloping seats are also available.

• Grab rails fixed to the wall near the toilet, or frames fixed around the toilet, will provide a firm grip for transfer. Again, many designs are available, including some which combine a toilet frame and raised seat.

• An individual must be able to cope with clothing, toilet paper and flushing the toilet as well as with transferring on and off the toilet.

• Where transfer onto the toilet presents great difficulty because of the person's disability, lack of space, distance to the toilet or other barriers, alternatives such as commodes, urinals, sanichairs

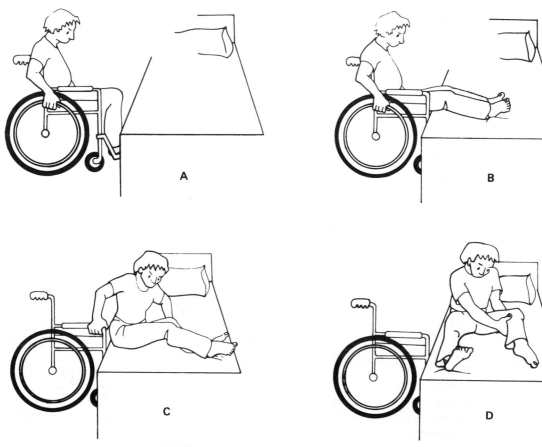

Fig. 9.8 Forward transfer onto a bed.

or sanitary facilities combined with wheelchairs or hoists must be considered.

• If a wheelchair is used the type selected should allow easy and close access to the toilet.

Standing up from and sitting down onto the toilet

The same principles are applied as for 'standing from sitting' and 'sitting from standing'.

Chair to toilet

The following methods may be employed:

• Corner transfer (see Fig. 9.2)
• Side transfer (see Fig. 9.3)
• Front transfer (see Fig. 9.5)
• Forward transfer (see Fig. 9.8). Note that for this transfer (for example, for a double lower limb amputee) the person uses the toilet facing the cistern with his legs on either side of the seat. Toilet rails are essential to assist transfer.

Bath transfers

Independent transfers into and out of the bath will require much practice and, frequently, considerable upper limb strength. Whenever bath transfers are being attempted it is advisable that the person be supervised until he is quite certain of his ability, so that assistance may be given if necessary. Where the bather, understandably, wishes to maintain his privacy it is advisable that someone remain within earshot in case the bather needs to shout for assistance. Alternatively a pull-cord alarm may be installed.

Where bath transfers create major problems that cannot be overcome by bath aids, an alternative method such as a shower, all-over wash or bed bath may be preferable for the sake of ease and safety. Where major expenditure is feasible, a specially designed bath such as one with opening sides may be considered as an alternative or in addition to the existing bath. It may be necessary to consider whether the person would prefer to expend the considerable time and energy required by bathing on activities which he sees as having greater priority.

Where aids such as bath boards, bath seats or grab rails are needed these should always be checked for security and safety and should, if at all possible, have a non-slip surface. It is also advisable that either a non-slip bath mat or some non-slip patches be placed in the bottom of the bath. Other bath transfer aids, such as those that work on an electrically operated bellows system, or a hoist, can also be considered. The therapist must also ensure that any aids selected will not cause damage to the bath/shower tray — especially if these are made of fibreglass.

Getting into and out of the bath from standing

Many types of grab rails are available for those who need a little help getting into and out of the bath. Two types are illustrated in Figures 9.9 and 9.10. Some baths are designed with integral grab rails.

Getting into and out of the bath from a sitting position

Transfers from a chair, stool, wheelchair, extended bath board, bath side or other seated position will now be described. For side transfer

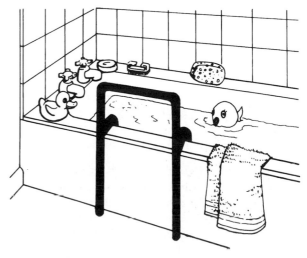

Fig. 9.9 Side-mounted rail

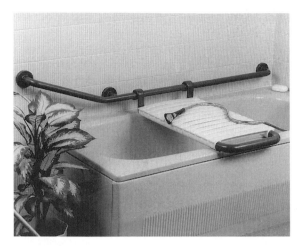

Fig. 9.10 Wall-mounted rail (used in conjunction with a bath board). (Reproduced by kind permission of Keep Able.)

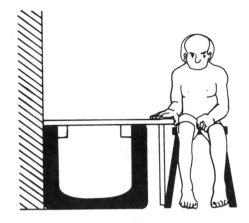

techniques with and without bath aids, see Figures 9.11–9.13. The following points should be noted:

- For those with a unilateral weakness it is advisable to have the stronger side nearest to the bath when getting in
- The person may take an all-over wash or shower while sitting over the bath on the bath board
- For many, the provision of a seat by the side of the bath, plus an inside bath seat, will suffice
- For those who need additional help the provision of an electrically or mechanically operated bath seat (Fig. 9.13) may be appropriate.

ASSISTED TRANSFERS

PRINCIPLES

For those whose disability does not allow them to move independently, assistance with transfers may be necessary. The therapist must be aware that under these circumstances both the disabled person and his assistant must have confidence in one another. Such confidence will come from the knowledge that each is sure of the moves the

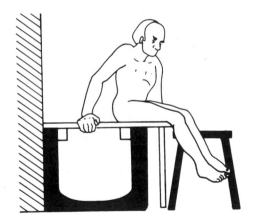

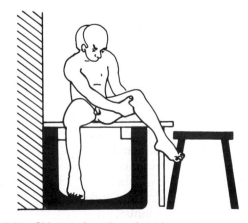

Fig. 9.11 Side transfer using a board.

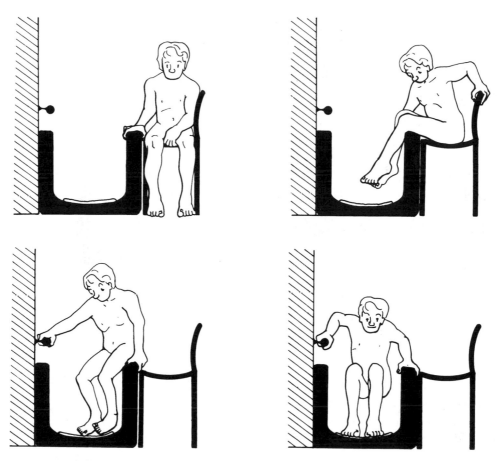

Fig. 9.12   Side transfer without aids.

other will carry out and that each person is sure of his own role in the procedure.

Legislation governing the therapist while undertaking manual handling manoeuvres

Under the EC Directive on Health and Safety at Work, implemented in 1992, one of the six regulations brought into effect related to the manual handling of loads (Health and Safety Executive 1992). These Manual Handling Operations Regulations (MHO Regulations) clarify the existing Health and Safety regulations and put responsibilities on both employers and employees to help prevent injury during manual handling manoeuvres.

Under the Regulations manual handling is defined as 'Movement of loads, by human effort, as opposed to mechanical handling' (MHO Regulations, p. 6). Within the directive a 'load' is described as any 'discrete movable object' and can therefore include people, equipment and materials. Manual handling includes transporting a load and/or supporting a load in a static posture. Lifting, putting down, pushing, pulling and carrying are also included in the definition. Lifting, within the directive, is defined as 'movement of a patient in which vertical displacement is a dominant feature', while transferring is defined as 'actions where movements are mainly horizontal, although there may be some vertical movement'. Assisted transfers involve the person being moved taking some of his own weight and helping towards the movement.

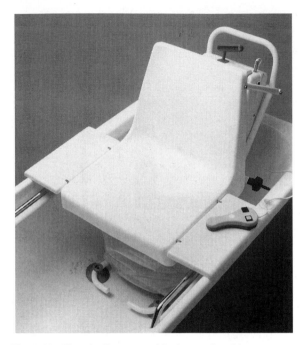

Fig. 9.13 Electrically operated bath transfer aid. (Reproduced by kind permission of Keep Able.)

The Regulations state that the employer has responsibility to assess the risks of injury to employees and, where a risk is identified, should ensure that:

- as far as is reasonably practical, the need to undertake any such manual handling operation is avoided
- any operations that cannot be avoided are assessed. Such an assessment should include information on the *load* (the person to be moved), the *individual* capability of the employee (for example knowledge and physical abilities), the *task* (the mechanics of the lift), and the working *environment* (space, heights, flooring, etc.) (*LITE*)
- the risk of injury is reduced as far as is reasonably practical.

The Directive's guidelines on how a hazardous manual handling operation could be assessed (see above) have, in many areas, formed the basis of assessment forms used within health and social services departments, and any occupational therapist whose work involves manual handling

should, therefore, acquaint herself with local interpretations of these assessment regulations.

The Directive also gives guidelines on how the risk of injury may be reduced. These guidelines, while not meant to be regarded as precise recommendations, give suggestions which could be considered during assessment. They give a recommended guideline weight for lifting by one person of no more that 25 kg (just under 4 stone), and thus for two people of 50 kg (just under 8 stone). Any person weighing more than 50 kg is deemed to be 'heavy' and alternatives to manual lifting should be considered. When considering assisted transfers, estimating how much weight is taken by the handler(s) and how much is taken through the person's foot is not a straightforward nor a wholly accurate process, and methods for estimating this will vary from service to service.

Responsibility for avoiding injury also lies with the employee. The Regulations state that each employee should make full and proper use of any system of work provided by the employer. This therefore puts responsibility on the occupational therapist to acquaint herself with, and use correctly, any specific regulations, systems, methods or equipment related to manual handling operations that are in operation at her place of work. The employee should, therefore:

- inform the employer of any condition which might affect her ability to undertake manual handling safely
- assist in making assessments or refer to a qualified risk assessor
- undertake training where provided
- keep precise records related to practice with individual patients.

Bearing the above in mind, various principles that apply when carrying out assisted transfers can be formulated.

- Before giving assistance the helper must be aware of, by means of assessment, the amount of help the person requires and how much assistance he is able to give.
- In some instances the person will be able to tell the helper how he is usually moved and/or

of any special needs which may affect the way he is moved.

• Giving assistance during transfer often demands considerable effort and the helper should therefore learn, practise and cultivate skill and technique rather than rely on strength. The helper should know her own capabilities and that of any assistant.

• The 'force' for assistance comes from the leg muscles. The helper should ensure that before and during the manoeuvre her hips and knees are flexed, her spine erect and untwisted, her head erect and her feet well spaced to give a firm base, and that balance is maintained throughout. She should use her body weight to balance and move the person.

• The helper should prepare the way, ensuring that any aids necessary are to hand and that the place the person is transferring to is prepared. There should be an obstacle-free passage through which both people can move.

• The helper should prepare herself, know exactly what help she is going to give and stand in the appropriate place to give it. She should ensure that she is suitably dressed — that shoes give firm support, that clothing allows adequate movement and that hair or jewellery do not dangle across the disabled person. The helper/therapist should also ensure that personal hygiene does not give offence!

• The helper should prepare the person, obtaining his permission and cooperation and explaining what she is going to do and how he can help. She should ask him to move into the position required to start the transfer or move him into that position if he cannot manage alone. She should ensure that he understands where he is transferring to and what method will be used to get him there.

• The helper should always lift towards herself and should hold the person as closely as possible.

• To facilitate movement the helper may rock the person backwards and forwards in the chair to help him gain enough impetus to stand. She should give clear instructions (such as 'one, two, three, GO') if appropriate.

As with independent transfers, there is no 'correct' way of giving assistance. When decid-

ing which transfer to use the therapist should consider:

• the person's abilities — balance, ability to bear weight, upper limb strength, cognition and whether the situation is static or changing
• the helper's abilities — her strength, fitness and cognitive ability
• the relative builds of the helper and disabled person
• the environment in which the transfer will be executed, including the relative heights and positions of surfaces, the space available and the floor covering
• legislation — policies determining which transfer methods are acceptable in any particular location.

Some basic holds are illustrated in Figures 9.14–9.18. The pelvic hold is described in some detail to explain some of the principles that apply to all assisted transfers.

The pelvic hold (Fig. 9.14)

• The person prepares for transfer by sitting towards the front of the chair, leaning slightly forward and placing one foot (the stronger where this is applicable, or the dominant) slightly behind the other. His feet should be apart.

• The helper faces the person and places one foot and knee against the person's forward leg and knee in order to 'block' the leg and prevent

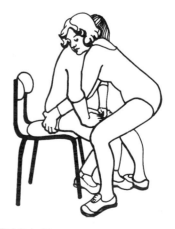

Fig. 9.14 Pelvic hold.

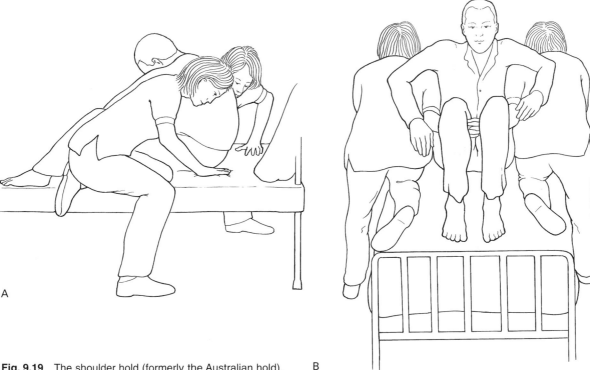

A

B

Fig. 9.19 The shoulder hold (formerly the Australian hold).

suitable slings or a static seat, from one place to another. A hoist is usually supplied in a person's home because:

- the person is unable to transfer himself independently. This inability may be total or may apply to just some situations such as transferring into and out of the bath
- assistance with transfers as previously described is not feasible, perhaps because of the carer's limitations of strength and/or stamina
- the carer and the disabled person prefer an alternative method of transfer to be available for all or some occasions.

SUPPLYING A HOIST

It is essential that an accurate assessment is made before a hoist is supplied, and that adequate training is given to all users once it is installed. Hoists and slings that are not suitable for a particular situation can be uncomfortable and, in-

deed, may be dangerous to use. Equally, if people are uncertain of how to use a hoist this may cause damage to the disabled person, the helper or the hoist itself. A bad experience when using a hoist can damage the users' confidence and make them apprehensive about or unwilling to use the hoist again. In order for a hoist to be used competently and regularly it must meet the needs of the disabled person and his helper to the extent that daily life is simpler with rather than without it. When a hoist is supplied it is essential that a maintenance contract is established so that both hoist and slings are checked regularly and assistance is readily available should the hoist break down. The users must be aware that they must *never* tamper with a hoist, try to adapt its slings or use another manufacturer's slings with that hoist.

ASSESSMENT

The therapist needs to consider the following when assessing for a hoist.

The user

- *Need for a hoist*. Is a hoist really necessary? Can the inability to transfer be more appropriately overcome by other means, such as a new transfer technique, a different wheelchair or an alteration to the environment?
- *Physical abilities and limitations*. These will influence the type of hoist supplied and the type of sling/seat to go with it. The therapist should look specifically at the user's head control, sitting balance, limb control, muscle tone and sensory abilities, especially related to visual and tactile appreciation. It is important to note that those people with amputations of the lower limb(s) will need special attention regarding the counterbalance of the slings. Do his physical abilities enable him to use a hoist or not?
- *Height and weight*. This must be taken into account in selecting the most suitable size of hoist and sling.
- *Clinical condition and prognosis*. This may indicate the period of time for which the hoist may be required and can be important when considering the feasibility of a permanent or temporary arrangement.
- *Cognitive abilities*. Can the person learn to use the hoist independently if he is physically able to do so? If not, has he the ability to cooperate with the carer by controlling his limbs and posture?
- *Specific needs*. For what purposes will the hoist be used? Do the slings need to be used for transferring on/off the toilet or in/out of the bath or car? Does the hoist have to transport the person from one place to another or is a static/fixed type more suitable?

The environment

- *Space available for use and storage*. This may dictate the size of the hoist chosen and whether it will be a mobile, floor- or ceiling-fixed or gantry type.
- *Construction of the building*. Certain types of building cannot support a fixed-track hoist. Similarly, if a hoist has to move the person from one room to another at different levels a mobile hoist would be unsuitable.

The carer/helper

- *Physical abilities and limitations*. These may affect decisions about the controls and sling attachments on the hoist, whether a mobile or track hoist, or manual or electric controls, should be supplied and how frequently a transfer can be carried out.
- *Cognitive abilities*. Is he able to learn to use the controls and slings safely?
- *Attitude*. Is he prepared to learn to use a hoist? Is he reluctant or over-confident? What type of hoist is most appropriate to him/his household?

Once the most suitable hoist has been chosen the therapist must ensure that the disabled person and his carer are instructed adequately in its use and care. A clearly written set of instructions and a rationale for decisions should be completed, especially if there is to be more than one carer. Teaching the use and care of a hoist should convey a sense of confidence and security so that the new users trust both the hoist and the therapist. The therapist must emphasise the importance of not trying to adapt or alter the slings or hoist in any way and to report any faults or problems as soon as possible. Any therapist, user or carer who wishes to try out a range of hoists and/or receive objective help in choosing the most suitable one should contact the nearest Disabled Living Centre.

TYPES OF HOIST

When the assessor has established the needs of the user and his carer and examined the features of the environment a choice of hoist must be made. The therapist needs to decide:

- which *type* of hoist is most appropriate
- which *model* of hoist within that group is most suitable.

The assessor must be aware, however, that a compromise may have to be made. Where necessary, she must decide which of the features and functions required in a hoist take priority. She may also, of course, be limited by factors such as existing contracts, cost and local policies.

Mobile hoists (Fig. 9.20)

These are the most commonly supplied type of hoist for home use and a wide variety is available. They are generally supplied where it is necessary to move a person over a distance, i.e. across a room or from one room to another, or where, for whatever reason, an overhead hoist is not appropriate. While a range of features is offered within the different models, all have certain features that need to be considered.

• *Castors.* These enable the hoist to be manoeuvred from place to place and vary in size on different models. Large castors will be easier to move over carpets or small thresholds but will require more clearance under a bed or car with which the hoist will be used.

• *They are helper operated.* The helper needs to be reasonably fit if he is to manoeuvre the hoist over carpets or around furniture.

• *Hoisting mechanism.* The boom may be raised or lowered by means of a hydraulic system, a pump handle, a hand screw mechanism or an electric motor. Motors add weight to the hoist but may make possible the use of a hoist by a frail carer who could not manage a hydraulic or pump control.

• *Safe working load.* All mobile hoists will safely lift people up to 127 kg (20 stone) in weight. Some models will guarantee to lift heavier weights.

• *Storage and/or transportation.* All mobile hoists can be dismantled for storage or transportation; however, some models are lighter and smaller than others.

Hoists fixed to the floor (Fig. 9.21)

These hoists may be permanently fixed to the floor or may be of a mobile type whose upright can be detached from the chassis and inserted into a floor socket as required. They are invariably used to transfer a person into and out of the bath. They are useful where space is limited or where the bath is unsuitable for use with a mobile hoist. Some models can be operated by the user or helper whereas others can be operated only by the helper. They can be side or end fixed depending on the space available.

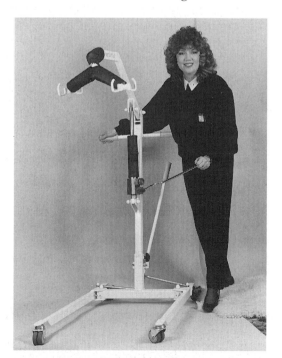
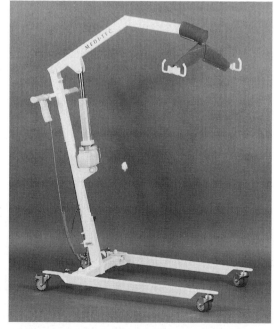

A
B

Fig. 9.20 (A) A manually operated mobile hoist. (B) An electrically operated mobile hoist. (Reproduced by kind permission of Aidserve Ltd.)

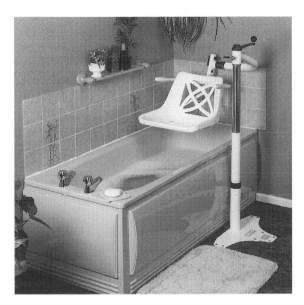

Fig. 9.21 Hoist fixed to the floor (Autolift). (Reproduced by kind permission of Arjo Ltd.)

Fixed overhead hoists (Figs 9.22, 9.23)

These hoists are fixed to an overhead mechanism by means of a retractable strap. They may be attached to a fixed point or to a track, enabling sideways movement over a distance. Points to take into account when considering an overhead hoist are:

● *Long-term or short-term need?* Most overhead hoists are supplied where a long-term need exists for assistance with transfers. Both practically and aesthetically a hoist fixed to the ceiling, either at a single point or on a track, will usually prove the most desirable means of help in the long term. Overhead hoists fixed to the ceiling occupy no floor space and the control box can be moved to one side when not in use. A ceiling track can be designed to run to one or more points specifically required by the user.

In some instances, however, an overhead hoist may be attached to a free-standing gantry. Such an arrangement may be appropriate in cases where:

— The structure of the accommodation is unsuitable to take a ceiling fixing point or a track

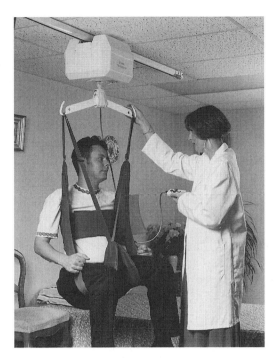

Fig. 9.22 An overhead hoist fixed to a ceiling-mounted track. (Reproduced by kind permission of Wessex Medical Ltd.)

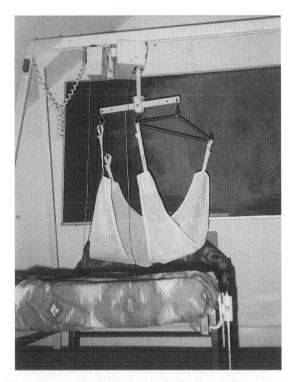

Fig. 9.23 An electrically operated hoist mounted on a gantry.

— The user may shortly be moving house or is being rehoused
— The user/carer wishes to try out an overhead hoist before committing himself to a permanent arrangement. He may, for example, be uncertain of the best layout of the room and wish to test his options
— The user may be terminally ill and/or a mobile hoist is unsuitable
— He may only need to use the hoist in one room, using a wheelchair or shower chair, for example, to transport him to living areas or bathroom.

• *Fixed point or track?* An overhead hoist may be fixed at one single point such that the person can be lifted straight up and down, or onto a track that enables him, additionally, to move sideways. The track may be short, for example to enable a transfer from bed to wheelchair, or it may run from one room to another on a straight or curved track to assist transfer from, say, bed to toilet. This, however, involves considerable alteration to the building, such as leaving gaps above the doors to allow for the passage of the track, and may, for this reason, prove impractical or unacceptable. Fixed-point hoists are also available which lift a person from the ground to the first floor.

• *Operation.* Overhead hoists are usually controlled by means of push buttons on a hand-set. Each button controls movement in one direction (up, down, left, right) (Fig. 9.24). The controls and hand-set should be clearly labelled so that the person is not moved in the wrong direction. Consideration should be given to who will operate the hoist. In some circumstances people who are unable to transfer themselves independently by other physical or mechanical means can do so by using an overhead hoist.

• *Installation.* If an overhead hoist is being considered the building will need to be assessed by an architect or the manufacturer of the hoist to ensure that the hoist can be used. A track must be attached to weight-bearing beams or joists or, if this is not possible, to bearers inserted between the joists. Electrically operated hoists will need a conveniently situated electricity supply.

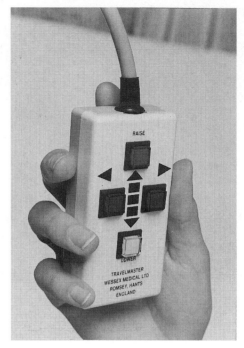

Fig. 9.24 A hand-set to control the movements of an electrically powered hoist. (Reproduced by kind permission of Wessex Medical Ltd.)

If such a hoist is to be used in a bathroom or toilet an isolating transformer is necessary so that it can be operated safely in a wet or damp area. The Electricity Board must be consulted in such circumstances.

Car hoists

These are fixed to a car roof by steel clamps and are helper operated. When considering the use of a car hoist the assessor must check that the car door is wide and high enough to allow easy access. Information about the suitability of the design of the car to take the hoist must also be obtained.

SLINGS

It is important that the assessor has a comprehensive knowledge of the slings available so that the most suitable type can be selected, taking into consideration the height, weight, comfort and physical and mental capabilities of the user.

Slings are available in a variety of materials, sizes and designs and are all washable. Manufacturers design their own range of slings to fit their particular hoists and it is important not to try to mix and match different manufacturers' slings and hoists. Most manufacturers now supply a range of slings which can be quickly fitted to the hoist without the use of metalware. Three basic types of sling are described below. All are available in small, medium and large sizes, or can be made to specific, individual requirements.

All-in-one slings

These are the most popular type of sling as they give overall support to the user. They are useful for carers who are themselves frail and/or may be concerned about correctly placing a sling. The sling may be left in place if the transfer takes place in a confined space or for a short time. Manufacturers produce a wide variety of all-in-one slings and while they all have their own particular features they can be regarded under the following headings.

Universal type (Fig. 9.25)

These slings are usually of the 'quick-fit' type and are used mostly to move a person from one seated position to another. They do not, generally, offer as much support as the hammock type. Designs with or without head supports are available. They can, however, be fitted and removed from sitting and lying positions. They provide good access for toileting and washing and when fitted with the leg bands crossed, provide very secure support. A more able user could possibly fit and remove the sling independently. Where more support is needed a deluxe type may be used.

Hammock slings (Fig. 9.26)

These slings give maximum support and security to more disabled users. They offer full support to the body and can also be ordered with a head support if required. They are generally used to lift a person from a lying position. Most manufacturers offer a commode aperture and/or divided leg options to assist with toileting. However these slings are relatively complex to put on and take off, and cannot be fitted independently by the user. They provide limited access for toileting or washing and the commode aperture, if present, may be difficult to line up. These and other disadvantages have made this type of sling less popular for regular use.

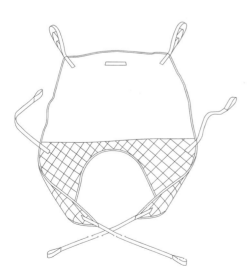

Fig. 9.25 A universal sling (Wispa universal sling). (Reproduced by kind permission of Chiltern Medical [Developments] Ltd.)

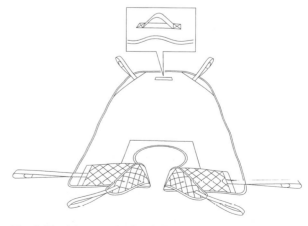

Fig. 9.26 A hammock sling (Wispa hammock sling). (Reproduced by kind permission of Chiltern Medical [Developments] Ltd.)

to overcome a specific physical problem or is he using it more as a 'prop' or a warning to others that he is unsteady on his feet?

THE MEASUREMENT AND USE OF WALKING AIDS

Walking aids can be divided into two main groups:

1. Aids based on a stick. Most of these aids are not free-standing. They include walking sticks, quadrupeds/tripods, forearm (gutter), elbow and axilla crutches.

2. Aids based on a frame. All these aids are free-standing. They include wheeled and non-wheeled frames based on a three- or four-legged frame.

WALKING STICKS (Fig. 9.29)

There are several types of walking stick available; these include:

- a crook handle wooden walking stick

- an adjustable metal walking stick
- a 'Bennett' type walking stick
- a 'Fischer' type walking stick
- those of individual design.

To measure the aid

Walking sticks can be measured:

1. Where a person is ambulant he is asked to stand erect with his weight evenly distributed on both feet, looking forward and with shoulders and arms relaxed. The therapist should ensure that he is not leaning forward or to one side and that he is wearing shoes of similar height to those he normally wears. If he requires support to stand the therapist must check that he is standing symmetrically. With the wooden or Fischer type walking stick the ferrule is removed, the stick turned upside down and the handle placed on the floor. Holding the stick vertically the shaft is marked at the point level with the ulnar styloid (Fig. 9.30). The shaft is then sawn off at this point and the ferrule replaced. For

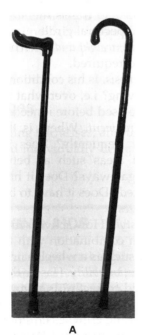

A

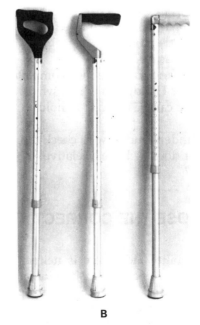

B

Fig. 9.29 Walking sticks. (A) (left) Fischer walking stick (right) Standard wooden stick. (B) Adjustable metal sticks (left) Bennett (centre) Swan neck (right) Standard.

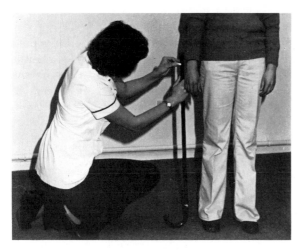

Fig. 9.30 Measuring a walking stick. The stick is held vertically and a mark is made on the shaft at the level of the ulnar styloid.

the adjustable walking stick the measurement is taken as above, but there is no need to turn the stick upside down as the adjustable shaft allows alterations to be carried out in situ.

2. If a person is non-ambulant he is asked to lie straight with his hands at his side and the distance between the ulnar styloid and the bottom of the heel is measured. An inch is then added to this measurement in order to allow for the height of the shoe. The measurement obtained will give the overall height of the stick.

With the stick measured correctly the user should be able to maintain an upright posture with the elbow slightly flexed. In this way he is able to lift his weight when walking by fully extending his elbow as he pushes down on the stick (Fig. 9.31).

Points of use

The user's wrist and grip must be strong enough to allow him to bear weight through this area when using the stick. If this is not possible an alternative aid, such as gutter crutches, should be chosen. When using the stick the person should be taught to look where he is going rather than at the ground and an even heel-toe gait should be encouraged.

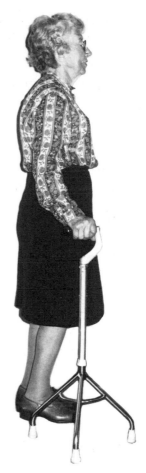

Fig. 9.31 A correctly fitted aid.

Occasions when walking sticks may be used

Walking sticks are used for a variety of reasons and may be required:

- to supplement power where there is muscular weakness, for example in cases of poliomyelitis or nerve injury to the lower limb
- to relieve pain, as in osteoarthrosis or following a fracture within the lower limb
- to widen the walking base in conditions of impaired balance, for example following a head injury or for those with multiple sclerosis
- to protect weak bones or damaged joints, for example in cases of osteoporosis or following a meniscectomy

- to compensate for deformity, for example where there is scoliosis or limb shortening
- as a feeler, for example for blind people or some with hemianopia
- for social reasons, for example to warn others of the user's slowness or lack of confidence in walking or — occasionally — as a 'fashion aid'.

THE QUADRUPED (Fig. 9.32)

This is a more stable version of the walking stick, having a four-footed base. Tripods with a three-footed base are also available but are considered by some to be rather unstable.

To measure the aid

These aids are measured in the same way as an adjustable walking stick. The therapist should ensure that, when the aid is in use, the open end of the handle is facing backwards and the flat side of the rectangle made by the feet is nearest the user; see Figure 9.31 for a similar example.

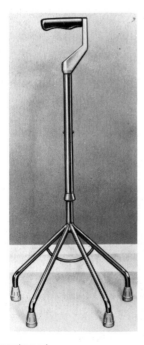

Fig. 9.32 A quadruped.

Points of use

These are as for the walking stick, but it is particularly important to ensure that the aid is neither so close to the user that he leans over it to balance when taking weight, nor so far away that the aid will tip inwards when weight is taken on it.

Occasions when quadrupeds may be used

These are usually issued singly for a weakness of one lower limb or a unilateral weakness of the whole body where more support is needed than can be obtained from the use of a walking stick, for example in some cases of hemiplegia.

N.B. The therapist may note that, where a 'bilateral' approach to treatment is followed, the use of such aids is discouraged by some practitioners, who feel that they raise muscle tone in the hemiplegic side by virtue of the effort involved in using them. Others, however, feel that where the rise in tone is slight, or if the provision of an aid offers independent mobility where this would not otherwise be possible, its value outweighs any disadvantages. The therapist, therefore, must weigh each situation individually and use her professional judgement as to whether such an aid is advisable or not. Quadrupeds may also be issued in pairs following bilateral amputation of the lower limbs or to young sufferers of cerebral palsy or spina bifida.

CRUTCHES
Elbow crutches (Fig. 9.33)

These aids, which are usually issued in pairs, provide an armband support which fits round the forearm thus bracing the wrist when the aid is in use.

To measure the aid

The height of the aid from the floor to the handle is measured as for the adjustable walking stick. The forearm band should be neither so tight that the aid is difficult to remove, nor so loose that it does not give enough support. The band should hold the forearm at a point slightly above mid-

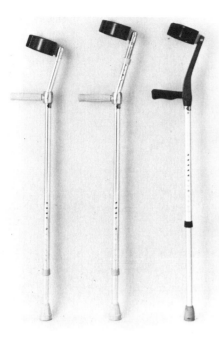

Fig. 9.33 Elbow crutches.

way between the wrist and elbow, for if it is too low it will not give sufficient support and if too high it may block the action of the elbow and/or rub on the ulnar nerve, causing bruising and subsequent tingling or loss of sensation in the fourth and fifth digits.

Points of use

The points of use of these aids are as for those of the walking stick. However, as elbow crutches can be awkward to handle, the user may need some practice in putting on and taking off the aids as well as in walking with them. It is essential that the user has good strength throughout his upper limbs as they support much of the body weight when walking on these aids.

Occasions when elbow crutches may be used

As elbow crutches offer a great deal of support to the lower limbs they can be used when the user's strength or balance has been severely affected. Elbow crutches may be issued to people with:

- bilateral weakness and/or incoordination of

the lower limbs, for example following spinal injury or in some cases of spina bifida
- unilateral weakness of a lower limb when the user is not permitted to bear his full weight through the injured limb, for example in the early stages following an ankle fracture or meniscectomy
- bilateral severe weakness and/or incoordination affecting the whole body and/or where the upper limbs are unable to provide sufficient support using walking sticks. This may occur in some cases of a progressive paralysis such as muscular dystrophy, or following brain damage.

Forearm or gutter crutches (Fig. 9.34)

This is another variety of a single stick aid, but one in which the weight is borne along the length of the forearm rather than through the wrist and hand.

To measure the aid

The user should stand as upright as possible with

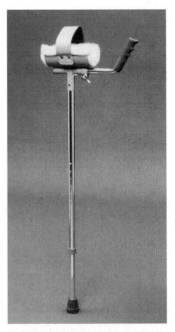

Fig. 9.34 Forearm or trough crutch. (Reproduced by kind permission of JMC Rehab Ltd.)

his arms and shoulders relaxed, looking forward and with his weight evenly distributed on both feet. Measurement is taken from the floor to the olecranon process. In some cases the user may have to be measured lying down, as he may have difficulty in standing without the use of an aid. In this instance the measurement should be taken from the olecranon process to the bottom of the heel and an inch added to allow for the height of the shoe. In both cases the measurement obtained will give the distance required from the ferrule to the bottom of the gutter padding.

When adjusting the handle the therapist should check that there is sufficient space between the front of the gutter and the handle to leave the wrist free from pressure, especially over the ulnar styloid. Similarly, she should check that the elbow is free at the back so that the gutter does not press on the ulnar nerve which, at this point, lies just under the skin with little protection from pressure.

Points of use

The crutches should not be placed too far in front of the body as this can unbalance the upright posture. It is important to ensure that the user's balance and coordination are adequate before he attempts to walk unsupervised, because the aids are strapped over the forearms and so cannot be discarded quickly in a crisis.

Occasions when forearm crutches may be used

These are usually issued in pairs and can be used for unilateral or bilateral weakness in the lower limbs in cases where the upper limbs are unable to bear weight through the wrists and hands. The most common example is the person with rheumatoid arthritis. Other examples include persons who, because of injury to both the lower and the upper limbs, find weight-bearing through the wrists and hands impossible.

Axilla crutches (Fig. 9.35)

These are aids in which weight is borne through the wrist and hand. The axilla pad, which is

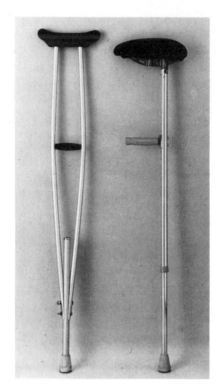

Fig. 9.35   Axilla crutches.

pressed against the chest wall, is not an area through which weight is taken but helps to stabilise the shoulder.

To measure the aid

The height of the hand grip is measured as for the walking stick, that is, it should be level with the user's ulnar styloid. The axilla pads should be adjusted so that there is a gap of approximately 2 inches (or three fingers' width) between the top of the pad and the axilla. If the aids are too long there is a danger of putting pressure on the brachial plexus, thus affecting the nerve supply to the upper limb. If they are too short, posture will be affected during walking and the user will have difficulty in keeping the pads pressed against the chest wall, as they will tend to slip out.

Points of use

It is essential that the user appreciates the importance of bearing weight through the handles of the aids and of not leaning on the axilla pads because of the danger of putting pressure on the brachial plexus. The axilla pads should be pressed against the chest wall in order to give support by bracing the shoulder and upper limb. The crutches should be used at an angle of approximately 15 degrees to the side of the body.

Occasions when axilla crutches may be used

These aids are issued in pairs and may be used where there is unilateral weakness of the lower limb through which only partial or no weight may be taken, for example following a fracture of the tibia and fibula or after a bone graft to a previously un-united fracture. The aids may also be used where there is bilateral dysfunction of the lower limbs for which a reciprocal gait is inappropriate, for example if the hips or spine are fixed in a hip spica plaster or if other supports fixing the hip are worn.

WALKING FRAMES

The lightweight walking frame
(Fig. 9.36)

This is the simplest style of walking frame and may be also referred to as a 'pulpit' or 'Zimmer' frame. A hinged version, known as a reciprocal walking frame, is also available.

To measure the frame

The height is measured as for the walking stick.

Points of use

It is important to ensure that the user does not step too closely into the frame as there is a danger that he may tip backwards. Where this is a persistent problem it may be practical to tie a piece of coloured tape or elastic across the back legs of the frame at knee level (not below, as this may trip those with poor sight or a high stepping gait) to prevent the user stepping in too closely to the frame. Similarly, the frame should not be placed

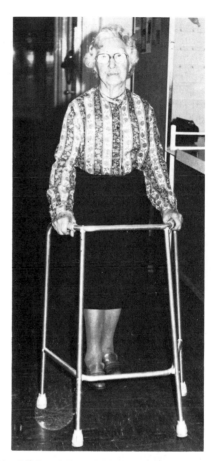

Fig. 9.36 A lightweight walking frame.

too far in front of the user when walking, for this may not only upset his balance but can also cause the frame to tip if all four legs are not placed firmly on the floor when weight is taken onto it.

Occasions when a lightweight walking frame may be used

This is a very popular aid and can be used for people with:

- unilateral weakness or amputation of the lower limb where general weakness or infirmity makes the greater support offered by the frame necessary, such as in osteoarthritis or a fractured femur in an elderly person

which has a padded resting platform on which the forearms are placed when walking.

To measure the aids

Both aids are initially measured as for the forearm crutches. However, depending upon the severity of disability of the user, some adjustment may have to be made in order to allow the most appropriate and comfortable posture.

Points of use

As both aids are rather cumbersome they can be difficult to manoeuvre in confined spaces or out of doors. However, many users are restricted to them as their only means of mobility and, therefore, will be obliged to adapt their activity to the limited manoeuvrability of the aid.

Occasions when forearm rest frames may be used

The forearm walker can be used in cases where a lightweight frame or gutter crutches are appropriate, but where weakness of the lower limbs, combined with weakness and/or incoordination of the upper limbs, make them impractical. The

aid is suitable, therefore, for some people with advanced rheumatoid arthritis or where injuries or deformities to both upper and lower limbs make weight-bearing through the wrist or hand impossible.

The standing aid may be used instead of the forearm walker when gutter attachments are inappropriate, for example in cases of upper limb deformity.

The therapist will notice, when looking through manufacturers' catalogues, that many variations and combinations of these aids are produced.

WALKING PATTERNS

All walking aids must be used correctly in order to provide adequate support and allow the user to maintain good posture, balance and gait. Walking aids, like all other aids, should never be issued unless full instruction for their use is provided. The walking patterns illustrated in Figures 9.40–9.55 below cover the use of aids already discussed. The therapist may find that the names given to the gaits vary from place to place. The types of aid with which each gait can be used are given in brackets.

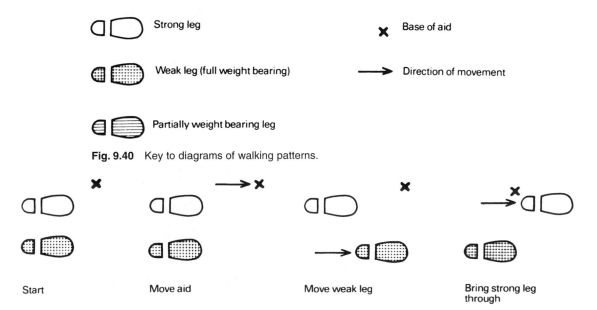

Fig. 9.40   Key to diagrams of walking patterns.

Start   Move aid   Move weak leg   Bring strong leg through

Fig. 9.41   The use of one walking aid in the early stages of recovery (tripod, quadruped or walking stick).

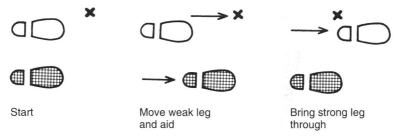

Start | Move weak leg and aid | Bring strong leg through

Fig. 9.42 The use of one walking aid in the later stages of recovery (tripod, quadruped or walking stick).

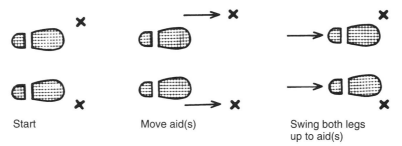

Start | Move aid(s) | Swing both legs up to aid(s)

Fig. 9.43 The swing-to gait (axilla crutches, elbow crutches or pick-up frame).

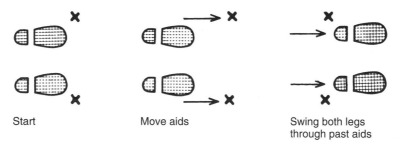

Start | Move aids | Swing both legs through past aids

Fig. 9.44 The swing-through gait (axilla crutches and elbow crutches).

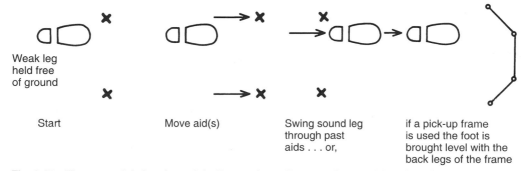

Weak leg held free of ground

Start | Move aid(s) | Swing sound leg through past aids . . . or, | if a pick-up frame is used the foot is brought level with the back legs of the frame

Fig. 9.45 The non-weight-bearing gait (axilla crutches, elbow crutches or pick-up frame).

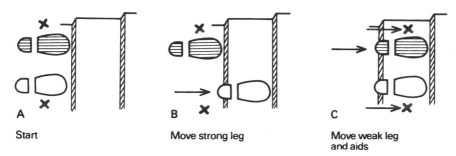

Fig. 9.52 Going up stairs using two aids (partial weight-bearing).

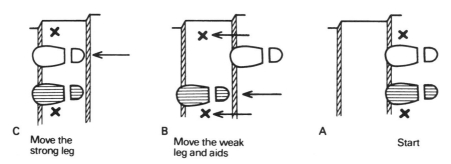

Fig. 9.53 Going down stairs using two aids (partial weight-bearing).

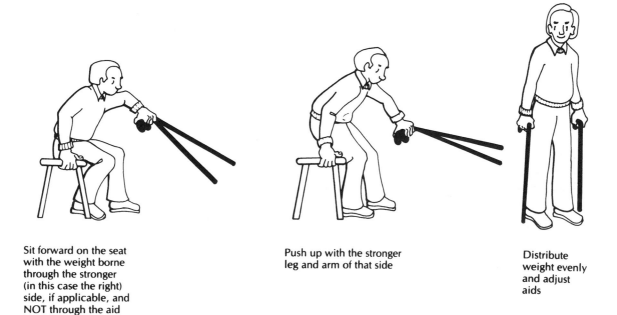

Sit forward on the seat with the weight borne through the stronger (in this case the right) side, if applicable, and NOT through the aid

Push up with the stronger leg and arm of that side

Distribute weight evenly and adjust aids

Fig. 9.54 Standing with a non-free-standing aid.

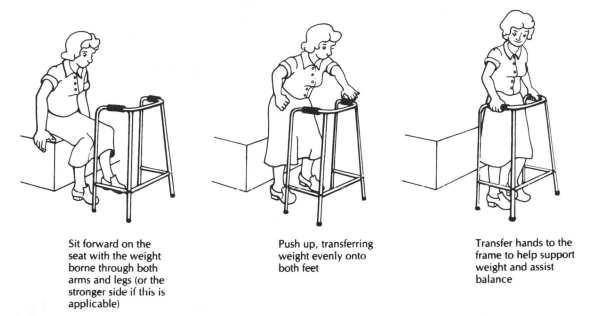

Sit forward on the seat with the weight borne through both arms and legs (or the stronger side if this is applicable)

Push up, transferring weight evenly onto both feet

Transfer hands to the frame to help support weight and assist balance

Fig. 9.55 Standing with a free-standing aid.

PART 3: WHEELCHAIR MOBILITY

There is more to wheelchairs than meets the eye. When, early in their training, occupational therapy students are asked to spend a day in a wheelchair in order to gain first-hand experience of disability their initial reaction is usually one of eager anticipation. However, the reports of their experiences invariably show that the novelty soon wears off (often around lunchtime when fellow students tend to get fed up with their slowness and incompetence) and they often sheepishly confess that their 'day' finished around 6 p.m. when they could stand the confines of the wheelchair no longer. Some have been ashamed to admit to wanting to throw the chair into the nearest river; others have been asked to leave restaurants, refused entrance to pubs, patted on the head, given sweets by elderly matrons and stared at by children and adults alike. Some have been infuriated to find, upon trying to buy a pair of shoes, that the shop assistant asked their partner what size feet they had!

Despite this love/hate relationship with an object that frequently provides mobility at the cost of anonymity and dignity, the occupational therapist needs to be aware of the wide variety of models that are available, their features and accessories, and how to assess for and obtain the most suitable model for the person in need of a chair.

AVAILABILITY AND SUPPLY

In 1986 McColl defined the objective of the wheelchair service within the NHS as being 'to meet the basic need for short-range mobility of all people of all ages who have serious and permanent difficulties in walking' (McColl 1986, p. 41). He stated that NHS wheelchairs are available on permanent free loan to anyone having a permanent disability which limits their short-range mobility.

Following the devolvement of responsibility for wheelchair provision to health care districts in 1991, each district has aimed to develop its service in a way that best meets the needs of its local population. Each health care district, therefore, has developed differently, with individual systems of referral, prescription priority and levels of responsibility. It is essential, therefore, that every occupational therapist is aware of the particular system which operates in her area.

A person who feels that he needs a wheelchair has the option of buying one himself from a private company, borrowing one (especially if it is only required for temporary use) or applying for one to be permanently lent to him from the local district wheelchair service. This last option is the one chosen by the majority of people. In order for a person to obtain a wheelchair in this way a referral has to be made to his local wheelchair service. People able to request the provision of a wheelchair vary from area to area but research (White 1993) shows that all services will accept referrals from general practitioners, the majority will accept them from accredited therapists (occupational therapists or physiotherapists), non-accredited therapists and hospital doctors, and certain services will accept self-referrals and referrals from other health workers such as district nurses or health visitors.

Each service has its own referral form, which requires accurate completion, and on receipt of the completed form the person may be further assessed by a therapist from the wheelchair service.

Services have also developed discrete criteria for eligibility of the supply of wheelchairs. White (1993) found that all services would supply wheelchairs to people suffering from a permanent disability, including terminal illness, who required use of a wheelchair at least once a week, while 43% of services would consider supplying those with a temporary disability of less than six months, and 51% would supply all occasional users who had a permanent need.

Supply

In theory services may provide any model of chair they deem most suitable to meet the person's need but, inevitably, choice remains limited by available resources. Time taken for the chair to be delivered will vary. A standard, popular wheelchair may be available for immediate delivery whereas a less common model, or one which requires additional features or alteration, will not be available straight away.

ASSESSMENT

Any therapist assessing a person for a wheelchair must be aware that a poorly prescribed chair may compromise independence and can cause fatigue, discomfort and deformity by affecting the user's posture, not offering correct support or not distributing weight effectively.

In order to determine the most suitable wheelchair for an individual the therapist should consider the following factors.

1. The user

The most important aspect of wheelchair provision is that the chair should meet the needs and expectations of the user. It should enhance the activities he wishes to perform at home, school or work and in his social/leisure pursuits. It should also relate to his level of function in personal and home-care activities.

Age. If he is young, is he likely to need room for growth? How much wear and tear is he likely to give the chair? For children cosmesis is very important. For some elderly people with diminishing faculties the provision of easily used and readily accessible features such as brakes and footplates may be necessary.

Size (Fig. 9.56). The size of the chair should enable the user to be comfortable and well supported when seated.

- *Hips*. Hips should be flexed at 90 degrees when the user is sitting at the back of the seat.
- *Knees and ankles*. There should be room to place a flat hand vertically between the back of the user's knees and the front edge of the seat/cushion, and also space to place a flat hand between the back of his knees and the top of the seat/cushion at the front when his ankles are resting securely at 90 degrees on the footplates. Footplates should support the feet securely and be at least 5 cm off the floor.
- *Back support*. The user should be able to reach the wheel-rims with ease while maintaining an

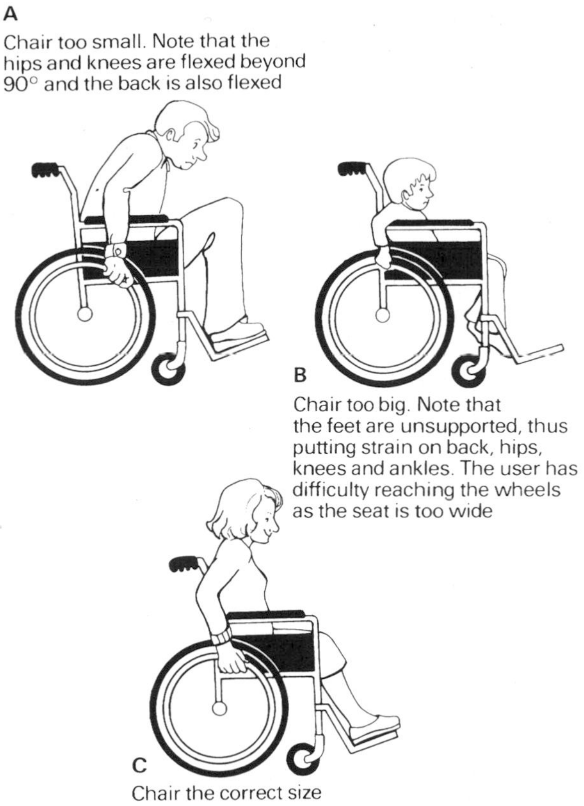

A

Chair too small. Note that the
hips and knees are flexed beyond
90° and the back is also flexed

B

Chair too big. Note that
the feet are unsupported, thus
putting strain on back, hips,
knees and ankles. The user has
difficulty reaching the wheels
as the seat is too wide

C

Chair the correct size

Fig. 9.56 Fitting a wheelchair.

upright posture. The backrest should offer sufficient support for his spine but not hinder his
ability to manoeuvre the chair. The 'correct' height
of backrest will vary according to the strength of
the person's trunk, i.e. the amount of support his
back needs to maintain a good posture, and the
use to which he puts the chair. For example, does
he need to twist his trunk to reach behind him
in the office or kitchen, is he an active sportsman
or does he need constant support to enable him
to sit comfortably at a computer?

• *Armrests.* Armrests should be 2.5 cm higher
than the distance from the seat/cushion to the
bottom of the flexed elbow.

• *Seat.* The seat should be wide enough to
allow a flat hand to be placed between either side
of the user's thighs/hips at their widest point
and the sides of the chair, remembering that if
the user is frequently going to wear bulky clothing or orthoses when using the chair, these should

be taken into account. A chair that is too narrow
can cause pressure sores and may inhibit transfers, while one that is too wide may affect the
ability to balance and propel the chair.

Weight. Different sizes of chair within each
range are available to take people only up to a
certain weight. If the user is too heavy for the
chair it will be under too much strain and will
wear out more quickly. However, if the chair is
too heavy for the user it will be hard and exhausting for him to push and manoeuvre, and may
be difficult for the carer to handle or lift.

Diagnosis. Whether the condition is static, progressive or likely to improve may determine
how long the chair will be in use, and indicate
how frequently it will be used. If the condition
is progressive is it possible to determine how long
the person will be able to control, manoeuvre and
use the chair before it will need to be modified
or replaced?

Physical abilities. The user's ability to physically cope with a chair should be carefully considered. Can he propel a chair himself, and if
so, can he do so over carpets, paths and rough
ground or only some of these? Can he cope with
slopes, tight corners and thresholds? Can he
balance sufficiently to open and close doors and
reach objects from a table or shelf? What type of
brakes can he operate? Can he remove armrests,
and swing and remove footrests?

If he cannot propel with standard hand-rims
can he manage a capstan type, or gain more
force if the propelling wheels are larger? If self-
propulsion is beyond him, has he the physical
and mental ability to cope with an electrically
propelled chair, and what method of control is
most suitable?

How will the user transfer into and out of the
chair? Do armrests and footrests need to be removable to allow this? If a hoist is needed to
assist transfer are the two compatible in size and
lifting height? Are the user's bed/bath/toilet of
the appropriate height to facilitate transfer from
the wheelchair?

Can any deformity, or any abnormality in
posture or balance, be accommodated in the
chair? For example, if the person suffers from

scoliosis will the chair being considered permit adequate support to be added?

Attitude and reason for supply. Has the person asked for a chair or has one been considered advisable? In the latter case, is the person prepared to accept a wheelchair? If he is reluctant to accept a chair can he explain why? Remember that for children, and some parents, cosmesis is extremely important.

Cognitive ability. Can the user understand when and how to use and maintain the chair? If not, will the attendant be confident in its use? Is a self-propelling chair appropriate if the user lacks cognitive skills, for example for those with brain damage or dementia?

2. The place of use

In the home. Consider the widths of the doors and corridors and the space for manoeuvring within them. What type of flooring has to be negotiated? Are there any steps that need to be negotiated and can they be ramped? If so, can the person manage the gradient of the slope? The angle and space available for transfers onto toilet, bed and easy chair should be noted. Can grab rails be fitted or will a hoist/assistant be needed?

Is there room to store the chair when not in use? Is the store dry and access to it easy?

Is there someone who can carry out routine maintenance to the chair? If an electrically propelled chair is being considered are battery charging facilities easily available and are these in a well-ventilated area? If the chair is to be charged overnight for a person who uses the chair constantly is there someone who can take it from the bedroom to the charging area and back?

Will the user's knees, when seated, fit under the sink, basin, desk or table as required?

Outside. Are paths, steps, gates and doors suitable for the chair or can they be made so?

At work or school. Is the chair suitable for use here? Can it be manoeuvred within the environment in which the person works? Is it compatible with any furniture or equipment he may need to use there? Does alternative provision need to be made by the Education Authority or Employment Service?

3. Other transport facilities

Is the chair going to be used in conjunction with any other transport? If so, can the user transfer in/out of the vehicle and can the chair be folded, lifted and stored in it, either by the user himself, an assistant or a roof-mounted hoist?

Will a hoist or any other equipment be necessary to help with transfer? Can the car be parked in a suitable place at home to allow room for (preferably sheltered) transfers?

4. Carers

Are carers able to accept the chair or will their attitude prevent the individual from using it? If carers do not accept the chair is it possible to ascertain why?

If help is needed for pushing, transfer or maintenance of the chair are carers willing and able to do this? In some cases carers' needs may equal or outweigh those of the user.

5. Stability

Several factors can alter a chair's stability and, therefore, make it less safe to use. Contributing factors include:

- excess movement, as when the user suffers from an athetoid or choreic condition or is an active sportsman
- an altered centre of gravity, for example when the user is a double lower limb amputee or has severe postural deformity
- the fitting of an angled backrest and/or cushions
- inappropriate controls on an electrically propelled chair which prevent the user from operating the chair smoothly
- an uneven environment such as an excessive camber on a pavement, drive or road, or a steep slope
- the fitting of a special seating system — a wheelchair fitted with a special seating system should always be tilt-tested for stability with the occupant in situ.

The user should be assessed using the chair in as wide a variety of circumstances as possible in order that stability can be checked before a final decision is made.

6. Cushions

Both the needs of the user and the chair in which it will be used should be carefully considered when deciding on a suitable cushion. The sitting posture and stability of the user can be helped or hindered by the cushion, and its height and firmness must be taken into account when considering transfers in and out of the chair. The therapist must also be aware that the use of a cushion will alter the internal dimensions of the chair, so it is imperative that the two are chosen together.

Additionally, the appearance, durability, weight, comfort, cost and purpose of the cushion, together with the user's continence and ability to care for the cushion, should also be taken into account.

7. Modifications and adaptations

Chairs supplied through the District Wheelchair Services can be modified according to need by the manufacturer or Service Rehabilitation Engineer. Where such adaptations cannot be made, or where a specially designed 'one-off' chair is required, specialist centres may be approached (see Special Seating, below).

When all those points have been considered the best size and model of chair, together with any additional features and accessories, can be decided upon. It is important to remember that the more standard the chair the more quickly it is likely to be delivered. (For further information on types of cushions available see p. 267.)

TYPES OF WHEELCHAIR AND FEATURES TO CONSIDER

While it is beyond the brief of this chapter to look at individual models of chairs it is essential that the therapist understands the different types of chair available and the main features to consider during assessment for the most suitable model.

Types

1. Non-powered wheelchairs

Ham (1987) showed that 93% of all referrals received are for basic, standard, non-powered chairs. Such chairs may be either:

- user-controlled (self-propelled), having two large wheels, generally with hand-rims, for self-propelling, and two small wheels which swivel freely for easy manoeuvre. These chairs are usually issued to long-term users who can undertake at least some degree of independent propulsion, although it must be remembered that this takes considerable stamina and strength
- attendant-controlled (transit) with four smaller wheels. These are usually issued to high-dependency users who cannot operate a self-propelling chair, or to occasional users who can walk indoors but not outdoors.

• Special chairs. When mobility needs cannot be met by a standard chair, chairs with special features, such as one-arm drive, foot-propelled 'Glideabout' chairs and recliner chairs, may be considered.

• Buggies. For children over 30 months of age a range of buggies is available.

• Children's wheelchairs. A range of standard and special chairs is available for children with moderate and severe disabilities.

• High performance chairs. McColl (1986) showed that provision of these chairs, which are designed for young, physically fit users, was governed more by finance than clinical need. However, with higher expectations and knowledge, and moves towards community living, requests to services (who, in theory, have no prescription bar on these chairs) will probably increase.

• Tricycles. Tricycles are theoretically still (1994) available for medical need (but not for social or therapeutic use), although many centres have ceased to supply these due to financial constraints.

or council warden-controlled (sheltered) accommodation; or exploring the feasibility of the individual moving to a Young Disabled Persons' Unit or into residential care or considering employing help within their existing home.

For social, personal and financial reasons the disabled person's preference is often to remain in his existing neighbourhood, and if possible in his present home, and it should be the therapist's aim to meet this wish in the most cost-effective way if it is at all practically and/or financially viable.

CREATING A 'USER-FRIENDLY' ENVIRONMENT

Almost the first statement emphasised by Pheasant (1987) is that an individual organising an environment must take account of the characteristics of the user. The adaptability of humans must not be the mainstay of returning a person to his or her home. The person who uses his home following a sudden or deteriorating condition is not the same person who used it before, and if the home is to become 'user friendly' again, change is necessary, with negotiation between therapist and resident as the guiding principle. The layout, contents and functions of a home evolve as the occupant progresses through life, and just as normal life events have changed some or all of these three aspects, so change in abilities following the onset of any dysfunction initiates another stage in the evolution of a home.

While it is clearly not often possible to start with the equivalent of 'a clean slate', the therapist must be aware of the dangers of accepting the status quo 'because the person can cope'. Rooms tend to be labelled by their use over the years — people will often still refer to a room as their son's room even though he has a family and home of his own. The therapist must be very careful not simply to try to fit the person back into the home. It is often helpful, therefore, to begin with the concept of a collection of spaces and then to distinguish between 'activity spaces' and 'circulation spaces' (Fig. 9.61). This will then lead on to the organisation of the spaces in order to permit the activities to be undertaken and to the pro-

vision of unobstructed routes for circulation. Modification of each, with specific regard to the needs of the occupant, will gradually result in an evolution towards maximal 'user friendliness', i.e. a maximally enabling home environment.

Levels, rooms and surfaces are three aspects which dominate an environment in which a person lives, so it is frequently useful to think in these terms, rather than by named rooms, as a starting point for an assessment of a home.

Levels

Horizontal surfaces will normally have many names — floors, seats, beds, work surfaces, shelves and so on. Once again the division into 'activity levels' and 'circulation levels' is useful to help clarify thinking and discussions. Pavements, footpaths, drives, hallways and landings clearly have circulation as their principle function. Kitchen worktops, desks, toilet seats and tables are all linked by their being levels on which activities take place. Other levels are less easily classified — the floor space around a bed or alongside a bath, for example, is used for the activity of dressing and also for circulation between activities.

Floor levels should ideally be continuous and horizontally the same; this is possible inside single-storey accommodation but over the threshold of the outer door the real world is far from having the ideal level, so slopes become necessary. Ambulant people will frequently find a series of low steps more easy to negotiate than a slope, especially if calipers are worn preventing plantarflexion. A grab rail may help stability. Wheelchair users naturally prefer slopes as the medium for changing levels (Fig. 9.62). A series of shallow steps is more easily converted into a suitable slope for the user with a changing dysfunction, so progression of the condition must be an important aspect for consideration by the therapist. For major changes in level, stairways, stairlifts, or through-floor lifts are necessary. Once again the principle of 'maximal enabling', not necessarily automatically meaning maximum provision, has to be the guide. For example, providing a chair near the head and foot of a

THREE BED SEMI DETACHED HOUSE

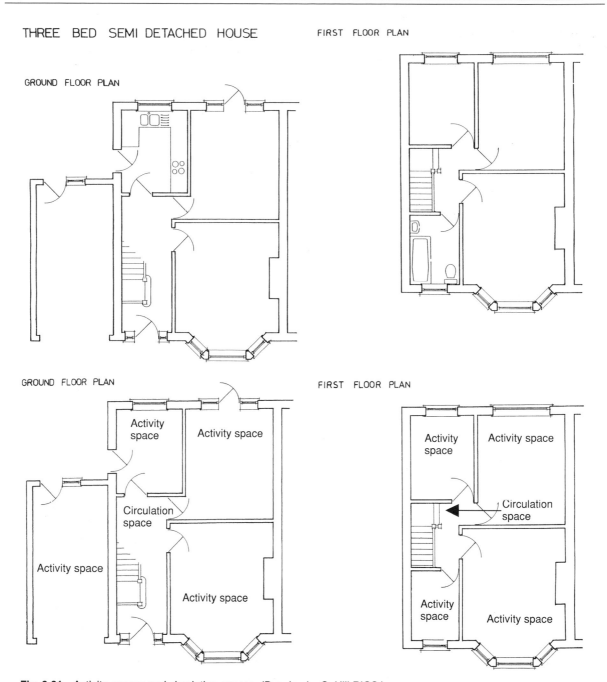

Fig. 9.61 Activity spaces and circulation spaces. (Drawing by S. Hill RICS.)

stairway may enable a person with respiratory dysfunction to ascend or descend and then rest before embarking on the next stage of circulation between activities. A person with locomotor dysfunction may need a system, e.g. a stairlift or through-floor lift, to compensate for that dysfunction. This is assuming that discussion with the therapist has not established that changing storeys may not really be necessary.

Furniture on which the person is to sit or lie

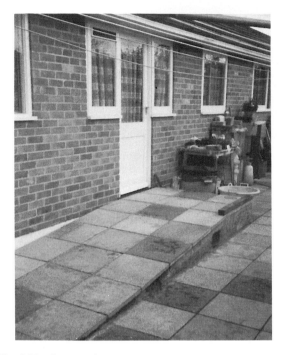

Fig. 9.62 A ramped access.

(or both, as on the edge of a bed) must be reviewed with respect to anthropomeric principles and medical precautions (e.g. limits to hip flexion following total hip replacement). There may be other constraints resulting from commercial decisions; the height of a wheelchair seat, for example, may mean an adaptation to the height of bed or toilet for transfers.

Shelving should be placed to maximise the occupational performance of the user, and in this context it may be appropriate to consider a kitchen worktop or a desktop as a large specialised shelf. Cupboards and sideboards are shelves with doors enclosing the contents. This means that the same principles which apply to shelf accessibility must apply to these variants. Once again anthropometry and medical precautions must guide the negotiations and decision-making. Marden (1987) in his section on ergonomics has some very useful diagrams, as does Goldsmith (1976).

One important consideration is the position of the bottom of sinks. Draining boards are normally placed level with kitchen worktops, but this means that the sink bottom will often be too low.

Placing an upturned baking tray or having a plastic-coated wire frame in the sink, upon which a washing bowl may be positioned, could be all that is necessary to prevent or overcome some dysfunction.

When considering the height of fixtures and fittings there are many reference sources. Diagrams illustrating recommended heights are to be found in Goldsmith (Fig. 9.63), and when specific environments are under consideration the publications of the Centre on Environment for the Handicapped are very useful. Once again the progression of a condition must be considered if ambulation is to progress to wheelchair mobility and the consequent reduction in reaching height of the individual.

Spaces

The word 'rooms' is usually used but this can lead into a trap of named rooms, specifying what happens therein rather than the activity organising the room. Within the room will be the 'activity space' with the necessary fittings, furniture or equipment for that activity. This may result in the need for negotiation about the furniture in a room (because it has always been there) when there are items which are more of a hindrance than a help.

Circulation spaces between activity spaces may be within the same room (in a kitchen/dining room for example) or between rooms, when the terms corridors or landings are commonly used. Circulation requires clear spaces through which to move and varies in relationship to the mobility aids which are required (or may be required in future). Once again Goldsmith offers many examples of the dimensions and layouts of circulation spaces. Although people may be able to 'cope', abilities change with age and changing dysfunction, and it may be more efficient to make one appropriate modification at the beginning than to be making a continual series of small changes over a long period. Placing items of furniture in circulation areas may not necessarily be problematical. A chair near the top and bottom of a stairway provides a resting place, as noted above; a sturdy hall table may be used as a handrest

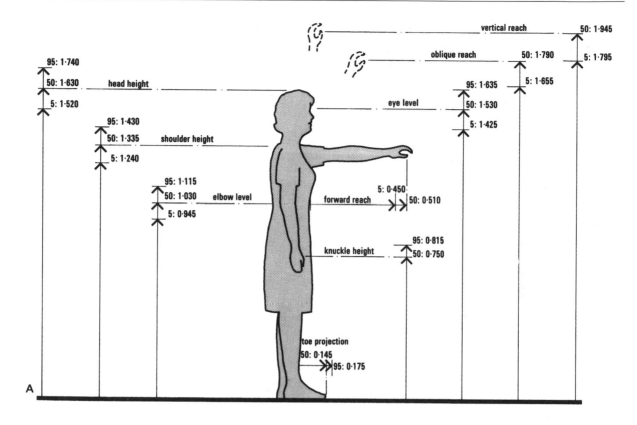

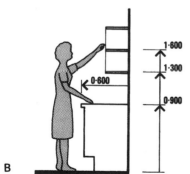

Fig. 9.63 A and B. Contrast of storage and working heights between ambulant and disabled women. (Reproduced from Goldsmith 1984 *Designing for the Disabled*, with kind permission.)

for balance on occasions. Care must be taken, however, to ensure that these items are more of a help than a hindrance.

It is important to remember that mobility and safety can be hampered by poor lighting. Switches, of optimum height and design for all users, should be available at the most frequently used entrance to an activity area.

Surfaces

Surface type is one of the properties of many of the 'levels' that needs to be considered. Floor covering must not impede the passage of the person. Many walking aids have small wheels that are difficult to run over many carpet finishes, so non-carpet flooring or very short-pile carpets may be necessary. Other people may need the slight friction provided by a carpet as part of a stable base to prevent slipping when walking or undertaking other activities. Once again the therapist must negotiate, and common sense should be the guide. Even where appropriate floor coverings are present, the surface may be made hazardous by loose rugs or even by the threshold bars where carpets join. If the therapist has the advantage of being able to advise on the floor covering before any fitting is undertaken, items such as carpet tiles have many advantages in rendering internal thresholds unnecessary. The thresholds of external doors provide problematical obstructions to the surface because of the need to make a weatherproof closure. There are some thresholds which drop automatically when the door is opened and rise when closed; this sort of fixture may be appropriate.

The surfaces on which activity takes place tend to be appropriate as a result of the designer's work. Occasionally a person's dysfunction may result in the need for variation, e.g. varying the colour or texture to help someone with a visual dysfunction, or emphasising the edges of steps to make changes of level more visible. The material of chair coverings may need to meet newly acquired demands, for example in a person for whom incontinence may result in the need for washable and/or waterproof materials. Similarly a high friction sheet on the bed may aid stability, while a low friction one may aid mobility. Non-slip materials placed on trays may compensate for recently acquired ataxia and still allow the use of a favoured tray.

Summary

Designers and manufacturers are constantly looking to produce new or improved products for all aspects of human activity. The therapist must also be using analytical methods in assessing the needs of a person returning home or wishing to remain at home. Visiting events such as National Aids Exhibition (NAIDEX) will maintain currency with products. Using 'models of practice' to provide a framework for organising the assessment is valuable to avoid overlooking important activities and roles within the life-style of the person. To this is added knowledge of the progression of dysfunction and anticipated life events, to enable outcomes that are both reasonable and appropriate.

CONCLUSION

As can be seen, restricted mobility can severely affect the life of a person and that of his family and friends. While it is not always possible to return the person to full mobility, the teaching of new techniques, the consideration of roles and dynamics within the family, the rearrangement of the environment, the supply of equipment and the alteration or adaptation of the home can go a long way towards reducing the impact such a disability may have. No one solution will be applicable to every circumstance, but careful consideration of priorities, needs, emotions and finances by the therapist, the individual and his family should enable the best solution to be found for a given situation.

ACKNOWLEDGEMENTS

Grateful thanks are extended to the following people for their help in the compilation of this chapter: Glynis Hill BA MA CertEd DipCOT, Senior Lecturer, St Andrew's School of Occupational Therapy, Nene College, Northampton; Allen Hinde BA MA MSCP DipTP GradDipPhys, Senior Lecturer, St Andrew's School of Occupational Therapy, Nene College, Northampton; Vivien Kilgour DipCOT, Lifting and Handling Advisor, Head Occupational Therapist, Northwing Hospital, Bedford; Kim Mellon, Lifting and Handling Advisor, Rockingham Forest Health Care Trust, Kettering; June Sutherland DipCOT, Head Occupational Therapist, Chelsea and Westminster Hospital, London; and Liz White DipCOT DKC (PhD registered), Senior Occupational Therapist, Wheelchair Assessment Unit, Kent and Canterbury Hospital, Canterbury.

ADDRESSES AND PUBLICATIONS

Disability Living Allowance Unit
Warbreck House
Warbreck Hill
Blackpool FY2 0YJ

The Disability Unit
Department of Transport
2 Marsham Street
London SW1P 3EB
Publishes booklet *Door to Door* offering advice to disabled travellers.

Disabled Drivers Association
Norwich NR16 1EX

Disabled Motorists Federation
National Mobility Centre
Unit 2A, Atcham Estate
Shrewsbury SY4 4UG
Publishes several booklets offering advice to disabled travellers.

Forum of Driving Assessment Centres
c/o Banstead Mobility Centre
Damson Way
Orchard Hill, Queen Mary's Avenue
Carshalton, Surrey SM5 4NR

Motability
Gate House
West Gate
Harlow, Essex CM20 1HR

RADAR
25 Mortimer St
London W1N 8AP
Publishes several booklets for disabled travellers including *Motoring and Mobility for Disabled People.*

REFERENCES

Goldsmith S 1976 Designing for the disabled. RIBA, London

Ham R 1987 Wheelchair provision in a London health authority. Physiotherapy 73(10): 576–578

Health and Safety Executive 1992 Manual handling guidance regulations. HMSO, London

Health and Safety Executive 1992 Essentials of health and safety at work. HMSO, London

Health Services Advisory Commission 1992 Guidance on manual handling of loads in the health service. HMSO, London

Heywood F 1994 Adaptations and the occupational therapist: an outsider's view. Occupational Therapy News, Dec 94: 6–7

McColl I 1986 A review of the artificial limb and appliance centre services, vol 1. Department of Health and Social Security, London

Marden A 1987 Design and realisation. Oxford University Press, Oxford

Pheasant S 1987 Ergonomics: standards and guidelines for designers. BSI, Milton Keynes

White E A 1993 An investigation into the requirements for an effective district-based wheelchair service. Thesis in progress (unpublished)

FURTHER READING

Chartered Society of Physiotherapists 1993 Standards of physiotherapy practice for trainees in moving and handling. Chartered Society of Physiotherapists, London

Corlett E N, Lloyd P V, Tarling C, Troup J D G, Wright B 1992 The guide to the handling of patients, 3rd edn. National Back Pain Association/Royal College of Nursing, Teddington

Disability Information Trust 1990 Hoists and lifts, equipment for disabled people. Disability Information Trust, Oxford

Disabled Living Foundation 1994 Handling people. DLF, London

Griffiths D, Wynne D 1986 How to push a wheelchair, 7th edn. Disabled Motorists Club, London

Griffiths D 1989 Wheels under you — a mobility handbook. National Mobility Centre, Shrewsbury

Maczka K 1990 Assessing physically disabled people at home. Chapman & Hall, London

Tarling C 1980 Hoists and their use. Heinemann/DLF, London

Wilshere E R 'Equipment for the Disabled' Series. Oxfordshire Health Authority, Oxford

LEAFLETS AND BOOKLETS

DS704 Disability Living Allowance 1994 Benefits Agency, DSS

FB28 Sick or disabled? 1993 Benefits Agency, DSS

HB5 A guide to non-contributory benefits for disabled people 1992 Benefits Agency, DSS

Housing Design Sheets. Available from Centre on the Environment for the Handicapped, 126 Albert Street, London NW1 7NF

The Housing Act 1988 HMSO, London

10

Orthotics

Pauline Rowe

INTRODUCTION

An orthosis is an externally applied device used to modify the structural and functional characteristics of the neuromusculoskeletal system (International Standards Organisation). It may be used to prevent deformity, support or protect a body segment and to assist in the restoration or improvement of function. In order to achieve these aims, it may be designed to assist or restrict movement of relevant body parts. The term 'orthosis' is often used in preference to the term 'splint', and the study of their design, manufacture and use is known as 'orthotics'. At present there is no universally accepted system of naming orthoses which unambiguously indicates the particular orthosis in question. In the past there was a tendency for orthoses to be given non-descriptive and arbitrary titles, such as 'paddle' and 'cock-up splint'. Now the nomenclature is a mixture of those terms which are based on the name of the designer or hospital of origin (eponyms) and those which indicate the area of the body over which the orthosis extends. Specific examples of these terms include the 'Capener' and an 'ankle–foot orthosis' respectively. The latter category of terms is more useful because they provide some basic anatomical information and are potentially more internationally understood.

While qualified orthotists undergo a specific course of training, other professionals, including occupational and physiotherapists, may be involved. An orthosis is prescribed within the context of a total treatment programme and not in isolation. Occupational therapists are well qualified to consider the principles of orthotics in relation to the physical and practical demands of every day life in addition to utilising clinical knowledge.

Orthoses are usually considered as part of a biomechanical approach, contributing to the maintenance and improvement of range of movement or muscle strength. However, in certain situations, the orthosis may be fulfilling a compensatory role. An example of this is the use of an enclosed support orthosis for a permanently weak joint which enables the person to use the limb functionally but does not change the biomechanics of the joint.

Depending on the reasons for prescribing an orthosis, it may be 'static' or 'dynamic' (see p. 288) and designed for permanent or temporary use. Although occupational therapists are more usually concerned with the design and fabrication of temporary orthoses, they may also assist the orthotist in the manufacture of permanent ones. Certainly, whether the orthosis is temporary or permanent, the occupational therapist should participate in the initial assessment and the subsequent education of the individual regarding its use and potential benefit.

In the following sections of this chapter, emphasis will be placed on the principles of orthotics rather than providing detailed methodological instructions for the manufacture of selected orthoses. Since occupational therapists are predominantly involved in the provision of orthoses for the hand, many of the examples used here will be of that type. However, where appropriate, some principles will be illustrated by referring to orthoses for other parts of the body.

ASSESSMENT

An occupational therapist or medical practitioner may decide that an orthosis is required. Indeed the occupational therapist may identify the need for an orthosis first since she works functionally with the client (Malick 1980), but an orthosis will not usually be supplied without appropriate consultation with and agreement of the supervising medical personnel. Some operative procedures necessitate a specific treatment regime, but the particular one utilised may vary from team to team. Therefore the occupational therapist will, as part of her work as a member of that team, recommend the most appropriate orthosis within the total treatment programme.

Before embarking on the selection, design and fabrication of an orthosis a thorough and holistic assessment of the person must be carried out. The aim of the assessment is to determine the individual's particular needs within the umbrella of clinical features common to the presenting condition. These points of general and specific information enable the therapist to determine which treatment aims may be satisfied or supported by the provision of an orthosis and which specific design and material would be the optimum choice in this instance.

Clinical and anatomical features

It is important to have clinical knowledge of the diagnosis and prognosis because these have implications for the aims of the orthosis, its design and the material chosen. Initially, information about the individual's medical history and current treatment can be gained from the case notes and through discussion with other personnel. If an orthosis is to become an effective and integral part of the person's total programme of treatment and rehabilitation, consideration must be given to any limiting or complementary factors which each regime imposes. Thus, if a priority of treatment is to provide active exercise to the dorsiflexors of the foot, it might be counter-productive to supply a static ankle-foot orthosis which passively supports the foot in dorsiflexion.

Although basic decisions about orthotic management can be made on the basis of the diagnosis, it is only by specific assessment of the individual that points of particular relevance may be focused upon and expanded.

A physical examination can supply important information about the current state of the individual and how the condition is affecting him. Since each person varies to some extent from the 'norm', it is often beneficial in unilateral conditions to compare the affected body part with the unaffected limb or side of the body. In this way, the therapist can determine what is the 'norm' for that person. Features which can be noted during this examination include:

- skin condition
- oedema
- range of movement.

Skin condition

Assessment of skin condition can indicate the current stage of the clinical condition and side-effects of medication, and contribute to the choice of splinting material and design. For example, if the skin is friable a softer more flexible material may be indicated, but this may need to be balanced with a need for a rigid material if the position of the limb part is to be maintained.

Observations of the skin can include its colour, temperature, texture and integrity, and the position and state of any scars and nodules. Assessment should also be made of the extent of any sensory loss. The therapist will not only need to examine the skin covering the part(s) directly involved, but also those areas over which the orthosis will extend for purposes of leverage, pressure reduction and strapping.

If an orthosis is supplied to a person with sensory impairment, it is particularly important to protect the person from warm materials while fabricating the orthosis. Furthermore, he must be instructed to check for early signs of pressure or skin irritation (see p. 291).

A useful example to illustrate potential skin changes is a peripheral nerve injury. Sympathetic nervous system involvement results in vaso-motor, sudomotor and trophic changes. The area of skin supplied by the damaged sympathetic fibres may initially become rosy, warm and dry but later become mottled or cyanotic and cool, and be either dry or moist. Sensory and motor function will be affected, the extent and nature of these being determined by which nerve has been damaged and the site and extent of the lesion. Wounds, possibly from the causal trauma or from reparative surgery, may be present.

Oedema

Oedema may present as a sign of a clinical condition, but the volume of even a healthy hand may change by 10% during any 24-hour period (Swan 1984). Wearing an orthosis will result in some immobilisation of the limb which in turn, through reduction in the pumping action of skeletal muscles, will decrease venous return and therefore produce some oedema. Whatever the cause, oedema may be transient, and therefore regular fittings must be arranged or a design must be chosen which encorporates potential for adjustments to accommodate fluctuations in size. To reduce the possibility or the degree of oedema resulting from wearing an orthosis, the client may be advised to elevate the limb for periods of time.

Comparison with the unaffected side can be of help in determining whether all the oedema has subsided. However, when comparing the upper limbs, one should allow for the possibility that slight differences may exist between the size of a dominant and non-dominant limb.

Range of movement

The alignment and range of active and passive movement at relevant joints should also be assessed. Range of movement may be limited by a variety of factors, e.g. pain, oedema and soft tissue or bony deformity. Conversely, movement may extend beyond a joint's normal range, for example when ligaments are lax.

Personal and social factors

An integral part of the assessment is to ascertain the individual's requirements and priorities with regard to his personal, social and work-related pursuits. Two individuals with the same clinical condition may require different orthoses when these factors are considered. Clearly, this aspect of the assessment can only be carried out with the full and active co-operation of the person. This involvement is important not only to help ensure that the orthosis meets the needs of the person, but also to facilitate correct usage and his acceptance of it.

It is important that the person understands the functions and limitations of the orthosis. If he has unrealistic expectations of an orthosis, seeing it as an instant or miraculous cure, or conversely considers it as an encumbrance, then it is very unlikely that he will gain the full potential benefit from its use.

The success of an orthosis depends on correct application by the therapist of biomechanical principles. At the same time an orthosis is an external device, and its weight, bulk and appearance, i.e. its cosmesis, will be important factors in determining whether it is worn. Some thermoplastics are now available in a range of colours which can enable choice by the client, and younger people often prefer the bright neon range.

'It may be necessary to compromise biomechanical effectiveness in order to make the orthosis acceptable. Better a partly effective compromise solution which is used than a technically brilliant one which lies in the cupboard under the stairs' (Bowker et al 1993, p. 2).

Similarly it is imperative that the orthosis is fitted and worn as prescribed. For this a certain level of cognitive and psychomotor skills is necessary. If it is not possible for the client to be independent in his orthotic management, the availability of relatives or other carers who are able to assist in this is an important point to consider.

THE FUNCTIONS OF ORTHOSES

Ultimately the aim of orthotics is to achieve an optimal position and physiological state, thereby maximising functional ability. In the case of the hand Duncan (1989) states the goal of any orthosis to be the maintainance of the balance of the hand.

In general orthoses may be protective, supportive or corrective (Malick 1980), the splint serving as the external force to counteract the imbalance of internal forces (Duncan 1989).

The means by which these aims are attained may not only vary between individuals but also at different stages of treatment. Indeed, the wearing of an orthosis may, on occasions, impede or totally inhibit function, but will enable greater mobility following its prescribed period of usage. However, whenever possible the orthosis should achieve the desired purposes while not creating dysfunction (Pedretti 1985).

During the initial assessment, specific aims and objectives will be identified, discussed and prioritised for each individual. Upon completion of the assessment, one or more orthoses can then be designed to meet the specific and often interdependent aims of treatment. These may include:

- pain relief, e.g. carpal tunnel syndrome
- facilitation of healing, e.g. ligament repair following whiplash injury
- prevention of development of soft tissue deformity or contractures, e.g. with burns (Cason 1981, Di Gregorio 1984)
- maintenance of improvements achieved by other forms of treatment, e.g. control of contractures between passive stretching (Barr & Swan 1988)
- protection of joint integrity by immobilisation, e.g. in rheumatoid arthritis
- improvement or maintenance of joint alignment, e.g. ulnar deviation in rheumatoid arthritis
- assistance of weakened muscles, e.g. peripheral nerve lesion
- substitution for lost muscle power, e.g. peripheral nerve lesion
- protection of vulnerable anatomical structures, e.g. meningomyelocele cyst.

Research and orthotics

The above are some of the proposed benefits of an orthotic regime. However, some of these are the subject of debate, with conflicting views being expressed by different clinicians. Although professionals involved in orthotics are and have been involved in research, more studies are needed. Methodological weaknesses, e.g. smallness of sample size and lack of comparison groups, are present in study designs, and contradictory results are presented by studies in the same area.

A particularly controversial area is that of the use of orthoses for conditions of spasticity. A useful review of literature and research pertaining to the use of hand orthoses and cerebral palsy is presented by Langlois et al (1989).

Falconer (1991) similarly considers the area of rheumatoid arthritis, and feels that observations and experiences of experts, case studies and reports are the primary sources of clinical evidence. She considers that only a small number of splints have been empirically studied, and theoretical support and indirect evidence for splinting are perhaps stronger than either clinical or empirical evidence of the efficacy, but are less well presented in the literature.

We need to question our use of orthoses and have a more sound basis for their prescription. Reid's (1992) survey of Canadian occupational therapists working with children with neuromuscular dysfunction illustrates a wide range of factors affecting use and choice of a particular orthosis in preference to another. The questions raised here serve as a basis for our self-questioning when considering the provision of an orthosis. More work is needed if current good practice is to be furthered.

Position of rest

Sometimes, symptoms can be alleviated by providing rest to the affected body parts. Rest is most effectively achieved by supporting the body part in a correct, yet comfortable position. The resultant effects of rest can include the reduction of pain and inflammation, as in the inflammatory stage of rheumatoid arthritis, and the facilitation of healing as, for example, following a whiplash injury.

A position of rest is based on the natural position the part assumes with normal muscle balance between antagonist muscle groups. When orthoses are constructed for the axial rather than appendicular regions, a prime objective is to achieve postural symmetry. In the case of the hand, the position of rest described by Malick (1980), is when the wrist is in 10 to 20 degrees of extension, the thumb is in partial opposition

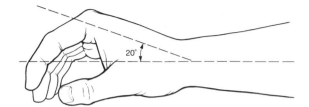

Fig. 10.1 Neutral or resting position of the hand. (Adapted from Malick 1980 with kind permission.)

and forward, and the distal and proximal interphalangeal and the metacarpophalangeal finger joints are slightly flexed (Fig. 10.1). While at rest the fingers adopt this flexed pattern because the flexor muscles are stronger than the extensors.

Position of function

On occasions, a body part can deteriorate as a result of impairment of neighbouring structures. If an orthosis supports an affected part in an appropriate position it can help to maintain function of structures at risk of this secondary involvement and thereby reduce the risk of deterioration of otherwise healthy tissues; for example, a position of some 20–30 degrees of wrist extension is necessary for full flexion of all the joints of the fingers and powerful prehension. Hence, a wrist extension orthosis has a direct and indirect effect upon upper limb function. Primarily, as stated earlier, it facilitates finger flexion and hand function, and secondarily, as a result of this increase in hand function, the more proximal joints of the upper limb are mobilised to enable a wide range of positioning of the hand.

According to Malick (1980), the position of function of the hand can generally be described as similar to that which it adopts when holding a ball (see Fig. 10.2). The wrist is in 20–30 degrees of extension, the thumb is abducted and opposed. The transverse arch at the level of the metacarpal heads is increased in curvature and the amount of flexion in the fingers is approximately 30 and 45 degrees at the metacarpophalangeal and proximal interphalangeal joints respectively.

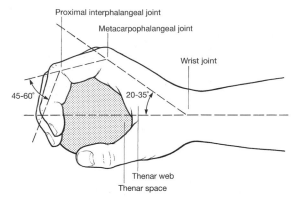

Fig. 10.2 Functional position of the hand. (Adapted from Malick 1980 with kind permission.)

Position of immobilisation

It may be necessary to immobilise a hand in order to allow healing to occur. Since this process may continue for a long period, it is important to maintain stretch on soft tissues to prevent contractures. An optimal position of immobilisation for the hand is illustrated in Figure 10.3. In this position, where the metacarpophalangeal joints are flexed to 90 degrees and the proximal and distal interphalangeal joints are extended, the collateral ligaments are taut. This ensures that if adhesions form in the ligaments during immobilisation of the hand, they will not restrict inextensible ligaments in a shortened position, which in turn would prevent movement of the fingers.

Dynamic orthoses

Some orthoses have moving sections, secured to a static base. These 'dynamic', as opposed to 'static', orthoses can support structures in an optimal position by their static base and also assist or produce movement by their moving, i.e. dynamic, portions. Dynamic orthoses may have the additional aim of substituting for lost muscle power, be it a partial or total loss. They also provide balance and exercise for unaffected muscles, which helps to maintain muscle condition and prevent contractures. In addition, the pumping action of muscle activity may help to reduce oedema. Furthermore, as dynamic orthoses encourage movement they help to prevent the formation of adhesions which would inhibit movement if left untreated.

The direction and size of the forces applied are paramount and must be mechanically and kinesiologically based. In general, 'dynamic' orthoses are more complex in design than 'static' orthoses; therefore it is advisable to develop expertise in the manufacture of static designs before progressing to dynamic ones. Although some basic points concerning the design of dynamic orthoses are given in the following section, more detailed guidelines can be obtained from such sources as Malick (1974) and Colditz (1983).

PRINCIPLES OF ORTHOTIC DESIGN

The general objective of the following discussion is to provide a theoretical framework and a checklist of criteria to assist in the design and fabrication of orthoses. As stated earlier, this approach has been adopted in preference to supplying descriptions of particular orthoses or details of their manufacture, because it was felt that this would be too restrictive and prescriptive. Furthermore, there are several specialist texts available which outline the orthotic management of specific conditions (see Malick & Kasch 1984, Clark et al 1993).

There are many anatomical, biomechanical and social factors which should be taken into consideration before designing an orthosis. In practice, these factors are often interrelated and dependent on each other. However, for the purposes of clarity, they will be discussed here under separate headings.

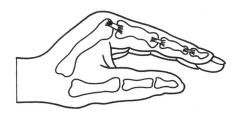

Fig. 10.3 Position of prolonged immobilisation (collateral ligaments of finger joints are taut).

Biological and biomechanical principles

A detailed description and application of biomechanical principles can be found in Bowker et al (1993). Basically external forces, e.g. gravity, and internal forces, e.g. muscle contraction and tension of ligaments, are constantly acting on the body. Following disease or injury the body's ability to produce appropriate forces across joints may be adversely affected or lost: e.g. flaccid paralysis of muscles following peripheral nerve injury with antagonist muscle groups producing normal tone, and lax joint capsules and ligaments in rheumatoid arthritis. Bowker et al (1993) suggest four ways in which an orthosis can modify the system of forces: by modifying the moments, normal forces and axial forces acting across a joint, and by controlling the line of action of ground reaction forces.

While it is not intended here to present a detailed coverage of the extensive and sometimes complex anatomical structures which an orthosis might encompass, reference will be made to the more salient anatomical and kinesiological features and some basic knowledge will be assumed. In particular, this section will focus on the surface anatomy of the body, methods of pressure reduction and management, and the protection of bony prominences.

Anatomical landmarks

The size and shape of an orthosis is partially determined by the body's anatomical structures and observable or palpable landmarks, such as bony prominences, joints and skin creases. These can provide a useful starting point when drawing a pattern or when trimming away excess material from a partially completed orthosis. Also, as these landmarks vary slightly from person to person in their size and exact location, correct fit and positioning will not be achieved unless they are taken into account when the orthosis is being shaped and moulded around the body part.

An orthosis for the foot will be more comfortable if the material conforms to the curved plantar surface, which is created by the medial and lateral longitudinal and transverse arches.

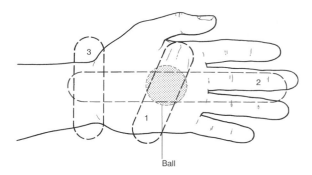

Fig. 10.4 Arches of the hand: palmar view, left hand. (1) Distal transverse arch. (2) Longitudinal arch. (3) Proximal transverse arch. (Adapted from Malick 1980 with permission.)

Three arches, the proximal and distal transverse arches and the longitudinal arch (Fig. 10.4), contribute to the prehensile abilities of the hand. The distal carpal bones of the proximal transverse arch form a strong, rigid base from which the hand can operate and provide mechanical advantage to the tendons of the finger flexors. The mobility of the distal transverse arch, its curvature increasing when grasping objects, is based primarily in movement of the fourth and fifth metacarpals at the carpometacarpal (CMC) joints. The longitudinal arch changes its curvature as flexion and extension occur at metacarpophalangeal (MCP) and interphalangeal (IP) joints. These arches are an essential consideration in hand orthoses if undue pressure and discomfort are to be avoided.

It is also important to note the position of an object held in the closed hand, its line being one of dual obliquity (Fig. 10.5). This is the result of the relative lengths of the metacarpals and the transverse arch being deepened primarily by movement of the 4th and 5th metacarpals. Any orthosis must incorporate this dual obliquity concept, and hence will extend more distally on the radial than ulnar side.

Skin creases on the palmar surface of the hand — digital, palmar, thenar and wrist (Fig. 10.6) — lie in relation to underlying joints (Fig. 10.7). Although these do not necessarily lie directly above the respective joints, they can be used to determine the position and boundaries of orthoses; i.e. creases must be included within an orthosis

of time is useful. The negative consequences of applying pressure will be minimised, or perhaps totally avoided, if the pressure is evenly distributed over a large surface area. For example, orthoses supplied to support the hand and wrist in a functional position extend proximally along two-thirds of the forearm, and this section should form a gutter, the height of which is half the depth of the arm. Nevertheless, a balance must be achieved between this reduction in pressure and the exposure of skin for sensory input, which is particularly important for hand function. Similarly, if an orthosis is supplied to change the alignment of a body segment, pressure will be applied more safely if correction is achieved in several consecutive steps.

In some circumstances, a deformity will only be reduced or corrected if pressure is simultaneously applied in diametrically opposed directions. This 'tri-point' principle can be illustrated by the swan-neck finger deformity, where the proximal interphalangeal (PIP) joint hyperextends and the distal interphalangeal (DIP) joint is flexed (Melvin 1989). Here, the finger can usually be corrected if pressure is simultaneously applied to the palmar surface of the PIP joint and the dorsum of the proximal and middle phalanges (see Fig. 10.9). The 'tri-point' principle of fixation could also be used to correct boutonnière finger deformity, knee hyperextension and spinal scoliosis.

When designing a 'dynamic' orthosis, although the principles which are listed above will apply to the static base, additional care will be needed to ensure that the dynamic components apply appropriate and controlled pressure. Finger slings should be sufficiently wide to comfortably support the weight of the fingers. It is desirable to apply a constant force over a longer period of time rather than a stronger force for a shorter time span. Any force applied to the dynamic

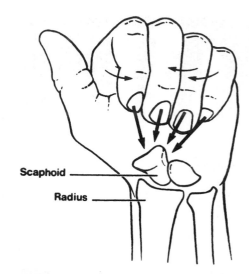

Fig. 10.10 Fingers' normal anatomical alignment in flexion is towards the scaphoid. (Reproduced from Cannon et al 1985 Manual of hand splinting with kind permission.)

section will be transferred to the limb part being moved and, via the static base, to the limb part covered by this. The force should be sufficient to correct the abnormal segment, but not so strong as to totally inhibit the opposing movement. Generally, as Malick (1989) and Cannon et al (1985) point out, the force should be applied at right angles to the part being mobilised, an angle of pull less than 90 degrees tending to transfer forces into the joint and one of more than 90 degrees tending to distract it. The direction of the force applied must also correspond with lines of movement. This can be illustrated by considering the movement of the fingers. When they flex, they follow an oblique line which incorporates an element of adduction. As a result, flexed fingers point towards the scaphoid carpal bone (see Fig. 10.10).

Protection of bony prominences

It has already been noted that bony prominences may require extra protection from the effects of pressure, particularly if the person is unlikely to detect points of pressure himself because of impaired sensation or cognitive function. Pressure may be relieved from a bony prominence in at least two ways. First, if the area of skin which is proximal and distal (or medial and lateral) to

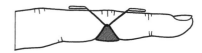

Fig. 10.9 Tri-point principle as applied to correct swan-neck deformity.

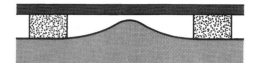

Fig. 10.11 Padding applied either side reduces pressure on prominence.

Fig. 10.12 Shape achieved when pre-padding is used in fabrication.

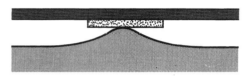

Fig. 10.13 Additional inner padding applied post fabrication merely increases pressure on prominence.

the protrusion is padded, this will prevent the material from rubbing the skin (Fig. 10.11). Alternatively, if the bony prominence is padded prior to moulding the orthosis, this will create sufficient space for the completed orthosis to be lined with a piece of soft material (Fig. 10.12). However, if the orthosis is moulded over the prominence without padding in situ, then any subsequent attempts to line the orthosis would merely exacerbate the problem because the thickness of the lining material would increase the pressure that is exerted over the bone and prevent the orthosis fitting correctly (Fig. 10.13).

Social factors

So far, the focus of attention has been towards the anatomy of the body and the biomechanical principles of pressure reduction and management. While these factors are important, it cannot be stressed enough that each orthosis should also be designed to accommodate the individual's needs and wishes.

In order to achieve this aim, the therapist should utilise the information which was gleaned during the initial assessment about the individual's personal, work and social circumstances, before designing and fabricating an orthosis. Consideration and integration of social factors can be important in ensuring compliance (see p. 285). The person's type of work and its associated demands must be considered, particularly in today's economic climate. An orthosis which limits the person's capacity to work rather than facilitating it might not be worn.

The therapist should explain and discuss with the person the range of orthotic solutions which are available before reaching a mutually acceptable decision about the choice of orthotic design and material.

Cosmesis and comfort

Research and personal experience suggest that orthoses are frequently abandoned if they are unsightly or uncomfortable. In view of this, it is essential that every reasonable effort is made to improve the appearance and comfort of orthoses, regardless of whether they are supplied for temporary or permanent use.

The cosmetic appearance of an orthosis will be improved if:

* there are no unsightly pen marks — patterns should be inscribed by a sharp instrument rather than a pen
* there are no finger or nail prints
* the edges are neatly finished
* the orthosis can be cleaned
* the straps are neatly attached
* the orthosis is as unobtrusive as possible.

The comfort of an orthosis will be improved if:

* it is not unnecessarily heavy or warm
* it does not enclose the body segment in such a way that it pinches the skin or impedes circulation
* pressure is not exerted over a bony prominence
* some air can circulate between the skin and orthotic material
* the edges and inside surface of the orthosis are smooth
* the straps are not placed over an area of sensitive skin nor over a bony prominence

of Paris and Neofract. The former can be applied to the skin following submersion in cold or tepid water, whereas the latter involves mixing two tins of resin (see below).

Although it is possible, if working in a community setting, to heat small pieces of low temperature thermoplastic material by pouring hot water into a bowl, it is safer to use an electric waterpan or 'Aquapan' which can be set to varying temperatures. Similarly, if purchasing an oven it is advisable to select a model which is fitted with a thermostat.

Some ovens also have a convector fan, which is particularly useful when heating large sheets of material as it helps to maintain an even temperature throughout the oven.

'Steam' and 'mixer' machines can be purchased from the respective suppliers of Fractomed and Neofract.

Miscellaneous equipment

In addition to the large pieces of equipment mentioned above, it may also be necessary to order a:

- heat gun
- glue gun
- soldering iron
- extractor fan
- plaster sink
- hole punch
- Stanley knife
- rolling pin
- spring wire jig
- pair of curved scissors
- tape measure
- rule
- plaster and wire cutters.

PREPARATION

Before making an orthosis, there are several practicalities to which an occupational therapist should attend:

1. It is advisable to check that all necessary materials and equipment are to hand and in good working order
2. The person should be given an explanation of

the manufacturing process and the opportunity to ask questions
3. If it is felt that assistance will be required from another person at some point during the manufacture, this should be arranged in advance
4. For the purposes of achieving optimal anatomical alignment, comfort and access, it is essential to check the positioning of the person
5. The occupational therapist should be aware of manual handling legislation (Health and Safety Commission 1992)
6. If manufacturing a number of orthoses, particularly ones requiring greater physical strength on the part of the therapist, rotation of roles within the manufacturing process helps reduce potential strain on the therapist.

METHOD OF MANUFACTURE

Over the years many orthotic materials have been marketed and this range continues to increase as new ones are developed. Some of these materials are rendered malleable by a chemical reaction resulting from the combination of two or more components, e.g. Neofract, and others by the external application of heat, i.e. thermoplastics.

Neofract utilises a chemical reaction between two components supplied in separate containers. To successfully combine these, specialist mixing equipment is needed along with adequate extraction and ventilation facilities. When thoroughly mixed the two components must then be poured into pre-formed stockinette moulds, rolled out to the desired size and then applied round the part and firmly held in position by an elastic bandage until the chemical reaction is complete and the compound material solidifies.

The majority of materials are thermoplastics, and an increasing number of these become malleable at temperatures low enough to allow them to be moulded directly onto the skin. From the three forms of dry, wet or steam heat, some thermoplastics can only be heated by one method whereas others can be heated by wet or dry heat, as summarised in Table 10.1.

Each material has a different working tem-

Table 10.1 Methods of heating thermoplastics

Heating method	Materials
Steam	Fractomed
Water	X-Lite (Hexcelite), Aquaplast, Orfit, Sansplint XR
Dry	Plastazote, Vitrathene
Water/dry	Orthoplast, Ezeform, Synergy, Polyform and Polyform lite

perature and some can be ruined by overheating. Also, some materials cannot be reheated. However, each supplier usually provides specific heating instructions for each product. Similarly, the particular properties of each material regarding conformability, rigidity (i.e. resistance to bending), strength (i.e. resistance to fracturing), strength:bulk ratio, elasticity, shrinkage, memory, setting time and flammability, can be gleaned from the suppliers and of course through individual experience. More formalised therapist evaluation of materials appears limited, but some work, e.g. Shimeld et al (1982) has been published. General useful tips for the handling of thermoplastics include:

* For those materials which in the raw state are very rigid, it may be helpful to use a Stanley knife or sharp scissors to cut out the approximate shape with as little wastage as possible. When cutting the material with scissors it is helpful to pull back one side of the material (see Fig. 10.14).

* The rough template of material can be partially heated, thus enabling an accurate shape to be cut, preferably using long, smooth scissor strokes. Cutting the accurate shape while the material is warm also produces a rounded edge which is neat and safer than the squarer edge of the raw material. Some therapists take the added precaution of rolling the edges of the orthosis. However, all edges against which movement occurs must be rolled to provide a smoother curved surface.

* A chemical solvent, as recommended by the materials supplier, can be used to remove the glossy surface of the material or grease and dust, thus increasing the material's self-adhesive properties. This may be useful, not only in fabricating the orthosis but also when utilising pieces of

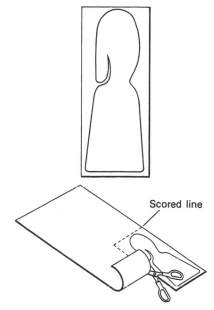

Fig. 10.14 Cutting an approximate template from cold materials.

material to attach straps or dynamic components. In order for bonding to be effective, both surfaces must be dry. Care should be taken in handling such chemicals, gloves or tweezers should be used, and attention should be paid to the Control of Substances Hazardous to Health (COSHH) Regulations (as amended 1994).

* Talcum or plaster powder may be sprinkled on the surface of the material to reduce its self-adherent properties. This is useful when, during the manufacture of an orthosis, parts of the material come into close proximity and could inadvertently self-adhere.

* For orthoses which have areas of marked curvature pre-stretching of the material of this part of the orthosis may be helpful.

* Spot heating by means of a heat gun, or by spooning water onto the material, can enable small adjustments to be made without the entire shape of the orthosis being affected.

* When moulding any orthosis the positioning of the client is important in terms of comfort and for correct alignment when tracing the limb outline for pattern manufacture, and for ease and accuracy of moulding the material.

* Do not rush. Even though some materials

11

Management and the occupational therapist

Sybil E. Johnson

We have available today the knowledge and experience needed for the successful practice of management. But there is probably no field of human endeavour where the always tremendous gap between the knowledge and performance of the average is wider or more intractable.

(Drucker 1968)

INTRODUCTION

How many times has the plea, 'Why do I need to learn about management? I don't want to be an occupational therapy manager, I want to treat clients' been heard, one wonders? Most of us, at one time or another, have had much of our educational and working life organised and managed for us; hence, there is a tendency to overlook the fact that management is an integral part of daily life. People need to organise themselves, to plan their working day, to communicate with others, to be in the right place at the appointed time and to prepare themselves for future tasks and activities. Therefore, whether the individual is a parent, an employee, a student or an employer, she requires management skills in order to achieve her goals.

It may be said that there are as many definitions of 'management' as there are managers. As Heller (1972) remarks: 'Any definition of management must be right, because almost any definition must fit something so amorphous and shifting'. Moreover, people's descriptions are influenced by background and personal viewpoint. However, any definition of management, whatever its origin, has common themes, e.g. that management is a *process* which involves achieving objectives through people, and thus cannot be carried out in isolation. A manager directs human resources and activities within the constraints of available finance, buildings, equipment and materials, with the purpose of achieving an organisation's overall aim.

Innumerable management texts debate the question of whether managers are born or made. Whichever belief is held, managers at all levels must have certain inherent qualities in addition to appropriate education and experience. This applies to occupational therapy as it does to any profession, workforce or organisation, and the intent of this chapter is to encourage the reader to formulate her own views and understanding of management and what it means.

All occupational therapy staff are involved in management to some extent. They all have to manage themselves and their daily allocated workload. For example, in certain settings a technical instructor may have day-to-day responsibility for a helper and will therefore need skills in supervising, directing, delegating and decision-making. A junior therapist will have to plan and organise her daily workload, communicate with colleagues and clients and, possibly, supervise a helper. An occupational therapy manager will be involved in all management processes in order to ensure that departmental aims and objectives are met, that resources are used effectively and efficiently to meet specific needs, that staff morale and motivation are sustained. Figure 11.1 sets out the management skills required by occupational therapy staff.

This chapter is organised into six sections. Section 1 discusses the concept of management in broad terms, outlining the basic components of the managerial process. Section 2 describes the framework within which occupational therapy management takes place by outlining the historical and legal context of present-day health and welfare services. This section also describes the regulatory framework for occupational therapy provided by professional bodies such as the Council for Professions Supplementary to Medi-

cine. Section 3 looks more closely at the legal and ethical principles that bear upon the therapist's professional practice.

Section 4 is intended to assist the occupational therapist in entering professional practice and developing her career. This includes discussion of: time management and prioritising; coping with pressure and stress; core skills and professionalism; and strategies for seeking and taking up a new post in an occupational therapy service.

Section 5 discusses the interpersonal skills that are necessary to occupational therapy managers and staff, outlining the essential components of successful communication as well as various approaches that can be used to enhance communication within an occupational therapy service. Particular attention is given to the dynamics of meetings and committees.

The final section of the chapter examines personnel and departmental management issues including: staff recruitment, supervision and development; managing change; planning, developing and marketing the service; resource management (including data); quality control, finance and caseload management; and day-to-day administration.

It is hoped that the new as well as the more experienced therapist will be able to apply many of the management principles described in this chapter to her own practice, and that she will welcome the challenges and opportunities offered by managerial responsibilities at all stages of her career.

SECTION 1: MANAGEMENT

THE MEANING OF MANAGEMENT

Approaches to the theory of management are many and varied and are described in the plethora of business studies and management texts now available. For the purposes of this text the understanding of management will be described within the ongoing cyclical *process* that enables an organisation to achieve its objectives by planning, organising and controlling its resources, and offering staff leadership (Fig. 11.2).

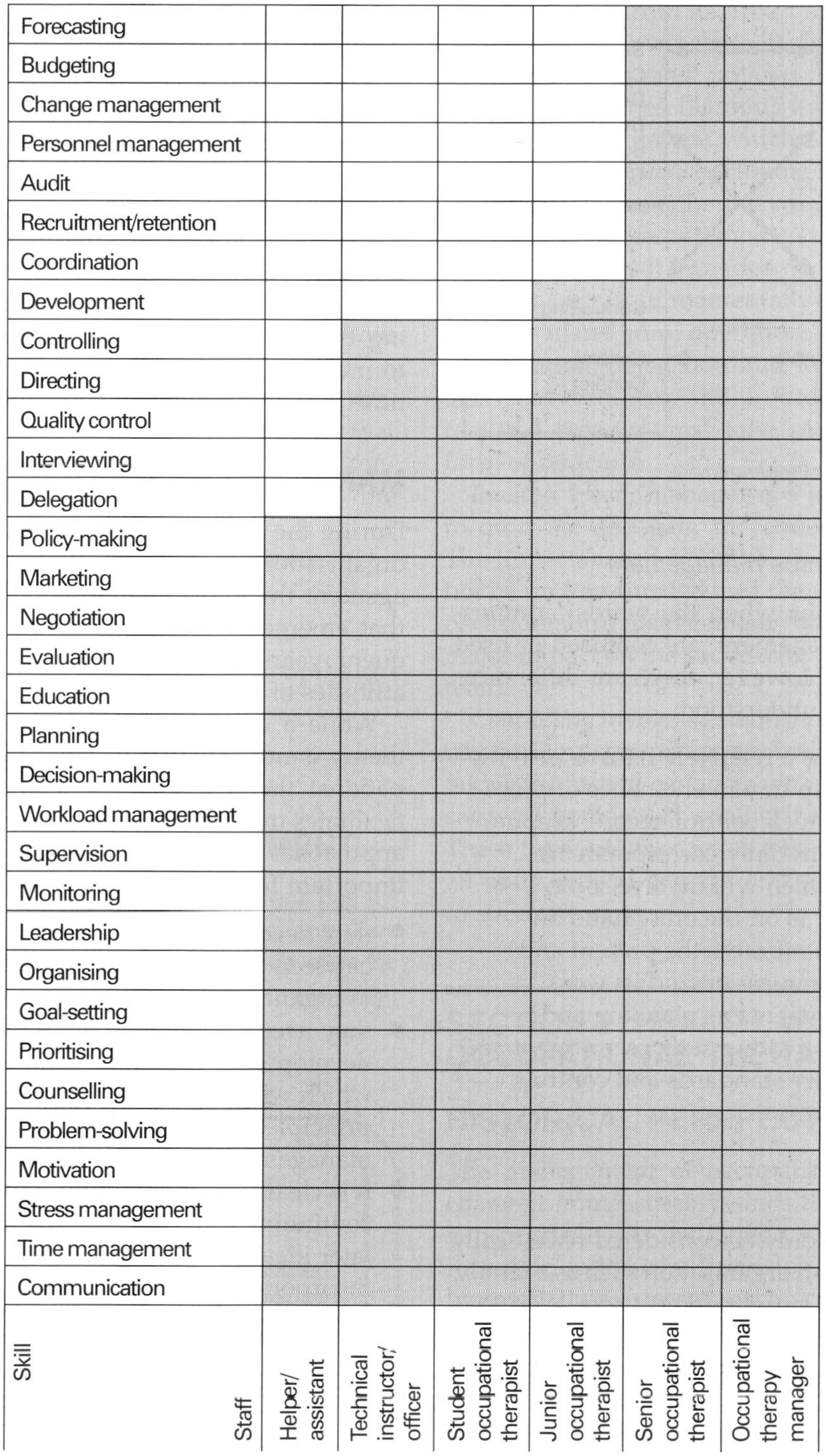

Skill	Helper/assistant	Technical instructor/officer	Student occupational therapist	Junior occupational therapist	Senior occupational therapist	Occupational therapy manager
Forecasting					▓	▓
Budgeting					▓	▓
Change management					▓	▓
Personnel management					▓	▓
Audit					▓	▓
Recruitment/retention					▓	▓
Coordination					▓	▓
Development				▓	▓	▓
Controlling		▓		▓	▓	▓
Directing		▓		▓	▓	▓
Quality control		▓	▓	▓	▓	▓
Interviewing		▓	▓	▓	▓	▓
Delegation		▓	▓	▓	▓	▓
Policy-making	▓	▓	▓	▓	▓	▓
Marketing	▓	▓	▓	▓	▓	▓
Negotiation	▓	▓	▓	▓	▓	▓
Evaluation	▓	▓	▓	▓	▓	▓
Education	▓	▓	▓	▓	▓	▓
Planning	▓	▓	▓	▓	▓	▓
Decision-making	▓	▓	▓	▓	▓	▓
Workload management	▓	▓	▓	▓	▓	▓
Supervision	▓	▓	▓	▓	▓	▓
Monitoring	▓	▓	▓	▓	▓	▓
Leadership	▓	▓	▓	▓	▓	▓
Organising	▓	▓	▓	▓	▓	▓
Goal-setting	▓	▓	▓	▓	▓	▓
Prioritising	▓	▓	▓	▓	▓	▓
Counselling	▓	▓	▓	▓	▓	▓
Problem-solving	▓	▓	▓	▓	▓	▓
Motivation	▓	▓	▓	▓	▓	▓
Stress management	▓	▓	▓	▓	▓	▓
Time management	▓	▓	▓	▓	▓	▓
Communication	▓	▓	▓	▓	▓	▓

Fig. 11.1 Management skills and occupational therapy staff.

social services from which most state provision can trace its origins. Generally it is accepted that the public sector services of today began with: the Education Act 1944, designed to provide equality of opportunity for children of all classes; the National Health Service Act 1946; legislation concerning family allowances and social security; the Town and Country Planning Act 1947, which enabled the government to control the physical environment in which people lived; and the National Assistance Act 1948.

The first NHS Act promoted the establishment of a 'comprehensive health service designed to secure improvement in the physical and mental health of the people', with free care, advice and treatment. In 1948 health care was divided into hospital services, teaching hospitals, community health (run by local authorities) and independent contractors. This cumbersome service remained in operation until 1974, when local authority health services were embraced by the NHS and a new management structure was established.

Other changes followed until, in 1983, the Government and the then Department of Health and Social Security (DHSS), still uncertain about management in the health service, commissioned Mr (now Sir) Roy Griffiths, to consider management practices. Griffiths was instrumental in introducing the idea of general management to the NHS — yet another significant change, which took effect in 1984/85. Devolution of responsibility, accountability and the resources to manage and provide services were introduced quickly, affecting all services and departments. In the late 1980s, government attention was still focused on health services. Consultative documents and a White Paper, subsequently to become part of the National Health Service and Community Care Act 1990, provided a framework for further internal change and gave new emphasis to community care for people living in their own homes.

While one upheaval in the NHS followed another, local government was not without its share of change. The 1948 National Assistance Act established the welfare role of local authorities, for example, residential care for elderly people and services for those with long-term and permanent disabilities. The Local Authority Social Services Act 1970 heralded new 'welfare' organisations — social service departments within local government. Coincidentally in the same year the first UK Act to deal solely with services for disabled people — The Chronically Sick and Disabled Persons Act (CSDP) — became law. In addition, the provisions made by housing departments, public and environmental health departments and education authorities had a far-reaching impact on personal social services. As services were modified to meet users' changing needs, the structure and management of local government services continued to change, the main focus being devolution.

During the early 1990s local government in the UK mainland counties (shires) was subject to an extensive review by a Local Government Commission. The outcome in many cases has been the formation of 'new' local authorities which have responsibility for and the capacity to deliver all or most of the principal local government services, the exceptions in some authorities being law and order, fire and other public protection services. No government blueprint was proffered, so the size and 'territory' of these authorities reflects the identities and interests of local communities and offers opportunities for improved coordination, quality and cost-effectiveness in service delivery. There is continuing emphasis on local government being enabling organisations, devolving day-to-day management responsibility to more local areas or external contractors.

While the public sector has been developing at a faster rate than its allocated resources have realistically permitted, voluntary organisations (non-statutory) have continued to make a substantial contribution to the care of people in need. Their involvement in care in the UK is of immeasurable value. They are not confined by legislation, accountability to the government or local electorates or by politics. While the statutory bodies have major responsibilities governed by law, voluntary agencies continue to attempt to fill the gaps left by the inadequacies of state provision, yet working in partnership with health and social services. They provide:

- direct services to individuals or groups of people in the form of information, advice, support and care, including contracted work from local authorities
- mutual aid and self-help centred on common interests or needs
- pressure group activity, coordinating information and debate related to specific causes or group interests and bringing these concerns to public attention through campaigning, advocacy and direct action
- resources, for example, services to other organisations both public and voluntary; research; expertise in specific areas such as disability and finance
- a coordinating function, i.e. representing the membership of other voluntary bodies, liaising and coordinating activities of common interest and lobbying the government, its ministers and departments, in order to influence local and national policies.

The health and community care changes of the 1990s will influence provision well into the 21st century, with extensive implications for all organisations and professions involved in care services. Increasingly, both statutory and non-statutory service providers work in partnership to enable the increasing numbers of less able and elderly people to remain in their own homes. The National Health Service and Community Care Act 1990, mentioned above, introduced new structures and internal organisation to health care, local social service authorities and general practitioner services.*

Health authorities act as commissioners (purchasers) of community health and hospital services on behalf of their resident population. Emphasis is placed on health promotion, accessibility, quality, equity, effective and efficient resource management and offering people choice.

Social service departments' provision for individuals and families emphasises assessment of need, care programmes, case management, the development of domiciliary, day and respite services, greater support for carers and the development of the independent care sector. The funding for certain social services has changed, particularly for people requiring residential care.

LEGISLATION RELEVANT TO OCCUPATIONAL THERAPY PRACTICE

Law affecting the professional practice of health and welfare workers is extensive, sometimes complex and warrants some explanation. Many aspects of an occupational therapist's work have their roots in legislation and, depending upon her specialisation, the therapist must have a working knowledge of those statutes. If she works in mental health, for example, she must have a thorough working knowledge of the relevant acts in order to contribute appropriately to her clients' care. If she works with people with physical disability, familiarity with laws making provision for personal assistance or home adaptations is important. Children receiving occupational therapy may need certain services within the auspices of educational legislation and the therapist must be *au fait* with such provisions.

Both local authorities and health services derive their powers and responsibilities from Acts of Parliament, certain sections of which 'require' them to undertake particular functions while others 'allow' them to do so. This legislation provides a framework within which occupational therapists and others function. Key statutes described in Box 11.1 are relevant to England and Wales. Readers in Scotland and Northern Ireland will need to refer to their own specific statutes, which differ from those listed*. In order to simplify reference, the relevant legislation is dealt with by subject i.e. Education, Employment, Health. For greater detail, reference should be made to the specific acts.

---

*Models of these revised structures and their organisation are not described as a variety of local models has emerged, precluding any description in this text.

*The author apologises to readers who work within a legislative framework which differs from that in England and Wales. Space precludes inclusion of every statute relevant to occupational therapy in the UK.

Box 11.1 Legislation relevant to the practice of occupational therapy

Act	Summary of relevant provisions	Act	Summary of relevant provisions
NHS			into a service which was community based and family orientated. With the reorganisation of Local Government in 1974, LASS provided social work support to NHS, which had previously supplied own service.
NHS 1946	Establishment of a comprehensive health service designed to secure improvement in the physical and mental health of the population; a free service of 'medical and ancillary care, advice and treatment for all'. Rehabilitation seen as an important element.	*Chronically Sick and Disabled Persons 1970*	Extended provision of National Assistance Act 1948. Describes specific services for people in the community, e.g. practical help, information, register of disabled people, access to public buildings, accommodation for under-65s, disabled drivers/passengers car badges.
NHS 1973	Reorganisation Act: all health services (community health previously with local authorities) to be provided by the NHS. Management arrangements very cumbersome. Between 1973 and 1989 there were numerous and substantial changes in the management structures and organisation of the NHS. These were initiated by the 1979 Royal Commission and documents such as 'Patients First' and health circulars.	*Disabled Persons 1981*	Amendments to CSDP Act 1970. Imposes duties on Highways and Planning authorities in particular, so that roads, new buildings and so on are planned and built to facilitate easy access for disabled people.
NHS 1986 (Amendment)	NHS lost its Crown Immunity, becoming subject to all Health and Safety legislation, including food hygiene.	*Disabled Persons (Services, Consultation and Representation) 1986*	Resulted from concern over deficiencies in CSDP Act 1970, the inability to enforce its provisions, and disquiet concerning community care. Considered an addition to the legal rights and protection of disabled people. Implemented sections 4,5,6,8,9,10, i.e. needs assessment for individual and carer(s), provision of information, meeting the needs of those leaving special education, authorised representatives (advocates) for individual disabled people.
NHS and Community Care 1990	Detailed in the White Papers 'Working for Patients' and 'Caring for People', this complementary combination provided a framework for health and community care for the 1990s and beyond. Includes: establishment of NHS Trusts, further devolution of responsibility, GP fund holding practices, audit, provision of welfare services, changes to nursing and residential care funding, planning, assessment of needs.		
		NHS and Community Care 1990	Refer to NHS section.
Local Authority Social Services (LASS)		**Local Government**	
		(Housing, Rating, Grants)	
National Assistance 1948	Local authorities given power to make arrangements for promoting the welfare of people with substantial and permanent handicaps, e.g. assistance in the home, residential accommodation.	*Housing 1957*	Introduced 'wheelchair' and 'mobility' housing.
		Local Government 1958	Introduced sheltered housing/warden schemes for elderly people.
LASS 1970	Preceded Local Government reorganisation in 1971. Described duties of new Social Services' departments and listed relevant legislation. United previously separate welfare services for elderly people, children, physically handicapped and mentally ill people	*Housing 1974*	Availability of grants for home improvements and adaptations for disabled people. Criteria re property's rateable value and age had to be met.
		Rating (Disabled Persons) 1978	Amended the law re rates relief in premises occupied by disabled people, i.e. own home, residential care.

Box 11.1 (cont'd)

Act	Summary of relevant provisions
Housing 1979	Housing authorities responsible for adaptations in their own housing stock.
Housing 1980	Criteria for grants (ref. Housing Act 1974) waived for disabled people.
Housing 1985	Section 8 consolidated provisions of previous legislation requiring Housing Authorities to have regard for the special needs of disabled people (made explicit in CSDP Act 1970).
Local Government and Housing 1989	Part VIII, 'House Adaptations for Disabled People', deals with new house renovation grant system, introducing Disabled Facilities Grant which replaced home improvement grant system. Seeks to build on established practice and reinforces community care philosophy by requiring housing and welfare services to cooperate. A summary of the Disabled Facilities Grant (Section 106) is offered in the Occupational Therapists Reference Book 1990 pp. 95–96.

Mental Health

Act	Summary of relevant provisions
Mental Health 1983	All previous mental health legislation repealed. Main changes include: establishing Mental Health Commission to protect interests of detained patients; new requirements regarding treatment of detained patients; changes in Mental Health Review Tribunal procedures; introduction of 'Approved Social Workers' in mental health; new powers for courts to remand people to hospital for reports or treatment; informal patients able to be included in electoral register.

Children

Act	Summary of relevant provisions
Children 1989	'The most comprehensive and far-reaching reform of child law . . . in living memory.' Includes child protection, assessment of children in need (including those with disabilities), registration of disabled children, provision of services designed to minimise effects of disabilities, working in partnership with families, parental responsibility.

Education

Act	Summary of relevant provisions
Education 1981	Followed 1978 Warnock Report re special educational needs with change in law on special education. All previous categories abolished and replaced by more general terms, e.g. 'learning difficulty' and 'special educational needs'. Children to be educated in mainstream schools as far as possible. Parents to be more involved in assessment, placement and reviews of their child. Introduction of statementing.
Education (Reform) 1988	In addition to introducing the National Curriculum and local management of schools, act offers advice to Local Education Authorities in reviewing their assessment and statementing procedures. Education for those with special educational needs up to 19 years.

Health and Safety

Act	Summary of relevant provisions
Health and Safety at Work 1974	Updated and clarified previous legislation. Responsibility of all to ensure the health and safety of themselves and others in their care or under their supervision. Now applies to *all* organisations.

Employment

Act	Summary of relevant provisions
Disabled Persons (Employment) 1944/1958	Introduced, and later reinforced, employment and training opportunities for disabled people of working age. Introduced quota scheme, Disablement Resettlement Officers, sheltered employment.
Employment and Training 1973	Services for disabled people of working age unchanged.

Readers should note that, at the time of writing, there is much discussion at government and non-statutory levels about disabled people's civil rights, carers, anti-discrimination (including employment), access to premises and services, including transport and its premises, housing grants, and recommendations that mental health legislation be overhauled in the wake of certain tragic events. Readers should therefore be alert to post-1995 statutes, regulations and guidance relevant to practice in these areas.

Legislation is supported directly and indirectly by significant numbers of Executive Letters, Health Service Guidelines, Local Authority Circulars and Notices. These are issued by government departments for a wide variety of administrative, managerial and guidance purposes. They frequently explain recent legislation or case law as it is likely to apply to health and local authority activities. In addition, authorities receive government reports and White Papers regarding specific services; for example, 'Promoting Better Health' (HMSO 1987) set out the government's plans for improving primary health care services.

Both the NHS and Local Authority Social Services (LASS) receive advisory visits from independent organisations. The Health Advisory Service (HAS), established in the early 1970s, advises authorities regarding services for mentally ill and elderly people. In the mid-1970s the National Development Team (NDT) was established to advise authorities about services for people with learning difficulties. Both the HAS and the NDT comprise people with experience of health and social service provision. Social service provision is usually represented by the Social Services Inspectorate (SSI). In addition the Audit Commission is developing a greater role within health care, to complement its long-standing functions within local government.

These frameworks are intended to be supportive, helpful and advisory and to assist authorities to monitor and audit the quality and quantity of their services, much as quality control might be managed in the private sector.

The plethora of statutes, reports, plans and so on are public documents. All are published and available to the general public through local libraries, community health councils and, for staff in particular, from medical and university libraries.

PROFESSIONAL FRAMEWORK FOR PRACTICE

Occupational therapy practice is affected not only by legislation relating to health, welfare and other public sector services but also by that concerning state registration, common and case law. As well as the law, there are ethical principles to which therapists are expected to adhere, such as maintaining confidentiality, updating clinical knowledge and skills, and managing resources appropriately.

A therapist's professional framework for practice commences with a recognised pre-registration course in occupational therapy. These courses must be approved by the Council for Professions Supplementary to Medicine (CPSM). The Joint Validation Committee, comprising members determined by both the CPSM Occupational Therapists' Board and the College of Occupational Therapists, ensures that courses meet statutory and professional practice requirements and that standards are enforced so that occupational therapists are safe, competent practitioners.

The CPSM

This body was established following the enactment of the Professions Supplementary to Medicine Act 1960. The Council is accountable to the Privy Council and its general function is to coordinate and supervise the activities of its nine Boards (Fig. 11.4). It includes representatives from the Privy Council, Northern Ireland, the

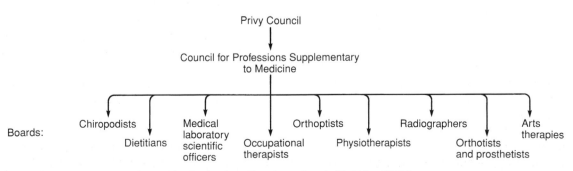

Fig. 11.4 Structure of the Council for Professions Supplementary to Medicine (1995).

Box 11.2 Functions of the Council for Professions Supplementary to Medicine

Statutory role: PSM Act 1960 (under review)

- *Aims.* To protect the public by regulating:
  - standards of pre-registration education
  - professional conduct
- *Functions.* Legal powers to:
  - register appropriately qualified individuals
  - approve standards of qualification, examination, education (i.e. the institution, course and final qualifying examination)
  - produce the Statement of Conduct and implement disciplinary procedures if necessary
- *Statutory visits*
  - a year following appointment of new head of course or as considered necessary
  - every five years with COT representation
  - tripartite validation in conjunction with COT and degree-awarding body
- *Visits include*:
  - tour of facilities
  - meeting with staff, students and managers
  - viewing the curriculum, coursework and assessments
  - visiting a selection of local and distant fieldwork placements
  - submission of report to relevant Board and the institution

---

Department of Health, several of the Royal Colleges (e.g. Physicians) and the General Medical Council. Box 11.2 summarises the functions of the Council and its Boards.

The Occupational Therapists' Board

This body comprises nine registered occupational therapists (who have alternates) who are elected by state registered therapists, and eight other members representing the medical profession and education. The three statutory responsibilities of the Board are to:

- approve training courses and be satisfied that educational institutions maintain standards for educating students
- regulate and maintain proper standards of professional behaviour through its disciplinary powers
- consider applications, including those from overseas, for registration and publish a

register annually of those approved for professional practice in the UK.

The Board is required to have both a Disciplinary and an Investigating Committee to regulate professional conduct issues. The Disciplinary Committee is independent of the Board and is responsible for preparing and circulating a statement of conduct to all registered occupational therapists. The Investigating Committee deals with allegations of professional misconduct made against registrants.

The College of Occupational Therapists (COT)

This body has a clearly defined role in pre-registration education and works closely with the CPSM. The COT is concerned with maintaining professional education standards in full- and part-time courses to enable newly qualified therapists to state register — a statutory requirement for public sector employment — and to facilitate the continuing education and development of all occupational therapy staff.

The British Association of Occupational Therapists

It is probably useful at this point to summarise the structure and activities of the British Association of Occupational Therapists (BAOT), as they have a bearing on both professional practice and employment conditions of service. The Association functions both as a union and as a professional body; hence, the BAOT, the parent organisation, consists of the BAOT Unison, dealing with employment and conditions of service matters, and the COT, which deals with issues of professional concern. An outline of the national structure of the Association is given in Figure 11.5. BAOT business is dealt with at all levels but is led and coordinated by Council and its boards and committees. This structure is shown in Figure 11.6.

The Association produces and updates a variety of codes, guidelines and standards, for example the Code of Professional Conduct, the 'Statement on Professional Negligence and Litigation' and

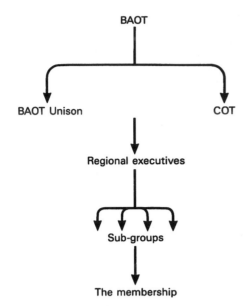

Fig. 11.5 Structure and organisation of the British Association of Occupational Therapists.

'Occupational Therapy Services for Consumers with Physical Disabilities'. While these documents do not impose any legal obligations on practitioners they do provide valuable sources of guidance and information. Further, more detailed, information about such publications and the work of the BAOT is described in the Occupational Therapists' Reference Books and Publications list, issued regularly by the Association.

SECTION 3: PRACTICE AND THE LAW

The upsurge in litigation in health and social care in recent years has resulted in the need for occupational therapists to raise their awareness and knowledge concerning their practice and how it relates to the law. The following discussion summarises legal issues relevant to the practice of occupational therapy. The reader is advised to refer also to the Association's 'Statement of Professional Negligence and Litigation' and 'Code of Professional Conduct' and to other professional literature for more detailed information.

Practising within the law implies that occupational therapy staff carry out their duties in a manner which 'takes account of current acceptable practice and professional standards' and that they 'record their actions clearly and routinely'. Staff have a duty to be 'careful, considered, responsible and educated in carrying out professional responsibilities', i.e. they have a 'duty of care' to those people accepted for treatment (BAOT 1990).

Duty of care

The duty of care to be undertaken by a person has been defined in law in the following manner:

You must take reasonable care to avoid acts and omissions which you can reasonably foresee would be likely to injure your neighbour. Who then, in law, is my neighbour? The answer seems to be persons who are so closely and directly affected by my act that I ought reasonably to have them in contemplation as being so affected, when I am directing my mind to the act or omissions which are called in question.

(Donoghue v. Stevenson, House of Lords 1932; Wilsher v. Essex AHA)

This means that the occupational therapist's duty of care demands responsible behaviour which is in keeping with the education and training she has received, her professional skill and the post she holds.

Professional judgement and standards

The fundamental requirement for a therapist is to act 'in accordance with the practice accepted at the time as proper by a responsible body of opinion in the field of occupational therapy' (BAOT 1990). Therefore, the practitioner is expected to continually update her knowledge and skills in keeping with the ongoing development of professional practice.

Negligence

Negligence can only be implied in circumstances where harm has been caused. Legal action can

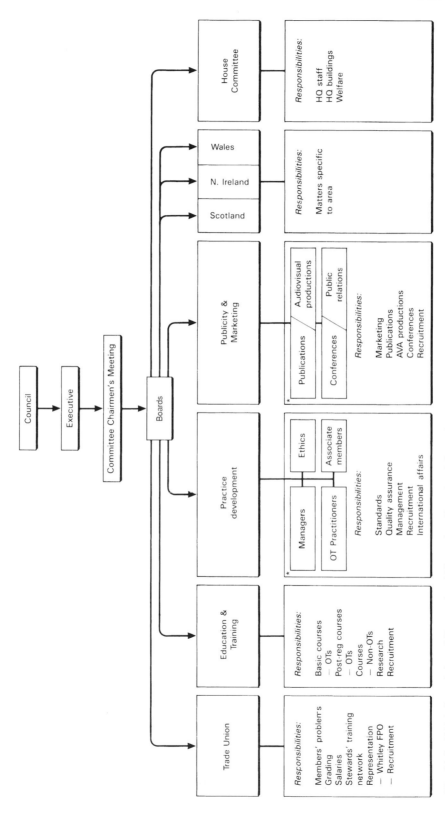

Fig. 11.6 British Association of Occupational Therapists: Board and Committee structure 1995.
* Committees.

also be defined as acting in pursuit or protection of the interests of one's profession.

In past decades, 'professionalism' was perceived largely as a matter of a therapist's behaviour and appearance — whether she was punctual, neatly dressed, had tidy hair, and so on. While these behaviours are still relevant, being professional is now interpreted rather more extensively and includes such considerations as the occupational therapist's clientele, education, behaviour and autonomy:

- *Clientele*:
  - the profession aims to provide a service for its clients
  - that service should be in the clients' best interests
  - interaction between client and therapist should be based on mutual trust and confidence
  - intervention should be conducted confidentially
  - the profession may be expected to make objective decisions about clients and to make decisions on their behalf
- *Education*. At an educational level, professionalism involves:
  - acquiring a systematic and scientific body of knowledge
  - undergoing a lengthy period of education
  - continuing to update knowledge and skills
  - setting one's own standards of competence to practise and auditing oneself
  - participating in the training of students and junior colleagues
- *Behaviour*. Behavioural standards are stated in the profession's Code of Professional Conduct, a set of rules which guide professional practice. The standards are described under the following headings:
  - relationships with, and responsibilities to, clients
  - professional integrity
  - professional relationships and responsibilities
  - professional standards

- *Autonomy*:
  - a profession forms a professional association and writes self-governing rules
  - it draws up a code of ethics to regulate members' standards of behaviour
  - it defines its own sanctions for members
  - it negotiates and collaborates with the state and other groups to maintain and extend its status
  - it may form pressure groups to initiate changes in social policy
  - it may monitor and evaluate the effects of changed policies.

Translating professionalism presents occupational therapists with a constant and worthwhile challenge, supported by their association's guidelines, statements and standards, which enables them to continually 'advance their expertise to the benefit not only of their clients but also of their field' (Wallis 1987).

PREPARATION FOR PRACTICE

The guidance offered in this section is intended to assist the individual to make the transition from student to therapist and to remind those returning to work following a break in service of a number of the procedures involved in identifying, applying for and accepting the ideal post.

Career opportunities in occupational therapy are extremely varied and numerous. Therefore, selecting the ideal job requires forethought, investigation and making choices. During the final year of a pre-registration course, most students will have formed an idea or plan for their first step on the career ladder. The choices available are considerable and may include:

- a post in a particular speciality, such as paediatrics or mental health
- a fixed rotation, for example two years divided into four six-month blocks, offering care of the elderly, orthopaedics, acute psychiatry and a younger disabled people's unit
- a negotiable rotation in which the first block may be allocated but where subsequent

blocks may be negotiated according to individual preference.

In the latter instance in particular, personal choice will have to be weighed against client and service needs, hence the need for the newly appointed therapist and her manager to negotiate the rotation. In addition to the *type* of post being sought, an individual will often have other criteria to consider, such as geographical area, reputation of the service, and further education opportunities in local higher education facilities. Whatever the individual circumstances, it is important that the therapist seek a position which will offer continuing development and support; this will enable her to make a valued and satisfying contribution to the profession. Lansdowne (1989) investigated rotations for basic grade therapists and identified ten points pertinent to the selection of a first post. These are listed in Box 11.4.

The next stage involves examination of advertisements for posts and/or following up offers made during fieldwork education placements. Advertisements in the profession's journal and other publications should be read carefully, as they may offer comparatively limited information and will raise a number of questions. They will describe the service and/or rotation, as well as specialities and the support and education available. Opportunities for obtaining further in-

formation and for making an informal visit are usually offered and it is advisable to pursue these offers prior to or in conjunction with requesting job descriptions and application forms.

Informal visits provide an opportunity to meet one's potential future colleagues, to view the facilities and resources available, to talk to junior staff, to ask questions and to obtain a 'feel' for the department and its philosophy. Such visits also benefit the potential employer, who can meet and talk with individuals informally and ascertain their possible suitability.

Job descriptions vary in format but the description of the function and main tasks of a particular grade of post will be broadly similar. One would expect to see the following tasks enumerated in a basic grade job description: assessment, treatment and resettlement of clients; administration associated with clinical work; liaison with colleagues; continuing education; contribution to departmental tasks; health and safety. Figure 11.9, a sample job description, also includes information regarding the post title and grade, its location, and to whom the individual is responsible. One should also expect to see a date indicating when it was last revised.

Applying for most junior posts will require the completion of application forms. These also vary in format but request similar information, e.g. personal details, a summary of education completed or nearing completion, relevant experience to date, the skills and qualities the applicant has to offer and the names of at least two referees.

An application form should be treated as an opportunity to market oneself on paper. It should be filled out neatly by hand or typed, offer information in a logical sequence and help the recipient to form a picture of the writer. Two of the most important sections will be 'relevant experience' and 'skills and qualities'. The former may include experience obtained prior to, as well as during, pre-registration education, for example a year's work as a volunteer in a residential home. The 'skills and qualities' section might include, for instance, information about a research study, the satisfaction gained when working with a particular age group or the additional

---

Box 11.4 Priorities: Preparation for practice. (After Lansdowne 1989)

1. Commitment of authority to provide continuing education, especially in developing specific skills
2. Commitment of occupational therapy service to the provision of planned rotations
3. Frequent supervision and support from senior staff; peer group support opportunities
4. Temporary accommodation
5. A pleasant location
6. Easy access/transport system to home area
7. Personal ties dictating location of first post
8. Prior knowledge of the service/department from clinical education block or peer group
9. An informal atmosphere in occupational therapy
10. Staffing structures within the authority for future career development.

development needs and discuss future potential prospects. Widely used as a stage in staff development programmes

- exit: to discover an individual's true reason(s) for leaving and to secure the employee's goodwill and the service or organisation's reputation
- consultation/fact finding: to gather facts and other relevant information from specific people in order to complete a particular task
- counselling: to listen to an individual and help her to consider options to solve or come to terms with a problem.

Interviews may be conducted with one or more of the following purposes in mind:

- to exchange information
- to seek behavioural change
- to solve problems
- to make decisions
- to gather new information.

Interviews may be described as a four-step process:

1. defining the purpose of the interview
2. preparing: selecting interviewees, choosing an appropriate environment, ensuring privacy, setting time, establishing any policies, procedures or rules needed
3. conducting the interview: stating its purpose, establishing rapport, listening, probing, measuring feelings/facts, using open questions, being impartial, deciding course of action
4. following up, to check that proposed action has been taken.

Interviewing, like any other skill, has to be learned and should improve with practice and experience. The checklist in Box 11.9 and the do's and don'ts of interviewing in Table 11.2 provide various rules of thumb for the objective and successful interviewing of clients, carers and staff (as well as advice for the interviewee).

Induction

Induction, or orientation, is usually a relatively formal programme designed and implemented

---

Box 11.9 Interviews: the key elements

I	Information
N	Naturalness
T	Technique
E	Eye contact
R	References
V	Verbal skills and fluency
I	Interaction
E	Experience
W	Weaknesses
I	Interests
N	Non-verbal communication
G	Getting to the interview
G	General impression
E	Effectiveness
N	Nervousness
E	Encouragement. Enquiries
R	Relaxation. Reception
A	Application. Attitudes. Attributes. Alertness
L	Listening
C	Communication
H	Humour. 'Homework'. Hypothetical questions
E	Environment
C	Control
K	Knowledge
L	Leading questions
I	Initiative
S	Skills. Selection/suitability. Selling. Smiling
T	Type (of interview)

---

by a manager to introduce a new employee to her job. The hours spent in induction are invaluable, as they offer new staff a starting-point for full participation in the service. During the induction period new staff should be given time to:

- familiarise themselves with the geography/layout of their work area
- read and understand information concerning the authority and service
- meet relevant colleagues, particularly those within their allocated team
- observe the service and the individuals and teams working within it
- understand the service's objectives
- discuss policies, procedures, paperwork, caseload management practices, support and supervision.

Induction programmes will vary according to local circumstances and individual needs. A sample induction programme is offered in Box 11.10.

Table 11.2 The do's and don'ts of interviewing: tips for the interviewee and interviewer (cont'd overleaf)

Checklist	Do	Do not	Checklist	Do	Do not
Information	Keep to the point Listen and absorb Ask for clarification	Waffle Try to bluff if you have misunderstood or were not listening	Interaction	Try to relate to interviewer by listening and making appropriate non-verbal signs	Try to 'take over' Overdo the 'listening' so that you give nothing
Naturalness	Aim to be yourself in your professional capacity	Overdo your intro/ extrovert tendencies	Experience	Ensure that interviewer is aware of relevant past experience: pre-, during and post-training	Waste time or effort on what you consider inappropriate information, *unless* you are asked
Technique	Practise — it helps if you appear relaxed, knowledgeable, interested Remember that interviewing and being interviewed should improve with experience	Ignore preparation — to do so is to fail Think that 'it'll be all right on the day' — nervousness will probably get the better of you	Weaknesses	Remember that everyone has them Know your own, and be able to admit them	Pretend that you are perfect Be afraid to admit a weakness, but follow it with an explanation of what you are doing/ going to do about it
Eye contact	Maintain it appropriately Remember non-verbal communication	Try to outstare interviewer Avoid eye contact by looking around room or at a point behind interviewer	Interests	Include these in your CV/ application. Both personal and professional interests provide information about you	Underestimate the value of personal interests — they show signs of the 'real you' Admit to having no professional interests
References	Choose your referees carefully Select those whom you know professionally, unless a 'personal' one is also requested Always ask if someone is prepared to give a reference	Ask friends to act as referees — they don't always say what the panel wishes to hear Assume, ever, that someone will act as referee. It may be inappropriate or they may not wish to act on your behalf	Non-verbal communication	Be aware of it — in yourself and others — and what it tells you, or the panel	Ignore your less endearing traits — do something positive to overcome them
			Getting to an interview	Allow ample time for travel, finding the right building/ office/department, and for freshening up	*Ever* arrive for an interview at a run, dishevelled, or late
Verbal skills and fluency	Be sure of your facts/reasons for application Practise your skills Try to predict what you may be asked so that you have an answer Prepare your questions if you are interviewing Pause before answering/asking a question — it gives you valuable seconds of 'thinking' time	Try to bluff; your fluency and skills will be lost Go unprepared (see Technique, above) Overdo the 'chatter' 'Dry up'; if you do, ask interviewer to clarify/ repeat question	General impression	Remember, first impressions can be lasting ones — what sort do you create?	Try to be clever and over-impress on first meeting, or withdraw and create no impression at all
			Effectiveness	Know yourself, both as an individual and as a therapist Convey this to your interviewer calmly, thoughtfully, objectively	Attempt to prove how effective you are by giving examples which indicate something else!

Table 11.2 (cont'd)

Checklist	Do	Do not	Checklist	Do	Do not
Nervousness	Remember everyone is nervous sometimes Learn to cope with the visible signs Remember that an interviewer will encourage you to talk and to relax	Admit that you are nervous to an interviewer Forget that the nervousness keeps the adrenaline flowing, which is good — so don't try to rid yourself of nervousness altogether	Attributes	Remember that personal and professional characteristics may have a bearing on the job for which you have applied Remember that your general health will be important too	Be sexist Be over-familiar
Encouragement	Encourage someone if you are interviewing them, i.e. help them where appropriate, give the right non-verbal signals	Discourage someone by being over-assertive, doing all the talking, giving no non-verbal response	Ambition	Admit to being ambitious, within reason. It shows that you are well motivated	Overdo it. You may need to tone down your true professional ambition(s) for the sake of the interview, i.e. don't tell the panel chair that you are aiming for her job in a year or two!
Enquiries (questions)	Use questions in a positive/specific way, even if some are hypothetical or reflective Remember that questions which could be construed as discriminative are unacceptable Prepare your questions beforehand, ensuring that they are sensible and relevant	Ask leading questions, or those which only require a 'yes/no' answer Be afraid to ask questions about the job, structure of department and so on Ask questions about salary, holidays. You should be told the answers to these	Alertness	Be alert throughout the interview, especially mentally	Look bored Yawn Fidget
			Listening	Really listen and understand what is being asked/said Learn to listen if it's not one of your strong points	'Switch off' — this can be fatal to your chances of a job
			Communication (written and verbal)	Be clear and concise Keep to the point Demonstrate that you are an efficient and effective communicator	Waffle, talk of irrelevant issues Distract others with non-verbal signals
Relaxation	Do give the appearance of being relaxed in manner and speech Practise the techniques which help you to relax *before* interview/trying situations	Relax, literally, by sprawling or sounding lackadaisical	Humour	Ensure that you have your sense of humour with you 'on the day'	Be flippant Tell jokes Appear miserable
Application	Ensure it's legible and to the point Apply yourself wholeheartedly to the interview Remember that short-listing is carried out on the basis of your written application	Ignore the importance of the first impression of a telephone enquiry or application form	'Homework'	Prepare yourself thoroughly for interviewing and being interviewed. This preparation shows interest, foresight and good sense	Try to get away with lack of preparation. It leads to failure because it creates a bad impression
Attitudes	Be positive Display a professional attitude throughout the interview	Try to impress with your personal attitude to any topic other than professional issues	Hypothetical questions (see Enquiries)	Be prepared for these. Interviews for OTs do not always include a practical assessment; therefore, the interviewer needs to ask you what you would do in a specific case	Rush your response or try to over-impress. Insist on telling of your experiences in 'X' hospital *ad nauseam*

Table 11.2   (cont'd)

Checklist	Do	Do not	Checklist	Do	Do not
Environment (see Reception)	Prepare the room for interview carefully. It must: be reasonably comfortable, have a pleasant atmosphere, afford absolute privacy and enable panel and candidate to observe behaviour and to see and hear Help the interviewee to be at ease	Accept any interruptions Blind the candidate with bright light Give her a creaky, uncomfortable chair Fill the room with distracting items		their professional development	
			Skills	Elaborate upon skills you possess (personal and professional) which are applicable, as asked Explain your particular interest in specific skill(s)	Undersell the skills you have Overstate. You may well be able to improve the level of skills in this post
Control	Be in control of yourself and the interview (as panel member) Be in control of yourself (as interviewee) physically and mentally	Ask questions which enable the interviewee to ramble at length; if this happens interrupt at a pause and say 'thank you' and ask your next question Take over the interview if you are being interviewed!	Selection/ suitability	Remember that the interviewer is trying to ascertain whether you are suitable for *this* job and *this* department. It is up to you to prove yourself Think carefully before applying — is the job right for you? Remember that there are always other chances and you will be successful	Expect success every time Be disappointed by failure — think of it in terms of experience and your own learning
Knowledge	Show that you are knowledgeable about OT Show that you have some knowledge re the job applied for, i.e. you have done your 'homework' Be modest, but sell yourself objectively	Blind everyone with science, e.g. by talking about a technique you've just learnt	Selling	Remember that you have to sell yourself at an interview. It is not just your qualifications, knowledge and skills which are being tested, it's also you as a person Remember that your 'performance' and your references 'sell' you	Be too modest or too outgoing so that you under- or oversell yourself 'Get on your soapbox' — it will not be appreciated!
Leading questions (see Enquiries)	Answer objectively if asked a leading question, e.g. how long would you stay if offered the job	Ask leading questions yourself. If you need an answer to a delicate subject, then phrase it accordingly, or seek the answer outside the interview	Smiling	Try to smile in a natural and relaxed way, and to appear at ease Remember to smile with your face and eyes not just with your mouth	Grin or pretend you are advertising toothpaste. It is highly suspect and your face will ache!
Initiative	Demonstrate that you possess it, in your application, in your replies to questions Remember that interviewers are seeking someone who has the initiative to 'get on with the job' and to continue	Over or underdo it Give the impression that you could undertake the manager's job tomorrow Be so reticent that you display no initiative at all	Type (of interview)	Remember the purpose of the interview you are attending/holding Be prepared	Underestimate the importance of interviews, be they formal or informal

---

Box 11.10 Example of an induction programme

Day 1

- Ensure contract has been signed
- Point out to new staff member location of: her desk, office and department facilities such as toilets, changing room, fire exits, refreshment areas
- Introduce her to immediate/team colleagues
- Conduct induction interview, discussing first two weeks of programme, establishing immediate needs
- Give tour of relevant facilities
- Describe structure of department and where new employee fits in
- Ensure that she has something positive to do if her line manager is called away
- Provide concise, clear, written information to support verbal input

Weeks 1–2

- Ensure programme is flexible so new staff member can contribute and gaps in knowledge/skills can begin to be addressed
- Encourage her to shadow appropriate colleagues in department and to meet and talk with other relevant colleagues e.g. team physiotherapist, social worker
- Clarify service objectives, priorities, expected standards
- Deal with departmental policies and procedures
- Clarify lines of accountability
- Establish ground rules, e.g. behaviour, dress, time
- Introduce employee to work schedules and own caseload
- Ensure that she attends organisation's induction course as soon as possible
- Begin to identify support network(s)
- Have line manager review induction with employee

Weeks 3–4

- Review induction to date
- Increase employee's contribution to caseload
- Plan to meet needs

Staff development and education

Staff development is an essential component of personnel management, offering many benefits to the organisation, the service and the individual.

To the organisation it offers:

- staff versatility, which will help the service to provide continuity in times of staff shortages
- increased quality of skills
- greater efficiency in meeting objectives

- the opportunity to produce senior staff
- enhanced competition and recruitment, particularly if the authority has a good reputation
- reduced turnover
- a continual flow of ideas
- cost-effectiveness in the short and long term.

Services benefit from developing their staff in an environment which:

- enhances the delegation process
- enables more effective decisions to be made at all levels
- offers opportunities to develop individual's potential
- promotes confidence in additional responsibilities when deputising.

Individuals benefit in a number of ways:

- Their skills, self-esteem and job satisfaction are enhanced
- Their confidence, security and interest are increased
- They develop specialist knowledge and skills
- Their career prospects are enhanced
- They feel valued.

After an induction programme and education to meet immediate needs, each employee should participate in a system of performance review (appraisal) which will form the basis of her continuing development.

Individual performance review (IPR)

In its present format IPR was initiated by Personnel Memorandum (86)10 which explained the process of IPR for NHS managers. IPR is now widespread in the NHS and is a *formal* means of reviewing and evaluating an individual's ongoing performance with the intention of discussing progress, locating strengths and weaknesses and setting goals to meet identified needs. IPR enables the manager to formally record staff performance on a regular (usually annual) basis and assists the individual to take a considerable degree of responsibility for her own career development.

The techniques used may vary but the process, essentially, is carried out in three stages — pre-interview, interview and post-interview — and is accompanied by documentation.

- *Pre-interview stage*: both manager and staff member will undertake preparation for the interview. This may entail the manager considering the individual's performance vis-à-vis the previous year's objectives or her job description if it is a first IPR. The individual may complete a time and task analysis (Fig. 11.8) as well as a review of her past twelve months' performance, explaining which tasks have given her the greatest or least satisfaction and why, and which have caused her most anxiety and why (Box 11.11). She will also identify her objectives for the forthcoming year. Her analysis and comments are forwarded to her manager, who will consider them prior to the interview.
- *Interview stage*. The interview is a continuation of the two-way dialogue. It should be conducted in privacy and relatively formally, offering both parties opportunities to review, discuss and plan ahead objectively, to consider the performance standards achieved, review accomplishments against objectives and agree on objectives and an action plan for them both.
- *Post-interview stage*: the agreed action should then be implemented by the manager and / or individual according to the actions and time-scales agreed. Interim reviews will enable both parties to modify objectives in response to changing circumstances. This may occur during supervision sessions.

In addition to IPR some organisations also encourage staff to review their manager's performance — an upward feedback / appraisal.

Education

Once a service has established an IPR system it is able to plan, systematically and objectively, a strategy for formal or informal staff education to meet identified needs. Ongoing education equips employees with the necessary knowledge, skills, behaviours and attitudes to meet standards, improve performance, and, if appropriate, prepare for the next grade. By applying a professional development framework, incorporating all staff grades, a manager can identify, very broadly, the key tasks required by grade, the competencies expected after, for example, six months, the knowledge and skills required to develop within a grade or to progress to the next level and how these needs might be met. This system can be utilised for individuals or for groups.

How do managers and staff meet these identified needs? Traditionally, courses have been considered the mainstay of continuing education, but experience demonstrates that there are other, more effective, means by which staff can develop skills. Examples include: being coached on the job by mentoring staff; job rotation (particularly in the case of junior therapists and helpers); undertaking research; working alongside a more experienced colleague; utilising opportunities offered by the Open University and other organisations; using self-development or learning packages developed in the service; and experiential learning, which provides new experiences in a practical setting.

Two particular areas of continuing education for therapists should be mentioned at this juncture: training staff to be trainers of others and fieldwork supervision training.

1. *Training the trainers*. All occupational

Box 11.11 Pre-interview questionnaires

A. Reviewing the past year
B. Considering the forthcoming year

A 1. What is the main purpose of the job I do?
2. What do I think is the main purpose of my manager's job?
3. What have I achieved or particularly enjoyed during the past year?
4. What has been difficult?
5. Have I had opportunities to improve my knowledge and skills and the way I do my job?

B. 1. In what areas of work/skill would I like to improve my performance in the coming year?
2. What opportunities and help am I looking for?
3. What aspects of my work do I (a) want and (b) need to concentrate on?
4. What objectives do I need to set myself for the next 3–6 to 12 months?

therapy staff adopt the role of teacher because they facilitate the learning of clients, carers and themselves. However, most staff will require specific, additional knowledge and skills to enable them to supervise and develop colleagues, particularly junior and support staff and students. Helping others to learn is a responsibility which should be taken seriously. The trainer will need:

- an understanding of the knowledge and skill competencies demanded by the area of work in question
- an understanding of the objectives of the development programme
- effective presentation skills and an understanding of the learning process
- sound evaluative techniques.

2. *Fieldwork supervision training* for occupational therapists who supervise the practice education of students is usually organised by pre-registration course staff with the object of enhancing the 'facilitation of learning' skills and role of supervising therapists. The content of this training includes: the purpose of fieldwork education, appreciation and application of learning theory and objectives; role-modelling; planning, implementing and evaluating fieldwork education; teaching and assessment techniques; coping with failure; developing and evaluating opportunities for learning; and partnership with course staff in the development of future colleagues.

Supervision

Supervision may be defined as regular, informal discussion between an individual and her manager. It is non-directive in that it encourages the therapist to take responsibility for her own practice, standards and development. It may be useful to consider the elements of supervision as follows:

- What is it? Supervision takes the form of free, unstructured discussion between two people. It is used at all grade levels to facilitate learning, offer guidance, promote the sharing of information, air concerns and problems and foster the maintenance of standards. It gives support and encouragement to staff as they develop skills and confidence. This particular management tool should not be confused with IPR.
- Who is involved? The individual therapist and her line manager.
- Why is it needed? Supervision is a valuable means of overseeing a therapist's caseload, enabling her to take responsibility for managing her current work and to measure her performance against established standards. It assists both people concerned to monitor the therapist's practices and procedures and to deal proactively with any potential difficulties with individual cases and with broader issues related to her daily work.
- Where does it occur? In the work place, in a private, quiet environment.
- When does it occur? Supervision discussions should take place for an hour or so at regular intervals, such as every week or month. The exact timing depends on the therapist's needs, grade and objectives.
- How does it take place? Supervision often commences on a case review basis. This offers security to both parties by focusing on the daily workload. For example, it may take the form of discussion of a particular case, in which the outcome of an initial interview, the aims established and the therapist's short-term plan for intervention are analysed and evaluated.

As both parties become more confident and comfortable with the supervision process the informal agenda may include discussion of more general issues such as working with carers of people with a certain disability, report writing, or standards for a given element of practice.

The object of supervision is to help staff to retain existing and develop further competencies, to facilitate their understanding of themselves and others, to monitor their progress and to encourage them to make the most of their strengths and consider their weaknesses. Although the two must not be confused, regular, positive supervision can complement and aid the IPR process.

Counselling

There are occasions when staff may need assistance with a particular problem which they are unable to resolve alone. One type of help offered by their manager or someone outside the service may be counselling.

Counselling should be a voluntary process by which the therapist can identify, explore and resolve problems and more clearly define her needs. It should enable her, in a supportive, non-authoritative and confidential environment, to seek reassurance, handle conflict, manage change, interpret her behaviour in particular circumstances, and cope with authority or power. It should give her the opportunity to express herself freely without fear of prejudice or repercussions. The manager should be as non-directive as possible; she should listen carefully, and endeavour to help the individual to seek a resolution for her difficulty and to set herself goals.

Having counselled a staff member, the manager should communicate regularly with the individual, helping her to revise her plans if necessary and to consider any additional needs or problems which may have arisen.

Leadership

The most vital element of any management job is leadership. A manager must obtain the commitment of her staff to the service and the tasks to be achieved. In doing so, she must consider her staff's need for cohesion as they work toward a common purpose, as well as the individual needs of staff members.

Managers' styles of leadership will relate to the task and to the group, but will also depend upon the environment and the leader's qualities. Management styles tend to be described in terms of extremes, i.e.

authoritarian v. democratic
autocratic   v. participative
job centred   v. people centred
directive   v. permissive.

In practice, an effective manager will develop an approach on the continuum between, say, authoritarianism and democracy which meets the demands of particular circumstances. She may need to be more authoritarian when a specific deadline is imminent; conversely, she will be more democratic when involving staff in standard-setting. Whatever the approach utilised, she needs to ensure that it facilitates team cohesion, loyalty, trust, confidence, respect and motivation.

In order to achieve results with the staff and other resources at her disposal, a leader must be capable of:

- setting certain standards and demonstrating them by example
- effective delegation
- accepting responsibility
- effective communication at all levels
- setting clear objectives
- praising, motivating and disciplining staff
- supervising and counselling
- selling ideas
- consulting others
- maintaining credibility, so that staff trust and respect her
- making the right decisions.

Many of the qualities expected in a good leader are summarised in Box 11.12.

Box 11.12 The qualities of a good leader

Personal	*Professional*
Approachability	Ability to delegate
Ability to accept criticism	Ability to facilitate learning
Decisiveness	Availability
Dependability	Conciliation/negotiation skills
Empathy	Confidence
Emotional stability	Dedication
Energy and drive	Democracy
Fairness	Effectiveness
Foresight	Innovation
Initiative	Judgement
Integrity	Loyalty
Interest in people	Objectivity
Interpersonal skills	Political acumen
Judgement	Recognition of others' abilities and limitations
Loyalty	Reliability
Recognition of own abilities and limitations	Skill as chairperson
Reliability	Skill as organiser
Sense of humour	Supportiveness
Sincerity	
Tolerance	
Trustworthiness	

Delegation

Delegation is the art and practice of giving a subordinate/delegate the necessary authority to make decisions in a specified area of her work while the delegator retains overall responsibility. Delegation is an essential component of successful leadership and, like other elements of management, may be described as a process. The steps in this process are as follows:

- goal-setting: identifying the task and its parameters
- programme planning: deciding how, when and where the task is to be implemented and completed
- the actual delegation to the staff member, ensuring that she is conversant with the task and how she is to fulfil her responsibility
- dealing with any issues which arise with the delegate
- monitoring and supporting the delegate, assisting her to reach a successful outcome.

Effective delegation has various benefits. It allows the manager to concentrate on major tasks without being distracted by lesser ones. It allows her to spend her time more creatively and to develop a more effective and motivated team.

Delegation offers team members rewarding challenges and a feeling of worth. It fosters the development of group decision-making skills and combined effort. It also accords to individuals appropriate recognition of their particular skills.

The involvement of groups and individual staff in delegation enhances job satisfaction, raises morale and ensures commitment to decisions which are made by those involved in the service's daily clinical work. Delegation fosters mutual trust and confidence, enhances the rate at which tasks are completed satisfactorily, and makes the service more effective overall.

However, delegating authority does carry a degree of risk; the manager should be fully aware of what is involved in tasks she is delegating and anticipate what might go wrong, bearing in mind that she retains overall responsibility.

The manager's role as delegator includes setting guidelines, providing parameters or limits, supporting staff and acknowledging their involvement. In order to delegate successfully and to accord an appropriate degree of authority to junior staff, the manager must know the members of her team in terms of:

- what motivates them
- their willingness to respond to challenge and opportunity
- their individual characteristics, knowledge, skills and competencies
- their creative abilities.

The following are essential elements in the manager's effective use of delegation:

- awareness that she retains overall accountability
- willingness to give staff freedom of action, usually within defined limits
- understanding of the responsibilities of her own job and that of the delegate's post
- realistic confidence that the delegate has the competence and potential to complete the task
- understanding of whether the task is of interest and whether it further develops the delegate's skills and knowledge
- effective communication
- realistic time-scales for task completion
- clear standards and targets set with the delegate
- programming review dates
- recognition of the abilities of the delegate and trust in her to complete the task, with support and review as required.

There are positive and negative aspects to delegation, as there are with any management tool; these are summarised in Box 11.13.

Managing change

We live in times which are constantly changing in one way or another. As individuals and as therapists we need to be able to manage change in order to retain our sanity and effectiveness. Any change — be it a client's terminal diagnosis or increased disability, a new manager, a new type of support worker, a revised grading structure, or an organisational modification — will

Box 11.13 Delegation: positive and potentially negative aspects

Positive aspects

- Can relieve pressure on leader
- Job enrichment for leader and delegate
- Utilises others' skills
- Enhances relationships
- Encourages maximum involvement
- Develops people
- Offers leader time for other tasks
- Decisions made closer to daily work of service
- Encourages group cohesion
- Enhances communication
- Can enhance quality of work and of decisions made
- Enables delegates to take on additional responsibility in a supportive environment
- Can reduce time taken to complete tasks

Potentially negative aspects

- Time leader spends training staff to cope with added responsibility
- Risk of losing control
- Over-delegation, i.e. staff over-loaded, leader underworked
- Anxiety/stress in delegate
- Time spent monitoring, supporting
- Sub-standard work
- Fragmentation of work or group if one person overloaded
- Poor briefing
- Lack of clarity re targets, standards, time-scale
- Slow (democracy is slower than autocracy)
- 'Buck-passing'

---

result in a number of reactions or stages through which one has to progress. These stages might be described as:

1. shock and disbelief
2. an emotional reaction: euphoria, anger, depression, denial
3. questioning: bitterness, anger, frustration
4. gradual acceptance
5. action to cope with the change.

Managing change can be likened to handling stress (see above). It entails being creative in finding ways to cope. It is helpful to understand the levels at which change can occur, and that there are different types of change, namely:

- that which is thrust upon people — the most difficult to manage
- that which is foreseen, and about which one

is consulted, although decision-making power is held by someone else
- that which one desires and about which one makes the decision.

Individuals are often able to contribute to debate and influence decisions concerning proposed change at a local level. They may be consulted about change at higher levels but are less likely to be able to influence the outcome.

Prior to considering managing change stages and strategies it is necessary to discuss the elements of creative management. First, one has to understand organisations (refer to Section 1.1) and individuals within them including their needs, drives and ambitions, and how the work is completed including planning, leadership and coordination. Second, one needs to comprehend the creative process, that is the development of insight into problems, recognising barriers and pre-conceptions, understanding entrepreneurship and the use of mentors. Third, there is the need to develop creative problem-solving techniques: lateral thinking, brain storming, experimenting with ideas, enabling through sensitivity, patience and the addressing of failure. Once these elements have been grasped, a manager should be able to initiate the 'change management' stages.

The successful management of change demands an understanding of: the need for and processes of change; the underlying conflicts and problems implied or created by change; methods of developing relevant responses and coping mechanisms. The individual will need to identify her own roles, needs and feelings within the change process:

- is change based on unmet/met needs, indicated by staff or clients?
- the skills required, i.e. problem-solving, communication, decision-making
- motivational factors such as leadership, support networks
- personal responses to fear, anger, aggression, uncertainty.

Managing one's own and others' responses to change entails:

- effective leadership and assertion

- very thorough and open communication
- support systems/networks for all staff
- making counselling available for those who request it
- analysing problems, options and decisions.

Change demands the development of coping mechanisms within the team. Initially, the leader of the team should never assume that others understand or interpret change in the same way. Change management must start with discussion and clarification of individual conceptions about the change. This will form the basis of a common understanding. Thereafter, coping mechanisms such as counselling, support and advice networks, or training can be agreed and established.

Managing change within a particular service such as occupational therapy is a task to which all staff can contribute. Small teams can research and evaluate ideas, review specific areas of the service, evaluate techniques utilised, review policies and procedures, monitor actual outcomes against agreed measures of quality and utilise their knowledge of human behaviour to understand how change will influence and affect groups and individuals. The service manager will facilitate and coordinate these efforts while undertaking her own analyses, review and evaluations of public sector legislation and policy and its influence on her department.

A service can prepare for change by establishing the nature and extent of existing services and their strengths and weaknesses. Visiting work areas, listening to staff and clients, reading relevant documents and undertaking surveys will enhance this preparation, which should be followed by a needs assessment and analysis based on client demand, market research and information analysis.

Planning for change

Strategies that might be used in planning for change include:

- examining current policy. This involves considering the implications of, e.g. current national trends in care, local demography and epidemiological patterns and trends, health gain targets, local planning proposals including community care plan objectives, consumer wants and needs and any issues regarding general service provision
- clarifying the service's vision of the future and agreeing on the steps required to turn this vision into reality. This may involve:
  — sharing aspirations, dreams, ideals
  — putting these ideals in a realistic perspective
  — agreeing on a common purpose
- identifying agents of change; these may include group discussion, planning, consumer and/or staff forums, partnerships with other services whose objectives are similar to one's own, networks, the political climate, local and national policy changes and pressure groups. Whichever change agents are used, they must be coordinated by an identified leader who can ensure that the object of the exercise remains clear and that change proceeds according to the agreed strategy
- designing a strategy (including time-scales, people involved) and, if the change is major, piloting the strategy
- implementing the strategy and following this with consultation with and participation of all staff on a continuous basis
- preparing to meet the resulting challenges and opportunities with the networks for support and counselling described above
- building in evaluation.

Managing change successfully presents many challenges and opportunities and requires managers and staff to utilise all of their personal and professional knowledge and skills. If change is planned, those concerned should agree its purpose and monitor changes in need and demand through consultation and review. They will also need to market their vision of the future, persuading consumers of the benefits of change and creating an environment conducive to creativity and innovation (see Marketing, below).

PLANNING AND DEVELOPMENT

Planning is one of the four major elements of

management. In health and social care it occurs within a national framework of legislation, government priorities and policies, circulars and economic constraints. It takes place within varying parameters, i.e. long-term, short-term and on a daily basis, utilising the same principles for each. In practical terms it involves: business planning, i.e. forecasting needs; defining objectives to meet those needs; making decisions, including how one deploys staff and other resources; negotiating change; and marketing the service.

The process of planning entails:

- reviewing existing services
- identifying gaps in services, the needs of the population and any particular characteristics affecting health and social care, such as the increase in people aged 85 and over
- participating in the development of draft plans or service agreements outlining care services
- identifying the resources to meet specific needs
- consulting with key health and/or local authority teams, other statutory and non-statutory organisations, unions and the public about the proposed plans
- developing aims and stages, including a timetable of implementation, the implementation itself and monitoring and evaluation.

It is also vital to consider the above within the context of the management of change. In order to review existing services and to identify needs, gaps and problems, the information available to planners must be carefully analysed and evaluated. All authorities collect information about their services, for instance:

- activity/resource use data
- needs assessment surveys conducted with the assistance of health and social care consumers, the general public, service providers, referral agents
- demographic studies
- epidemiological studies and reports
- ongoing organisational changes which have implications for how and where services may be delivered
- performance indicators (see p. 357)

- the result of work undertaken by specific task groups, which include a user/consumer contribution.

Planning for health and social care now operates within the framework described in the NHS and Community Care Act 1990. Fundamentally, this means that health and local authorities, with local users, plan together to meet the needs of their resident population. For example, the planning of community based health services should consider comprehensive primary health and social care needs including after-care and support required by people on discharge from hospital and collaborative care arrangements among all agencies. This process applies to any client group and will occur within local purchaser/provider roles and frameworks; its outcome will often depend on the co-terminosity of authority boundaries, local pressure groups and the pattern of existing services.

Planning a service

Planning, developing and coordinating an occupational therapy service take place within the frameworks described above and in Section 2. Occupational therapy managers examine the relevant statutes, priorities, policies, business and care plans and establish the implications of these for their particular service. For instance, if the joint community care plan states that health care for elderly people or treatment at home for young people with physical handicaps are priority areas, occupational therapy plans must reflect this.

When planning her service a manager must consider the following elements:

- definition of the service's aims and how action can be unified in order to achieve those set goals. For instance, occupational therapy's aims for neurological services may include the formation of an informal yet effective cross-organisation team of therapists, whose expertise will ensure that individuals transfer from acute care to the rehabilitation unit and subsequently to community care with minimum disruption to their intervention programme

relevant issues are considered thoroughly. One decision-making process, described as the five 'C's — i.e. Consider, Consult, Crunch, Communicate and Check — may provide a useful guide:

1. Consider
   — First clarify the issue or problem. Is it genuinely a problem? Does it need specific action?
   — If it requires action, define the objective(s) to be achieved
   — Decide who should make the ultimate decision
   — Clarify a time-scale, including a date by which a decision must be made
2. Consult
   — Collect all relevant information in the time available. This may include local, regional or national information gleaned from colleagues
   — Organise and analyse the information
   — Call a meeting of those involved, if appropriate, to identify causes, to consult and to seek options and ideas
   — Determine when any discussion about the issue has to cease due to time constraints
3. Crunch
   — Weigh up the options and, if time permits, think about them for a day or so
   — Select an option, i.e. make the decision
   — If the arguments of those involved are balanced the decision-maker must take her own reasoned course to the decision, having listed the pros and cons, examined the consequences, and measured them against the objective(s)
4. Communicate
   — Write an implementation plan, if applicable
   — Brief all those involved or affected on the action and subsequent outcomes
   — Aim to obtain acceptance of the decision. Agreement will not always be forthcoming or vital
5. Check
   — The decision-maker must check that the decision has been implemented
   — This will be followed by monitoring and

review and, if necessary, by further corrective action
   — The decision-maker should bear in mind that it is not possible to please everyone involved all the time.

Negotiation

Negotiation forms a part of the decision-making process and is another personal skill which is learned and used by people in their daily lives. Fundamentally, it concerns influencing other people through the exchange of ideas or something of material value, such as salaries. It is used to satisfy one team's or individual's needs when someone else controls what they want or need. 'Bargaining' and 'persuading' are other words used to describe negotiation. The term used may be influenced by particular circumstances; for instance, one may 'bargain' with an employer for a pay rise in return for increased productivity, 'persuade' a colleague to undertake a particular task for the status it offers or 'negotiate' a treatment contract with a client. Regardless of the term used or the circumstances, negotiation will usually follow a particular pattern. Brewster (1984) describes negotiation succinctly and offers practical suggestions which are summarised in Box 11.14. In addition, therapists should utilise their knowledge of motivation theory to enhance their negotiation skills.

RESOURCE MANAGEMENT

Resources in any setting include staff, their skills and expertise, accommodation, equipment, materials, information and finance. Effective and efficient management of these resources should facilitate the provision of a quality service or product to an organisation's clients and enable a manager to make more informed decisions about how the resources she controls can be used to maximum effect, while relating service activity to running costs. This section describes the key areas of resource management within occupational therapy; these are summarised in Figure 11.11.

Box 11.14 The four stages of negotiation

Before

- Aim for a positive atmosphere
- Collect relevant information
- Assess strengths and weaknesses of both parties
- Identify own objectives
- Consider possible tactics
- Select your negotiating team
- Allocate roles to team members
- Ensure everyone is clear about both objectives and tactics

During

- Listen carefully
- Take your time
- Ask questions
- Keep calm
- Use summaries
- Clarify stage of negotiation reached periodically
- Use adjournments if necessary
- Make concessions and obtain concessions in return

At the end

- Proceed with caution on 'final' offers
- Ensure both parties can claim success
- Summarise
- Put agreement in writing
- Congratulate both parties

After

- Ensure agreement is communicated
- Implement the agreement
- Monitor its results
- Review with your team

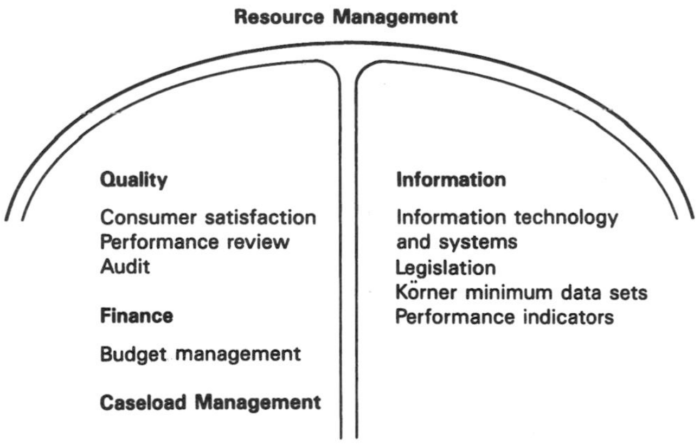

Resource Management

Quality

Consumer satisfaction
Performance review
Audit

Finance

Budget management

Caseload Management

Information

Information technology and systems
Legislation
Körner minimum data sets
Performance indicators

Fig. 11.11 Components of resource management.

Information

Data concerning local populations, their health and ill health, welfare needs, birth and death rates and predominant illnesses have been collected by health and local authorities for many years. This information has enabled the DoH, the Regions and local providers of services to plan services in a very general way, but it has never provided an adequate basis upon which therapists, nurses, doctors, home care or social work services could monitor, evaluate, plan and develop services to meet identified needs. This state of affairs has hindered the management of static or decreasing resources, which are now unable to match increasing and/or changing demands.

Since the late 1980s the collection, collation and storage of health and social care information has changed radically, because of the need to provide evidence of cost-effectiveness, efficiency, quality, effective resource deployment and the changing needs of the population.

If information is to form the basis for all planning, development and service coordination, managers will need to make use of various kinds of data. Information may be needed with reference to:

- diagnostically related groups (a system for coding people by diagnosis and identifying a cost for examination and treatment for a particular condition)
- other groups, classified by, for instance, history, diagnostic procedures, drugs, appliances, preventive procedures and health status
- performance indicators such as cost of occupational therapy by client type, outcomes of intervention
- priorities at all levels
- national and local strategies and joint plans
- local epidemiological and demographic trends
- financial position of the health and local authorities
- alternative funding sources such as Joint Finance
- modern treatment methods and future trends
- educational needs and methods at pre- and post-registration levels
- the effectiveness of existing services
- future staff recruitment and retention
- staff, i.e. motivation, job satisfaction, attendance, special skills/qualifications,

requirements. Quality assurance is regarded as an ongoing process. Some of the terms used in this area are defined in Box 11.16.

Three basic components of quality assurance are applicable to occupational therapy:

Box 11.16 Quality assurance: glossary of terms

Audit: a methodical clinical and managerial review or investigation of resources and activities

Concurrent review: a method of reviewing process and outcome of client care during an episode of care

Criteria: predetermined elements of care against which quality and appropriateness are measured

Effectiveness: performance and level of benefit under normal conditions by average practitioner for typical client

Efficiency: the probable benefit expected/intended in ideal circumstances for a defined population

Frame of reference: theoretical and moral basis upon which a particular intervention is founded

Indicator: professionally developed, clinically valid and reliable dimension of the quality and appropriateness of intervention

Input: see Structure

Monitoring: planned, systematic and ongoing collection and organisation of information and comparison with predetermined performance levels

Outcome: results of structure and process related to improved health, restored or improved function and client satisfaction

Process: intervention/management activities, e.g. assessment, treatment, preventative input, documentation

Quality: the degree or standard of excellence

Quality assurance: a process in which desirable and achievable quality levels are described along with the extent to which they are achieved and the action taken to enable them to be reached

Reliability: reproducibility of findings

Retrospective review: review which focuses on data collection and analysis from clients' records and after discharge

Standard: an accepted/approved statement of something against which measurement and/or judgement take place

Structure (input): resources used to provide a service and the manner in which they are organised

Validity: the ability of a test to measure what it purports to measure

---

1. technical quality, which can be equated with professional performance
2. efficiency of resource use
3. consumer satisfaction vis-à-vis stated and unstated needs.

Quality must be viewed in its totality, taking account of available resources, the environment, staff needs, professional opinion, local and national health care targets, public opinion and the needs of the individual. This approach is called Total Quality Management (TQM). Authorities throughout the UK have produced TQM documentation to assist their staff to provide, monitor, review and evaluate quality. This approach also gives one discipline the opportunity to learn from another.

Professional performance and standards

Quality assurance comprises a range of procedures undertaken in order to promote better quality services. It requires an analytical and evaluative approach within which a manager and staff can analyse, appraise, review, evaluate, modify, observe, ensure equity of provision, consider client and staff needs, question, audit and identify satisfaction levels. It is a process which begins with general principles or the setting of standards. Its purpose is to:

- define acceptable minimum levels of performance and service delivery
- develop policies, procedures and administrative systems
- define goals for service delivery and set realistic objectives
- define goals for personal development and set realistic targets
- review performance and achievements
- consult with those involved.

In practice, the following procedure can be helpful:

1. Staff select a topic, for instance assessment of the person with hand dysfunction.
2. A care group is defined, i.e. outpatients.
3. Staff decide on their objective and justify it, for example the standardisation of hand assess-

ment in the authority's outpatient occupational therapy units, which will aid evaluation and research.

4. They identify the process structure required in terms of input (the resources needed), the process (how intervention is to be conducted) and the outcomes (measurable and observable treatment results).

5. They prepare a standard statement about their agreed quality measure.

6. They agree a date by which the standard is to be achieved, using a realistic time scale.

7. They agree a review date, e.g. three months following acceptance of the standard.

8. Staff commit themselves to the standard, e.g. by signing it.

9. They begin to index standards in order to code them and to avoid duplication.

10. As they commence measurement of outcomes they identify the need for changes, if any.

Both staff and their managers have to assess the quality of the service provided and should select a method which best meets their needs, remembering that no one method is ideal. Broadly, assessment will entail asking questions about input, process, outcome (Box 11.17) and satisfaction and may include random sampling, measuring against agreed criteria and standards, and monitoring information about client and staff activity. Preliminary questions include (Graham 1990):

- What do we mean by 'quality'?
- What are the evaluation objectives?
- What sources of information are available and reliable?
- What resources are available and justified for inclusion in an assessment?
- Is a particular time-scale being used, i.e. retrospective, concurrent or prospective?
- What kind of treatment problems are envisaged?

In addition, the manager will consider:

- practitioner performance, i.e. knowledge, skills, qualifications, judgement, interpersonal skills
- the appropriateness of the service to the client group
- client participation (which is difficult to measure but is none the less important)
- accessibility of the service i.e. time, location
- continuity of care between home and hospital and vice versa
- the intervention recording system
- costs
- client satisfaction.

A manager should influence and implement change in order to provide better quality services. She can facilitate this change by developing her staff using some of the following methods:

- actively encouraging support systems, staff advocacy and consumer forums
- improving organisation and communication skills
- developing caring approaches in her team
- improving the environment when and wherever practicable
- encouraging staff to set up quality circles
- helping them to learn how to monitor and audit their own performance.

Efficiency and effectiveness

An efficient and effective service is one that provides value for money, using measures that ensure that the service offered is the best within current available resources. It is also one with sufficient flexibility to cope with social, environ-

---

Box 11.17	Example of a general quality standard	
Input	***Process***	***Outcome***
Staff grade, time, facilities and equipment to undertake a specific assessment	Therapist will administer assessment(s) as appropriate to client group/individual, e.g. — personal daily living — life roles — community living skills — cognitive function	Time and ease of completion during and after assessment — Ease of analysis — Relevance of information obtained from analysis — Value of assessments in current use

1. Budget adjustments are required periodically to take account of service changes or monetary factors, such as pay awards, on costs and inflation. The two former categories are generally added to a budget automatically. However, inflation and price rises affecting non-pay items may be adjusted in accordance with the Hospital Services Price Index (HSPI) or with the percentage calculated for authorities for a particular year (i.e. local authorities work on a base percentage rate for supplementing budgets which operates in a similar way to the HSPI). There will be instances in which adjustments are not made, usually due to an organisation's financial status, which leads to a devaluing of a budget over time.

2. The manager must monitor expenditure against income. Although pay is automatically charged to the appropriate service's budget, a manager also needs to monitor expenditure in relation to recruitment, resignations, maternity leave, vacancies and frozen posts.

Under the non-pay heading the manager needs to monitor orders and requisitions for goods and services. Additionally, she will consider income generated by the service to ensure that this is credited against planned expenditure.

3. Overall, budget management relies on the regular receipt of information about the state of a budget, issued on the statements mentioned above. The manager will check the staffing position against the agreed pay allocation, bearing in mind any vacancies or maternity leave. Non-pay expenditure will be monitored by comparing expenditure-to-date against the allocation-to-date, allowing for any orders and requisitions as yet unpaid. Each manager will develop a system of ensuring that the non-pay budget is expended in such a way as to avoid underspending or year-end panic purchasing. Overspendings in any part of the budget need to be corrected; this may be done through virement from underspent areas, providing the organisation does not recover such surpluses to balance overspendings elsewhere.

Occupational therapists are well able to monitor, review and control their budgets providing they receive accurate and regularly updated budget statements and seek advice and support from their finance colleagues who appreciate the finer nuances of health and social care funding and budgets.

Caseload management

Pressure on services in which demand outstrips available resources frequently means that work has to be prioritised. Caseload management (not to be confused with care management) is a system or tool for facilitating prioritisation. It helps an individual to manage her time in relation to her caseload and a manager to monitor and manage the service, thus ensuring that agreed quality standards are maintained and that staff do not suffer from overload.

Before describing the process of caseload management it is necessary to define certain terminology:

- referral: any request for assistance or a service which requires face-to-face contact and interaction of some sort
- case: a client *accepted* for assessment and/or intervention. The client remains a case until discharged from the service
- waiting list: people who have been referred who are awaiting allocation to a therapist
- caseload:
  — annual: total cases dealt with in a particular year
  — current: cases for which the service has ongoing responsibility
  — potential (contained): in a particular work area such as a ward where all people could be potential but not actual cases
  — potential (very large): e.g. people living in a particular geographical area
- workload: daily work with current caseload, including related administration, liaison, teaching and managerial tasks
- case mix: the type and complexity of cases on a therapist's caseload
- priority: a person who comes before other clients when his needs are analysed against set criteria
- weighting: the weighting allocated to a client will depend on the complexity of his needs, the input required at the caseload review date and the resources needed to meet his

current needs. Criteria for weighting within a caseload may vary according to speciality and/or location but, in essence, will depend on professional judgement re the level of input per case from simple/minimal to complex, the time and skill mix required over a weekly or monthly time-scale *and* the inclusion of other vital caseload-related duties.

The system or process of caseload management employed by a service needs to be simple to use, take as little time as possible to operate and be sufficiently refined to identify the optimum number of clients each therapist can manage in view of her grade, experience and need for supervision.

Caseload management has become increasingly important in the context of more recent legislation, quality standards, audit and costings. Service agreements need to identify the available resources which can be used to assess and treat a certain number of people with varying needs at an agreed standard at a particular time. Managers can then also identify and justify the difference between actual and estimated shortfalls in service provision in relation to their existing resources.

The ultimate outcome of improved resource management systems is to enable government departments, the SSI, Regional Offices and local health and social service authorities to monitor, review, evaluate and analyse data with a view to obtaining the highest quality of service for the greatest number of people within available resources. Health care and social services operate within ongoing and significant change; as resource management becomes more sophisticated, managers will be better informed and will be able to make more informed judgements.

ADMINISTRATION

In contrast to the proactive nature of management, administration is a reactive activity which deals with the day-to-day tasks which support the overall function of a service or department. Administrative activities are dealt with by managers, therapy staff and any clerical support allocated to the service. These activities include record-keeping and report writing, stock and equipment control, monitoring staff absences, collecting and collating information, coordinating staff rotas for particular duties and organising clerical support for typing, filing and telephone reception.

Record-keeping

Records are administration's memory bank. They contain information about a service, its clients and staff, supplies, equipment and so on. They take a number of forms, for instance files, written reports, charts, tapes and discs, and are important in the control and assessment of work. They assist a manager, and others, to monitor what is happening or has happened, to make effective decisions and to assess progress towards goals. They must be accurate, accessible and informative and each manager needs to consider the following questions when deciding whether or not to keep records:

- Will the information be useful? How? When? To whom?
- What part will it play in decision-making and evaluation?
- Can it be collected accurately enough to serve its purpose?
- Will it be accessible?
- Will it be available when and where it is required?
- Can it be stored at a reasonable cost?

Having decided it *is* appropriate to keep a particular record, the form it will take must be considered, e.g. manual, computerised, with or without back-up.

Rather than describing types of records in detail in this text we refer the reader to Creek (1990) which provides a thorough overview of record keeping generally, occupational therapy records in particular and the systems which are commonly used.

Report writing

Reports contain information which has to be communicated to clinical colleagues, others in

involve the occupational/staff health department's assistance and advice and assistance from medical and other colleagues in cases of sickness or injury.

Staff rotas

Rotas are time plans by which certain activities are distributed among staff members such that each takes responsibility for a specific task for a particular period. Rotas in occupational therapy departments may be drawn up for tasks such as end-of-day security; printing press preparation and cleaning; general tidying/storage; refrigerator checking, cleaning and defrosting; collection of in-service training programme contributions; selected maintenance of equipment. They are common in most if not all organisations and are needed for the following reasons:

- to distribute work fairly and evenly during normal working hours
- to distribute uninteresting and interesting work equally among staff
- to provide staff with the opportunity to contribute to the overall function of the service, including daily housekeeping.

There are two clear rules for drawing up rotas. First, the period of time for each allocated duty must be the same for all staff. Second, if groups of staff are allocated a task, that task must be subdivided equitably.

Clerical duties

All occupational therapy staff have to undertake clerical tasks during the course of their work, whether or not clerical staff are available to support the service. If clerical support is available, tasks may be allocated specifically or be performed by a pool of clerical staff. Where support is provided, therapy staff will obtain assistance with typing, filing and telephone duties. However, there are still services which have to function with little or no support; therefore, therapists need to be able to devise clerical systems which facilitate rather than hinder their clinical duties.

Written communications

Most services will have assistance, however limited, for the typing of letters, reports and the like. However, staff may have to hand-write clients' treatment notes, memoranda and so on.

Filing

It is essential that all services and their work areas have an efficient filing system for clinical and managerial records. A filing system must be simple so that it is easily maintained and facilitates easy retrieval of papers. It should include a place for every type of record normally found within the service and organisation. Three key methods are commonly used in filing systems:

- alphabetical: files are arranged in alphabetical order regardless of subject. This is probably the most straightforward system in use
- numerical: this requires each file to be allocated a number. This requires a master index which can be cross-referenced, if necessary, to a subject index
- by subject: this is useful for general purposes and for small filing systems, but requires some type of indexing for easy reference and retrieval.

Whichever method is selected, all staff with access to it must learn how to use it correctly so that it maintains its effectiveness.

Telephone duties

Therapists may spend many hours each week on the telephone dealing with matters regarding particular clients. However, they may also find that they take calls and messages for colleagues, and that this works satisfactorily providing those colleagues reciprocate. Calls can be screened by reception or clerical staff if this support is available; otherwise, each service or work area will need an appropriate and foolproof message relaying system which will enable staff to continue their clinical work with as few interruptions as possible.

Administration is not a popular task with occupational therapy staff, but if a service and its resources are to function at an optimum level of efficiency and effectiveness simple and reliable administrative procedures, practices and systems are indispensable.

RESEARCH

Research involves planned observation or experimentation using particular methods of recording and measurement. It is an essential component of clinical and managerial work. Informally, it may entail discussing cases with colleagues, thus stimulating discussion and speculation. Formally, it is undertaken to answer clearly defined questions, for example whether a particular technique is effective or an information system meets current and future needs.

The process of research includes:

- identifying a broad area of study
- undertaking a literature search and review
- specifying the question to be answered
- designing the appropriate methodology
- collecting appropriate data
- analysing the data
- disseminating the findings to colleagues.

Its overall purpose is to further the individual's and the profession's knowledge in a particular area.

While all pre-registration occupational therapy courses include research, therapists at all levels find that courses offered by higher education provide additional learning opportunities, advice and support. The reader is also referred to the plethora of information now available, e.g. from the BAOT, its Education and Research Board, the DoH and Regional documents on research and funding and the Medical Research Council.

CONCLUSION

Management in all areas of public service has changed and continues to develop apace, not only as a result of legislation and government policies but as a direct result of the developments and trends in health and social care and the increasing need to use resources in a way which provides high-quality, cost-effective services.

This chapter has, it is hoped, placed management in a realistic and practical perspective, offering background information about the history, theory, legislation and practice of management and describing many of the day-to-day tasks which face staff at all levels. People's management skills, like their clinical abilities, develop over time and with experience. Most skills are learned 'on the job', with occasional injections of theory from specific courses. Few, if any, managers are born. Most are *made*, and are shaped by their own personalities, knowledge, skills and attitudes, whatever their level of responsibility. Occupational therapists have an advantage over some other professionals in that the intervention processes they use give them the opportunity to develop many management skills (see Fig. 11.2). Therapists should remember that Cole's (1984) description still rings true — 'management is not an activity that exists in its own right. It is rather a description of a variety of activities carried out by those members of organisations whose role is that of a manager'. All occupational therapy staff are managers of something or someone, and most especially of themselves.

USEFUL ADDRESS

British Association of Occupational Therapists
6–8 Marshalsea Road
Southwark
London SE1 1HL

REFERENCES

Armstrong M 1991 A handbook of personnel management practice, 4th edn. Kogan Page, London

Brewster C 1984 Understanding industrial relations. Pan Books, London

British Association of Occupational Therapists 1990 Statement on professional negligence and litigation (SPP 135). BAOT, London (under review)

British Association of Occupational Therapists 1990 Code of professional conduct. BAOT, London (under revision)

Cole G A 1984 Management theory and practice. D.P. Publications, London

Council for Professions Supplementary to Medicine 1990 Statement of conduct. CPSM, London

Creek J (ed) 1990 Occupational therapy and mental health: principles, skills and practice. Churchill Livingstone, Edinburgh

Dale E, Michelon L C 1966 Modern management methods. Penguin, Harmondsworth

Drucker P F 1968 The practice of management. Pan Books, London

Graham N O 1990 Quality assurance in hospitals: strategies for assessment and implementation. Aspen, Rockville, MD

Handy C B 1985 Understanding organisations, 3rd edn. Penguin, Harmondsworth

Heller R 1972 The naked manager. Barrie & Jenkins, London

HMSO 1944 Education act. HMSO, London

HMSO 1944/58 Disabled persons (employment) acts. HMSO, London

HMSO 1946 National Health Service act. HMSO, London

HMSO 1948 National assistance act. HMSO, London

HMSO 1957 Housing act. HMSO, London

HMSO 1958 Local Government act. HMSO, London

HMSO 1960 Professions supplementary to medicine act. HMSO, London

HMSO 1970 Chronically sick and disabled persons act. HMSO, London

HMSO 1970 Equal pay act. HMSO, London

HMSO 1970 Local authority social services act. HMSO, London

HMSO 1973 Employment and training act. HMSO, London

HMSO 1973 National Health Service act. HMSO, London

HMSO 1974 Health and safety at work act. HMSO, London

HMSO 1974 Housing act. HMSO, London

HMSO 1974 National Health Service (PSM) regulation act. HMSO, London

HMSO 1975 Employment act. HMSO, London

HMSO 1975/86 Sex discrimination act. HMSO, London

HMSO 1976 Race relations act. HMSO, London

HMSO 1978 Employment protection (consolidation) act. HMSO, London

HMSO 1978 Rating (disabled persons) act. HMSO, London

HMSO 1979 Housing act. HMSO, London

HMSO 1980 Housing act. HMSO, London

HMSO 1981 Disabled persons act. HMSO, London

HMSO 1981 Education act. HMSO, London

HMSO 1983 Mental health act. HMSO, London

HMSO 1984 Data protection act, HMSO, London

HMSO 1985 Housing act. HMSO, London

HMSO 1986 Disabled persons (services, consultation and representation) act. HMSO, London

HMSO 1986 National Health Service (amendment) act. HMSO, London

HMSO 1987 Access to personal files act. HMSO, London

HMSO 1987 Consumer protection act. HMSO, London

HMSO 1987 Promoting better health. White Paper. HMSO, London

HMSO 1988 Access to medical reports act. HMSO, London

HMSO 1988 Education (Reform). HMSO, London

HMSO 1989 Local government and housing act. HMSO, London

HMSO 1989 Working for patients. White Paper. HMSO, London

HMSO 1990 Access to health records. HMSO, London

HMSO 1990 National Health Service and community care act. HMSO, London

Lansdowne J 1989 To rotate or not to rotate. British Journal of Occupational Therapy 52(1): 4–7

Mullins L J 1985 Management and organisational behaviour. Pitman, London

Penn B, Penn J 1990 Marketing occupational therapy: imperative for the future? British Journal of Occupational Therapy 53(2): 64–66

Wallis M A 1987 'Profession' and 'professionalism' and the emerging profession of occupational therapy. British Journal of Occupational Therapy 50(8): 264–265; 50(9): 300–302

Wilson M 1984 Occupational therapy in short term psychiatry. Churchill Livingstone, Edinburgh

FURTHER READING

Adair J 1985 Effective decision making. Pan, London

Broadbent M, Cullen J 1993 Managing financial resources. Butterworth Heinemann, London

College of Occupational Therapists Research: how to do it. COT, London

College of Occupational Therapists Standards, policies and proceedings: standards of practice for occupational therapy services. COT, London

Cooke S, Spreadbury P 1995 Trent Region Occupational Therapy Clinical Audit & Outcomes project. Available from: Nottingham City Hospital NHS Trust Occupational Therapy Department

De Gilio S; Bowden R, Burrows H 1989 The management manual for health care professionals. Winslow Press, Bicester, Oxon

Finch J D 1984 Aspects of law affecting the paramedical professions. Faber & Faber, London

Fletcher W 1983 Meetings, meetings. Hodder & Stoughton, London

Handy C 1990 The age of unreason. Arrow, London

Haylock S 1989 A method of caseload management. British Journal of Occupational Therapy 52(10): 380–382

HMSO 1989 Caring for people. White Paper. HMSO, London

HMSO 1993 (Dec.) The local government commission for England — reviewing local government in the English Shires — a progress report

Katz D 1964 The motivation basis of organisational behaviour. Behavioural Science 9: 131–136

Kingston W, Rowbottom R 1989 Making general management work in the NHS: a guide to general management for NHS managers. Brunel University, Uxbridge

Maddux R B 1988 Successful negotiation. Kogan Page, London

Mays J, Forder A, Keidan O 1983 Penelope Hall's Social Service of England and Wales. Routledge & Kegan Paul, London

NHS Management Executive 1990 (HC(90)22) A guide to consent for examination or treatment. NHSME, London

NHSTA 1985 Better management, better health. NHSTA, London

Ouvreteit J 1986 Organisation of multidisciplinary teams. Brunel University, Uxbridge

Partridge C, Barnitt R 1986 Research guidelines: a handbook for therapists. Heinemann, London

Scott J, Rochester A 1984 Effective management skills: what's a manager? Sphere, London

Practice

Practice is the culmination of the professional and personal philosophies we adopt: it is the principles, theories, knowledge and skills we learn and develop with experience and the passage of time. Part 3 illustrates this well by following the logical sequence of 'principles–skills–practice' and demonstrating occupational therapists' application of Parts 1 and 2 in relation to individuals who have innate abilities, skills and experience, widely varying problems and subsequent needs, and who may 'suffer from' any one of a seemingly increasing range of conditions. Readers will see that Parts 1 and 2 offer a wealth of information, observation and discussion about our foundations, i.e. history and philosophy, theoretical frameworks and life development, and our skills, i.e. the practice process, activity analysis, the therapeutic use of activity, assessment, life skills, mobility, orthotics and management.

Part 3 is the next step in the sequence, offering the reader the opportunity to share the extensive range and depth of applied knowledge and skills, tried and tested by expert occupational therapists. This part of the text is subdivided into four sections: neurology, musculoskeletal and vascular problems, coronary care and AIDS and cancer. The first two sections comprise the bulk of Part 3, with the latter significant, yet small, number of conditions 'bringing up the rear'.

Each section begins with an introductory chapter that gives an overview and summary of what follows, including philosophy, principles of occupational therapy, comparisons and contrasts of, for example, causes, features, incidence by age, gender and geography, theories of occupational therapy, and the current thinking and research concerning diagnosis, prevention and/or cure.

The contents' grouping, devised for the previous edition of this book, has been retained, as this approach is logical and appropriate, enabling the reader to make quick reference or undertake in-depth study of a particular group of conditions. The chapters within each section are written by experienced occupational therapists, all experts in their specialist areas of practice and in fieldwork or course-based student education.

Each chapter offers relevant underpinning knowledge on the condition, philosophy and models. In the interpretation and application it also discusses and justifies appropriate frames of reference, approaches and techniques that may be adopted in particular instances, and how these may be modified during a period of intervention. Each chapter closes with the contributor's conclusion, references and suggested further reading, which readers are encouraged to pursue, as this extensive text cannot cater for every need and still be portable and affordable.

each response pattern. Mistakes or seemingly useless responses are 'forgotten' but not erased. They are 'in limbo' and can be retrieved if necessary.

An example, of this mechanism of development is the smile (Fig. 12.2). After a baby has been fed, he may get 'wind'; this discomfort produces the so-called windy smile. It is a reflex response and thus involuntary. However, his mother may choose to receive this stimulus as a social smile and think that it reflects affection and pleasure, so returns the smile (providing a visual stimulus), possibly accompanied by talking (auditory stimulus) and a tickle under the chin (tactile stimulus). This process is repeated many times until the baby recognises this combination of stimuli and produces a voluntary smile response. Thus, a new and more complex program is established. However, the smile (grin or grimace) is still produced in response to 'wind' (indigestion, burping or colonic movement), even as an adult.

Often-repeated programs move from the voluntary, conscious level to the voluntary, subconscious level of control. They may be initiated at a cortical level, but the actual running and monitoring of the program is at a sub-cortical level (without thinking). Examples are walking,

eating (hand to mouth), riding a bike and driving a car.

This movement down the hierarchy of control frees the higher, conscious level of the brain to concentrate on 'thinking', to, for example, create new programs, imagine, dream, forward plan and reflect. However, should an 'unexpected' stimulus occur within the subconsciously controlled program, thinking is interrupted so that control of the program is at a conscious level, allowing instant decision-making and a change in response. For example:

- walking — tripping over an obstacle on the pavement
- eating — food too hot or falling into lap
- bike riding — a flat tyre or a shout from a friend
- driving — a child running into the road or brake lights in front.

Another example of nervous system development is the bladder emptying reflex (Box 12.1).

The computer was designed to emulate the nervous system, each part of a personal computer corresponding to a part of the nervous system and functioning in a similar way. It provides a suitable illustration for describing the somatosensory-motor components and their layout

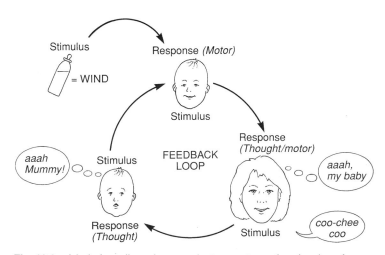

Fig. 12.2 A baby's smile — how a voluntary motor action develops from a complex stimulus/response feedback loop that is initiated by the involuntary motor response of a simple reflex arc.

Box 12.1 Nervous system development – the bladder emptying reflex

- *Reflex arc.* The bladder is primarily under unconscious, involuntary control; i.e. receptors in the bladder wall detect changes in pressure as the bladder fills, receptors in the abdominal muscles detect stretch, and when a certain level of stimulation is reached, the response is initiated (relaxation of the sphincter and contraction of the abdominal muscles), thus expelling urine.
- *Feedback loop.* The changes are detected and evaluated: relief of pressure versus wet legs.
- *Immature control.* Stimuli are recognised at a conscious level, and the reflex response is inhibited until the child is on the potty (voluntary response). However, when the conscious level is busy concentrating on a task, the response is again involuntary: he has an 'accident'.
- *Mature control.* Stimuli are recognised at a subconscious level and are brought to the conscious level by further stimuli, e.g. sees 'toilet' sign, before going out or with a very full bladder.
- *Survival reflex.* Mature control can inhibit or override the response until the system is in danger, at which point the unconscious, involuntary level regains control to prevent the bladder from bursting.
- *Nervous system dysfunction.* Interruption of the arc results in a flaccid bladder (distension); interruption of the loop results in a reflex bladder (loss of voluntary control, i.e. reflex emptying).

(Fig. 12.3). The functions of these components are detailed in Box 12.2.

As the nervous system consists of, and functions through, a multitude of interrelated and interdependent feedback loops, the result of breakdown anywhere along the loop(s), for whatever reason(s), is system dysfunction or failure.

Within the human body there are many systems (cardiovascular, respiratory, digestive, reproductive, endocrine, musculoskeletal, excretory and immune) that may be considered as discrete, but which must be integrated if the human body is to function as a single integral unit. The nervous system controls, monitors and integrates the various systems; its dysfunction will cause dysfunction of one or more of these systems. Continued dysfunction will eventually affect all body systems. Complete cessation results in death of the system, the body part or the human being.

DYSFUNCTION OF THE NERVOUS SYSTEM

WHAT CAN GO WRONG?

The impulse fails to be initiated, transmitted, conducted, received and/or interpreted, either at all or correctly. Failure can be sub-divided into two types:

1. structural or mechanical failure or dysfunction, i.e. of the anatomy of the nervous system
2. electrochemical failure or dysfunction, i.e. of the physiology of the nervous system.

Structural failure

The most obvious illustration of structural failure is absence of an essential part of the nervous system, either from failure to develop, for example:

- anencephaly — usually affecting the cerebral hemispheres
- anophthalmia — the eyes fail to develop
- amelia — congenital limb absence
- sacral agenesis — the lower body fails to develop,

or because it is lost later in life through, for example, burns, frostbite, gangrene, amputation, gunshot or surgical removal. Less obvious, but more common, is when the structures are present but non-functional, or dead through genetic aberration or disease, or following haemorrhage, compression or ischaemia.

Electrochemical failure

Electrochemical failure occurs when structures are intact but the impulse still fails to get through. The electrolyte balance may be disturbed following, for example, severe vomiting, diarrhoea or starvation. Thus, the chemical components essential for the action potential and impulse conduction (e.g. sodium and potassium) are in insufficient quantities or of the wrong proportions.

Chemical transmission of the impulse at the

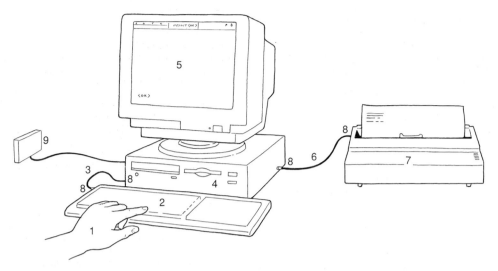

Fig. 12.3 Computer system/nervous system analogy.

Computer

1. Stimulus (able to accept various but has to suit (2))
2. Access device (keyboard — designed to receive touch typing)
3. Flexible electrical wiring (input)
4. Central processor (CP) (pre-programmed and blank for customised programs)
5. Visual display unit (VDU) (shows covert CP activity)
6. Flexible electrical wiring (output)
7. Printer (produces hard copy of selected CP activity)
8. Connectors/jack plugs (transmit current)
9. Power supply

Nervous system

1. Stimulus (able to accept various modalities, but has to suit receptor)
2. Sensory receptors (mechanoceptors, baroceptors, thermoceptors, chemoceptors, nociceptors)
3. Sensory (afferent) neurones
4. Central nervous system (pre-programmed reflexes and blank for voluntary customised programs)
5. Facial expressions and body postures show covert brain activity*
6. Motor (efferent) neurones
7. Muscles (tangible demonstration of selected brain activity)*
8. Synapses (transmit electrical impulse)
9. Oxygen, food, electrolytes*

*Although these are not strictly parts of the nervous system these are included for completeness.

synapses can be blocked by drugs, as in anaesthetics and pain relief, by poisons, such as curare and strychnine, and by disease, for example myasthenia gravis.

Some disorders result in a combination of the two types of failure. A peripheral nerve lesion in the form of a cut will damage the structure, thereby blocking the message transfer. Multiple sclerosis (MS) damages the myelin sheath (actually a support structure), thereby disturbing or slowing the message transfer.

WHERE?

There computer analogy again provides a suitable illustration of the possible sites of nervous system dysfunction (Fig. 12.3 above). When either system fails to function, each and every component needs to be investigated for possible fault or site of dysfunction (the numbers refer to the components of Fig. 12.3):

• *Sensory receptors* (2). Any of these may be absent (e.g. anophthalmia) or damaged (e.g. burns).

Box 12.2 Components of the nervous system and their functions

---

The numbers refer to Fig. 12.3.
- *Sensory receptors* (2) — detect changes in the internal and external environment and provide access to the nervous system. Each is designed to detect a specific stimulus, for example mechanoceptors detect movement or structural change, thermoceptors sense a change in temperature, baroceptors respond to a change in pressure, and chemoceptors detect a change in chemical composition. Great changes in any of these will stimulate the nociceptors (pain). Stimulus is coverted to an electrical impulse for conduction.
- *Sensory neurones* (3) — provide a pathway for the conduction of the electrical impulse from the sensory receptor along either (a) a spinal nerve to the cell body in the dorsal root ganglion along the dorsal root to the spinal cord, where it may proceed through the posterior columns, or (b) a cranial nerve to the cell body in the brain stem nuclei.
- *Central nervous system — spinal cord* (4) — provides:
  - pathways for ascending and descending neurones, which are grouped with similar neurones into tracts (white matter)
  - sites for the cell bodies of motor neurones (grey matter)
  - small connector neurones (within the grey matter), which connect the tracts and facilitate the ipsilateral, contralateral and bilateral spinal cord reflexes.
- *Central nervous system — brain* (4) — various structures from the cerebral cortex to the brain stem with the cerebellum attached inferiorly and posteriorly.

First, it is responsible for the interpretation and integration of sensory information; the control and coordination of body systems; the initiation, control, monitoring and evaluation of responses; the storage of programs and memories; and the production of emotions, behaviours and thought processes.

Second, it provides pathways for both sensory and motor neurones, with numerous connector neurones. UMNs are usually classified as those which conduct the electrical impulse via the pyramidal (corticospinal) tract. The majority of these neurones cross within the pyramids of the medulla oblongata (in the brain stem), thus innervating the contralateral side of the body.
- *Motor neurones* (6) — the LMNs provide a pathway for the conduction of the electrical impulse from the cell body in either (a) the anterior horn of the spinal cord or (b) the brain stem, via the anterior root along a spinal or cranial nerve to the motor end plate.
- *Synapses* (8) — these are the connection points between neurones. The electrical impulse is transmitted across the synaptic gap by chemicals known as neurotransmitters.
- *Motor unit* — consists of a single anterior horn cell, its motor neurone and the muscle fibres it innervates. Motor unit activity is initiated, inhibited or modified at the anterior horn cell by impulses from motor neurones of the pyramidal and extrapyramidal tracts, and by the sensory neurones of the posterior columns.
- *System integrity* — a system needs all of its components to be functional and connected for the system to function as a unit.

- *Sensory neurones* (3). These may be damaged anywhere from the receptor to the posterior columns in the spinal cord, i.e. in the peripheral nerve (e.g. a lesion), dorsal root ganglion (e.g. Herpes zoster), dorsal root (e.g. compression by prolapsed intervertebral disc) or posterior column (e.g. tumour).
- *Central nervous system* (brain/spinal cord) (4). Cells of the cortex may be damaged (e.g. encephalitis), as may the basal ganglia (e.g. Parkinson's and Huntington's diseases), anywhere in the brain (e.g. stroke, head injury and cerebral palsy), anywhere along the spinal cord (e.g. lesion or spina bifida) or in areas throughout the central nervous system (e.g. MS and tumour).
- *Motor neurone* (6). Lesions affecting the upper motor neurone (UMN), interrupting the passage of a motor impulse, can occur anywhere along the pyramidal (corticospinal) tract, i.e. from the

cerebral cortex to the synaptic junction prior to the anterior horn cell. Examples are those from head injury, stroke, cerebral palsy, encephalitis, meningitis and spinal cord lesions above L1. Lesions affecting the lower motor neurone (LMN) interrupt the motor impulse anywhere along the motor unit, i.e. from the cell body (anterior horn cell for spinal nerves, brain stem for cranial nerves) to the muscle fibres. Such lesions may be caused by poliomyelitis, motor neurone disease, nerve root compression, plexus lesion, peripheral nerve lesion, peripheral neuropathy, muscular dystrophy or a spinal lesion below L1 (cauda equina).
- *Synapses* (8). The neuromuscular junction is affected in myasthenia gravis, where there is destruction of the acetylcholine receptors on the post-synaptic membrane (muscle).

Although not strictly part of the nervous

ACQUISITION OF SKILLS

The acquisition of each new skill or activity occurs in three phases:

- trial and error
- consolidation
- acquisition.

- Trial and error. At this stage a new skill is emerging. It may lead directly from a previously acquired skill (for example, as walking follows from standing) or it may be accidental or spontaneous (for example, discovering that pulling at a sock will make it come off the foot).
- Consolidation. Once the correct movement or effect has been achieved it is repeated until it has been perfected.
- Acquisition. Here the skill or activity is executed in an easy and relaxed manner and can be used for play and pleasure and as a basis for new skills.

Thus, in the trial and error phase of walking, the child takes a tentative step forwards, usually lifting his leg too high or taking too long a step, and falls. In the consolidation phase, he manages three or four steps and enjoys practising but will revert to the previously acquired skill of crawling for speed and pleasure. In the acquisition phase, walking becomes the preferred method of locomotion.

It must be recognised that the acquisition of various skills is interrelated. Being able to feed oneself depends upon motor skills (head control, trunk control, hand function, hand-eye coordination), intellectual ability (understanding what food is and what it is for) and perceptual skills (knowing where one's mouth is and where one's hand is in relation to mouth and food). If one is asked to feed oneself, the understanding of language is also a prerequisite.

THEORETICAL FRAMEWORKS

CP is a condition which occurs early in life, is static and is, therefore, present throughout the person's lifetime. It can affect any or all aspects of the person's development through life, so a

fundamental and encompassing theoretical basis or framework is required. The involvement of many professionals who will assess, provide intervention and evaluate necessitates the use of a model which not only allows for but also encourages integration. The most obvious choice is the Model of Human Development, which offers a lifetime perspective on all areas of development. It views the person as an integrated entity and his life as a continually changing process.

The Model of Human Development regards life as a continuum, from conception to death, which may be divided into life stages and subdivided into areas of development. These divisions are necessary to render the complexities of life and the whole person into simpler, more manageable portions. The way in which the whole is divided, and the content and subsequent labelling of the areas, depends upon the theorist(s). For example, the stages suggested by Dworetzky & Davis (1989) are:

- Beginnings (0–1 year of age)
- Early childhood (1–6 years of age)
- Middle childhood (6–12 years of age)
- Adolescence (12–18 years of age)
- Early adulthood (18–40 years of age)
- Middle adulthood (40–65 years of age)
- Late adulthood (65+ years of age)

with developmental areas as:

- Physical
- Cognitive
- Personality
- Social–emotional
- Sexual
- Moral.

These theorists offer an overview of human development which forms the basic model for assessment, goal-setting and evaluation. Identified problem areas will require a more detailed, stage-by-stage breakdown, such as those by Klein (1983) for dressing skills and Erhardt (1982) for prehension.

The occupational therapist may use a model of her own preference or she may have to work within the framework of one selected by the multidisciplinary team.

However, she will need to refer constantly to

the overall model so that no developmental area either leaps ahead or is left behind. Development must be regarded as a whole, or else intervention becomes fragmented rather than holistic, and insular rather than integrated.

The Model of Human Development is inappropriate for the very young, or the severely affected, person with CP. His level of function is so low, and his rate of progress along the developmental sequence so slow, that it barely registers on the developmental scale. In such circumstances it is suggested that Maslow's Hierarchy of Motivational Needs (see Ch. 12) provides a sound framework for assessment, intervention and evaluation. The baseline identifies physiological needs which must be satisfied for survival and for progression to higher functional levels, i.e. the need to breathe, eat, drink, sleep, eliminate waste, reproduce (menstruation), keep an even temperature and be free of pain.

The occupational therapist will assess the person with CP using her professional skills or tools: observation, handling, activity analysis, interview (of person, family and other professionals), play (Burke 1993) and, possibly, standardised checklists and assessment batteries. The resulting information will detail the person's abilities and problem areas. The priority of areas for intervention and objective setting will be negotiated with the person and / or his family.

Following the assessment, which will be both initial and on-going, the occupational therapist will select an appropriate frame (or frames) of reference as the theoretical basis of her intervention and approaches with which to put the theory into practice. The frame(s) of reference and approach(es) may depend upon the developmental area in which there is a problem and / or upon the knowledge and experience of the occupational therapist. The frames of reference and approaches most often used with those who have CP, and therefore of which the occupational therapist should have a working knowledge, are as follows:

● *Developmental: neurodevelopmental (or neurophysiological)*, which is based upon the developmental sequence from involuntary, reflex nervous activity through to voluntary, mature nervous activity, i.e. the sequential progression from a predetermined motor response to a sensory stimulus, to controlled, coordinated voluntary movements in response to integrated multisensory stimulation. If primitive reflexes predominate they will inhibit mature movement patterns and therefore impede function. The approaches facilitate the desired motor response through sensory stimulation and / or reflex inhibition, for example using techniques such as total reflex inhibiting postures and gravity to reduce the tonic reflex activity, combined with proprioceptive stimulation (Bobath 1967, 1975, 1980), and cutaneous stimulation, temperature (hot and cold) and rhythmical movement (Rood 1962).

● *Sensory integrative*, which focuses on sensory system integration, especially at a sub-cortical level, as being essential for the development of function and skills. The important sensory systems are vestibular, proprioceptive, tactile, visual and auditory, the first three being precursors to the development of the last two (Ayres 1972, 1979). The approach uses techniques which provide and control sensory stimuli, to facilitate sensory system integration, and thus promote normal reflex responses and voluntary movements.

N.B. The approaches and techniques outlined above are used by occupational therapists as 'a means to an end' rather than an end in themselves. They change muscle tone, improve balance and posture and increase voluntary motor control, thus enabling functional activity.

● *Compensatory*, using the adaptive approach whereby the lack of, or reduced, ability to perform an activity or skill is compensated for by adapting one or more of the following:

— the person (e.g. positioning, orthosis)
— the activity or skill itself (part or whole)
— the method or technique employed
— the equipment used
— the environment.

● *Biomechanical*, which uses the laws of physical nature and the principles of mechanics as related to the human body, such as gravity, forces, levers, equilibrium, weight, density, stability, inertia and momentum with muscle work, joint angles, base of support, weight distribution and position in space. The approach focuses on the posture, position and handling of the person using himself, the therapist and others, orthoses, equipment and the immediate environment.

- *Learning*, which focuses on the human ability to change: to develop within, or adapt to, his environment. The cognitive approach concentrates on the 'thinking' aspects of learning, which include planning, decision-making and choice. It uses techniques which promote the understanding of that which is learned so that the new skills can be transferred to different situations, and/or used as a foundation for more complex skills, and/or used as a stepping stone to allied skills. The behavioural approach does not necessarily need 'thinking' or understanding, and is not therefore generally used by occupational therapists as it does not adhere to the humanistic philosophy. However, some of the techniques have been successfully adapted and incorporated as the skills or tools of the occupational therapist. There are also intervention programmes which broadly follow the behavioural approach to learning, with which the person with CP may be involved and the occupational therapist should be familiar. Conductive education, as developed by Dr Andras Peto, and patterning for the brain-injured child, developed by Glen Doman and Carl Delacato, are examples.

The theory and practice within this chapter is biased towards the young person with CP and those who are severely affected. The older person with CP who is mildly to moderately affected will generally require less intervention from the occupational therapist. Such intervention will be problem initiated, probably based within the compensatory frame of reference and utilising the adaptive approach, or the rehabilitative approach if previously gained skills have been lost through the ageing process or from disuse.

THE ROLE OF THE OCCUPATIONAL THERAPIST

The person with CP may be referred to the occu-

pational therapist at any time during his development from infancy to adulthood. If the diagnosis of CP is made at or soon after birth, intervention will probably commence while the baby is in the special care baby unit (SCBU). Diagnosis might not be made, however, until it is evident that certain developmental milestones such as rolling over, sitting and standing have not been reached within normal limits. This is most likely to occur with the milder forms of CP. On rare occasions, a child or adolescent who has 'slipped through the net', moved to a new area or arrived from another country will be referred to the occupational therapist for the first time (Box 13.1). Most people with CP will receive advice and support from an occupational therapist throughout their lives, sometimes in the foreground as new problems arise, often in the background as the person adapts to his handicap and life-style. In the early years, intervention is usually frequent and intensive, gradually tapering off as the child moves through school age into adolescence and adulthood. As an adult, the person with CP may call upon the services of the occupational therapist as life changes occur — for example, a new job, new home, marriage and children. The holistic approach taken by the occupational therapist will involve her not only with the individual but also with his family (mother, father, siblings, grandparents), teachers, employers and partner.

Intervention cannot be rigidly subdivided into early, middle and late stages of treatment, as the form it takes will be determined largely by the severity of the CP, the personality of the individual and the support he receives from others. Some people with severe CP will require the multisensory input of early intervention throughout their lives; others will attain independence in many areas as their chronological age allows.

EARLY INTERVENTION

The occupational therapist may be involved with a moderately or severely affected baby during the neonatal period (Box 13.2) and the first contact may take place in the special care baby unit (SCBU). The initial aim will be to support and advise the parents; this will be the aim not only

Box 13.1   Case study

Jan is 39 years old; she has severe CP of the athetoid type, and an IQ within the normal range and lives in a residential care home. She has expressed the desire to live within the community, with support but as independently as possible.

Presenting picture

Jan uses an unmodified standard 9L wheelchair with the footrests removed. Her position is: semi-reclined with weight transferred through the right side (thigh, buttock and lower back), head and shoulders against the backrest, buttock and upper thigh at the front of the seat, both upper arms over the armrests to maintain the position. Jan propels the wheelchair backwards using her left foot on the floor (hence the removal of the footrests). She communicates 'yes' and 'no' answers as appropriate to questions. She is dependent upon others for her personal care (toileting, bathing, feminine hygiene, feeding and so on). She can indicate need and control the timing if given the opportunity (which is not always possible in the home). Jan has no special equipment for her own use or to meet her individual needs. She is unable to read or write.

Assessment

Using the Model of Human Development (Dworetzky & Davis 1989) a person of Jan's age and intellectual ability should have achieved the young adulthood life stage in all developmental areas. However, Jan's physical skills (locomotion, manipulation, oral control and functional posture) are at the Beginnings (0–1 years) stage. Other areas, which are dependent upon motor function (personal care, communication, cognition, domestic tasks, education/work), are at the Early childhood (1–6 years) stage, although assistance from, or facilitation by, a carer is often essential to reach this stage.

With assistance from a carer, Jan reaches the Adolescent stage in the social, leisure, sexual and relationship areas. Development in personality, emotional and moral areas is probably at the Adolescent stage, as they are closely related to the other areas at this stage, but possibly at the Young adulthood stage.

Overall aim

To enable Jan to achieve her personal goals of each developmental area within the life stage commensurate with her age and intellectual ability.

Aims

To enable activity by:

- modifying her body posture to facilitate function
- supporting these functional postures
- modifying or changing the method or technique employed during the activity
- modifying or changing the equipment with which the activity is undertaken
- modifying or changing the environment in which the activity takes place.

Theoretical basis of intervention

Jan's current body posture has developed over a number of years; therefore it is inappropriate to consider correction except in peripheral ways. However, her posture requires modification depending upon her functional requirements, so the biomechanical approach within the biomechanical frame of reference is selected.

For Jan's inability to maintain such functional postures and to achieve the required level of activity without modification or change, the adaptive approach within the compensatory frame of reference is selected.

Examples of intervention

- Re-positioning so that more weight is transferred through the pelvis and lower limbs and is symmetrically distributed, thus freeing the head, shoulder girdle and upper trunk for function.
- The use of an adjustable, customised seat, for example a Matrix, to support the head, neck, trunk, pelvis and thighs, thus releasing the upper limbs for function.
- Adapting the remote control unit and attaching it to the wheelchair so that Jan can operate the TV, video, radio and cassette and CD players without waiting for her carer.
- Attaching the customised seat to an electric wheelchair to achieve independent locomotion.
- The use of a simple communication aid, for example, a 'picture' book with a colour-coded index for developmental/subject areas. This can be attached to the wheelchair for easy access.
- Re-arranging Jan's room and the communal rooms so that objects and equipment are accessible from a wheelchair. Similarly, changing the layout of the rooms so that Jan can negotiate her way around independently.

of the occupational therapist but of all the members of the multidisciplinary team involved in the SCBU.

The arrival of a new baby is a time of great change for any family, particularly if he is the first baby. The baby will have been looked forward to for a number of months. If there has been a history of miscarriage or difficulty in conceiving, the baby will be especially precious. The relationship between the parents will have changed and will continue to change as they adjust to the baby's arrival and their relationships with him. The news that their baby has problems which will affect his development (the diagnosis of CP may not be initially apparent) will be devastating. The parents will experience shock,

---

Box 13.2 Case study

Sean is three weeks old, cerebral palsy is suspected. He lives at home with his parents.

Presenting picture

Sean is a floppy baby who cries and becomes rigid when he is touched or moved. He startles, screams and goes stiff to unexpected or loud noises, to sudden visual changes (light turned on, face in front) and when his cot is bumped. Thus Sean is exhibiting extreme motor responses to sensory stimuli. This sudden change in muscle tone, body position and the loud cry further frightens and startles Sean. It produces an upward spiral which is apparently impossible to stop until he is exhausted.

Assessment

Sean's low level of function indicates the use of Maslow's Hierarchy of Motivational Needs, beginning at the bottom line: physiological or survival needs.

- *Respiration* — breathing is arrhythmic because of frequent startling, which produces a momentary cessation of breathing and then a sudden intake of breath, followed by rapid breathing.
- *Food* — feeding is difficult as the change in position makes Sean fretful and restless.
- *Elimination* — nappy changing is very difficult as Sean screams and becomes stiff throughout the process.
- *Sleep* — periods of sleep are very short, being constantly disturbed by sudden starts and crying.
- *Warmth* — the changes in body position when he is dressed/undressed cause stiffness and crying, which makes this process extremely difficult.
- *Lack of pain* — the changes in muscle tone and breathing probably cause physical pain and emotional distress.
- *Cleanliness* — washing and bathing are virtually impossible because of the changes in body position and temperature.

Clearly, none of Sean's basic physiological needs can be provided in the normal way, so intervention is required.

Overall aim

To re-establish a state of equilibrium, by breaking the increasing spiral of stimulus/response, thus providing a foundation for development.

Aims

- To control the levels of sensory stimulation
- To inhibit the reflex responses.

Theoretical basis of intervention

The above treatment aims lead to the selection of the sensory stimulatory/reflex inhibitory approach within the neurodevelopmental/physiological (developmental frame of reference) and sensory integrative approaches. With a baby of Sean's age a state of equilibrium can be achieved by replicating the 'womb' conditions, so a combination of techniques suggested by Rood and by Ayres is utilised.

Examples of intervention

- Close swaddling of the body, including the head, provides a constant cutaneous stimulation and inhibits gross reflex response. It stabilises the head against the body so that tonic neck reflexes are not stimulated when the baby is turned or lifted. In this fully supported state rocking can be introduced either within the cot or by holding him close to the body while the parent sways. The use of a baby sling which securely fastens the baby to the parent's chest allows movement through space, similar to that experienced in the womb, when the mother changes position.
- The change in tactile stimulation when the baby is handled is reduced as the skin is already receiving stimulation. Gentle but firm rubbing and massage can be started through the cloth layers.
- Swaddling alleviates the need for clothing to keep the baby warm. Nappies can be changed by loosening the lower part of the swaddling only so that the head and upper body remain stable and comfortably supported. It is possible to free individual body parts for cleansing so that movement and temperature changes are reduced.
- There should be a background of sounds rather than silence, so that changes are presented as a gradual increase in volume and pitch rather than a startling change from quiet to noise. A background of sounds also dampens any unavoidable sudden noises, for example telephone rings, doorbell chimes or toilet flushes. Music, the singing of nursery rhymes, tapes of womb sounds or relaxation themes and talking in a low, soothing voice when feeding, changing and washing the baby all provide controlled auditory stimulation.
- Visual stimulation can be controlled by keeping lighting constant, for example using a nursery lamp so that the main light does not need switching on at night. The sight of a face close to the baby need not be unexpected if it is preceeded by a quiet, low voice and the gradual emergence of the person.

---

disbelief, anger and guilt. They will have to pass through the grieving process and mourn for their lost normal baby before they can accept their handicapped baby.

During this period the therapist's role is to support the parents; in doing so she must work closely with the other team members. The mother/baby and father/baby bonds are vitally important at this stage; therefore, the occupational therapist should encourage the parents to actively participate in all treatment programmes (Holloway 1993).

Parents are anxious and unsure when handling and caring for their new baby and a handicapped baby brings additional worries; therefore, advice and encouragement are of paramount importance. Advice on handling and stimulating the baby should be coupled with encouragement and praise to help the parents become more confident. A 'normal' baby has no voluntary motor control and requires total support of head and trunk, while his arms and legs usually adopt the flexed posture and so look after themselves. The baby with CP, however, may be floppy or stiff and is therefore more difficult to hold and care for. Floppy arms and legs need to be remembered and supported. Arms and legs which are stiff make nappy changing and dressing difficult. Slow, smooth movements are required as quick, jerky movements will increase the spasticity. Parents will need to be taught how to decrease the spasticity, for example by flexing the baby's hips and knees before attempting to abduct the thighs at nappy change.

Babies develop spontaneously, i.e. without apparent intervention, in many areas. Vision and hearing gain voluntary control as a baby learns to turn his head to look and listen in response to a variety of auditory and visual stimuli. A baby with CP will need help in this regard however; because he is unable to turn his head, stimulation must be brought to him. A SCBU is full of sights and sounds but not those which normally surround a developing baby (Langer 1990). If the baby requires this specialist medical support for more than a few days, multisensory stimulation must commence before he goes home. The parents should be encouraged to bring in items from home, particularly all the usual baby paraphernalia, which is preferable to that used by the hospital. His mother's choice of soap and talc, for example, will enable the baby to know his own smell. As the parents wash and clean their baby and massage lotion onto his body they will quickly learn how to handle him, forge bonds with him, and build their own confidence. As they cuddle him he will learn their personal smells and recognise them apart from the professionals who also handle him.

Toys to stimulate the senses are also important.

Musical and squeaky toys encourage location of sounds and bright or reflective toys stimulate vision. Communication is vital and parents should be encouraged to talk to their baby and to tell him what they are doing to him. A baby with spastic CP will relax and anticipate movement if he is spoken to and stroked before handling; if he is touched or picked up unexpectedly, he will jump and stiffen. Talking to a handicapped baby is often difficult, as he may not respond. Parents may become discouraged. The occupational therapist can provide support and encouragement by setting an example. The way in which she handles, stimulates and communicates with the baby is often the model which parents imitate and adopt.

POSITIONING

Positioning is used in the treatment of CP to prevent contractures and deformity, to facilitate movement, and to enable function. A given position may further any or all of these aims. The basic positions used are lying (supine, prone, side), sitting (floor, side, chair), and standing. Most positions can be supported with one's own body (i.e. with the mother's, therapist's or teacher's body), with everyday furniture and objects, or with specialised furniture and equipment.

When positioning the person with CP the therapist uses principles from three treatment approaches:

- reflex inhibitory — to inhibit involuntary movements and facilitate the voluntary control of movement
- biomechanical — in calculating joint angles, weight distribution, centre of gravity and gravitational pull or resistance
- adaptive — the use of external support (human or non-human) in maintaining the position if the person's bodily control is insufficient to hold it.

Lying

Supine

The supine position is the least used, as stimulation to the back of the head may trigger a full

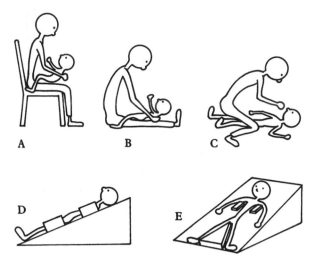

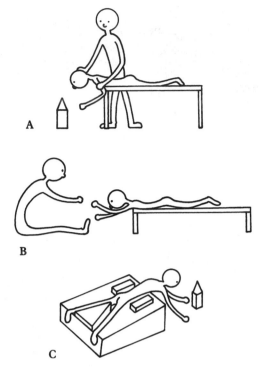

Fig. 13.5 Positioning: supine lying.

Fig. 13.6 Positioning: prone lying.

extension pattern and it is difficult to use the upper limbs against gravity. However, this position can be used to stretch those in a total flexion pattern or when encouraging eye contact and early communication skills in the young or severely affected person. Supine lying can be supported as follows:

- own body: babies and small children can be positioned on an adult's lap (Figs 13.5A, B)
- everyday: for use with people of any age; the adult can position herself astride the person on the floor (Fig. 13.5C)
- special: for the moderately or severely affected person wedges made from foam or wood with harnesses and supports (Figs 13.5D,E) can be used.

Prone

This position is used to prevent flexion contractures of the lower limbs, encourage head control and enable upper limb function. It can be assisted as follows:

- own body: lying supine (on the floor, bed or sofa) the adult can position a baby or small child on her chest. The adult supports the baby's head; a slight bouncing movement will stimulate the neck extensors and allow some weight to be taken by the baby. This

position is particularly successful with floppy babies. With the adult standing, the person with CP can be positioned at right angles, e.g. on a plinth, facilitating both head control and upper limb function (Fig. 13.6A)

- everyday: the person can be supported in the prone position using a bed, sofa, cushions from the sofa or pillows (Fig. 13.6B)
- special: a wedge made from foam or wood with harnesses and supports will hold a person securely in the prone position (Figs 13.6C, 13.7).

Side lying

This position provides total body support, including the head; facilitates shoulder protraction and brings hands into the midline; enables upper limb function (lower arm is in midline with gravity eliminated and upper arm is brought to midline, assisted by gravity); and inhibits spastic posturing of the lower limbs. It is particularly

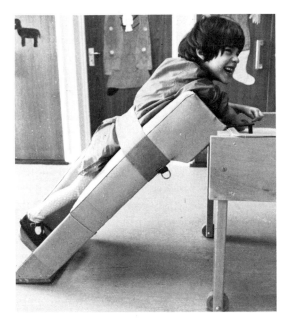

Fig. 13.7 Positioning: prone board enabling hand function.

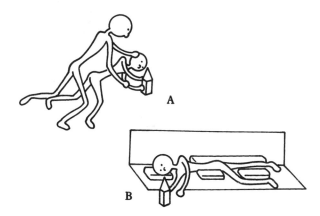

Fig. 13.8 Positioning: side lying.

from heavy density foam or orthotic materials such as Plastazote and Hexcelite. The boards should be adjustable, if possible, so that alternate sides can be used (Fig. 13.8B).

beneficial for the person who experiences difficulty in maintaining a symmetrical posture prone or supine. In itself, side lying is not a supportive position; therefore, support must be provided, especially to the head, trunk and the uppermost lower limb. Side lying can be facilitated as follows:

- own body: this position is tiring for the adult so should only be used for short periods of time. The baby or small child is positioned in side lying on the floor, protected by a rug or foam mattress. The adult is positioned on all fours astride the child, with one arm supporting the head and spine and the other facilitating play, one leg behind the child to support the lower back and under leg, and the other between the child's legs to position and support the uppermost leg (Fig. 13.8A)
- everyday: as above, but the position can be used with a person of any age. Support is provided by foam blocks, cushions or pillows
- special: side lying boards are available in many forms from various manufacturers and custom-made boards can also be fashioned

Sitting

The main aim of the sitting position is to enable function, for example: learning — play, reading, writing; personal tasks — eating, toileting, dressing, applying make-up, shaving; communication — looking, listening, talking; leisure activities — games and hobbies, watching television.

However, it has been shown that a good sitting position enhances pulmonary function (Nwaobi & Smith 1986) and has a positive effect on feeding and general health.

Throughout the day we change our sitting postures according to the desired function. For hand–eye coordination the trunk is inclined (we lean forwards) to bring the head/eyes over the hands. The elbows and forearms are often supported by a table to increase control and reduce tiredness. For hand to mouth coordination, as in eating, the upright trunk position is adopted. This frees the elbows and forearms to bring the hand to the mouth and promotes good digestive function. For more relaxed function (watching TV, reading, listening to music or conversing) the trunk is reclined, usually with the head supported.

These postures should be considered when seating the person with CP and/or providing adapted seating. It is unlikely that any one position or chair will provide a satisfactory posture to facilitate function throughout the day.

The sitting position provides a stable base from which head, upper trunk and upper limb movement is made easier. The two main types of sitting are floor sitting and chair sitting.

Floor sitting

'W' sitting (Fig. 13.9A) and 'tailor' sitting (Fig. 13.9B) should be discouraged, as both encourage backward pelvic tilt (sacral sitting) and flexion con-

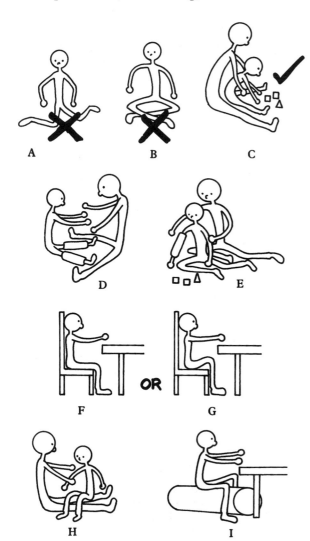

Fig. 13.9 Positioning: sitting.

tractures of the lower limbs. Floor sitting can be further subdivided into long-legged sitting and side sitting.

Long-legged sitting provides stretch to the hamstrings and Achilles tendon with hip abduction and lateral rotation and enables hand function by bringing the hands into the midline assisted by gravity. This position can be supported as follows:

- own body: the adult sits on the floor with legs astride; the person with CP sits in the same direction, close to the adult's body, thus obtaining support for the trunk and pelvis. The legs can be supported in extension and lateral rotation by the hands (if not needed for the head and arms), leg gaiters (see p. 426) or by the adult's legs. With the adult's arms free, upper limb function can be assisted (Fig. 13.9C)
- everyday: the person may require trunk support to the rear, so sitting with his back to a wall, corner or sofa will help. Leg extension supported by gaiters will leave the adult free to face the individual for play, eye contact and communication (Fig. 13.9D)
- special: various floor sitters are available, with or without trays or tables, harnesses, head supports and pommels (to encourage abduction and lateral rotation at the hips) (Fig. 13.10).

Side sitting: although an asymmetrical posture, this is used to provide a position in which weight-bearing through one upper limb is encouraged while the other limb is kept free for function. It is particularly useful for those with spastic hemiplegia. Side sitting can be supported by:

- own body: a person can be supported by an adult sitting behind in a similar position, providing support for and weight through the shoulder and elbow joints. An arm gaiter may be utilised to hold the elbow in extension (Fig. 13.9E).

Chair sitting

The correct posture is one in which the head is

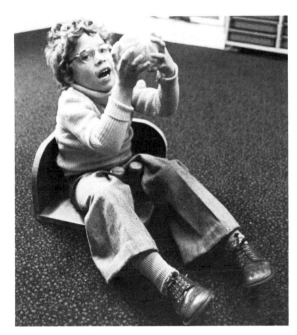

Fig. 13.10 Positioning: corner floor sitter; supported sitting to enable hand function.

upright, the spinal curves supported, the person's weight distributed evenly through the buttocks and thighs, the knees at 90 degrees and the feet plantigrade. Some people may require their hips and knees to be more flexed in order to inhibit spastic posturing (Fig. 13.9F,G). Support can take the following forms:

- own body: a small child can be supported in the sitting position on an adult's thighs. This is especially useful for undressing and dressing (Fig. 13.9H)
- everyday: baby chairs, high chairs, kiddy chairs, dining chairs, pushchairs and armchairs can all be successfully utilised by most individuals. The addition of cushions, foot stools or tables will often suffice maintaining a good sitting position
- special: the severely affected person often requires more support in the sitting position, either to prevent deformity or to enable function. Many variations are available; therefore assessment, selection and fitting are of vital importance. For people with tightness of the hip adductors, an astride or

bolster chair may be the most suitable (Fig. 13.9I). Extra support can be provided using foam wedges, harnesses or moulded inserts.

Standing

Standing positions should encourage an upright posture (enabling perception of height and distance), prevent flexion contractures, ensure weight-bearing through the hip joints (essential for bony joint development), and facilitate stability of the knee and ankle joints prior to independent standing and walking. The following support can be provided:

- own body and everyday: while the child stands at a sofa, chair or table the adult supports his hips and knees in extension (Fig. 13.11). This is particularly useful for those with spastic diplegia who can use their upper limbs but require support for their lower limbs. Gaiters can be used to hold the knees in extension, thereby freeing the adult's hands to facilitate function in the upper limbs for those with more severe CP
- special: prone standers, flexistands and standing frames are available, providing a wide range of positions and support (Fig. 13.12).

Table or tray position

The position of a table or tray greatly influences function. A table sited close to the trunk enables the person to reach objects without leaning forwards, especially if an upright trunk position is desired. Siting the table just below axilla height supports the arms, thus eliminating the need to

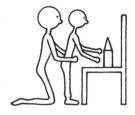

Fig. 13.11 Positioning: standing.

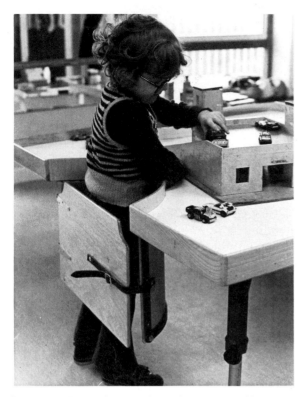

Fig. 13.12 Positioning: special equipment to enable standing (The Amesbury Quadra table).

raise the arms against gravity. Inclining the working surface brings the hands to eye level, thus promoting hand–eye coordination. This is particularly important if by flexing the neck, to bring the eyes towards the hands, a flexed body pattern is initiated and/or reduction in muscle tone is produced.

Relative positioning

The position adopted by the individual and adult relative to each other has important implications. The ideal positions are:

- face to face, as this promotes symmetry and eye contact
- one behind the other, which removes distraction and enables the adult use of her own movement patterns when facilitating movement, as in feeding and dressing.

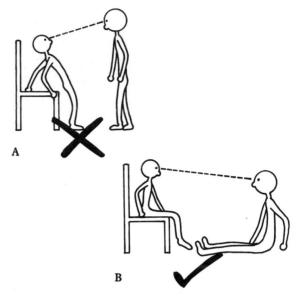

Fig. 13.13 Relative positioning.

Looking upwards may stimulate the total extension pattern (Fig. 13.13A); in this case relative positions must be taken such that eye contact is on a downward gradient from the individual to the adult (Fig. 13.13B). Positioning oneself to the side of a person with CP encourages asymmetrical posturing, as it forces him to turn, stimulating the asymmetrical tonic neck reflex and making swallowing, chewing and vocalisation extremely difficult.

PERSONAL SKILLS

Independence in personal care is dependent upon the successful integration and interpretation of sensory stimuli, combined with coordinated voluntary movements (both gross and fine). The person with CP will have problems with these skills and may, therefore, show a delay in the area of personal care. Early consideration should be given to the adaptive approach, i.e. adapting the technique, equipment and/or environment to achieve independence as close to that of the normal developmental sequence as possible. By adopting this treatment approach the occupational therapist can minimise the frustration of the person with mild or moderate CP, and maximise the ease of care for a person with moderate or severe CP.

Toileting

Problem areas include:

- sitting on the potty/toilet
- getting onto and off the toilet
- wiping
- bladder and bowel control
- toilet training
- removing and replacing clothing
- menstruation.

Sitting on the potty/toilet

Various toilet aids are available. Whether these are used in the short or long term will depend upon the individual's degree of success in acquiring head and trunk control and balance. The young child may be secure on a potty which has a large base with back and side supports. The standard Watford potty chair has a higher back and sides with a removable front bar which prevents the child falling forwards. If the person is thin and bony, and thus finds the toilet aperture too large and uncomfortable, an insert with or without sides will help. Special toilet chairs which are either attached to the lavatory pan or slide over the pan are suitable for more severely affected people. These chairs have various accessories, for example head and trunk supports, harnesses and footrests, which can be added and adjusted to suit the individual.

Getting onto and off the toilet

Appropriately sited handrails will assist the person who is unsteady but otherwise independent and a step or platform around the base of the toilet will help if the toilet is too high. The dependent older child or adult may be too heavy to transfer onto the toilet, especially if the area is small, and in such circumstances a commode in the bathroom or bedroom will make toilet times easier.

Wiping

This is always an awkward task, requiring good hand function, balance and body perception. If tearing paper from a roll is difficult, a flat-pack of single sheets or wet-wipes may be easier. Wiping aids are available but these are often not suitable for a person with CP; an automatic washer or bidet can give the individual total independence.

Bladder and bowel control

People with severe CP are unlikely to achieve full control or to be able to make their needs known. If bowel habits are regular, routine toileting using the previously described aids can help the carer. Shop-bought terry or disposable nappies are adequate for the young incontinent child, but the older child and adult will need special pads, pants or larger nappies. The type of protection will depend upon the individual's needs and the availability of supplies from the local continence service. The help of the continence adviser should be sought.

Toilet training

The occupational therapist is unlikely to be directly involved with the routine of toilet training but she can assist by ensuring that the physical aspects of toileting, as described above, are appropriate for the individual.

Removing and replacing clothing

Mastering this aspect of toileting is of vital importance in giving the person with mild CP confidence and independence in using the toilet at school, work and in social settings. Clothing should be loose and limited to a few layers. It should have elasticated waistbands, which are easier to manage than belts, buttons and zips. Adapted clothing using Velcro fastenings is especially suitable for those in wheelchairs.

Menstruation

Menarche is always a time of change for the

Cutting food

While it is appropriate for a small child to have his food cut up for him, the older child and adult will want to be independent. Special cutlery, such as the combined fork/knife or rocker knife may be suitable. If such items are unacceptable away from home, the person should be encouraged to take packed lunches to work or school and to select foods from restaurant menus which do not require cutting.

Controlling liquids

Problems with controlling the lips and tongue often lead to liquids dribbling back out of the mouth. In the early stages, thickened liquids such as soups, custards and thick milkshakes can help the person to gain control. The difficulty may be in controlling the flow of liquids (i.e. tipping too much into the mouth); this can be eliminated by using a straw or a cup with a lid, or by putting only a small amount of liquid into the cup. Both hands can be used with a double-handled cup, thus promoting symmetry and better control. People with an intention tremor often find a cup with a weighted bottom easier to use.

Mealtimes are an important social occasion in which the person with CP should be included, even if he is not actually fed at this time. This enables him to take part in family discussions and provides an ideal opportunity to learn social skills and mealtime etiquette.

The occupational therapist can provide the more independent person with opportunities to acquire skills related to mealtimes, for example food preparation, cooking, laying the table, nutrition and shopping. This can be started with the young child by using 'make-believe' play such as dolls' tea parties, setting up a shop, cooking in a Wendy House, or making dinner with Play-Doh; these activities also provide practice in gross motor control, hand function, perception, communication and social skills.

Sleeping

Problems associated with sleeping include:

- too much sleep
- too little sleep, disturbed sleep patterns, hyperactivity
- waking during the night, possibly having fits
- restlessness, falling out of bed
- inability to move or turn over in bed
- adopting abnormal postures.

Too much sleep

Often associated with severe forms of CP, this problem is sometimes found in the child who is described as 'very good' or 'no bother at all'. If the child sleeps for long periods during the day, opportunities for exploration, learning and play are severely limited and motivation may be very low. The aim is to provide frequent stimulation to discourage unwanted sleep. Waking periods should be gradually increased and a regular routine of sleep and wakefulness established. A programme of multisensory stimulation and varied activities of short duration supervised by a number of people and in different environments should be implemented.

Too little sleep

A person who does not sleep through the night should be provided with a very active day, with physical activity as well as mental stimulation. Naps should be avoided and a wind-down routine before bedtime (e.g. taking a warm bath, having a milky drink and listening to a bedtime story) will help to establish a healthy sleep pattern. If these measures fail to induce a full night's sleep other action will be required, given that parents or carers need to 'recharge their batteries' overnight. Sedatives may be prescribed, but these may affect alertness the following day. Arranging for a night-sitter or periods of respite care with a link family may be more appropriate.

Waking

Some people with CP are wakened during the night by cramps, spasms or fits. The new listening devices which plug into the household electrical circuit are an ideal way to alert parents or carers to the individual's distress.

Restlessness

For any child, outgrowing the security of a cot and learning to sleep in a bed can be a difficult process. The person with CP may have particular problems with physical security, and it may be easier to achieve the process in stages, for example by placing the mattress directly onto the floor, then onto the divan base and, finally, fitting the legs. Placing the bed in a corner, against the walls and using two or three 'baby-shop' bedsides should safely contain most individuals. Those with greater problems may need a sleeping harness attached under the mattress or an 'all-in-one' bottom sheet and duvet cover, which functions as a large sleeping bag attached to the bed.

Inability to move

If a person is unable to change position during sleep, stiffness, cramps, spasms and pressure sores can develop. It is impractical to expect the parents or carer to get up frequently during the night to reposition the individual. Turning beds or mattresses which automatically and regularly change the areas of pressure may be necessary. Sheepskins and polystyrene bead-filled mattresses also help to prevent pressure sores.

Abnormal postures

During sleep a person with CP may adopt positions which encourage deformity or contractures. Night splintage (see p. 425), foam wedges and bean-bags, in various combinations, can be used to support limbs or the whole body in a more satisfactory position.

Dressing

Problems with dressing may be of a physical, psychological or perceptual nature:

- physical: difficulty in controlling the limbs, maintaining balance, and holding gaze on the task to hand
- psychological: poor motivation, concentration, understanding, memory
- perceptual: apraxia, inaccurate body image,

difficulty with sequencing and with understanding position in space and orientation of self and clothing.

The person with severe CP will be dependent upon someone else to dress and undress; therefore, the aims of intervention will be to teach the helper useful techniques and to advise on clothing which makes dressing and undressing easier and quicker. Positioning the individual on the floor, bed or specially fitted work surface is safer than using one's lap, a chair or a wheelchair. Techniques to inhibit spastic postures will facilitate the movement of limbs into and out of clothing. Clothing should be loose, free from unnecessary fastenings and limited to a few layers.

Physical

A good sitting position (see p. 410) is essential to trunk control and balance; it also facilitates head control, thus enabling the person to look at what he is doing.

Psychological

Problems in this area require the activity to be analysed (see Ch. 6) and the broken-down task to be taught using the backward chaining technique (Box 13.3). This method enables the therapist to monitor very small achievements rather than the whole task, which may not show any progress. These small but important improvements also motivate and encourage the individual to continue. If motivation is a problem the activity should be made more interesting and/or rewarding. With children and those with low intellectual ability the ideal motivator is that of dressing up either in adults' clothes (to be like Mummy or Daddy) or in costumes. Undressing can be rewarded by playing in the splash pool or body painting.

Perceptual

Various activities can be used to help the person to grasp the dressing/undressing process. Large dolls can be used at first to show the differences between front and back — face/tummy/knees/

A

B

C

D

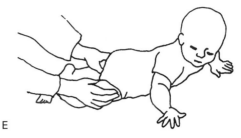

E

Fig. 13.17 The child with spastic diplegia moving from supine to prone position. Compare with Fig. 13.2A–E. (Drawings by Sarah Denvir reproduced from Griffiths & Clegg 1988 *Cerebral Palsy: Problems and Practice*, by kind permission.)

play (Fig. 13.17A). He needs to roll over onto his stomach to free his hands but even when his head is turned he is unable to roll over (Fig. 13.17B). The therapist will need to facilitate this manoeuvre either from the upper limb (Fig. 13.17C) or the lower limb (Fig. 13.17D), so that when lying prone the child has his hands free for play (Fig. 13.17E).

The child with athetosis is able to roll over but the movement pattern is uncontrolled and abnormal, taking much effort and often ending in frustration (as he ends up, for example, even further away from the toy he was trying to reach) (Fig. 13.18). It may be a long time before he is able to sit unsupported and therefore use his hands for play; the therapist can support this position while facilitating or encouraging hand function (Fig. 13.19).

MOBILITY

Locomotion

Children acquire independent locomotion through creeping, crawling and walking at an early age. They use this skill to move through space, explore, play and socialise. It is a major component of experiential learning. A child with CP is reliant upon others for his locomotion and, may therefore miss out on these important aids to development. Choice, spontaneity and motivation are similarly reduced. A passive, dependent life-style can become the norm. The early use of mechanical or powered locomotion promotes an active, independent life-style for the young child with

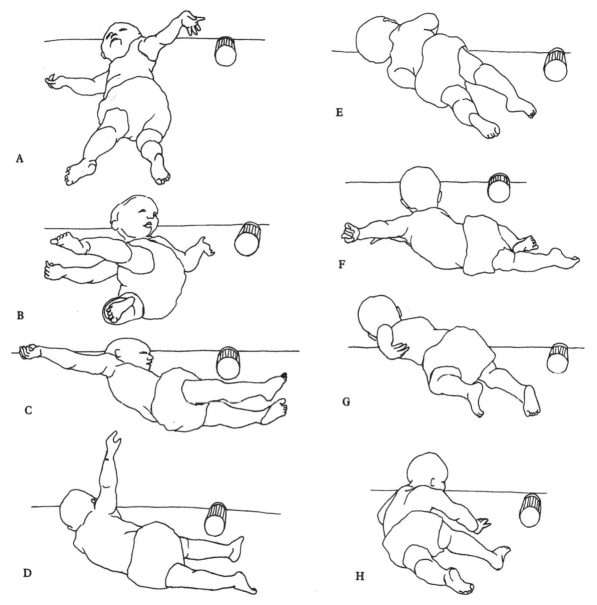

Fig. 13.18 The child with athetosis rolling over towards a toy. Compare with Fig. 13.2A-G. (Drawings by Sarah Denvir reproduced from Griffiths & Clegg 1988 *Cerebral Palsy: Problems and Practice*, by kind permission.)

CP. He can move freely around the home, play with siblings and peers, and actively join in family outings.

The benefits of this early independence have been recognised (Butler 1986), and many trollies, scooters, buggies and wheelchairs are available. It is important to note that the use of this equipment is supplementary to, and not a replacement

for, the skills of creeping, crawling and walking. It follows the developmental model of regarding each area of development separately as well as a part of the whole; thus locomotion should not be delayed by a problem within another area of development.

The person with severe CP will be dependent upon wheelchairs and someone to propel them.

skills, hand function, mobility, homecraft and education, and must be considered when planning intervention in any area.

Visual perception is the ability to interpret accurately that which is seen. It is dependent upon good visual function, which is, briefly, oculomotor control (tracking, scanning), visual attention (looking), near/distant vision, binocular control (using the eyes together for depth and dimension), full visual field and colour perception. The person with CP may have one or more problems with visual function and he can be difficult to assess because of his other problems (motor, cognitive, communication). However, it is essential for the therapist to know the extent of the visual function/dysfunction before visual perception can be assessed. As the assessment and treatment of visual perception is detailed and specialised the reader is directed to Todd (1993).

MICROTECHNOLOGY

The advances in microtechnology have enhanced the lives of many people with CP. Environmental control systems, communication aids, home office systems, kitchen 'gadgets' and leisure electronics have brought the world to disabled people and enabled them to become active participants in virtually all aspects of life. It is sometimes difficult to keep abreast of innovations, so therapists need to liaise with experts who know of and understand the applications of appropriate devices.

Microtechnology can compensate for lack of motor function provided that the person with CP has voluntary control over one movement, no matter how slight. This ability can be used to gain access into, and control, the various systems. Microtechnology cannot, as yet, compensate for sensory, integrative and cognitive disabilities.

Microcomputers

The use of the microcomputer has grown rapidly over the last few years in the workplace, in education and in the home. Children and adults alike have found them invaluable as tools and as play-things and occupational therapists use computers for assessment, treatment and administration. The microcomputer has opened many doors for the person with CP — literally, by means of environmental control systems, and metaphorically, as communication aids. The occupational therapist may advise the person with CP on the suitability of a system, the position in which to use the computer and the means of access to the computer. A number of devices are available for access; these include pointers attached to headbands, mercury switches, light-sensitive switches, suck and blow devices, touch-sensitive pads, joysticks, mice and concept keyboards. The occupational therapist, working with an electronics engineer, can usually design and construct special individual access devices if the above switches fail to meet the needs of the person with CP. In this way even the most severely physically handicapped person can be accommodated (see p. 425).

BEHAVIOUR

The person with severe or moderate CP may exhibit the following behaviours:

- self-stimulation or self-mutilation: rocking, head-banging, eye-gouging, teeth-grinding, hand-biting, masturbation
- aggression towards others
- screaming, breath-holding.

Management and behaviour modification programmes, within the learning frame of reference, are usually directed by a clinical or educational psychologist but must be agreed to and implemented by parents, therapists and teaching staff so that the approach is consistent. Preventive or protective measures may be necessary but must be accompanied by a programme to change or modify unwanted behaviours. For example, if hand-biting is a problem splints may prevent the hands from getting to the mouth (see p. 425) but this behaviour is often replaced by mouth-biting or head-banging. The person with mild CP may exhibit behaviours associated with a handicapped person trying to compete with peers;

these include attention-seeking and immature behaviours, temper tantrums and over-dependency. Parents and teachers will need advice, reassurance and support through these episodes. If problems persist, referral to the psychology service will be appropriate.

ORTHOSES

Orthoses can be used to facilitate function (compensatory frame of reference), inhibit reflex activity (developmental frame of reference) (Bohannon 1987, Tona & Schneck 1993) and/or to prevent or correct deformity (biomechanical frame of refer-

Table 13.3 Orthoses for persons with cerebral palsy

Problem	Aim	Orthosis	Material	Other treatment	CP type
Head banging: intentional — self-stimulation/ mutilation; accidental — falls from fits or incoordination	To protect the face and head	Helmet (A)	Plastazote, leather, skate-boarder's crash helmet	Psychologist, behaviour modification	Severe intellectual impairment
				Physiotherapy, balance, gross motor coordination	All types
Mouth open: continual drooling, difficulty with feeding, speech	To facilitate mouth closure	Chin cup attached by elastic to lightweight head bands (B)	Canvas and elastic webbing, chin-cup — thermoplastic	Speech therapy, voluntary control	Athetosis
Access to computer required, only head control possible	To facilitate computer access	Helmet as above, attach pointing stick, mercury switch, light control			Athetosis, spastic quadriplegia
Tightly fisted hand, passively correctable	To maintain functional hand position (C)	Mitten-shaped paddle, supporting full palmar surface of forearm, wrist, hand, fingers and thumb. Serial orthosis (D)	Thermoplastics	Physiotherapy, passive stretching	Spastic hemiplegia, quadriplegia, baby in SCBU, older child or adult
Fixed flexion deformity of wrist and hand — pressure sores likely	To achieve a satisfactory position or to prevent further deformity			Surgery — tendon lengthening	
Fixed flexion deformity of elbow		Serial orthosis, full-length arm cylinder	POP, fibreglass casting tape		All types
Inability to maintain elbow extension	To support elbow in extension for weight-bearing (see p. 410)	Full-length arm cylinder, wrap-around arm gaiter (E)	Reinforced Plastazote, canvas with steel staves		
Hand function marred by inability to actively abduct thumb	To facilitate thumb abduction to enable controlled grasp and release	Working or active orthosis to dorsal aspect of hand and base of thumb	Thermoplastics	Physiotherapy, towards voluntary control of movement	Athetosis, spastic diplegia, hemiplegia
Hand function marred by inability to actively extend wrist	To facilitate wrist extension to enable hand function	Wrist cock-up orthosis	Thermoplastics, off-the shelf canvas, Plastazote		
Intention tremor restricts hand function	To reduce tremor to enable function, writing, feeding, shaving, putting on make-up	Weighted wrist band	Close-woven cloth holding lead shot in compartments		Ataxia

preparing and supporting the child before he starts school or when he changes schools. She will need to visit the school well in advance to assess and advise on the environment, i.e. on access, stairs, lifts, ramps and the equipment needed for the child to participate in all parts of the National Curriculum. Preparation and support for teachers and peers is also vital.

Personal skills

The child will not want to stand out from his peers; therefore, great emphasis must be placed on achieving independence before integration. He should be able to take himself to the toilet and manage by himself (adaptations may be necessary), to feed himself (a packed lunch may be suitable if he has difficulty with cutlery), to serve himself if hot meals are supplied and to dress and undress for PE and playtime. The therapist should also give consideration to the following:

- Positioning/seating: a good position at desks, tables and workbenches is essential to enable function in the classroom, laboratory, workshop (metal and woodwork) and kitchen
- Mobility: around the classroom, in all of the above rooms, from the classroom to the playground and around the playground and school campus
- Hand function: intervention may be required to enable the child to participate in all activities, from early skills, e.g. using scissors, pasting, to the later skills used in fine arts, science experiments and vocational activities
- Gross motor control: practice in balance and coordination will facilitate participation in games, drama, movement to music, crafts and kitchen activities
- Handwriting: this may require specific intervention or, if it is too great a problem and delays the child's learning, the provision of an alternative, such as a typewriter or word processor
- Perceptual problems: these may affect many areas of learning and will need constant monitoring and intervention as difficulties arise.

Liaison

Exchange of information between the therapist and the classroom teacher is of vital importance. The therapist should discuss her aims with the teacher and describe how they might be achieved. Often the teacher will be able to incorporate some of these objectives within her curriculum for the class as a whole. If the teacher finds a task with which the child is experiencing difficulty, for example drawing lines with a ruler, the occupational therapist can give the child a short, intensive programme either at school or at home, out of sight of his peers, so that he does not fall behind. Problems should not be pessimistically anticipated, as often a child, especially one who has initiative and perseverance, will overcome problems in his own way; this gives the therapist an ideal opportunity to learn methods of overcoming difficulties to use with other children.

HOME SKILLS

The person with moderate CP is expected to be partially independent. He is unlikely to live alone but will need to perform some household tasks himself. Basic home skills should form part of the occupational therapy programme for the adolescent. These should include: making a hot drink, getting a snack meal, cleaning and tidying his room, answering the telephone and, possibly, visiting the local shops. Those with less severe dysfunction who are expected to live independently should be able to manage all home skills, from cooking, cleaning, laundry, budgeting and nutrition to opening a bank account and selecting suitable accommodation and furnishing. The occupational therapist should ensure that all aspects are assessed and that information, advice and intervention is supplied as necessary. Aids and equipment may be required to achieve independence.

Home environment

The baby or young child with CP is unlikely to require major alterations to the home environment, but as he grows older and heavier and his needs change the accommodation may become unsuitable. As the effects of CP are lifelong, it is possible to anticipate some future needs. The person with severe or moderate CP will be safer, easier to care for (or more independent) in ground-floor accommodation. This may be in an unmodified bungalow, a purpose-built bungalow or a ground-floor extension. Accommodation should have access and manoeuvrability suitable for a wheelchair, a bathroom and bedroom with suitable adaptations and an area for leisure or play. Any alterations to the home should be considered well in advance and discussed with the family so that changes are acceptable and as unobtrusive as possible. The person with mild CP may be able to become completely independent only in a 'user-friendly' environment; he will need the occupational therapist's assistance in arranging his home to best advantage.

EMPLOYMENT

The person with mild CP should be able to manage full employment, although he may require assistance in choosing suitable work and help with adapting the work environment. The occupational therapist will need to liaise with the person and his employer and with the special services available for people with disabilities in employment. The Youth Employment Officer will liaise with the school careers officer in providing vocational guidance and information on job and educational opportunities. He or she can be contacted through the local Careers Office. Those who wish to continue their education or to enrol in vocational training colleges will find provision for people with disabilities at many centres of further and higher education; individual prospectuses will give details. There are also a number of residential colleges around the country which offer special facilities for the more physically handicapped person as well as various vocational training and further education courses. The Disability Employment Advisor (DEA), based at Job Centres, can help the person to find suitable employment and can offer support to the employed. He or she may refer the person to a training college specialising in the assessment and training

of people with disabilities. The Disablement Advisory Service helps with access and alteration to the worksite and the installation of special equipment such as ramps, toilets, lifts and occupational aids. The Rehabilitation Engineering Movement Advisory Panels (REMAP) can advise on the design and supply of special items of equipment which will help individuals to overcome specific problems at work.

The person with moderate CP is more likely to need sheltered or supported employment. Workshops vary from open employment to those provided by the social services or non-statutory sector. The previously mentioned services may also offer information, advice and support.

The person with severe CP will usually transfer from school to a local authority training centre offering sheltered work with continuing education in personal, independent living and social skills. Special Needs Units attached to training centres offer placement for people with severe physical and mental handicaps, with input from therapists so that intervention programmes are continued. SCOPE run industrial units around the country, some with residential hostel accommodation, specifically for people with CP; referral is made directly to SCOPE.

ADVICE AND SUPPORT

The long-term effects of CP on the family depend upon their attitude to handicap and to the affected individual. Some parents are unable to come to terms with or accept their handicapped child. For some, who feel unable to cope in the long term, the only answer is adoption. Often adoption takes place early in the child's life; the therapist will be involved throughout this process with both the foster or adoptive parents and the original family. Other parents accept the child as a member of the family but refuse to believe the diagnosis or recognise its implications. Another difficulty occurs when one parent accepts the child and the other does not; relationships between the parents and between the parents and child are affected and the therapist should be aware of the effects on the child in particular. Such difficulties may remain unresolved, resulting in divorce or in one parent immersing himself in work while the other's life revolves around the handicapped person.

The majority of parents of children affected with CP accept them as individuals and encourage independence. However, the transition from childhood to adolescence and adolescence to adulthood will be no less problematic than in any other family. As life changes occur the person with CP may lack self-confidence and become frustrated or bewildered. These emotions are not exclusive to people with CP, but the presence of a disability may make these feelings occur more frequently or more strongly. The emergence of self-identity and the development of social and sexual relationships are trying processes in which the occupational therapist can offer advice and support. Parents, siblings, grandparents and partners need to understand all aspects of the individual's handicap, problems and treatment programme if they are to help and support the person. Their main role, however, is that of family member — mother, father, brother, sister, and so on.

The occupational therapist can also provide advice about holidays and social and leisure activities and can make referrals to other agencies such as social security, SCOPE, local support groups and counselling services.

CONCLUSION

Cerebral palsy is a lifelong disorder which affects many areas of function. It is not, however, an unchanging condition and the occupational therapist can play a major role in facilitating improvement. She must work closely with the affected person, his family and with other professionals; she must be prepared to offer advice, support, education and intervention in widely ranging areas of function. The occupational therapist is instrumental in enabling the person with CP to become 'his own person' and to achieve his full potential.

USEFUL ADDRESSES

SCOPE (formerly The Spastics Society)
12 Park Crescent
London W1N 4EQ
Tel: 0171–636 5020

DFE Publications Centre
PO Box 2193
London E15 2EU
Tel: 0181–533 2000

Equipment for Disabled People
The Disability Information Trust
Mary Marlborough Lodge
Nuffield Orthopaedic Centre
Headington
Oxford OX3 7LD
Tel: (01865) 750103

Sensory Integration Association (UK)
PO Box 149
Wolverhampton WV1 1AA

REFERENCES

Ayres A J 1972 Sensory integration and learning disorders. Western Psychological Services, Los Angeles
Ayres A J 1979 Sensory integration and the child. Western Psychological Services, Los Angeles
Bobath B 1967 The very early treatment of cerebral palsy. Developmental Medicine and Child Neurology 9(4): 373–390
Bobath B 1975 Motor development in the different types of cerebral palsy. William Heinemann, New York
Bobath K 1980 A neurophysiological basis for the treatment of cerebral palsy. Clinics in Developmental Medicine, 75. William Heinemann, London

Bohannon R 1987 Inhibitive casting for cerebral palsied children. Developmental Medicine and Child Neurology 29: 122–123
Burke J P 1993 Play: the life role of the infant and young child. In: Case-Smith J (ed.) Pediatric occupational therapy and early intervention. Butterworth-Heinemann, Stoneham, MD, pp 198–224
Butler C 1986 Effects of powered mobility on self-initiated behaviors of very young children with locomotor disability. Developmental Medicine and Child Neurology 28: 325–332

Dworetzky J P, Davis N J 1989 Human development — a lifespan approach. West Publishing Company, St Paul, MN

Erhardt R P 1982 Developmental hand dysfunction. Ramsco, Laurel, MD

Griffiths M, Clegg M 1988 Cerebral palsy: problems and practice. Souvenir, London

Hagberg B, Hagberg G 1984 Prenatal and perinatal risk factors in a survey of 681 Swedish cases. In: Stanley F, Alberman E (eds) The epidemiology of the cerebral palsies. J B Lippincott, Philadelphia, pp 116–134

Holloway E 1993 Early emotional development and sensory processing. In: Case-Smith J (ed.) Pediatric occupational therapy and early intervention. Butterworth-Heinemann, Stoneham, MD, pp 163–197

Holm V A 1982 The causes of cerebral palsy. Journal of the American Medical Association 247: 1473–1477

Hughes I, Newton R 1992 Genetic aspects of cerebral palsy. Developmental Medicine and Child Neurology 34: 80–86

Johnson A, Townshend P, Yudkin P, Bull D, Wilkinson A R 1993 Functional abilities at age 4 years of children born before 29 weeks of gestation. British Medical Journal 306 (6894): 1715–1718

Klein M D 1983 Pre-dressing skills. Communication Skill Builders, Tucson

Langer V S 1990 Minimal handling protocol for the intensive care nursery. Neonatal Network 9(3): 23–27

Nwaobi O M, Smith P D 1986 Effect of adaptive seating on pulmonary function of children with cerebral palsy. Developmental Medicine and Child Neurology 28: 351–354

Paneth N, Kiely J 1984 The frequency of cerebral palsy: a review of population studies in industrialized nations since 1950. In: Stanley F, Alberman E (eds) The epidemiology of the cerebral palsies. J B Lippincott, Philadelphia, pp 46–56

Robinson R O 1973 The frequency of other handicaps in children with cerebral palsy. Developmental Medicine and Child Neurology 15: 305–312

Rood M 1962 The use of sensory receptors to activate, facilitate and inhibit motor response, autonomic and somatic, in developmental sequence. In: Scattely C (ed.) Approaches to treatment of patients with neuromuscular dysfunction. William Brown, Dubuque, IO

SCOPE 1994 What is cerebral palsy? Leaflets and Information Service, SCOPE, London

Stanley F J, Blair E 1984 Postnatal risk factors among the cerebral palsies. In: Stanley F, Alberman E (eds) The epidemiology of the cerebral palsies. J B Lippincott, Philadephia, pp 135–149

Todd V R 1993 Visual perceptual frame of reference: an information processing approach. In: Kramer P, Hinojosa J (eds) Frames of reference for pediatric occupational therapy. Williams & Wilkins, Baltimore, pp 177–229

Tona J L, Schneck C M 1993 The efficacy of upper extremity inhibitive casting: a single subject case study. American Journal of Occupational Therapy 47(10): 901–910

Warnock Report 1978 HMSO, London

FURTHER READING

Development

Bee H 1992 The developing child, 6th edn. HarperCollins, New York

Illingworth R 1991 The normal child — Some problems of the early years and their treatment, 10th edn. Churchill Livingstone, Edinburgh

Sheridan M D 1975 Children's developmental progress — from birth to 5 years. NFER, Windsor

Sugarman L 1986 Life-span development — concepts, theories and interventions. Routledge, London

Cerebral palsy

Cogher L, Savage E, Smith M (eds) 1992 Cerebral palsy — the child and young person. Management of Disability Series, 1. Chapman & Hall, London

Finnie N R 1977 Handling the young cerebral palsy child at home. Heinemann, London

Scrutton D 1984 Management of the motor disorders of children with cerebral palsy. Spastics International Medical Publications, Oxford

Occupational therapy

Case-Smith J (ed.) 1993 Pediatric occupational therapy and early intervention. Andover Medical, Butterworth-Heinemann, Stoneham, MD

Clancy H, Clark M 1990 Occupational therapy with children. Churchill Livingstone, Edinburgh

Eckersley P, Clegg M, Robinson P 1986 The 1981 Education Act — guidelines for physiotherapists and other paediatric professionals. Chartered Society of Physiotherapists, London

Erhardt R P 1982 Developmental hand dysfunction. Ramsco, Laurel, MD

Klein M D 1983 Pre-dressing skills. Communication Skills Builders, Tucson (published in UK by Winslow Press, Oxon)

Klein M D 1982 Pre-writing skills. Communication Skills Builders, Tucson (published in UK by Winslow Press, Oxon)

Klein M D 1987 Pre-scissor skills. Communication Skills Builders, Tucson, (published in UK by Winslow Press, Oxon)

Kramer P, Hinojosa J (eds) 1993 Frames of reference for pediatric occupational therapy. Williams & Wilkins, Baltimore

Levitt S 1984 Paediatric developmental therapy. Blackwell, Oxford

Pratt P N, Allen A S 1989 Occupational therapy for children. C V Mosby, St Louis

Semmler C, Hunter J 1990 Early occupational therapy intervention — neonates to three years. Aspen, Gaithersburg, MD

Ward D E 1984 Positioning the handicapped child for function. Phoenix Press, St Louis

14

Cerebrovascular accident

Sue Jackson

INTRODUCTION

This chapter discusses the particular challenges faced by the occupational therapist in helping individuals who have suffered a cerebrovascular accident (CVA) or stroke.

The first section of the chapter describes CVA, its incidence, prognosis and causation. A brief introduction to neuroanatomy follows, aiming to explain the neurological damage that can result from CVA. Characteristics of normal movement and posture are also outlined, together with the possible effects of CVA on motor control. The chapter then turns to other clinical effects of CVA, such as sensory deficit, spasticity, emotional disturbance, altered cognition, speech disorders, and perceptual dysfunction.

Next, the chapter describes in detail the specific role taken by the occupational therapist in facilitating rehabilitation, beginning with assessment of the impact of the CVA upon the individual's motor, sensory, perceptual, and cognitive function, and upon his ability to resume his former level of independence. Likely aims of the rehabilitation programme are outlined, along with practical suggestions for treatment in such areas as the prevention of deformity, reduction of spasticity, enhancement of independence in personal and home care, management of perceptual problems, and resettlement at home and work.

Finally, specific physical problems that may present obstacles to rehabilitation are briefly described; these are the 'pusher' syndrome, shoulder and ankle problems, and multiple diagnoses.

The presenting problems of CVA are many and varied, and no one approach can offer solutions to them all.

However, a developmental frame of reference is most commonly used, with a primarily neuro-developmental approach based on the concept that after brain damage improvements in movement control follow a developmental pattern, and therefore treatment should follow those same steps. This approach requires analysis of normal patterns of movement and of deviation from that norm in the individual, followed by facilitation of improvement using the techniques specific to the approach. This involves inhibiting abnormal movement, and relearning through experiencing normal movement. While a neurodevelopmental approach is usually utilised, others, for instance humanistic, compensatory and/or problem-solving, may also be introduced alongside or independently. Therefore, the therapist must be flexible in her interventions, always keeping the individual's own priorities firmly in mind, and ensuring that her treatment complements that provided by the other members of the multidisciplinary team.

CHARACTERISTICS OF CVA

'A cerebrovascular accident is a rapidly developed clinical sign of a focal disturbance of cerebral function of presumed vascular origin and of more than 24 hours duration' (WHO 1986).

Excluded from this definition are episodes which resolve spontaneously within 24 hours. These, termed transient ischaemic attacks (TIAs), may precede a completed stroke; a predisposing medical condition such as hypertension may be present.

Stroke syndromes of slow, insidious onset are more likely to be due to another cause, such as a cerebral tumour. A full medical history is vital in order to establish an accurate diagnosis.

INCIDENCE AND PROGNOSIS

The incidence of strokes is about 1.8–2.0 per 1000 of population per annum. About 70% of all strokes occur in people over 70 years of age.

Approximately 80% show some useful recovery and are able to return home; 60% of the total number regain independence in activities of daily living (ADL) and 30% are able to resume normal activities. The risk of mortality increases with age and the presence of associated conditions such as heart disease.

AETIOLOGY
Ischaemia

Occlusion of either of the carotid arteries, one of the major cerebral arteries (middle, posterior, anterior), or of one of their smaller branches is the most common cause of CVA; 70–75% of all strokes are attributable to occlusion.

Atherosclerosis

Intracranial arteries which have degenerative atherosclerotic changes may become occluded if platelets adhere to the damaged endothelial lining, forming a thrombus. The tissue beyond the occlusion is consequently deprived of blood which carries oxygen, and so becomes infarcted. The function normally performed by that area of the brain is lost or reduced, depending on the severity of the lesion. This type of CVA is most common in elderly people.

Embolus/thrombus

Occlusion may also be caused by an embolus, a part of a thrombus which breaks away and is carried by the circulation into the smaller vessels of the brain, where it becomes lodged, thus depriving distal brain tissue of its vital blood supply. Particularly susceptible to this type of stroke are people with cardiac disease in which emboli arise from the left atrium or ventricle and cause problems in the middle cerebral arteries in particular.

Haemorrhage

A smaller percentage of strokes is caused by cerebral haemorrhage and may occur at any age due to a rupture of abnormal blood vessels. In elderly people, hypertension, particularly in combination with arterial degeneration, may result in the rupture of small intracranial arteries. Sites prone to this are the internal capsule, pons, thalamus and cerebellum.

In younger people the presence of aneurysms or, more rarely, arteriovenous malformations (angiomas) may lead to haemorrhage; the Circle of Willis is a particularly susceptible site.

Pathology

In the case of haemorrhage, as with occlusive strokes, the area of the brain normally supplied by the ruptured vessel will be deprived of its oxygen supply. Additionally, function will be reduced in the area of the brain into which blood has leaked. This area, however, may regain function if the blood is reabsorbed or the resulting haematoma surgically evacuated.

Medication

Medication may be prescribed to increase the uptake of oxygen by damaged cells to attempt to maintain their function. Other medication to normalise blood pressure, reduce platelet aggregation or increase blood flow may also be given, depending on the cause of the CVA.

NEUROANATOMY

The following is a brief introduction to the neurological consequences of CVA. A knowledge of the mechanisms of neuroplasticity is also useful as it forms the theory underpinning the nervous system's adaptability following damage. The reader is advised to consult appropriate texts of neuroanatomy and physiology for more detailed information.

Blood supply to the brain

The brain obtains its blood supply from two main pairs of arteries: the internal carotid and the vertebral arteries. These, together with other arteries, form the Circle of Willis (Fig. 14.1).

The Circle of Willis can act as a safeguard, allowing blood to flow to an infarcted area via an alternative route if a vessel is occluded, but where there is severe degenerative arterial change this may not be possible.

Nerve pathways

Sensory nerves

Sensory information from the trunk and limbs is conveyed via sensory nerve fibres in the peripheral nerves to cell bodies in the dorsal root ganglia and on into the spinal cord. From here, different types of sensory information are conveyed to the sensory cortex via separate pathways (Fig. 14.2).

Nerve fibres conveying information about *light, touch, vibration* and *joint position* travel up the ipsilateral side of the spinal cord (i.e. the same side on which they entered) along the dorsal columns to the brain stem dorsal column nuclei. There, they synapse with secondary neurones, which send nerve fibres to the opposite side to ascend to the thalamus in the medial lemniscus. From there, tertiary neurones send nerve fibres to the sensory cortex of the central hemisphere on that side.

Fibres carrying information about *pain* and *temperature* pass their impulses to second sensory neurones, which then cross to the opposite (contralateral) side of the cord. These then travel up to the thalamus in the spinothalamic tract, where they synapse with other neurones to convey the impulse to the sensory cortex in the parietal lobe.

Motor nerves

Weakness on one side of the body occurs as a result of injury to upper motor neurones in the opposite side of the brain. The motor nerve fibres, axons or pyramidal tracts arise from the motor cortex on one side of the brain, passing down through the internal capsule to the medulla, where about 90% cross to the opposite side to form the lateral corticospinal tracts. They then continue down the spinal cord to the appropriate level, where they synapse with a second (lower motor) neurone. This passes out as a peripheral

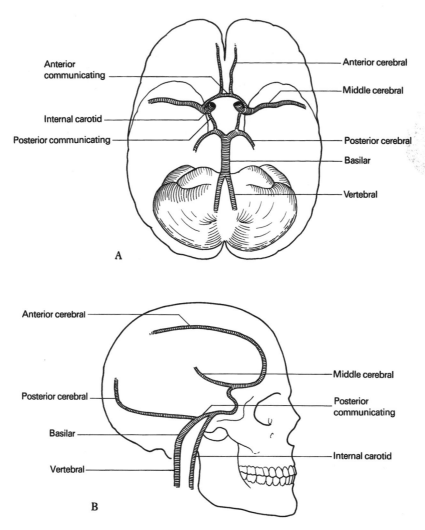

Fig. 14.1   The Circle of Willis: (A) basal view and (B) lateral view.

motor nerve fibre in a mixed peripheral nerve to skeletal muscle on that side of the body (Fig. 14.3).

The deficits resulting from CVA will depend on which area of the motor cortex is affected (Fig. 14.4).

Optic nerves

Some of the optic tract fibres cross at the optic chiasma, while others do not. The area of any visual field deficit will depend on the lesion site. In CVAs the most common lesion produces homonymous hemianopia with loss of vision in half of each eye on the same side as the lesion.

However, as the retina receives visual information from the opposite side of the environment, the net effect is the inability to see information on the opposite side to that of the lesion (Fig. 14.5).

Facial sensation

Sensory fibres in the trigeminal (5th cranial) nerve serving the face enter the spinal nucleus of the trigeminal nerve, where they synapse with secondary neurones. Their axons cross the midline to ascend on the opposite side in the trigeminothalamic tract to the thalamus. There,

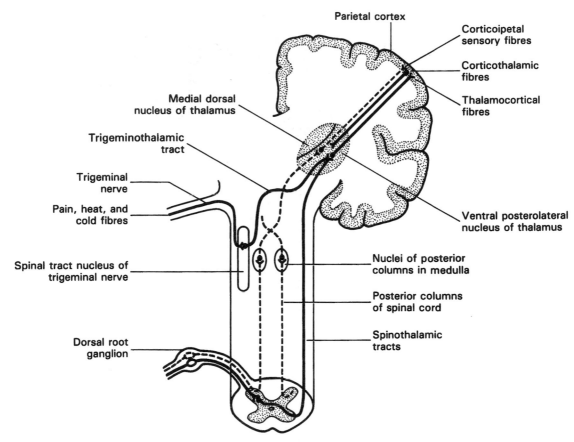

Fig. 14.2 Ascending sensory pathways in the brain and spinal cord. (Reproduced from Walton 1977 Brain's diseases of the nervous system, 8th edn, by permission of Oxford University Press.)

they synapse with neurones which send axons to the sensory cortex of the cerebral hemisphere on that side (see Fig. 14.2).

It can be seen, therefore, that the pathways for both sensory and motor function cross over, so that a lesion in one hemisphere of the brain results in disability on the opposite side of the body.

Location of lesions

Internal capsule

The internal capsule within the hemispheres is the site where bundles of motor nerves, sensory nerves and the optic tract fibres pass in close proximity to one another. Lesions in this region may cause loss of motor ability, sensory appreciation and hemianopia.

Cerebellar and brain stem CVAs

The pyramidal system works in conjunction with the extrapyramidal system to produce smooth movements. The extrapyramidal system (which consists of fibres from the premotor area, the basal ganglia and the brain stem) and the cerebellum are jointly responsible for coordinating the smooth contraction and relaxation of muscle groups and the maintenance of posture and body equilibrium. Lesions in these areas result in impairment of posture and righting reflexes and loss of control of voluntary movement, with intention tremor if the person attempts to move his affected limb (ataxia). Ataxia may involve one or more limbs, be unilateral or bilateral, and may involve the trunk, causing unsteadiness when standing and walking (truncal ataxia).

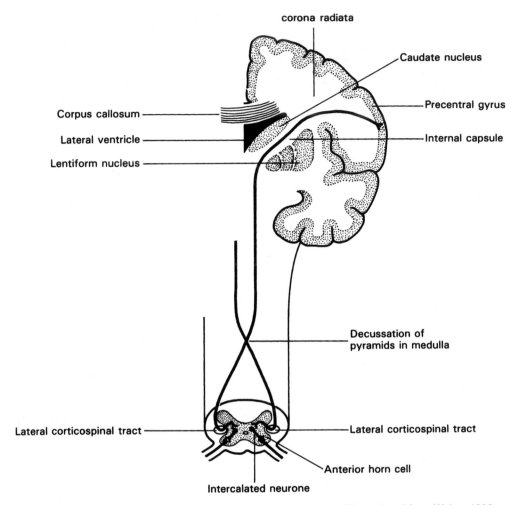

Fig. 14.3 Descending motor pathways in the brain and spinal cord. (Reproduced from Walton 1993 Brain's diseases of the nervous system, 10th edn, by permission of Oxford University Press.)

Vertigo and vomiting may occur at the onset of a brain stem stroke and are common with obstruction of the posterior inferior cerebellar artery. Nystagmus (jerking of the eyes during voluntary eye movements) and disturbance of coordination of simultaneous eye movement (conjugate gaze) can also occur.

If the nuclei and nerve tracts controlling extra-ocular movements are affected, strabismus (squint) or diplopia (double vision) may be present. With lesions low in the brain stem (e.g. in the medulla), the lower cranial nerve nuclei and axons may be affected, giving rise to bulbar palsy with dysphagia (difficulty swallowing), dysarthria (slurred speech) and difficulty with coughing.

This should be distinguished from pseudobulbar palsy, which has similar symptoms, but is due to bilateral upper motor neurone lesions within the motor cortex.

NORMAL MOVEMENT

The therapist needs a thorough understanding of normal movement in order to treat the motor and sensory manifestations of CVA. Normal movement occurs automatically; for example, the individual does not generally think consciously about moving from a sitting to a standing position. However, individuals move in patterns

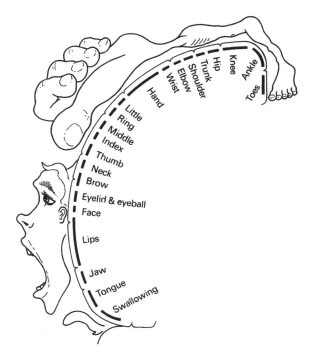

Fig. 14.4 The motor homunculus, showing the origins of the neurones controlling movement in different parts of the body on the motor cortex of the frontal lobe of the brain.

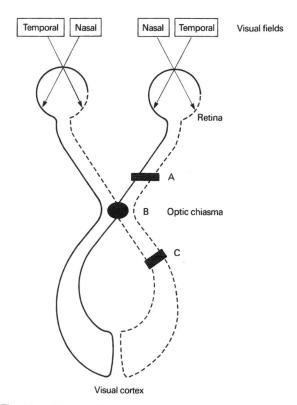

Fig. 14.5 Visual pathways and lesion sites. Lesions at site A result in total blindness in one eye; at B–bitemporal hemianopia; at C–homonymous hemianopia.

which vary slightly according to factors such as build, personality, habits and pain.

In order to move normally, the central postural control mechanism is needed, accompanied by normal sensation, tone, balance, righting and equilibrium reactions and a combination of reciprocal innervation and co-contraction.

Patterns of movement

When an individual moves deliberately he chooses how to do so by selecting the movement and controlling it; he does not move in gross motor patterns but in refined, highly selective patterns of movements.

Sensation

Everyone is aware of pain, temperature, pressure and proprioception. All these are integrated from the periphery and transmitted to the centre, providing feedback to facilitate normal movement and balance.

Normal muscle tone

This provides a background for normal movement. Normal tone allows freedom of movement without conscious thought. Tone needs to be sufficiently high to support the body and to enable it to move against gravity but not so high that it impedes movement. It is normal for tone to vary between individuals. It is affected by emotion, pain and effort and also varies in different positions/postural sets of the *same* person. For example when lying prone, tone is lower than when standing, because more muscle contraction is needed to maintain the body upright against gravity.

Balance, equilibrium and righting reactions

During everyday activity the body's tone and posture adjust automatically to take account of

Abilities usually retained include:

- singing (this is controlled by the non-dominant hemisphere)
- automatic and social speech — counting by rote and greetings
- swearing — usually unintentional.

Verbal dyspraxia

Verbal dyspraxia is a disorder of the *purposeful* coordination of muscle movement for the production of speech. It is characterised by numerous attempts to achieve the correct sounds for the word, awareness of the errors and some speech produced automatically without thinking. The muscles themselves are not weak and automatic movements are retained.

These three forms of communication disorder can present in isolation; however, they often occur together, in differing severities. Dyspraxia, in particular, is rarely dissociated from any dysphasia.

Visual disturbances

The most common visual disturbance is homonymous hemianopia resulting from trauma to the optic tract or visual cortex in the occipital lobe (see Fig. 14.5). The person is unable to see half of their visual field on the same side as the hemiplegia. However vision may be peripheral, sparing central sight, or lost in only one quadrant (quadrantanopia) (Fig. 14.8).

Functional difficulties associated with visual disturbance are often related to safety e.g. in the kitchen, negotiating stairs and crossing roads.

Perceptual deficits

Perception is 'the ability to interpret sensory messages from the environment such that the sensation has meaning' (Zoltan et al 1986).

Following a CVA perceptual deficits may be present, their type combination and extent depending upon the site of the lesion. Perceptual dysfunction occurs when the sensory end organ

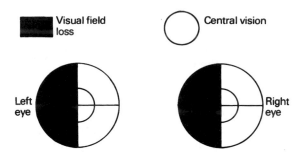

A Left homonymous hemianopia splitting central vision

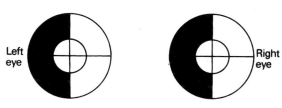

B Left homonymous hemianopia sparing central vision

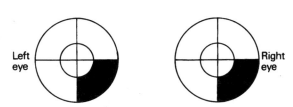

C Right lower quadrantanopia sparing central vision

Fig. 14.8 Homonymous hemianopia.

is intact but the area within the cortex concerned with interpretation of the stimuli is damaged.

The main categories of perceptual disturbance are outlined briefly below; again, the reader is encouraged to gain a deeper understanding from specialised texts.

Agnosia

A person is unable to recognise familiar objects using a given sense although the corresponding sense organ is undamaged. For example, a person with visual agnosia may fail to recognise personal objects such as hairbrushes or combs using sight but may identify them correctly through touch. If a person has problems with agnosia he may put himself at risk from injury, for example by inadvertently putting a knife in his mouth.

Spatial relationship disorders

- *Figure/ground.* The individual has difficulty differentiating foreground from background. He may have difficulty finding his matching shoe in a wardrobe.
- *Position in space.* The person has difficulty orientating himself or objects within the surroundings; for example, he may look on top of the bed when told his shoes are under it.
- *Form constancy.* The individual may have difficulty recognising everyday objects when viewed from unusual angles, in unusual positions, or when they are of different sizes but similar in design, for example a hairbrush and a toothbrush.
- *Depth/distance perception.* The person may misjudge depth and distance and so have difficulty negotiating stairs or trying to fill a cup.

Apraxia

This is loss of ability to perform a previously learned movement although the individual retains the motor power, sensation and coordination essential to the action. Apraxia is a problem of sequencing or of initiation. In ideomotor apraxia the person may be unable to initiate an action on request but may still be able to carry out the task automatically, whereas in ideational apraxia the concept of the task is lost and even automatic performance is affected. Apraxia denotes total loss of an ability; **dys**praxia denotes partial loss of a skill.

Body image/body scheme disorders

Body image is the mental representation of one's body that expresses one's feelings and thoughts whereas body scheme is the postural model of the body's physical structure.

Included in body image and body scheme disorders are unilateral neglect/inattention and failure of right/left discrimination.

Unilateral neglect/inattention is the inability to respond appropriately and consistently to stimuli from one side of the body. An individual may bump into objects on one side or may only eat the food on one side of his plate.

When right/left discrimination is affected the concepts of right and left are no longer understood and the individual is unable to identify the right and left sides of his body.

THE ROLE OF THE OCCUPATIONAL THERAPIST

The occupational therapist works alongside the individual who has suffered a CVA and his carers, as part of the multidisciplinary team. Her work will complement that of other members of the team in enabling the individual to achieve his personal goals and maximise his independence.

At various stages of the rehabilitation programme the therapist's role will change considerably in accordance with the findings of continuous assessment; for example, in the early stages of treatment good positioning may be the most important aim, whereas safety in the kitchen may take priority later on.

ASSESSMENT

Assessment forms an integral part of intervention and is a component of each treatment session.

Due to the complexity of the information required to form an accurate assessment it may not be possible to build a full picture of the individual's abilities and problems in one session. Therefore sources of information such as medical notes and the observations of team colleagues and relatives should be used to complement information gained from the person himself. Medical prognosis should also be considered, because pain, poor stamina or drowsiness are factors that may improve with surgery or medication rather than with rehabilitation. A full and accurate assessment is needed before priorities for the treatment programme are established. This assessment should include information about the person's home environment, previous and present level of health, independence and life-style, the likely support available to him short and long term and his attitude towards his stroke — all will affect the outlook for rehabilitation.

level of independence in ADL as this often forms the baseline for treatment. Only skills relevant to the individual need be considered. For example, if someone did not cook his meals prior to stroke, his assessment in this area is of little value. Continual assessment will indicate areas of improvement as well as areas in which the individual may need support in the longer term.

In addressing functional problems the cause of the difficulty needs to be ascertained. For example, if the individual is unable to wash his face it may be because he cannot cross the midline, has an inattention, has extensive loss of postural control or lacks understanding or motivation.

Home assessment

If the individual is being treated at home, problems can be addressed as they arise. If, however, the person is being treated in hospital a home assessment may be necessary, either to ensure that the transition from hospital to home is as trouble-free as possible or to ascertain the feasibility of returning home. The visit is often also used as the venue for confirming support services, e.g. a home help.

Assessment in a person's home environment is described in Chapter 7, but four areas which may be of particular importance for those who have had a CVA are briefly summarised below:

- *Access*. If the person is unable to manage the access with any mobility aids, e.g. a wheelchair or walking frame, then adaptations such as a ramp, half steps or rails may be indicated
- *Doors and corridors*. The width of these may hamper mobility around the house if the individual is dependent on a wheelchair or walking frame. Widening or rehanging doors and removing thresholds may enhance mobility
- *Stairs*. Problems ascending or descending may indicate the need for a second banister and two walking aids, one situated upstairs, the other downstairs. More major adaptations may include a stairlift or

through-floor lift as an alternative to bringing a bed downstairs
- *Transfers*. If the individual is having difficulty with any transfers furniture heights may need adjusting to make standing easier; for example, a raised seat and rail in the toilet.

It may prove impossible to adapt existing accommodation to suit the needs of the individual. Rehousing to more suitable premises may be an alternative but this may have far-reaching effects on the person and his family. The convenience of more suitable accommodation needs to be weighed against the disadvantages of being removed from familiar surroundings and local support networks. It may also be more difficult for relatives and carers to visit the individual in a new location and provide the necessary levels of support.

APPROACHES TO TREATMENT

Within a neurodevelopmental framework a wide variety of approaches is available to the therapist treating individuals who have suffered a stroke. These include Rood, Bobath, Brunnstrom, Proprioceptive Neuromuscular Facilitation (PNF) and Conductive Education. Each has its own particular emphasis and for this reason it is essential that people from different disciplines agree on a broad base of treatment. This will ensure that the individual being treated is approached in a consistent manner by all concerned.

The merits of each approach need to be considered in conjunction with the aims of the individual. This may result in the adoption of components from several approaches; for example, the principles of a neurodevelopmental approach could be applied to an adapted rehabilitative technique to ensure that the latter does not permit any undue increase in tone. As no single approach will solve all individuals' problems, the therapist needs a good working knowledge of a wide range of approaches.

AIMS OF TREATMENT

Although the individual may present with a

number of problems which can be treated separately, the therapist should maintain an holistic outlook, as it is the *combination* of the individual's problems which prevents him from being independent. For example, resolving body scheme problems may not make someone independent in dressing if he also has problems sequencing the activity.

After assessment a treatment programme should be formulated, taking into account the individual's needs and priorities.

Broad aims of treatment, and subsequent goals, may include the following:

- prevention of deformity
- reduction of spasticity and promotion of normal movement
- maximisation of personal independence
- maximisation of independence in domestic activities
- exploration of coping mechanisms for psychological problems
- management of perceptual problems

- resettlement within the family
- reestablishment of work and leisure roles
- all aims and goals to include inbuilt review.

Preventing deformity

Good positioning is essential in both the early hypotonic stage and the later hypertonic stage of muscle tone. All joints which have their supporting structures affected should be supported, to avoid damage to soft tissues, pain and joint misalignment. The individual needs to be encouraged to take responsibility for his own positioning as early as possible. Education for relatives should also be provided. The individual should be taught to recognise increase in tone, what causes it and how he can reduce it himself. Good positioning should be constantly reinforced by all members of the multidisciplinary team so that it is maintained for as great a part of the day as possible.

Positioning should aim to break up any abnormal patterns and inhibit increased tone such as

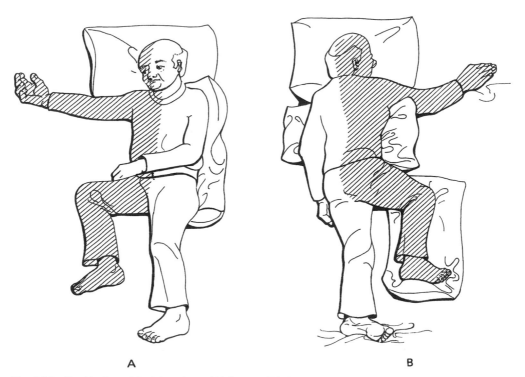

A   B

Fig. 14.9 Positioning while lying down. (A) Supine. (B) Prone.

rehabilitation both as an inpatient and, where facilities exist as an outpatient, and in the community. Rehabilitation may last several years and focus on improving levels of self-care and independence, as well as on meeting vocational needs, generally at a much later date. Those able to return to employment generally do so in a much reduced capacity and many severely injured people may only be able to work in sheltered employment. They often remain dependent on their families and/or social service agencies for care or at least regular supervision and support.

Very severe injuries

These people have coma lasting weeks or months, after which the persistent vegetative state emerges. In this coma-like state they have sleep/wake cycles, in which they allow themselves to be fed but usually do not speak, follow commands or indicate any ability to understand what is said to them. If this state persists very long after coma has ended, it is unlikely that any real improvements will ever be made.

CLINICAL FEATURES

The clinical features resulting from head injury are as varied as the physical, cognitive and psychosocial functions that the brain itself supports. The focus in this section is on the relatively common features resulting from moderate and severe injuries.

Physical deficits

- *Paralysis* may involve all limbs. Muscle tone may be lost, reduced or increased as a result of damage to higher centres of the brain responsible for the regulation of muscle tone and the integration of muscular reflexes. The initial loss of tone, i.e. hypotonus or flaccidity, is usually replaced by an increase in tone, i.e. hypertonus or spasticity. Where higher centres are damaged reflex activity will predominate.
- *Ataxia* implies disturbance of muscular contraction and tone leading to an inability to co-ordinate movements. Ataxia is caused by damage to the cerebellum, which regulates muscle contraction and joint position, thus affecting and controlling balance. Muscle power, however, is not usually affected. Damage to the cerebellum will lead to incoordination of movement with inaccuracies in speed, timing and direction. Loss of sensation and of proprioception, i.e. the ability to feel the position of joints and limbs in space, will considerably exacerbate the situation and the person will try to compensate through vision.
- *Extrapyramidal tremor* is due to damage to the extrapyramidal system, in particular to the basal ganglia, and manifests itself by continued tremor, caused by fluctuating tone in opposing muscle groups.
- *Disturbances of equilibrium and righting reactions* are caused when the centres of the brain concerned with these mechanisms are damaged, resulting in the inability to place and maintain the body in the required position against gravity. Postural adjustments to maintain balance are upset.
- *Sensory disturbance* may be caused by damage to the sensory area of the cerebral cortex and posterior column tracts in the brain, causing lack of appreciation or distortion of sensation. There may be disturbances in tactile discrimination (pain, temperature, texture) and/or proprioception.

There may also be disturbances in the functions of the other special senses as a result of damage to the central processing centres of the brain rather than to the sensory organs (e.g. eyes, ears) *per se*, although these may also be damaged. There can thus be disturbances in visual, auditory, gustatory and olfactory perception.

- *Disturbances in speech* (see ch. 14) may occur while language comprehension remains intact. Two common deficits are:
  - *Dysarthria* — difficulty in articulation of speech due to injury to the motor speech nerves
  - *Apraxia* — impairment of articulatory programming in the cortex.

It must be stressed that these are purely motor problems and are not caused by impairment of the cognitive processes of interpretation and understanding of written and spoken language.

Cognitive deficits

• *Attention and concentration* difficulties may manifest themselves as an inability to filter out irrelevant background stimuli. The person responds to the most salient stimulus even though it may not be the most relevant and thus he is very distractable.

• *Memory and learning* deficits are very common. Invariably, head-injured people do not remember events around the time of the injury and for a variable period immediately before it; this is known as *retrograde traumatic amnesia*. Memory for these events is very unlikely to ever return. Memory for events prior to the injury may be disturbed although deeply ingrained material generally remains intact. Perhaps most significant is the difficulty most head-injured people face in their ability to learn and remember new material.

• *Perceptual deficits* occur when there is a disruption in the process of organisation and interpretation of incoming stimuli leading to an inappropriate response. Such deficits may include spatial relationship problems, body-image disorders and an inability to recognise familiar objects.

• *Language deficits* imply a disruption of linguistic competence and performance in contrast to speech deficits, which are purely motor. *Dysphasia* is the most common and is described in Chapter 14.

Psychosocial deficits

In the early stages of recovery from head injury, the person may exhibit behavioural disturbances and poor psychosocial function. Such disturbances may include emotional lability, aggressive outbursts, disorientation, impulsiveness and agitation. Typically there is an improvement in psychosocial functioning, although irritability, impulsiveness, poor frustration tolerance, denial, anxiety and depression may persist. It is arguable whether such symptoms are a direct result of brain damage or a psychological reaction to the situation in which the person finds himself.

THE ROLE OF THE OCCUPATIONAL THERAPIST

The common clinical features following head injury outlined above might be conceived as 'micro-deficits'. Micro-deficits such as ataxia, poor concentration and memory problems may combine in innumerable ways to form larger patterns of dysfunction or 'macro-deficits'. For example, a partial paralysis would certainly impede independent living activities, but when a paralysis is combined with a memory or attention difficulty an entirely different picture emerges. Such macro-deficits produced by particular combinations of micro-deficits can produce substantial handicaps in any of the following areas: activities of daily living (ADL), social involvements, educational/vocational activities and family relationships. Rehabilitation for the head-injured person must focus on both the micro-deficit level and, perhaps more importantly, on the more holistic macro-deficit level.

THEORETICAL FOUNDATIONS

The complexity and diversity of deficits experienced by head-injured people as a direct result of the injury, together with the widely differing combinations of deficits, necessitates the therapist drawing on a wide range of theoretical frameworks in order to select the most appropriate treatment techniques for each individual.

There is no one frame of reference which would be applicable to every case but rather a combination of approaches is generally used, particular approaches being more appropriate at certain times during the treatment process as the individual progresses from one stage to the next.

For example, in the early stages of intervention, while attempting to facilitate recovery and integration of motor function, the therapist might use approaches derived from the developmental frame of reference. Several 'purist' techniques (or more frequently a combination of these) might be used at this stage within the neurodevelopmental approach. Techniques used include: Bobath and Rood, which emphasise normalisation of muscle tone, inhibition of abnormal reflex activity and facilitation of normal movement patterns through skilled handling and positioning; proprioceptive neuromuscular facilitation (PNF), which aims to promote neuromuscular activity through the stimulation of the proprioceptors; and the sensorimotor approach which is based on the principle that motor output is dependent on sensory input, so sensory stimuli can be used to activate or inhibit motor responses. The underpinning principle relating to these approaches is that the acquisition of integrated voluntary movement occurs in a developmental sequence, so they are based within the developmental frame of reference.

Subsequently behavioural and cognitive approaches from the learning frame of reference might be utilised in, for example, addressing social skills training and memory management techniques. Based on the theory that an individual learns through experience and education, a behavioural approach might be used in attempting to extinguish patterns of antisocial behaviour. Likewise a behavioural approach might be used in skill building through the use of modelling and chaining techniques.

At the later stages of treatment the therapist might employ approaches from the compensatory or rehabilitative frame of reference, whereby the individual with persisting disability adopts compensatory strategies to overcome functional problems.

All this might seem quite complicated at this stage but theoretical applications will hopefully become more clear as the stages of recovery are considered.

It is also worth noting that while therapists draw from several frames of reference in treating head injured people, there are those Centres whose approaches to treatment are very much based on a particular frame of reference, such as a behavioural approach, although this is usually in response to persisting behavioural difficulties experienced by the individual.

PRINCIPLES OF TREATMENT

1. Therapeutic intervention should commence as early after injury as is feasible.

2. Treatment should be provided in an holistic manner. The person should not be regarded as someone with a collection of particular deficits but rather as a whole person whose multiple needs require an integrated response.

3. Since the occupational therapist works as a member of a team, treatment approaches should be well coordinated with the other team members and treatments should complement one another.

4. Therapy should focus on micro-deficits and macro-deficits simultaneously. While it is important to try to rectify specific problems such as concentration/attention difficulties within the treatment setting, it is equally important, if not more so, to focus on the person's functional abilities, for example daily living skills. Therefore, attempts to overcome a cognitive problem should be made on both 'fronts' simultaneously.

THE OCCUPATIONAL THERAPY PROCESS

The following points should be considered by the occupational therapist when assessing and planning treatment at any stage after head injury. Refer also to Chapter 4 for more detailed information.

Gathering information

1. About the individual. It is important to know as much about the individual as possible before setting overall aims and planning treatment. Relatives, friends, employers and teachers, for example, are all sources of information.

Information should be requested regarding family circumstances: for example, names, ages, relationships, educational/work background, hobbies and interests, personality, likes and dislikes.

2. About the injury. It is also necessary to understand the individual's condition in detail in order to establish a baseline from which to plan

treatment. Medical notes, doctors, nurses and other professionals are important sources of information.

Information is needed regarding: date of injury; circumstances of injury, e.g. driver, pedestrian, industrial accident, assault; extent and location of damage, e.g. open or closed injury, temporal or frontal damage; any other injuries; any other relevant previous illness/disability.

Assessment

Assessment of the head-injured person may need to take place over several sessions as the individual's concentration span may be greatly reduced and he may tire easily. The environment in which he is assessed is also important. It should be quiet, well lit, comfortable and free from distractions.

Assessment should be through both observation of and interaction with the individual. Careful notes should be taken to record all responses, including duration, strength, quality and consistency of response.

As well as functional capabilities, areas to be assessed may include physical ability, cognitive function and behaviour. In the early stages of recovery it may not be realistic to attempt formal assessment; however, information about the person's abilities can be gleaned through careful observation. The therapist should observe his position and posture, motor control, eye and head movements, communication ability and response to commands.

For those people who are more alert or who are at a later stage of recovery it may be relevant to use more standardised assessment procedures such as the Rivermead Behavioural Memory Test (RBMT) (Wilson et al 1985) and the Chessington Occupational Therapy Neurological Assessment Battery (COTNAB) (Tyerman et al 1986). The RBMT is an assessment of functional memory in areas where the head-injured person is likely to encounter problems, e.g. remembering names, recognising faces, remembering an appointment. The COTNAB assesses four broad functional areas, i.e. visual perception, construc-

tional ability, sensorimotor ability and ability to follow instructions. Both these assessments are valuable tools in obtaining a baseline from which to plan and evaluate treatment.

Treatment planning and evaluation

The following points should be considered in treatment planning.

- Different types of injuries produce different patterns of disabilities and rates of recovery. Therefore, the knowledge of the type of injury will help determine treatment priorities.
- Treatment should be directed towards improving functional abilities and social skills.
- Targets for therapy should be established on the basis of short- and long-term goals. Short-term goals can be considered as priorities for treatment and usually comprise some aspect of disability or behaviour which, if not improved, will become a major obstacle preventing rehabilitation in other areas.
- Continuous evaluation and modification of treatment is essential.

Progression of treatment

Rehabilitation of the head-injured person is a continuous and prolonged process and can be divided into three phases. The first is the acute phase, which takes place in the hospital, generally in the intensive care unit or neurosurgical ward. The second is the post-acute inpatient rehabilitation phase which may take place in a specialised ward or inpatient rehabilitation centre where available. The third phase is the long-term follow-up care shared by outpatient facilities and the community.

As the person progresses through these phases, treatment goals will probably change in accordance with progress. Initially, long-term goals may be quite unforeseeable, as the early short-term goals, such as encouraging the individual to swallow or to participate minimally in an activity, are very basic. Later the long-term goals may be to enable him to be as independent as possible with a view to returning home, so that the short-term goals at this stage would be, for example, to aim for balance and coordination and for independence in relevant ADL. Later still, the long-term goals may be to return the person to some form of employment or other productive activity, in which case the short-term goals would be to develop relevant skills such as speed, manual dexterity or accuracy.

TREATMENT IN THE ACUTE PHASE

The occupational therapist has an important part to play even in the very early stages of recovery from head injury, when treatment would take place on the ward (Garner 1990).

Aims of treatment

- Increase the level of awareness by using controlled stimulation
- Promote orientation and reduce confusion
- Prevent deformity and promote good positioning and posture
- Facilitate family involvement in rehabilitation and offer support.

During the acute phase therapeutic intervention draws from the developmental and learning frames of reference. The head-injured person has essentially regressed, owing to the effects of the injury, to an earlier developmental stage and through adopting a sensorimotor approach combined with a cognitive approach to orientation, the therapist can begin to facilitate the recovery process.

Stimulation and activity promote recovery of the injured brain. Deliberate and therapeutic stimulation is the beginning of the process of restoring the integrative action of the nervous system. The individual should be encouraged to respond appropriately to direct stimulation and environmental influences. All five senses should be stimulated in order to promote recovery but the therapist must be careful not to over-stimulate or flood the system, which will lead to either withdrawal or agitation. Any interaction with the person must be accompanied by slow, clear and precise words of explanation, orientation and encouragement.

- Tactile stimulation can be used with contrasting stimuli — heat/cold, roughness/smoothness, hardness/softness, deep pressure/light touch — on various parts of the body to encourage tactile discrimination and appropriate responses.
- Auditory stimulation involving familiar sounds such as voices, music or animal calls can be used to stimulate him, allowing periods of rest.
- Visual stimulation involves having familiar objects such as photographs and personal belongings within the person's visual field. It is better to have isolated objects in strategic places where they can be utilised specifically rather than to have a collection of things together.
- The senses of taste and smell should not be forgotten. The familiar smells of perfumes, polish, foods and so on, can be used in stimulation. Before attempting gustatory stimulation using bitter, sweet, salty and sour sensations, it must be ensured that the individual has an effective swallow and gag reflex.

As suggested above, the occupational therapist should encourage orientation by giving clear and precise explanations as to what is happening. Orientation can be further encouraged by keeping familiar objects near the individual, having a clock and calendar in view, and by facilitating as normal a wake/rest routine as possible.

The occurrence of a head injury in one family member has a devastating effect on the others, who in the early stages will feel bewildered and helpless and will need much support, guidance and encouragement. The therapist would adopt the role of counsellor and educator and encourage the family and significant others to participate in rehabilitation. The individual often responds more positively to a relative, and as it is often the relatives who will be responsible for continued care and support in the community, they need education and the opportunity to share their fears and anxieties. It often helps them to share their feelings with others who have experienced similar circumstances, and the national head injuries association, Headway, may be of value to them.

TREATMENT IN THE POST-ACUTE PHASE

Once the individual has begun to recover consciousness and his condition has stabilised, the intensive and prolonged programme of rehabilitation begins. The post-acute phase is the most active rehabilitation phase, encompassing a wide range of treatment aims and approaches.

Aims of treatment

- Facilitate normal movement patterns and inhibit abnormal reflex activity
- Increase independence in ADL
- Facilitate adaptation to perceptual deficits
- Promote strategies for managing memory and overcoming learning difficulties
- Facilitate socially acceptable behaviour and social competence
- Ensure appropriate community resettlement.

These aims of treatment are obviously very broad and by no means exhaustive. The complexity of deficits following head injury necessitates individualised treatment planning and it is perhaps better to consider how the occupational therapist can assist with some of the most common problems.

The typical pattern of motor recovery following head injury is that, in the majority of cases, the person initially has reduced muscle tone which gradually returns to normal, although it often develops into patterns of spasticity (hypertonus). Motor deficits can affect any or all four limbs and trunk muscles. In promoting recovery the therapist's treatment is based on a developmental frame of reference and may utilise various treatment approaches, as outlined below.

Paralysis

When paralysis is present it is essential to maintain range of movement of the joints and to prevent contractures. It is also important to ensure that affected parts are not neglected: the individual should be encouraged to take responsibility for them. This can be facilitated by using bilateral activities and by ensuring that the affected

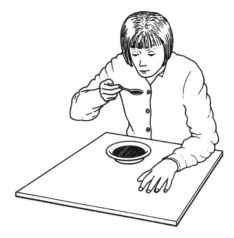

Fig. 15.3 The left (affected) arm is brought forward into a spasticity inhibiting position.

parts are always within the person's visual field; for example, the affected arm should be positioned on the table in front of him at meal times (Fig. 15.3). Further activities should encourage weight-bearing in order to stimulate the proprioceptors and should aim towards stability of the affected joints (PNF approach). For example, with the affected arm positioned on a chair or plinth at his side, the person can be encouraged to cross the midline with the unaffected hand in playing solitaire, using a guillotine or printing. The therapist may need to support the elbow in the weight-bearing position (Fig. 15.4).

Spasticity

Treatment of spasticity should aim at normalisation of muscle tone and the inhibition of spastic patterns (neurodevelopmental approach). Good positioning of the body is vital in inhibiting spasticity and forms a firm base from which normal movement can be facilitated. It must be remembered that normal movement cannot be superimposed on patterns of spasticity and, therefore, before any attempt to facilitate movement is made, the spastic pattern must be broken down, working proximally to distally, that is, from the centre of the spasticity outwards. Several factors will encourage spasticity and should therefore be avoided, such as increased effort or working against resistance, fear, anxiety and pain.

Loss of memory can be aggravated by hospital routine, as the person tends to be told what to do, and when and where to go, so that he need not think for himself. Even though the head-injured person's memory problem may persist, there are many ways in which the occupational therapist can help him increase his independence. In planning treatment, however, the therapist should bear in mind that there is no evidence to suggest that practice on memory games, such as Kim's game, generalises to improvement of memory in all aspects of function.

Management of memory deficits may include use of both internal and external aids. The use of internal aids might include forming a visual image associated with a name to be remembered (Fig. 15.7), learning rhymes or stories in order to remember and recall information, and devising first-letter mnemonics. External aids include diaries, notebooks, calendars and lists (Wilson & Moffatt 19884). In encouraging the individual to adopt memory management techniques the therapist again draws from learning theory as the individual learns to use those techniques which are successful for him in managing his problems.

Difficulties may arise in teaching the person to use memory aids in that he may not acknowledge that he has a deficit, may not wish to use memory aids, or may forget to use them. The therapist must be persistent, and encourage him to incorporate memory prompts into his daily routine — for example, looking at his diary of the day's events at a particular time of day, in a particular place.

Personality/behavioural changes

Both personality and behavioural changes are common after head injury. An individual's personality consists of a complex combination of the idiosyncratic characteristics which make up his distinctive character. Following head injury any such characteristics may change and such symptoms as lability of mood, inability to control emotions, apathy and euphoria are common. Likewise, behavioural traits such as aggression, sexual disinhibition and other attention-seeking behaviours are common. It is arguable whether such changes are a direct result of brain damage or secondary to it in the respect that they may be born out of frustration. Whatever the cause it is possible to control behaviour in the right circumstances by using behaviour modification techniques (Fussey & Muir-Giles 1988).

Based in the behavioural frame of reference, behavioural techniques can be utilised to extinguish unwanted behaviour or shape existing behaviour into a more socially acceptable pattern, and are based on the principle that if desired behaviour is rewarded then the use of that behaviour will be encouraged. They need to be very carefully structured and well coordinated for them to be successful. The following points should be borne in mind:

- A common response must be adopted by the whole team, including family and friends.
- The reasons for therapy must be clearly understood by all concerned, including the individual.
- Targets should be set as low as possible

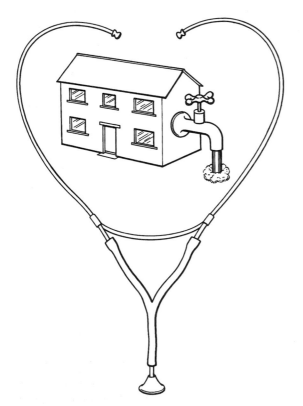

Fig. 15.7 A typical visual image which might be used to remember the name of Dr Waterhouse.

and raised gradually. If the individual does not achieve success initially he will become discouraged and perhaps cease to cooperate.

• Rewards for desired behaviour must be given as soon as possible after the behaviour has occurred.

Rewards should be appropriate for the particular person. Material rewards may be more acceptable in the early stages, but later they should be replaced by social rewards. A points system may be more suitable: i.e. points can be awarded for achieving the target or deducted for unacceptable behaviour; they can then be exchanged for rewards when a set target has been reached. Whatever form of reward is chosen, it must be easily controlled within the intervention setting. Every care must be taken by all members of the team that the programme is strictly adhered to and the individual is not manipulating events.

LATE STAGE TREATMENT

Unfortunately it is often the case that once the head-injured person is sufficiently mobile and orientated to return home, he is discharged from hospital with little support and follow-up. At this stage his problems are often only just beginning. Both the individual and his family feel abandoned, experiencing increasing social isolation. For the head-injured person, rehabilitation may well be required over many years if he is to maximise his potential for recovery and adjustment; in this late stage of treatment, the occupational therapist has an important part to play (Warnock et al 1992).

Aims of treatment

• Continue to address specific 'micro' deficits
• Maximise level of social re-integration
• Maximise independent living skills
• Facilitate strategies to assist with new learning
• Resettle into productive use of time and energy
• Offer continued family support

Again, these are broad aims and therapeutic intervention may be based on several frames of reference such as learning — using cognitive and/or behavioural approaches in social skills training, and developing independent living skills; and rehabilitative — enabling the individual with persisting physical difficulties to use compensatory techniques to overcome functional problems. Late stage rehabilitation should aim to equip the person with the skills needed to live in the least restrictive environment possible. This may involve work in a diversity of areas, ranging from meal planning, shopping and cooking to community orientation and the effective use of community resources. The occupational therapist can also help in retraining social skills and competences. Rehabilitation within the community entails the development of a programme with the individual by the different professionals involved, supplemented where necessary and possible by other carers. These other carers will include the family as important key workers who need to be trained and helped to cope with the stresses of long-term rehabilitation.

Community-based rehabilitation enables the team to capitalise on the available resources to be found in the area, such as training schemes, schools and leisure facilities. The community approach allows the individual to remain a part of the community while the last stages of rehabilitation are completed and thus there is less chance of the individual and his family becoming socially isolated.

At this stage post-injury the occupational therapist's holistic perspective, and the Model of Human Occupation in particular, is well suited to addressing the complexity of ongoing needs of the head-injured person and his family (Series 1992).

RESETTLEMENT

At some point the individual will reach a stage where no further dramatic improvement is likely. There are many possible alternatives to be considered when this stage is reached. The individual's physical, cognitive, emotional and social abilities need to be considered before he and his family are counselled on his future prospects (Jackson 1994).

her to choose and use the most relevant approaches and techniques for each individual while ensuring that there is consistency and coordination within the multidisciplinary team.

A number of models are currently used to underpin practice with people who have progressive disorders. The example used here to illustrate those principles is Kathlyn Reed's Adaptation through Occupation (Reed 1984) because of its emphasis on flexibility of approach and the significant effect of the environment on independence.

Reed subscribes to the theory that an human being is an open system, i.e. he affects and is affected by the environment. This leads to change, an ability to adapt and to learn new skills, which in turn leads to further learning. Reed subdivides the environment into the physical, the individual himself and the sociocultural environments. The model illustrates the interrelationship between each of these subdivisions and their influence on occupational skills, i.e. self-maintenance, leisure and productivity (Reed 1984).

Several frames of reference may be used depending on the person's initial needs and desires, and his changing priorities as the disease progresses. For instance a learning frame of reference may well be utilised with a cognitive approach so that the individual and his carers learn, through specific education if required, how to manage living with multiple sclerosis, e.g. time management in relation to daily routines, energy conservation and to help families invest in planning ahead. It may be appropriate to introduce a cognitive/behavioural approach if particular preventitive techniques are indicated, e.g. back care for the family or anxiety management. These guide the occupational therapist's intervention and interaction throughout her contact with the individual. The other key frame of reference would be compensatory, with its rehabilitative and adaptive approaches. The sequence in which these two approaches is used will vary according to individual needs. In the initial stages, functional techniques may need modifying, but as the condition progresses alternative support will be needed, e.g. daily living equipment, and changes to the personal, family and physical environ-

ment, e.g. role modification or home/workspace adaptation.

Woven through these approaches is that of problem-solving, adopted to identify strengths and needs and to select, modify and teach differing ways of management and living.

The overall object of intervention is to enable optimum function, self-satisfaction and accomplishment within a person's usual living environment. Incorporating a model, frames of reference, and particular approaches with their respective techniques, into the mutually agreed goals and subsequent programme will enable the therapist and the individual to understand the impact of multiple sclerosis on himself, his family and carers, his home and other relevant environments.

PATHOLOGY

MS is the most common progressive disease affecting the central nervous system. The disease affects the white matter in the brain and spinal cord leading to progressive weakness and disability. During the course of the condition demyelination occurs, which is the destruction of the myelin sheath (protective covering of the nerves) in patches both in the brain and spinal cord. These patches become sclerotic, can vary in size, and occur irregularly through the brain and spinal cord. They become shrunken in appearance resulting in the conductivity being seriously affected.

AETIOLOGY

The main causes of multiple sclerosis are now believed to be environmental (a virus) and genetic. Intensive research continues, including a three-year study involving 20 000 people with multiple sclerosis, to examine further the possible genetic cause.

COURSE

The disease is characterised by remissions and relapses. During a remission, temporary or prolonged improvement may take place. There is never a set pattern between one remission and another and there is no way of foreseeing when a relapse will occur. No two cases ever present the same pattern but some factors, such as trauma, surgery, influenza, pregnancy and stress, are known to precipitate a relapse, and a more progressive course has been associated with late age onset.

DIAGNOSIS

The disease is usually diagnosed in young adults between 20 and 40 years of age and is slightly more common in women than in men. Occasionally it may be diagnosed later in life but this is often in hindsight, on examination of a person's past medical history.

CLINICAL FEATURES

The clinical features from the onset will vary from one individual to another. There may only be an isolated symptom or a combination of several, for example nystagmus and paraesthesia. The initial episode may only last for a short period of time and be followed by a remission. However, as the condition progresses, the subsequent disturbances will become apparent, depending on the areas of the brain and central nervous system affected.

Visual

Involvement of the optic nerve may give rise to blurred vision, severe pain and tenderness of either one or both eyes. Diplopia (double vision) and nystagmus (oscillatory eye movement) or ptosis (drooping of the eyelid) may be present. In some severe onsets, blindness in one or both eyes has been known to occur on a temporary basis.

Motor and sensory

General weakness and 'clumsiness' in one or both lower limbs in the early stages are common, indicated, for example, by toes catching on ir-

regularities in the ground causing tripping. This may also be associated with a feeling of heaviness. Paraesthesia gives rise to numbness and tingling in the extremities. Ataxia (muscular incoordination) and hypotonus (diminished muscle tone) will be present if the cerebellum is affected; and with pyramidal involvement, spasticity can lead to flexor spasm, contracture and exaggerated reflexes.

Bladder and bowel

Frequency, urgency and incontinence of urine cause particular concern to the individual. Retention of urine and constipation may also occur.

Sexual problems

Partial or complete impotence may be experienced. Lack of sensation and vaginal lubrication will also cause distress, and fear of incontinence can reduce libido.

Psychological/emotional

Prior to diagnosis, there is often a long period of uncertainty regarding the problem — feelings of 'I must be going mad' or of being labelled neurotic or hysterical. When a definite diagnosis is finally given it is often greeted with relief. Feelings of anger — 'why me?', denial, sorrow and grief may also be experienced. The individual may have to go through all these emotions as part of coming to terms with multiple sclerosis. Emotional lability is common. Euphoria when it occurs is quite significant. Depression is often present as a reaction to the diagnosis and the prospect of increasing disability, and can in some cases become severe enough to require specific treatment. In addition, poor body image and feelings of uselessness can lead to fear of isolation and rejection by family and friends.

Communication impairment

Slurred speech is not uncommon and will occur if the bulbar area of the brain is affected. The speech may become slow and deliberate with emphasis on each syllable.

A common picture of multiple sclerosis is one of a variety of symptoms, such as an ataxic gait, intention tremor, incoordination and loss of dexterity. The person will become weak and quickly fatigued, taking a long time to recover.

TREATMENT

As the causes of multiple sclerosis are still being explored treatment is symptom alleviation and condition management focused as opposed to curative.

Acute episodes can be treated with intravenous methyl prednisolone or a high dose of oral therapy. This helps to shorten the episode but does not prevent relapses. The spasticity may be treated with baclofen (Lioresal) or dantrolene (Dantrium). Oxybutymin (Ditropan) is sometimes helpful with bladder problems, especially frequency.

Research continues in the field of treatment; for example in 1993 a new drug, Betaseron or Beta Interferon was formally licensed in the USA. This drug has been developed through genetic engineering and is based on human interferon-beta. Evidence has shown that it decreases the severity and frequency of relapse, but it is not a cure and it is not clear whether it helps people with chronic, progressive multiple sclerosis.

Physiotherapy is essential in helping the individual to maintain balance, normal patterns of movement and mobility skills. Occupational therapy is also essential for the maintenance of mobility, personal independence, social and leisure interests. District nurses, social workers and speech therapists play an important role in the overall management of the individual.

PROGNOSIS

People with multiple sclerosis may live for two to three decades with the disease, but eventually extreme weakness, ataxia and loss of movement render them totally wheelchair or bed bound.

The cause of death is usually as a result of intercurrent infection.

THE ROLE OF THE OCCUPATIONAL THERAPIST

This progressive disorder requires a flexible approach from the therapist, enabling her to utilise relevant frames of reference to guide her through her contribution at all stages. Following diagnosis the individual will need to be educated about the disease and may also need to relearn skills or learn new ones in order to manage his condition. The learning frame of reference offers a basis from which the therapist teaches, advises and informs the individual and his family, enabling them to find ways of overcoming difficulties and to encourage as normal a life-style as possible.

In the long term, maintenance of or improvement in functional ability may only be achieved by changing the environment (Reed & Sanderson 1992). The therapist would use the compensatory frame of reference within which to advise about daily living equipment and any adaptations to the external environment that may be needed to maintain an optimum level of independence.

In fact, the learning and compensatory frames of reference are used throughout the course of the disease, although the emphasis is initially on learning skills without the use of any assistive aids, but these may be introduced when further barriers to independence are met.

The role of the occupational therapist will therefore include those of teacher, advisor, information giver and problem-solver, but she will also need to build a good working relationship with the individual and his family to provide continuing assistance and support over potentially a long period of time.

Following an initial assessment the therapist should aim to solve any immediate problems, i.e. those of particular concern to the individual. Further contact will depend on the course of the condition but should be maintained on a regular basis.

It is essential that the therapist works closely with other members of the team at all times to ensure that an overall coordinated approach is both made and maintained. For instance, the community occupational therapist must work alongside the treatment team in the hospital where the person may be admitted periodically for a re-assessment of chemotherapy or intensive rehabilitation. She must also be aware of all the relevant resources available.

These resources may include:

- appropriate financial benefits such as Disability Living Allowance (both mobility and personal care components), Disability Working Allowance and Invalid Care Allowance
- help at work through the Disability Employment Advisor (DEA)
- appropriate support networks, for example home care, meals on wheels and voluntary organisations.

OVERALL AIMS OF INTERVENTION

In the context of current research and medical treatments, the general management of the condition and the intervention by the occupational therapist should aim to:

- assess and maintain the person's optimum level of personal independence in accordance with their priorities
- advise and support both the individual, family and/or carers
- maintain and restore where possible the person's optimum physical, mental and social capacity
- enable the person to maintain his dignity despite increasing disability
- advise and assist the person regarding employment or alternative productive use of time
- advise about caring for the home and family
- introduce other resources at appropriate times (see Fig. 17.1 Chart of resource needs).

THE INITIAL INTERVIEW

The initial interview between the therapist and the individual will be of extreme importance and it is imperative, therefore, that the occupational therapist plans the interview and gives the person sufficient time to discuss problems, fears and anxieties. The therapist must be a good listener as this will enable her to gain a clear picture of the immediate family set-up, home and work circumstances, if appropriate, and social networks and interests.

It is important that the therapist discovers the individual's attitude to his disability and what, if anything, he knows of the condition.

In the early stages, the person may not have been informed of the diagnosis, as the results of tests are awaited or because his doctor has decided not to tell him. If, however, he is aware of the diagnosis, he may still be going through the grieving process. The pace at which the therapist can begin to work through problems will depend upon the ability of the individual to discuss issues. It is important, however, that he and his family are helped towards adopting a realistic attitude to the future.

Recording a baseline for intervention following the initial assessment can be achieved by returning to Reed's model (p. 498) in which she suggests that each area of occupation, i.e. self-maintenance, productivity and leisure, can be analysed in terms of five performance areas or skills — motor, sensory, cognitive, intrapersonal and interpersonal (Fig. 17.2).

Interventions

Specific activity programmes may be appropriate for some people and occupational therapy should include graded activities to increase range of movement, strength, coordination and balance, and improve mobility and endurance. The individual will need to learn problem-solving skills to find ways of conserving energy and simplifying tasks. These strategies, which could include keeping a diary to help identify levels of fatigue following exertion, can then be applied to any environment and routines adapted accordingly.

Shaving can become difficult due to poor grip and incoordination. Wet shaving may be made easier with a loop-handle grip fixed to a razor. Electric and battery-operated razors are not always a suitable remedy as they are heavier to hold. A razor holder, or strapping in conjunction with the elbow being supported, may be helpful.

Hair care problems may be overcome with the use of a long-handled comb or brush. A change in hair style which is both easy to manage and falls into place could be suggested. A shower spray, either over a bath or attached to basin taps, will help with the management of hair washing.

Make-up application could become a problem due to the finer movements required to hold and control items such as lipsticks, mascara and eye shadow. Again, enlarged handles may help, but often a change, for example to an all-in-one liquid make-up base, may be a more effective way of overcoming such difficulties.

The therapist may also advise on suitable protection and ways of coping with hygiene during menstruation. The use of self-adhesive pads and a portable bidet may allow continuing independence and dignity.

Use of the toilet

Initially, the person may only experience difficulty in using the toilet when rising from the seat. Thus it is important that the height of the toilet is correct for the individual; if a change in technique is not possible, the correct toilet height and possible installation and positioning of grab rails may be sufficient to help the person overcome any difficulties. As the condition progresses, the use of a commode on wheels, for example the Mayfair (Fig. 17.3) which can be pushed over the toilet, may help to eliminate the need for some transfers. A reacher for toilet paper can extend the reach. Where grip and coordination are poor, single sheet toilet paper is a good alternative.

When the condition reaches a stage where transfers are becoming a more obvious problem, the therapist will need to consider:

* the general layout of the toilet and bathroom

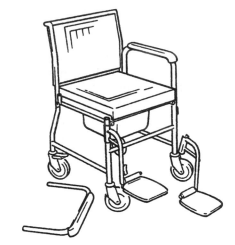

Fig. 17.3 The Mayfair commode.

and the space which will be needed for wheelchair use

* alternative means of transfer, i.e. with assistance
* the possible installation of an overhead hoist or use of a mobile hoist.

Bathing/showering

General weakness, lack of coordination and fatigue will make it increasingly difficult for the individual to get in and out of the bath. However, the use of a combination of bathboard, seat, non-slip mat and well-positioned grab rails may be all that is required. If he gets too tired, strip washing while sitting may be advisable. When taking a bath, it is important that the therapist advises the individual not to have the water too hot as heat will weaken and fatigue him and, therefore, exaggerate the difficulties of getting out. As balance and coordination deteriorate, more complex equipment may need to be considered, such as an in-bath lift, an exterior-to-bath lift e.g. Auto lift (Fig. 17.4) or a hoist.

Showering may well be an acceptable alternative and, if this is the case, a specially designed shower tray for a wheeled shower chair or a 'dished' floor finished with a slip-resistant surface would need to be considered. A thermostati-

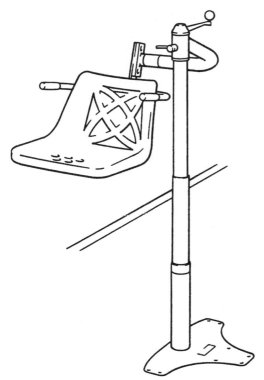

Fig. 17.4   The Auto Lift.

cally controlled shower unit will be imperative as loss of sensation could lead to scalding.

HOME MANAGEMENT

All aspects of general home management will need discussion, including household cleaning, food preparation, cooking and shopping, and general mobility around the home environment.

It is important that the normal role of the individual be maintained as far as possible as the psychological and emotional effects of role loss will have a detrimental effect on well-being and performance; for instance, if a housewife is unable to continue her usual routine in the preparation of family meals and depends on her husband, she will feel inadequate and that she is becoming a burden to her family. The general problems of fatigue will be in evidence with all daily routines so it is important that the therapist advises and encourages each person to plan

his days, allowing time for activity and rest alternately.

Food preparation/cooking

As far as possible all food preparation should be undertaken sitting down. This will help the individual to overcome problems of balance and fatigue. Various alternatives regarding the position of work surfaces, layouts of kitchens, aids to independence, e.g. a perching stool (Fig. 17.5), and labour-saving techniques will need to be considered in conjunction with all family members who use the kitchen and its facilities. Safety aspects in the kitchen must be highlighted at all times. The large number of available labour-saving items and kitchen aids makes it impossible to mention them all, but a few well-chosen pieces such as a stable vegetable slicer/peeler, electric

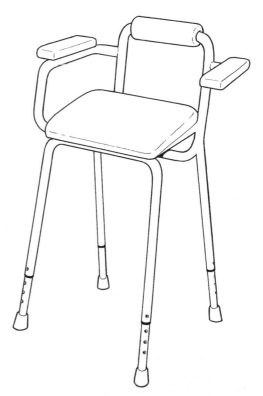

Fig. 17.5   An adjustable perching stool can be used for many tasks, e.g. ironing.

tin opener and a spread board may be sufficient. The therapist can advise on labour-saving and safe techniques, such as using a chip basket in a saucepan for boiling vegetables to make draining easier and eliminate the risks of burning from the boiling water.

The general layout of the kitchen must be considered to ensure safety for the individual. It may not always be possible to achieve an ideal layout as this will depend largely on the space available and finances. However, problems of mobility around the kitchen and moving articles from one area to another can be solved by sliding items over continuous surfaces or moving them on a trolley. Suitable and accessible cupboards and shelving and their proximity to working surfaces may need attention. If visual disturbances are present, ways of identifying the contents of storage jars and marking cooker controls, for instance, will need to be considered.

The individual's lack of coordination and loss of sensation may make cooking difficult. Saucepans which are light and have wooden handles may be an answer, and guards to cookers and adapted control knobs, such as those advised by both Gas and Electricity companies, may be appropriate.

Convenience meals may be an acceptable alternative for some people, combined with the use of a microwave oven. Other electrical appliances, such as food processors and drink dispensers, may not only be labour saving but also help the individual keep his independence for a longer period of time. However, an adequately balanced diet will be vital, and input from a dietitian should offer both general *and* specialist dietary advice.

Floor surfaces should be as far as possible slip resistant as spills will be dangerous. If or when the individual uses a wheelchair, the layout of the kitchen will need to take into account the height of work surfaces. It is usually prudent to have an area suitable for wheelchair use as well as one suitable for other members of the family.

Cleaning

As mentioned above, it is important for the therapist to help the individual decide how to tackle household tasks and plan the day or week in order to avoid fatigue. She may recommend that he continues with lighter tasks but that heavier tasks are managed by other family members or an agency.

Laundry

Most households these days have a washing machine; nevertheless it is advisable to split the weekly washing and ironing so that a little can be undertaken at a time rather than all at once. If a washing machine is not available, local alternatives need exploring. Some health and social service authorities provide a separate laundry service, primarily for people who are incontinent. Ironing should be carried out in a seated position and, as previously mentioned, when buying new clothes it is advisable to buy those which need minimum ironing. Likewise, sheets which are crease resistant are invaluable.

Shopping

General weekly shopping may gradually be taken over by other members of the family or carers, but it is important that this is not done too rapidly to the extent that the individual acquires a sense of uselessness. Supermarkets with wheelchair access make it feasible for the person with multiple sclerosis to continue to participate. Other retail outlets are becoming more conscious of the need to provide facilities for wheelchair users and the therapist should be aware of these to encourage the individual to continue with smaller and more personal shopping for as long as possible.

Transport

Transport will become more of a problem as the condition progresses. Various methods of transport may be appropriate, depending on the locality: for example, if the home is within easy reach of local shops, the person may be able to cope with an outdoor powered chair and be able to undertake some shopping. There are national schemes to facilitate easy transport, such as the car badge scheme, the mobility component of the Disability Living Allowance and Motability. Where local schemes such as Dial a Ride, Dial a Bus and parking concessions exist, the therapist should advise accordingly. The National Key Scheme for public toilets also needs a mention as any anxiety the individual may have about toileting when going out can be easily overcome with this facility.

GENERAL MOBILITY/MOBILITY AIDS

In the early stages, the use of simple walking aids may be required. While the individual is still ambulant, the normal heel–toe gait should be maintained and good posture encouraged. Walking should be encouraged for as long as possible but, whereas it may still be safe to walk in the home, the use of a wheelchair outdoors may be appropriate to avoid fatigue and the risk of falling on uneven surfaces.

The timing of the introduction of a wheelchair is crucial, not only in terms of safety but also from the psychological point of view. Very often people with multiple sclerosis see the introduction of a wheelchair as depressing. However, if the approach is both tactful and well timed, with the benefits of using a wheelchair stressed, it may be easier for the person to accept: for example, the use of a wheelchair will enable him to continue to carry out activities he enjoys such as outings, general shopping and holidays.

Other areas of general mobility which need to be assessed will include the heights and accessibility of bed, chair and toilet. The length of time the person will be able to maintain his independence may be increased with a technique change or the provision of bed-raisers, high chairs, appropriately positioned grab rails and raised toilet seats. Once a wheelchair is introduced, the heights must ideally be the same as the wheelchair seat to facilitate transfers. General instructions for safe, assisted transfers while the person is still weight-bearing will need to be given to his carers. As general weakness, lack of coordination and non weight-bearing occur, the need for mechanical assistance from a wheelchair to all areas may become necessary, but through all stages the

therapist should advise about supportive seating and posture which enhances cardiac and respiratory functions, discourages potential deformity and offers pressure relief and adequate skin care.

SOCIAL INTERACTION

It is important from the outset that the individual and his family are encouraged to maintain social contacts of all kinds for as long as possible. Problems of mobility and incoordination, speech impairments and difficulties with bladder control make it difficult for him to anticipate his ability to 'carry on as normal'. The therapist will need to give him help and guidance to overcome these problems and allay his fears in order to avoid isolation; for example, a toileting programme may be worked out to ensure a regular routine and the continence adviser will be able to give expert advice.

Leisure activities

Special interests and leisure activities will become increasingly important as the condition progresses. If the individual is unable to continue to work, he will have more time to fill. This will be particularly important for the person who may not be able to continue in the role of breadwinner. Activities which can involve the family unit as a whole, for example ornithology, outings focused on studying wild life and other outdoor interests will be the most rewarding as these will prevent the individual from feeling isolated or that he is becoming a burden. Pursuing new interests will not only depend on the individual's physical abilities and interests but also on local amenities and financial resources. For the person who has been a Do-It-Yourself enthusiast, such activities as light carpentry may still be enjoyed if a work area is made suitable for wheelchair use with correct work-bench height and fixed tools.

Gardening can still be encouraged with built-up borders or suitable greenhouse layouts. Some people may benefit from attending Further Education classes, for example in languages, accountancy, art, music and word processing. Involvement in local societies and clubs should always be encouraged, and very often they are keen to involve people with disabilities.

Day centres run by social services may provide a good outlet for some people where new skills can be learnt to maximise ability. The introduction to such centres should be approached with the same tact as the introduction of a wheelchair, as some people could respond badly to seeing people who are more disabled than themselves or they may not be interested in this facility.

A young mother who has multiple sclerosis may benefit from a baby sitting circle or child minding, not only for social contacts but also to allow her time during the day for rest periods.

The divorce and separation rates in families where one member has multiple sclerosis are high, and this needs to be borne in mind by the therapist at all times when advising on leisure pursuits to encourage interaction between the family unit.

Where couples coping with multiple sclerosis are experiencing difficulties with interpersonal relationships, it may be appropriate for the therapist to be involved in counselling to allow feelings, thoughts and issues to be explored. This may need to be undertaken with or alongside other organisations, for example, the Association to Aid Sexual and Personal Relationships of People with Disability (SPOD).

Communication

As social contacts become more difficult for the individual to maintain, he will become more dependent on other means of contact to keep him in touch with family and friends.

If he has a specific impairment, assessment and advice from a speech and language therapist is required, and the occupational therapist can reinforce her advice regarding communication in several ways, for example built-up pens and writing boards to help eliminate difficulties with grip and the use of an electric typewriter, computer or word processor to enable written communication *and* to facilitate work and leisure interests. The Aidis Trust and Sequal are possible resources for obtaining long-term loans of computers and word processors for disabled people.

Telephones designed with disability in mind are available from British Telecom and other telecommunication manufacturers; for example, there are telephones with large buttons which make it easier to dial if tremor is a particular difficulty. There are a multitude of alarm systems on the market and, again, financial help may be available through social services or local housing departments, or people can be advised on suitable models to purchase.

If the person does not have a telephone, financial help may be provided by social services for its installation, especially if he is left alone, living alone or could be at risk without a telephone.

As the condition progresses and the individual is unable to use a telephone, a 'hands off' telephone linked to an environmental control system may well be appropriate. These environmental controls are available through the NHS and need to be approved by the local assessor.

Work

If the individual can continue to work, it will be of great benefit to him, not only physically but also because he will maintain his normal role of wage/salary earner and breadwinner. This is especially important as it helps him keep his self-respect, dignity and one of the key adult roles.

It is often possible for large firms or organisations to transfer an employee internally to an alternative job. This is advantageous to the employer and the individual as he will be familiar with the type of work, surroundings and colleagues, and can also retain any pensionable rights. If a change of employment and employer is necessary, where the existing one is unsuitable, the individual may need the advice and guidance of the Disability Employment Advisor (DEA) and the Placing, Assessment and Counselling Team (PACT), both of which can be contacted via the local Job Centre.

Financial help to enable him to get to work, adaptations at the place of work, for example ramping, access to the toilet and adapted tools may all be needed and are available via the DEA.

GENERAL HOUSING NEEDS

From the early stages of multiple sclerosis, the occupational therapist must be aware of the problems which may arise from the layout of the home and its locality. Reed emphasises that a person is affected by and can change the environment, and while initially a change in approach or technique may be sufficient, this may need to be considered in conjunction with early advice and help with minor alterations which will enable the individual to remain mobile and independent at home for as long as possible. For instance, the installation and correct positioning of grab rails in the toilet and bathroom have already been mentioned, but the use of rails in hallways and extra bannister rails on the stairs will help to give him support in more open spaces. The positioning of furniture will become important. Stable furniture strategically placed will give support and may eliminate the need for walking aids early on, but at a later stage the furniture may need to be rearranged to allow maximum space for a walking frame and subsequently for wheelchair manoeuvrability. If the person lives in a house, a day's routine will need to be planned so that he does not have to climb stairs more than once a day in order to avoid fatigue. It may be necessary to consider the need for a ground floor toilet, if one is not already available.

Long-term planning for eventual wheelchair use will need to be broached at a time when the individual and family are psychologically attuned to accepting that he will need a wheelchair. It is imperative that the physical needs of the individual are taken into account, but not in isolation from the whole family. When considering major adaptations, the therapist will need to discuss what is the usual practice and routine of the household in order to maintain normality as far as possible. For instance, if the major problem is one of gaining access to a first floor bedroom, a single bedroom on the ground floor would immediately split partners which would not only be detrimental to their relationship but enforce feelings of isolation on them both. If they have young children, it would also lead to the person's exclusion from normal bed-time reading and seeing children 'tucked up'. The consideration of a through-floor lift which would give general access to the whole house might be more appropriate.

General access to the home and garden, as well as changes to internal fixtures such as the height of electric sockets, light switches, window openers and appropriate door handles, will all need to be considered.

The therapist will need to advise the family of all possible financial help available to assist with adaptations, whether it be a disabled facilities grant from the local authority, and/or local social services schemes or other national and local sources of assistance e.g. other housing funds or the voluntary sector.

If the person lives in a local council property, recommendations for adaptations under the Joint Circular from the Department of the Environment 10/90 'House Adaptations for People with Disabilities' will need to be made. If, however, the property is not totally suitable, it may be necessary to consider re-housing, bearing in mind that the proximity of friends, good neighbours, schools and work may be of equal if not greater importance.

SUPPORT NETWORKS

The therapist cannot provide all the services which may be required by a person suffering from multiple sclerosis, so it is vital that she is aware of supporting organisations and other professionals who can contribute to the family's overall management and support in order to introduce them at appropriate stages as the condition progresses. If some services are introduced at too early a stage, the outcome may be one of dependency rather than independence, and the individual may become overwhelmed, frustrated and morose concerning the future. Therefore, the therapist must be adept at introducing assistance and other agencies' and organisations' support at the pscyhologically 'right' time for the individual and his carers.

Statutory agencies and professional helpers other than occupational therapists need to be mentioned — these include the physiotherapist, social worker, district nurse, home carer and DEA — as does the importance of those networks supplied by the voluntary organisations.

1. Multiple Sclerosis Society

The Society was set up in 1953 for the sole purpose of:

a. promoting and encouraging research into the cause of the condition
b. providing welfare and support for both sufferers and families.

Local branches have been set up nationally to provide practical help within their own community, for example social functions, fund raising for research, respite care and holidays.

2. Carers Association

This association has local branches which give support to the carers, not only of people with multiple sclerosis but of all disabled persons.

3. The Association to Aid Sexual and Personal Relationships of People with Disability

This association provides advice, practical assistance and counselling.

CONCLUSION

The therapist will play a key role in the management of an individual with multiple sclerosis but must also be aware of the need for appropriate input from other professionals and voluntary organisations.

A model of practice has been suggested which encompasses an humanistic, problem-solving, client-centered approach compatible with the complex problems faced by the multiple sclerosis sufferer and his family. It is not intended to be the definitive guide to practice, more a tool which clarifies the ongoing assessment and evaluation necessary to cope with changing needs experienced over a long period of time. The therapist will need to take into account the requirements of the family in all aspects of daily living, be a good listener and planner, and above all be resourceful.

ACKNOWLEDGEMENT

Grateful acknowledgement is made to Mrs Jenny Goulter, friend and mentor, whose chapter this is.

USEFUL ADDRESSES

Multiple Sclerosis Society
25 Effie Road
Fulham
London SW6 1EE
Tel: 0171–736 6267

(Scotland)
27 Castle Street
Edinburgh EH2 3DN
Tel: 0131–225 3600

(N. Ireland)
34 Annadale Avenue
Belfast BT7 3JJ
Tel: 01232 644 914

Aidis Trust
18a Fallwood Avenue
Bear Cross
Bournemouth BH11 9NJ
Tel: 01202 571188

The Association to Aid Sexual and Personal Relationships of People with Disability
286 Camden Road
London N7 0BJ
Tel: 0171–607 8851

Carers National Association
29 Chilworth Mews
London W2 3RG
Tel: 0181–742 7776

SEQUAL (Special Equipment and Aids for Living)
Welfare and Administration Office,
Ddol Hir
Glyn Ceiriog
Llangollen
Clwyd LL20 7NP
Tel: 01691 718331

Environmental control systems can be accessed via the Director of Public Health in local health commissions. Addresses and telephone numbers will be found in the local telephone directory

REFERENCES

Reed K L 1984 Models of practice in occupational therapy. Williams & Wilkins, Baltimore
Reed K L, Sanderson S 1992 Concepts of occupational therapy. Williams & Wilkins, Baltimore

Sanderson S, Reed K L 1980 Concepts of occupational therapy. Williams & Wilkins, Baltimore

FURTHER READING

Bickerstaff E 1987 Neurology. Hodder and Stoughton, London
Bumphrey E 1987 Occupational therapy in the community. Woodhead–Faulkner, Cambridge
Department of the Environment 1988 Housing adaptations for people with physical disabilities. HMSO, London
Hagedorn R 1992 Occupational therapy: foundation for practice. Churchill Livingstone, Edinburgh

Matthews W B 1991 McAlpine's Multiple sclerosis. Churchill Livingstone, Edinburgh
Macleod J, Edwards C, Bouchier I 1988 Davidson's principles and practice of medicine. Churchill Livingstone, Edinburgh
Multiple Sclerosis Society 1990 Information pack for professional carers. H&M Printing Company, London
Pedretti L W 1990 Occupational therapy — practical skills for physical dysfunction. C V Mosby, New York

18

Muscular dystrophy

Jenny Wilsdon

INTRODUCTION

'Muscular dystrophy', a term first coined in the 1890s, refers to certain hereditary diseases which are characterised by progressive degeneration of muscle. It is classified within the group of neuromuscular diseases, that is, among those diseases which involve one or more parts of the 'motor unit'.

A basic motor unit consists of:

- the motor nerve cells (neurones) in the anterior horns of the spinal cord
- their nerve fibres (axons), which run from the spinal cord to the muscles
- the neuromuscular junctions, the points at which nerve impulses are chemically transmitted to muscle fibres
- muscle fibres, highly specialised contractile cells.

Disease or abnormality of function can occur at any of these levels. Myopathies, of which muscular dystrophies are the most significant, develop when failure occurs at the muscle fibres and the muscle fibres gradually die. Some regeneration takes place but cannot combat the amount or rate of destruction; eventually, the muscle fibres are replaced by fibrous tissue and fat.

Not all muscles are uniformly involved. Muscular dystrophies are classified according to their presenting pattern of affected muscles, as well as by their mode of inheritance (Box 18.1). Many of the muscular dystrophies are rare and unlikely to be seen by occupational therapists other than

---

Box 18.2 (cont'd)

For the intervention to be successful it is important that there is close and regular liaison between the occupational therapist, Michael, his family and his school. Many schools have a designated liaison teacher who coordinates and supervises the requirements of children with special educational needs. As Michael may come into contact with a number of teachers, classroom assistants and support staff, the liaison teacher provides a convenient link between the occupational therapist and the school. Her services can be particularly useful in supervising any alterations to the school environment. She is also on hand to be notified of any new developments and/or difficulties which may arise during day-to-day school activities. Her assistance in planning for Michael's future needs within the school environment will be invaluable.

---

sented by other theorists (Hurlock 1978, Mussen et al 1990, Bee 1992), but whichever model is selected it will offer the basis for assessment, goal-setting and evaluation. During the disease process the occupational therapist will probably view each developmental area individually, but she will need to refer constantly to the overall model so that no developmental area either forges ahead or is left behind. Development must be regarded as a whole, otherwise intervention becomes fragmented rather than holistic, and insular rather than integrated.

Towards the end of the course of the disease the Model of Human Development becomes less appropriate as the level of independent function decreases rapidly. At this stage the basic physiological needs and their satisfaction predominate. Maslow's hierarchy of motivational needs provides a comprehensive framework for assessment, goal-setting and evaluation (Box 18.3). The baseline identifies physiological needs — the need to breathe, eat, drink, sleep, eliminate waste, reproduce, keep an even temperature and be free from pain — which must be satisfied for survival and for progression to higher functional levels. It is possible that both models will be used concurrently if the basic physiological needs are satisfied; then there may be sufficient motivation to enable function at a more cerebral or intellectual level, particularly in the area of social–emotional development.

The occupational therapist will assess the person with DMD using her professional skills or tools: observation, handling, activity analysis, interview (of person, family, other professionals), play and, possibly, standardised checklists and assessment batteries. The resulting information will detail the person's abilities and problem areas. The priority of areas for intervention and objective setting will be negotiated with the person and his family.

Following the assessment, which will be both initial and ongoing, the occupational therapist will select an appropriate frame (or frames) of reference as the theoretical basis of her intervention, and approaches with which to put the theory into practice, The frame(s) of reference, approaches and techniques will depend upon the problem areas and the knowledge and experience of the occupational therapist. Those most often used with those who have DMD and with which the occupational therapist should have a working knowledge are:

- *Biomechanical*, which uses the laws of physical nature and the principles of mechanics as related to the human body: e.g. gravity, forces, levers, equilibrium, weight, density, stability, inertia and momentum with muscle work, joint angles, base of support, weight distribution and position in space. The approach focuses on the posture, position and handling of the person, using the person himself, the therapist and others, orthoses, equipment and the immediate environment.
- *Compensatory*, using the adaptive approach, whereby the lack of, or reduced, ability to perform an activity or skill is compensated for by adapting one or more of the following:

  — the person (e.g. positioning, orthosis)
  — the activity or skill itself (part or whole)
  — the method of technique used
  — the equipment used
  — the environment.

Box 18.3   Case study: David is 17 years old. DMD was diagnosed when he was aged six. He no longer attends school, spending all his time at home with his family.

Presenting picture

David looks crumpled, both in his posture and in his facial expression. He sits cross-legged (tailor sitting); his trunk is folded forwards, leaning more to his right side, with a twist which brings his right shoulder more forwards than his left; his lower ribs are resting on his pelvis. His face shows a tense, pained grimace. David sits quietly with his head down; it is difficult to get him to talk or answer questions; after a brief pause his mum usually answers for him. She reports that David is usually like this, showing little interest in what happens to him or is going on around him. He spends most of the day in front of the TV without really paying attention to the programmes. He is sitting in a standard adult indoor electric wheelchair with a joystick control attached to the right armrest; mum has added a few cushions for comfort.

Assessment

David's low level of function suggests the use of Maslow's hierarchy of motivational needs as the model for assessment, goal-setting and evaluation. His lack of motivation indicates that his basic physiological needs are not satisfied, so the base line of the model is used for assessment.

If these needs are satisfied it should be possible to incorporate the social–emotional developmental area at the adolescent stage within the Model of Human Development.

- *Respiration*. David has difficulty in breathing and is prone to chest infections. His current sitting posture further restricts his limited respiratory muscle power.
- *Food*. Although David has some movement in his hands he is unable to get his hands to his mouth, so he relies on others to feed him or give him drinks.
- *Elimination*. David finds his current toilet aid too hard and uncomfortable, so it is not used. Instead he is in nappies/incontinence pads, although he has control over both bladder and bowel.
- *Sleep*. David is unable to change his position in bed, which causes pain (see below), so relies on his mum to change his position. She comes in every two hours throughout the night.
- *Temperature*. As David's motor skills are severely limited he is unable to generate heat through movement and is susceptible to the cold. Areas of constant skin contact make him prone to sweat rashes and sores.
- *Cleanliness*. David would love a good soak in the bath but he finds it too hard and slippery. He has to make do with a strip wash.
- *Pain*. David is in constant pain, mostly caused by his posture and inability to move, which gives rise to areas of constant pressure and muscle cramps.

Overall aim

To improve David's quality of life by satisfying his basic physiological needs, restoring personal control over his life and enabling social–emotional function and development.

Aims

To facilitate personal control over activity by:

- modifying his body posture according to activity
- supporting these postures
- modifying or changing the equipment required during the activity
- adapting or changing the environment in which the activity occurs.

To facilitate age-appropriate social skills and leisure activities.

Theoretical basis of intervention

The above treatment aims lead to the selection of the biomechanical approach within the biomechanical frame of reference, in combination with the adaptive approach within the compensatory frame of reference.

Examples of intervention

The extent of David's spinal curvature precludes internal support, and rigid external bracing is too harsh in his present state. A lightweight cloth or canvas corset which is partially reinforced with a mouldable splinting material (e.g. Hexcelite, Neofract, Orthoplast) may prevent further collapse, reduce pain and offer trunk support while allowing unrestricted respiration, thus enabling function.

The use of an adjustable, customised seat (e.g. Matrix) to support the modified body posture, including the arms and legs, will allow even distribution and transference of body weight, thus avoiding points of pressure. The back of the seat can be extended to provide support for the neck and head if required.

Independent locomotion can be regained by attaching the moulded seat to the existing electric wheelchair, re-siting the control unit and modifying or changing the access switch. The home should be assessed for wheelchair accessibility and modifications made as appropriate.

Participation in family outings will be possible if an outdoor wheelchair (pushchair) is provided which will accommodate the moulded seat. The seat may also be used as a car seat if attachments are made to suitable anchorage points and the seat belt can be adjusted accordingly.

A pressure diffusing mattress is a priority so that both David and his mum can sleep through the night. An adjustable bed, preferably operated by an electric hand control, would enable changes in body position as required and provide a more upright sleeping position to facilitate respiration.

A length of foam rubber (e.g. as used under a sleeping bag when camping) attached to a suction bath mat (with rubber adhesive) to line the back and bottom or the bath gives padding and reduces slippage. A hoist should be considered if one is not already available.

A toilet aid which has a padded seat, back and armrests is required to enable David to use the toilet,

---

Box 18.3 (cont'd)

reducing the need for nappies and thus restoring his dignity. This may be a free-standing commode type, one which slides over the toilet pan or one which is attached to the toilet pan, depending on the availability and access of the toilet.

When David's posture has been modified and supported he will need a table which can be positioned close to his chest at axilla height. This will support his upper arms, enabling David to feed himself.

As David's senses are intact but his motor function is poor, modern microtechnology can be exploited to the full to allow him to control and manipulate his immediate environment. Examples are remote control switches for the TV, video and music systems, computers, an environmental control system and a free-standing telephone. The use of these devices will enable David's independence, social development, emotional expression and leisure pursuits.

● *Learning*, which focuses on the human ability to change: to develop within, or adapt to, the environment. The cognitive approach concentrates on the 'thinking' aspects of learning, which include planning, decision-making and choice. It uses techniques which promote the understanding of that which is learned, so that the new skills can be transferred to different situations, and/or as a foundation for more complex skills, and/or used as a stepping stone to allied skills.

PSYCHOLOGICAL AND EMOTIONAL WELL-BEING

After diagnosis the family will have to come to terms with the disease and its implications. The acceptance of the diagnosis will depend upon many factors, among which foreknowledge of the previous family history of the disease will be the most important. As DMD is inherited from the mother there will be disturbances in the family dynamics. Relationships between the parents, affected child, siblings and extended family will change, and the occupational therapist must be prepared to be involved with the whole family at various stages during the course of the disease.

The occupational therapist can provide support, advice and encouragement and offer opportunities to express emotions as they arise. She must, however, be aware of her own limitations and make referrals to other professionals as necessary.

Regional and local branches of the Muscular Dystrophy Group (see p. 532) can offer information, support and contact with families in similar circumstances. The occupational therapist should be able to provide her clients with appropriate contact names and addresses.

Early stages

The child

It is unlikely that the child will be aware of the course and eventual outcome of his disease at this stage, unless a relative is or was similarly affected. However, it is important that he is fully involved in all aspects of his treatment so that he feels in control of the situation. He will feel frustration at his inability to perform certain tasks and confusion as to the reasons why. He may be bewildered by changing family dynamics. Play therapy and creative therapies offer outlets for these emotions in a structured, protective environment. The occupational therapist can also reinforce information and treatment given by other professionals.

Parents

Parents will be emotionally shattered by the diagnosis of DMD and its implications, both for the child and the family as a whole. Before the diagnosis is accepted they will go through the bereavement process, mourning the loss of their 'normal', healthy son and of their hopes and aspirations for him and his future. Their relationships with him will change and they may become over-protective. However, they must be encouraged to allow the child to do as much as possible for as long as possible. Once the diagnosis is accepted the future must be anticipated and planned for. This is hard but necessary and the occupational therapist should be honest and factual in order to allow the parents to make well-informed decisions. However, while she should provide information, advice and support, plans and decisions must ultimately be made by the parents themselves.

The relationship between the parents will be strained, particularly if the husband blames his wife for 'giving' the disease to their son. The occupational therapist is often used as an impartial third party in discussions about their relationship; this is a difficult role, however, and may require a more experienced counsellor.

The parents may experience antagonism from the extended family. The paternal side may express anger and detachment: 'It did not come from *our* side of the family.' The maternal side may feel guilt at having passed on the abnormal gene, as well as apprehension that the disease may occur again within the family. All of these emotions will strain family relationships at the very time when support and closeness are needed. Although the prognosis is poor the parents should always be allowed hope and optimism.

Siblings

The early stages of DMD can be very frightening for brothers and sisters, who may not understand the changes that are becoming evident in their brother and in family relationships. They will want to know what is going on, what is wrong with their brother, whether they will catch the disease and what to tell their friends. The Muscular Dystrophy Group produce an excellent booklet for siblings which answers many such questions. Brothers and sisters can offer a great deal of support and should be encouraged to do so.

Middle stages

The young person

The transition from walking to using a wheel-chair for mobility will have a great impact on the young person with DMD. The occupational therapist must be positive in her support and encouragement, emphasising the increased independence and new opportunities which a wheelchair can afford. It is important that the person's self-esteem is kept high, possibly by changing objectives and concentrating on what he can do and not on what he can no longer achieve. The change to a wheelchair may also necessitate a change in school, which will bring additional emotional changes and demand the occupational therapist's further support and encouragement. It is important that the home environment is ready for this transition and is 'wheelchair-user friendly'.

During this stage the person will also undergo the transition from child to adolescent (and possibly to adult) and experience the normal physical and emotional changes which this entails. For anyone, this is a time of uncertainty and insecurity, but the person with DMD will also have to cope with the progress of his disease. The occupational therapist must be aware of his development and be ready to offer opportunities to express related anxieties.

Parents

The wheelchair that becomes necessary in the middle stages of DMD presents parents with a constant visual reminder of the eventual outcome of the disease. Again, the occupational therapist must be positive in her approach, emphasising the young person's independence in his wheelchair. She can help the person and his family to set objectives which take into account his change in mobility. There may be a tendency for the parents to look upon their son as a baby, the wheelchair reminding them of the pushchair stage of development. The occupational therapist can make the parents aware of such pitfalls and encourage them to see their son as an emerging adolescent or adult.

Although the young person will require an increasing amount of care and attention, his parents should be encouraged to allow him privacy, both alone and with his friends. It is important for the parents to help in maintaining their son's social circle so that he does not become isolated.

Later stages

By this stage the future will look bleak and it will be difficult for the person and his family to think positively. A reassessment of the overall situation will be required and the occupational therapist can help to set short-term objectives.

Often, two contradictory thoughts are present within the family: first, that time is running out and they have much to do, to talk and to think about; second, that the inevitable is dragging on and that it would be better for the end to come quickly. This creates emotional conflict and may present as anger, guilt, depression or detachment. The occupational therapist must be aware of these emotions and provide opportunities for their expression and discussion in order for the family to feel as comfortable and secure as possible when death occurs.

The person and the family will need support while they plan for the final few weeks. The majority of families wish to have the person with them until the end and therefore may require night- or day-time support care. Occasionally, family wishes or circumstances will dictate that the person is within hospital or similar care during these final stages. Whatever the situation, the person and his family will require a great deal of the occupational therapist's time and support.

Aftercare

The person's death does not signal the end of the family's need for help and advice. Support is often provided by a Family Care officer from the Muscular Dystrophy Group; if not, this role should be undertaken by the occupational therapist, who will have been involved with the family throughout the course of the illness and will be well acquainted with their outlook and needs.

Removal of the deceased person's belongings is an important part of coming to terms with his death. The timing of the return of equipment which has been on loan should be considered carefully. Returning equipment too soon or after too great an interval will cause the family unnecessary distress.

Many parents who have received support from the Muscular Dystrophy Group find great comfort in remaining active in the organisation and providing support for others.

HOME ENVIRONMENT

In general, houses are not designed to accommodate wheelchairs. Consequently, turning a home into a place in which a wheelchair user can be independent almost always involves major structural alterations and/or additions. The MD group currently offers a Housing Adaptation service which provides assessment by an occupational therapist, architectural plans, building supervision and assistance with grant applications.

It is important that the subject of major alterations to the home is broached well before the need for them is apparent. Alterations take time and money and thus require advanced planning. Although this may seem hard and can be distressing for the family, it is essential if the person is to remain independent. The parents will need to know the requirements of a wheelchair user well in advance so that decisions with regard to major alterations or moving house can be made in good time. It is advisable for long-term needs to be addressed in the early stages, as short-term, temporary measures can be costly.

Once a decision to build an extension has been made, approximately two years should be allowed to obtain architects' and builders' plans and planning permission, make financial arrangements, complete building, decorating and equipping, and finally move in.

A ground-floor conversion or extension are the ideal alternatives but alteration to first-floor accommodation with a through-floor lift may be the only practicable solution. Whatever alteration is made must be acceptable to the family after the person has died. An extra ground floor bathroom and toilet are always useful and the bed/sitting room may be used for another child or as an extra living room, playroom or study.

The adaptations to the home should provide a bed/living room which allows the person privacy. This is very important for an adolescent or young adult who needs his own place in which to be alone or to entertain his friends. There should also be an adjoining bathroom and toilet. Access around the ground floor of the home is also important in enabling the person to remain an integral part of the family. Easy access to and from the house is also vital. Early in the designing of an extension or alteration to ground-floor accommodation the suitability of the ceiling for bearing an overhead tracking hoist system should be considered. This type of system will greatly assist in the care of the person in the later stages.

The family may in fact prefer to move house before major alterations become necessary. The present home may be unsuitable for adaptation. The family may wish to be nearer to a particular school or hospital, or closer to relatives. The family may have been intending to move anyway. In any event, the occupational therapist should be available to advise on the suitability of a new house so that costly mistakes are not made.

Whether the family opts for alterations or for a change of home, the occupational therapist's primary aim will be to ensure that a safe environment (including safe access) is provided. Second, she will aim to ensure that the home environment is one in which the person can remain independent for as long as possible. Third, she will try to ensure that the environment offers carers maximum ease of management.

Early stages

The occupational therapist can advise the family on how to make the home easier for the person to move around in freely and safely. A spacious, clutter-free environment will reduce the possibility of falls, and of injury should falls occur. Non-slip floor coverings are more suitable than rugs and deep pile carpets, which may catch the person's feet. Furniture may be used for support as the person moves around, and so should be solid, stable and without castors.

The person should be encouraged to sit on chairs rather than the floor so that he is supported in a good position and can rise and sit down more easily. He may have difficulty in negotiating the stairs; hand rails should be fixed to both sides. Alternatively, the person may prefer to revert to sitting (bottom-shuffling), especially to come downstairs. Stairlifts are not advisable as they are expensive for such a short-term solution. A through-floor lift which accommodates a wheelchair may be suitable if the first floor is to be adapted.

Hand rails by the toilet and bath will provide additional support. Outside steps should be fitted with interim hand rails and replaced by ramps as soon as possible in readiness for wheelchair use.

Middle stages

Space should be sufficient to allow easy manoeuvrability of the wheelchair, with room for transfers to bed, toilet, bath and chair. Light switches and power points should be situated at a height which enables the person to use them with his arms supported by the wheelchair armrests. For safety, alarm cords may be fitted in the bathroom and bedroom, or baby monitors which can be plugged into the mains supply may be used to enable the person to call for assistance.

Work surfaces must be suitable for use from a wheelchair, standing frame or prone stander. Storage cupboards, shelving, wardrobes and drawers should all be accessible from the wheelchair. Room should be available for fitting orthoses and doing exercises. A small, thin, foldable mattress may be helpful.

The bathroom should provide a toilet, basin, bath, shelving and storage facilities. Taps should be of the lever type, as these require less effort to operate and are more easily reached. Further suggestions for equipment can be found on p. 526.

Good heating is essential, as limited mobility reduces the production of body heat and the person will feel the cold more quickly than others do.

Later stages

A ceiling-track hoist is most suitable at this stage as it will provide ease of transfer between bed, toilet, bath and wheelchair. If this is not possible

In the early stages, participation in selected sports such as swimming and horseback riding is beneficial in maintaining function and providing exercise. Organisations such as the Physically Handicapped and Able Bodied Clubs (PHAB) and therapeutic riding associations may offer local facilities.

The importance of holidays should not be overlooked; libraries and social services departments hold literature about places which cater for the wheelchair-dependent person. Some charitable organisations also offer holiday chalets which have been adapted to accommodate wheelchairs. Social services departments and libraries can also furnish information on access to public buildings, swimming pools and restaurants.

FINANCE

A chronically sick or disabled family member always places additional strain on the family budget. In the case of DMD, financial pressure will build quickly, allowing the family no time to plan or save. In the early stages expenses may relate to frequent visits to the regional treatment centre. During the middle and later stages adaptations to the home and special equipment will be costly. One parent may also need to give up work to care for the person, further restricting resources. Early contact with a social worker from the local hospital, regional centre or the Muscular Dystrophy Group will ensure that advice on allowances and grants is obtained in good time. Fund-raising groups and charities may be called upon to provide expensive equipment such as computers, environmental control systems, electric wheelchairs and special beds. The family will already be under great emotional strain, given the diagnosis and its implications; therefore, money worries should be alleviated as far as possible.

ORTHOSES AND SURGICAL INTERVENTION

The aims of orthotic and surgical treatment in DMD are:

- to maintain mobility

- to maintain a functional position for as long as possible
- to reduce the development of contractures and deformities to a minimum
- to support weakened areas.

Early stages

Weakness of the muscles around the pelvic area will cause a forward tilting of the pelvis with accompanying increase of the lumbar curve. This means that the body's centre and line of gravity will be pushed forwards. In order to counteract this displacement and maintain balance in standing and walking the child will flex at the knees and transfer weight through the ball of the foot. As walking on 'tip-toes' is in itself unstable, intervention is necessary to hold the foot plantigrade. Footwear which extends over the ankle joint is essential; Piedro-type boots or 'bumper'-type trainers, for example, are suitable. An ankle-foot orthosis (AFO) which extends from the base of the toes to above the bulk of the calf muscles can be used in conjunction with footwear. Night-time AFOs help to maintain the stretch on the Achilles tendon. In some cases it has been found that the restriction of the feet to the plantigrade position (heel down) actually inhibits mobility because balance is upset by the displacement of the line of gravity backwards and outside the body (see Fig. 18.2) (Thompson 1993). In these instances the child should be allowed to continue 'toe walking', but special emphasis should be placed upon the compliance with night splints and physiotherapy to maintain the resting length of the Achilles tendon. As the muscle weakness progresses the child will require knee-ankle-foot orthoses (KAFO) extending from the upper thigh to the foot, followed by hip-knee-ankle-foot orthoses (HKAFO) which combine the former orthoses with a pelvic band, or an ischial seating KAFO, in which body weight is transferred through the ischial tuberosities. Surgical lengthening of the Achilles tendons is often required at this stage. Finally, a full set bracing system attached to a thoraco-lumbar corset may be necessary if walking is to continue. The extent of the bracing used should be closely monitored and discussed with the person and his parents. The use of orthoses requires great motivation, patience and application; therefore, their provision should not be automatic. It is important to bear in mind that the above-mentioned orthoses are not suitable for all persons with DMD.

Middle stages

When walking becomes too difficult, too tiring or unsafe, even with extensive external support, a wheelchair will be necessary. At this time the trunk muscles are greatly affected; this, combined with limited mobility, produces spinal deformity. The lumbar lordosis becomes fixed with compensatory thoracic kyphosis, often with a scoliosis as the person slumps to one side. As spinal deformities may restrict lung capacity and limit lung function, spinal support will be necessary to reduce the amount of deformity and allow unrestricted breathing. As previously stated, the main cause of death in DMD is recurrent chest infections; therefore, the maintenance of correct spinal position is highly important. There are two main alternatives: external support using a corset, or internal fixation through surgery.

There are many types of surgical corset available but the most commonly used are the lightweight thermoplastic and Neofract types. All corsets are moulded individually to achieve as much correction as possible and are remoulded or replaced as necessary. Body bracing is introduced as soon as scoliosis is detected. The control of the scoliosis is variable; once the curve exceeds 40–50 degrees, body bracing is usually ineffective in preventing further deformity.

The second alternative is surgical intervention in the form of internal fixation of the vertebral column. The decision to pursue this course is made by the individual, his family and the consultant. It should be remembered that the younger child is more able to cope physically and mentally with major surgery than the older child, and that in earlier stages the curves can be more easily straightened.

The benefits of having a straight spine are not only physical (i.e. concerned with breathing and better sitting and lying posture) but psychological. With a straight spine the individual will be able to look the world 'straight in the eye' again, and his self-confidence will be enhanced by a 'normal' body image.

Later stages

During the final stages of DMD, orthoses and surgery are used to reduce pain and ease management of the person. Special inserts may be required for comfort in sitting and/or lying. These can be made from a variety of materials, for example Hexcelite, vacuum bean bags, Matrix and foam rubber.

OTHER TREATMENT

The physiotherapist plays an important role in the treatment and maintenance of the person with DMD. Contractures frequently occur at the ankles, knees and hips, partly because of increasing muscle weakness and muscle imbalance and partly because children with DMD tend to spend more time in the sitting position than other children of a similar age. The development of contractures is further exacerbated by the child walking on his toes in an effort to keep his balance. Physiotherapy is started before tightness and deformity occur, as a preventative measure.

Initially, a detailed assessment of muscle strength and joint range of movement (both passive and active) is undertaken to provide a precise baseline for treatment planning. The principal aims of the physiotherapist's intervention are:

- to minimise the development of contractures (through frequent passive stretching)
- to prolong muscle strength (through exercise and hydrotherapy)
- to prolong mobility and function (using various orthoses)
- to maintain adequate lung capacity and function (through breathing exercises).

These treatment aims are similar to those of the occupational therapist; therefore, close liaison between therapists is essential.

Another area in which the physiotherapist

and occupational therapist must work closely is in the provision of certain equipment. Postural drainage is often necessary in the later stages and the occupational therapist can advise and supply suitable equipment, ranging from foam wedges and tilt frames to a tilting facility on the person's bed. Prone lying boards and standing frames are often used to promote a straight posture and to stretch the spine, hips and knees. These items can be used in conjunction with various activities; for example, the person can use a prone lying board while watching television or reading, and a standing frame at a table or work surface of suitable height while writing, doing homework or using a computer.

As weight gain can be a problem, a dietitian is often involved with the person with DMD. The person will have enough difficulty in moving without the burden of excess weight. The dietitian will advise the person, his family and appropriate school staff with regard to diet. The occupational therapist can help by reinforcing this advice and encouraging the person if he experiences difficulty in following the diet.

CONCLUSION

Of the many neuromuscular diseases which manifest as muscular weakness, almost all are progressive in nature. Apart from the muscular dystrophies previously mentioned, these diseases include: polymyositis, dermatomyositis, myasthenia gravis, the spinal muscular atrophies, the glycogen storage diseases, myotonia congenita and the peripheral neuropathies.

Problems associated with the neuromuscular diseases which commence in childhood will be similar to those resulting from Duchenne muscular dystrophy, thus giving rise to similar treatment aims and strategies.

Those neuromuscular diseases which become apparent in adolescence or early adulthood may also give rise to some of the problems typical of DMD and thus to similar management aims. Specific treatment strategies, however, will more closely resemble those suggested for persons with motor neurone disease and multiple sclerosis (see Chs 16 and 17).

USEFUL ADDRESSES

Information, literature and advice are available from:

Muscular Dystrophy Group of Great Britain and Northern Ireland
7–11 Prescott Place
London SW4 6BS
Tel: 0171–720 8055

National Occupational Therapy Advisor
Muscular Dystrophy Research Labs
Newcastle General Hospital
Westgate Road

Newcastle upon Tyne NE4 6BE
Tel: (01661) 842605
or 0191–2738811 × 22461 (sec.)

Equipment for Disabled People
The Disability Trust
Mary Marlborough Lodge
Nuffield Orthopaedic Centre
Headington
Oxford OX3 7LD
Tel: (01865) 750103

REFERENCES

Bee H 1992 The developing child, 6th edn. HarperCollins, New York
DMD Factsheet 1993 Muscular Dystrophy Group, London
Dworetzky J P, Davis N J 1989 Human development — a lifespan approach. West Publishing Company, St Paul, MN
Emery A E H 1967 The use of serum creatine kinase for detecting carriers of Duchenne muscular dystrophy. In: Milhorat A T (ed) Exploratory concepts in muscular dystrophy and related disorders. Excerpta Medica, Amsterdam

Hoffman E P, Brown R H, Kunkel L M 1987 Dystrophin, the protein product of the Duchenne muscular dystrophy locus. Cell 51: 919–928
Hurlock E B 1978 Child development, 6th edn. McGraw-Hill, Tokyo
Inkley S R, Oldenburg F C, Vignos P J 1974 Pulmonary function in Duchenne muscular dystrophy related to stage of disease. American Journal of Medicine 56: 297–306
Khan Y 1993 Respiratory support. Paper presented at a

symposium on Advances in the practical management of childhood neuromuscular disease, Pinderfields Hospital, Wakefield, West Yorkshire

Martin A J, Stern L, Yeates J, Lepp D, Little J 1986 Respiratory muscle training in Duchenne muscular dystrophy. Developmental Medicine and Child Neurology 28: 314–318

Miller G, Tunnecliffe M, Douglas P 1985 IQ, prognosis and development in muscular dystrophy. Brain and Development 7: 7

Muntoni F, Mateddu A, Marrosu M G et al 1992 Variable dystrophin expression in different muscles of a Duchenne muscular dystrophy carrier. Clinical Genetics 42: 35–38

Muntoni F, Mateddu A, Cau M et al 1993 Diagnosis of DMD carrier status in a family with no known affected males.

Developmental Medicine and Child Neurology 35: 65–78

Mussen P H , Conger J J, Kagan J, Huston A C 1990 Child development and personality, 7th edn. HarperCollins, New York

Newsom-Davis J 1980 The respiratory system in muscular dystrophy. British Medical Bulletin 36: 135–138

Roberts R G, Cole C G, Hart K A, Bobrow M, Bentley D R 1989 Rapid carrier and prenatal diagnosis of Duchenne and Becker muscular dystrophy. Nucleic Acid Research 17: 811–816

Thompson N 1993 Orthotic and physiotherapy management of Duchenne muscular dystrophy. Paper presented at a symposium on Advances in the practical management of childhood neuromuscular disease, Pinderfields Hospital, Wakefield, West Yorkshire

FURTHER READING

Development

Bee H 1992 The developing child, 6th edn. HarperCollins, New York

Dworetzky J P, David N J 1989 Human development — a lifespan approach. West Publishing Company, St Paul, MN

Llorens L A 1991 Performance tasks and roles throughout the lifespan. In: Christiansen C, Baum C (eds) Occupational therapy overcoming human performance deficits. Slack, New Jersey, pp 44–66

Shortridge S D 1989 The developmental process: prenatal to adolescence. In: Pratt P N, Allen A S (eds) Occupational therapy for children, 2nd edn C V Mosby, St Louis, pp 48–64

Sugarman L 1986 Life-span development — concepts, theories and interventions. Routledge, London

Muscular dystrophy

Bethlem J, Knobbout C E 1987 Neuromuscular diseases. Oxford University Press, Oxford

Brooke M H 1986 A clinician's view of neuromuscular diseases, 2nd edn. Williams & Wilkins, Baltimore

Dubowitz V 1987 The colour atlas of muscle disorders in childhood. Times Mirror International, London

Emery A 1988 Duchenne muscular dystrophy, 2nd edn. Oxford University Press, Oxford

Emery A E H 1994 Muscular dystrophy, the facts. Oxford University Press, Oxford

Harris S R, Toda W L 1985 Genetic disorders in children. In: Umphred D A (ed.) Neurological rehabilitation, vol. 3. C V Mosby, St Louis, pp 184–206

Harper P S 1989 Myotonic dystrophy, 2nd edn. Baillière Tindall, London

Walton J (ed) 1988 Disorders of voluntary muscle, 5th edn. Churchill Livingstone, Edinburgh

Occupational therapy

Case-Smith J (ed.) 1993 Pediatric occupational therapy and early intervention. Andover, Butterworth-Heinemann, Stoneham, MA

Clancy H, Clark M 1990 Occupational therapy with children. Churchill Livingstone, Edinburgh

Eckersley P, Clegg M, Robinson P 1986 The 1981 Education Act — guidelines for physiotherapists and other paediatric professionals. Chartered Society of Physiotherapy, London

Kramer P, Hinojosa J (eds) 1993 Frames of reference for pediatric occupational therapy. Williams & Wilkins, Baltimore

Pratt P N, Allen A S 1989 Occupational therapy for children, 2nd edn. C V Mosby, St Louis

Ward D E 1984 Positioning the handicapped child for function. Phoenix Press, St Louis

Early death

Barnstoff P 1989 The dying child. In: Pratt P N, Allen A S (eds) Occupational therapy for children, 2nd edn. C V Mosby, St Louis, pp 580–589

Kubler-Ross E 1983 On children and death. Macmillan, New York

19

Parkinson's disease

Alison Beattie

INTRODUCTION

Parkinsonism is a chronic progressive disorder of the central nervous system characterised by hypokinesia or bradykinesia (poverty of movement), tremor and rigidity, often with postural instability. It is caused by dysfunction of the basal ganglia. Various disorders may produce this syndrome (Box 19.1) but the cause of the most common form of parkinsonism (widely known as paralysis agitans or Parkinson's disease) remains unknown. This is generally referred to as idiopathic parkinsonism. The disorder takes its name from Dr James Parkinson who described six cases in 'an essay on the shaking palsy' in 1817.

Box 19.1   Parkinsonism and Parkinson's disease

Parkinsonism

Idiopathic (Parkinson's disease)
Drug induced (e.g. phenothiazines)
MPTP toxicity
Post-encephalitic
Wilson's disease

Parkinsonism plus

Progressive supranuclear palsy (Steele Richardson syndrome)
Multiple system atrophies
— Olivopontocerebellar atrophy
— Striatonigral degeneration
— Progressive autonomic failure (Shy–Drager syndrome)

Parkinsonian 'features' occur in
● Alzheimer's disease
● Head trauma (e.g. boxers)
● Multiple cerebral infarcts

This chapter begins by describing the pathology and aetiology of Parkinson's disease, as well as its principal clinical features, diagnosis, and treatment. The important contribution that chemotherapy has made to alleviating the symptoms of parkinsonism is considered, as well as the much more limited application of surgical intervention. The contribution of the physiotherapist and speech therapist to rehabilitation is then outlined.

There is as yet no cure for the condition, so the occupational therapist's involvement with people with parkinsonism is likely to take place over a period of many years. This chapter describes the aims and approach of this ongoing intervention, first in general terms and then in the context of the 'initial' and 'later' stages of the disease. The various facets of the person's needs as they relate to each stage are described in detail; these include personal care, mobility, home-care and safety, communication, activity etc.

The needs of family members and carers, especially for respite provision, are given increased attention in the discussion of late-stage intervention, as difficulties in coping are likely to increase as the person's condition deteriorates. However, it is stressed throughout the chapter that Parkinson's disease has profound consequences not only for the person suffering from the condition but also for his family, and that the occupational therapist must plan her intervention with a sensitive awareness and understanding of the challenge that Parkinson's disease poses to all concerned.

PATHOPHYSIOLOGY

Idiopathic Parkinson's disease is associated with a disturbance of the neurotransmitter systems and accompanying cell degeneration in the dopaminergic pathways in the basal ganglia, primarily in the substantia nigra (Fig. 19.1). There is loss of pigmentation in the substantia nigra and to a lesser extent in other pigmented nuclei. This is associated with depletion of the neuromelanin-containing cells at these sites, and shrinkage of surviving neurones. By the time of presentation of disease, approximately 80% of dopaminergic neurones in the substantia nigra have degenerated, with a proportional decrease in striatal dopamine. This disturbance upsets the balance

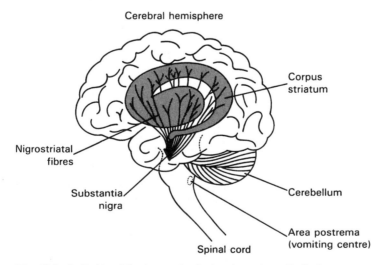

Fig. 19.1 Left side of the human brain showing schematically the substantia nigra and the corpus striatum (shaded area) lying deep within the cerebral hemisphere. For simplicity, only one side is shown. Nerve fibres extend upward from the substantia nigra and, dividing into many branches, carry dopamine to all regions of the corpus striatum. (Reproduced from Duvoisin 1978 Parkinson's Disease — a Guide for Patient and Family, with kind permission.)

between the cholinergic and dopaminergic transmission systems.

The neuropathological hallmark of Parkinson's disease is the Lewy body. This is a type of intraneuronal inclusion body which is characteristic of Parkinson's disease, although not specific since it can also be found in other disorders such as motor neurone disease and Alzheimer's disease. Lewy bodies are invariably found in the substantia nigra and other regions of the central nervous system, autonomic nervous system and gastrointestinal tract. Their relationship to the aetiology and pathophysiology of Parkinson's disease is unknown. Lewy bodies may be found in up to 10% of apparently asymptomatic individuals over the age of 50 at the time of death. These may represent the picture of pre-clinical Parkinson's disease.

The symptoms of parkinsonism reflect the dysfunction within the basal ganglia (Fig. 19.2), particularly in the system of nerve cells forming the substantia nigra which produce and store dopamine. The substantia nigra's nerve cells connect with the corpus striatum via long fibres along which dopamine travels. Within the corpus striatum the dopamine acts as a transmitter of chemical messages. When the substantia nigra nerve cells are unable to produce or store dopamine, the striatum suffers a deficiency which, if sufficiently severe, gives rise to parkinsonian symptoms.

EPIDEMIOLOGY

The exact prevalence of Parkinson's disease is difficult to determine since the diagnosis is entirely clinical. The prevalence of idiopathic Parkinson's in Europe and North America is approximately 1.5 per 1000, although in Asia prevalence is reported to be around 0.75 per 1000. Men may be affected slightly more often than women. There is a marked rise in prevalence with age which is consistent throughout the world. This may approach more than 1% of individuals aged 60 years or over. Some reports have suggested a plateau in prevalence after the eighth decade. This may be artefactual because of poor clinical diagnosis, or because the absolute number of cases in the very

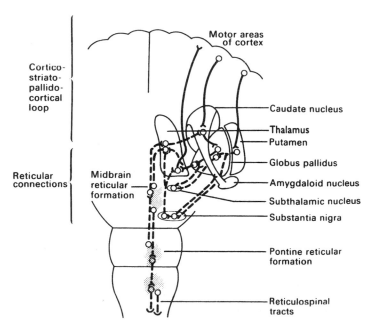

Fig. 19.2 Diagram of the principal connections of the basal ganglia (Reproduced by kind permission from Bannister 1986 Brain's Clinical Neurology. Oxford University Press, 1986, p 336).

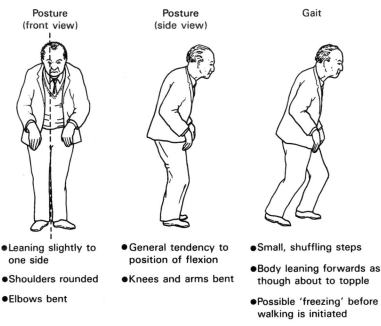

Posture (front view)	Posture (side view)	Gait
•Leaning slightly to one side	•General tendency to position of flexion	•Small, shuffling steps
•Shoulders rounded	•Knees and arms bent	•Body leaning forwards as though about to topple
•Elbows bent		•Possible 'freezing' before walking is initiated

Fig. 19.3 The characteristic stooped posture and hurrying gait of Parkinson's disease.

to a cog wheel. Cog-wheel rigidity is not simply parkinsonian rigidity superimposed on parkinsonian tremor, as it may be observed in the absence of resting tremor. Rigidity increases with anxiety and concentration. As the disease progresses such rigidity may lead to contractures and muscle atrophy.

The flexed attitude of individuals contributes to the festinant (hurrying) gait. When they are pushed from behind they demonstrate increasingly rapid steps. This was described by James Parkinson as 'an almost invincible propensity to run when wishing only to walk'.

Tremor

Tremor is the presenting complaint in approximately 70% of people with idiopathic parkinsonism. It is often intermittent and usually affects distal muscle groups such as those in the hand, forearm or foot. It is often initially one sided, spreading to the ipsilateral lower limb and then affecting the other side of the body.

The tremor is characteristically present at rest and has a rate of approximately 4–6 cycles per second. It is exacerbated by anxiety or fatigue and may be elicited by asking the individual to perform mental arithmetic. Voluntary movement of the limb may partly inhibit the tremor. Tremor of the fingers is often characteristically described as 'pill rolling'. The jaw or tongue may be affected but a tremor confined to the head is probably not parkinsonism. Postural tremor may also appear in Parkinson's disease.

The most common diagnostic error is to attribute essential tremor to Parkinson's disease. This tremor increases with age and in approximately half of all cases there is a family history. It may affect different parts of the body but most often the hands; it is usually bilateral, although asymmetrical in severity. It can be detected by asking the person to hold his arms outstretched. Movement of the head (titubation) or tremor of the voice may occur. This tremor is also worsened by anxiety but is alleviated with alcohol.

Hypokinesia

Hypokinesia or bradykinesia refers to a slowness and poverty of voluntary movement. This results in difficulty initiating and carrying out coordinated movements, e.g. fastening buttons, writing and turning. There is general poverty of automatic and associated movements. Hypokinesia accounts in part for a variety of parkinsonian symptoms and signs, such as a mask-like fixed facial expression with staring eyes and apparent diminution of emotional responses. A reduction in arm swinging while walking, micrographia (small writing; Fig. 19.4), reduced frequency of blinking and impaired ocular convergence of the eyes are other features which may occur.

The individual's general activity level may be reduced, with slow actions and difficulty maintaining independence. Repeated effort may lead to fatigue, aching muscles and, in some cases,

actual muscular pain. Difficulty in initiating movement will frequently cause a delay between a stimulus, such as a request to sit down, and the subsequent response. The mobility problems caused by bradykinesia include difficulties in rising from a bed or chair and in getting into or out of the bath. The individual's walking pattern may be grossly impaired, with an accelerated gait (festination) in association with short, shuffling steps and a tendency to lurch. He may give the appearance, with a flexed posture, of trying to catch up with his centre of gravity. He will stop slowly, will find it difficult to turn to the left or right and may 'freeze' when he meets a minor obstacle, for example a door threshold.

An interesting phenomenon in Parkinson's

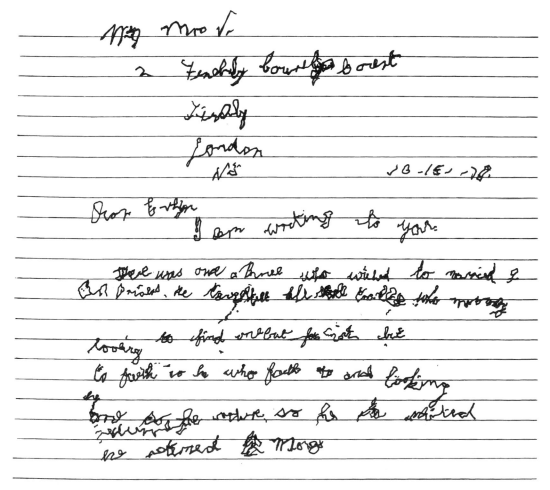

Fig. 19.4 Tremulous handwriting: letter written by a 63-year-old.

referral to speech and language therapy for appropriate assessment, it is not possible to determine the level of activity belied by the mask-like face. Even swallowing medication can be a problem. Pharmaceutical companies, aware of this, are exploring the use of medication in a syrup-like consistency.

● Enhancement of non-verbal communication. This may include: more emphasis on gesture and facial expression; communication boards (particularly in the later stages) adapted to suit individual needs; electronic typewriters with assisted keyboards; amplification aids, especially where volume loss is the only disorder; lightwriter (a speech replacement aid with a light touch keyboard and visual display). Speech therapists will utilise exercises for verbal communication along with non-verbal alternatives at all stages of the disease, dependent upon individual needs.

Dementia can occur in Parkinson's disease, and again the speech and language therapist can help. Strategies exist to facilitate orientation, communication and carer support.

GENERAL HEALTH

The basic rules for general health and fitness are the same for people with parkinsonism as they are for everyone, but they are additionally important for the former group if some of the effects of the disease are to be minimised. The individual should be advised and encouraged to include general health routines in his daily programme. These may include:

● maintaining a sensible, well-balanced diet which includes plenty of fluids and fibre
● eating at regular intervals throughout the day and, if his appetite is poor, taking smaller, more frequent meals
● maintaining the tone and bulk of his musculature, joint mobility, the efficient function of his cardiovascular and respiratory systems and a good posture. This will require regular exercise, preferably of a type he enjoys, which will encourage him to remain as physically active as possible
● continuing with activity which he finds

mentally stimulating, such as the daily crossword or a favourite quiz show
● negotiating medication times to suit his daily routine
● interspersing activity with rest to avoid becoming overtired
● attempting to avoid upper respiratory tract ailments as these will take him longer to recover from, slow him down, and make him extremely tired.

PSYCHOLOGICAL CONSIDERATIONS

By its nature, Parkinson's disease makes the individual vulnerable to depression, anxiety, embarrassment, confusion, loss of motivation, changes in attitude and fear. These feelings, if and when they occur, will also affect his family to a greater or lesser degree.

If he is treated in a positive manner — i.e. if the effects of the disease are explained to him, and if he is encouraged to participate actively in planning his treatment regime and permitted to voice his fears — then his attitude and general emotional state are more likely to remain objective and positive. It is important to identify the person's interests and his key sources of motivation while, simultaneously, identifying concerns or problems. In this way a balance can be established which will be realistic, and acceptable, for most people.

Anxiety should be expected and dealt with appropriately. Any anxiety or nervous tension may increase the individual's tremor temporarily and if this is permitted to continue the resulting 'tension equals tremor' pattern will be difficult to overcome. Many people find that relaxation techniques which can be used in a variety of environments can offset the need for further medication.

Depression is a common feature of Parkinson's disease. It should be discussed openly with the individual and his carers and means of counteracting it initiated. It is usually best coped with by maintaining and/or developing interests and activities around and outside the home, as companionship and stimulation often alleviate the depression.

Absent-mindedness and thought block are experienced by most people at some time or another and minor levels of both are found in people with parkinsonism. However, evidence of absent-mindedness or mild confusion does not necessarily mean that the individual's mental function is deteriorating, nor do these 'episodes' lead to serious memory disturbance. Some drugs may cause confusion in older people but, for the majority, making notes or accepting prompts will alleviate the problem.

Fear is usually overcome by encouraging and supporting the individual in his search for information and knowledge about the disease. This enables him to place his fears in perspective, and to make informed choices about course(s) of action which will motivate him, increase his self-esteem, and help him to remain active in his local community.

Embarrassment is another effect of the disease for some people. This, and other problems, must be dealt with on an individual basis in a sensitive and empathetic manner. Establishing the exact cause of the person's embarrassment and utilising a problem-solving, self-help approach with therapy support will often ease the effects.

Learning new skills and recalling what has been learned may be difficult for some. The therapist should use her skill and ingenuity to provide an optimum learning environment, methods which suit the individual, a pace which is realistic and associations which are meaningful. We all learn in different ways and at different speeds; therefore, some experimentation by the individual and the therapist may be needed to ascertain optimum learning conditions.

OCCUPATIONAL THERAPY

Despite advances in chemotherapy and research into fetal implants, the progressive nature of Parkinson's disease will probably require that a person and his family maintain contact with the occupational therapist over a period of many years. Clearly, it is impractical and unnecessary for the individual to receive continuous therapy throughout the course of the disease. Often, following a period of initial assessment, goal-setting and appropriate intervention, the individual should receive regular re-assessment, advice and/or short periods of intensive therapy at regular intervals. This pattern should enable him to continue to maximise his functional ability in relation to his life-style and interests and to learn, over a period of time, how to adjust himself to any limitations and to manage life with the disease.

It should be noted that the disease will produce a wide variation in the degree of disability. Some people may have minor symptoms for many years and never become severely impaired, while others may become severely disabled and require full nursing care. The treatment required will vary and the therapist must maintain a realistic outlook in relation to the condition's progression and its effect on the individual and organise the intervention programme accordingly. She must also remember that some types of parkinsonism respond more readily to medical intervention than others and that this will affect the outcome of rehabilitation. People with idiopathic parkinsonism, for example, respond relatively well to chemotherapy and are therefore more likely to benefit from rehabilitation. In contrast, those with other forms of parkinsonism may gain less benefit from drug therapy.

THEORETICAL FRAMEWORK

The occupational therapist and the person with Parkinson's disease jointly identify and analyse what the latter can manage, his functional problems and the possible resolution of these. The therapist and the individual will most frequently be working with the symptoms of the disease and the problems posed by these rather than applying specific neurological theories to treatment; their concern will be to find ways in which the person can live with, or in spite of, his progressive disorder. There are several frames of reference and approaches which can be effectively utilised.

Learning frame of reference

This is based on the person's ability to learn/

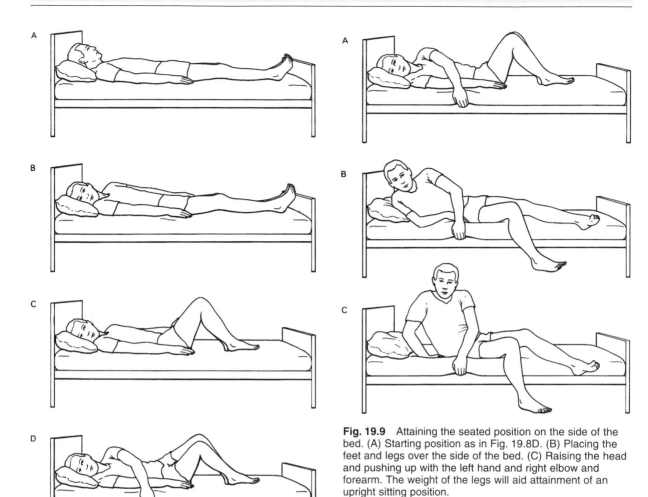

Fig. 19.8 Turning over in bed. (A) Starting position, supine in bed, arms by sides, legs uncrossed. (B) Turning the head towards the direction of the required total movement. (C) Raising the knees and placing the feet flat on the bed. (D) Moving the left arm over the body, towards the direction of the turn.

Fig. 19.9 Attaining the seated position on the side of the bed. (A) Starting position as in Fig. 19.8D. (B) Placing the feet and legs over the side of the bed. (C) Raising the head and pushing up with the left hand and right elbow and forearm. The weight of the legs will aid attainment of an upright sitting position.

lies down, bringing his legs up onto the mattress. In all transfers, the individual should be taught to move his head first as this will influence the position of his trunk and the rest of his body will follow.

Transport

If the person drives he must report his condition to the Driver and Vehicle Licensing Centre. He will have to undergo a medical assessment of his fitness to drive and will be given a licence for fixed periods. His condition will be reviewed regularly and assessment at a specialist driving centre may be advisable. It may be wiser for his carer to drive as the condition progresses.

Home-care and safety

Managing and caring for the home, in safety, requires a planned and flexible routine which will maximise the effects of the individual's chemotherapy and conserve his energy for those activities he *wants* to do as well as those he *has* to do to care for himself. He should be advised to remain active and independent at home, maintaining the routines to which he is accustomed when and wherever possible. He must learn to balance his activity so that self-care, home-care, leisure and/or work retain the right proportions.

The routines of shopping and cooking, cleaning and laundry, Do-It-Yourself and gardening, for example, will need planning in advance and tasks may be reallocated among family members. General advice will probably suffice at this stage and will relate to an individual's abilities and needs. Advice offered may include the following points:

- Ensure that hallways, stairs and work areas are well lit
- Eliminate dangerous floor coverings or provide visual reminders of potential hazards to mobility
- Maintain a warm home for comfort and general health
- Sit rather than stand to avoid overtiring
- Utilise labour-saving appliances for food preparation, laundry, cleaning
- If tremor hinders activity, particularly food preparation, stabilising food or food preparation tools with non-slip mats or clamps may help.

Communication

The Speech and Language Therapy section, above, offers a summary of specific interventions. The occupational therapist can augment formal speech therapy in several ways, and assist the individual to avoid the isolation which may be caused by communication and language deficits in the following areas:

- Verbal
  - Give the person time to express himself
  - Encourage him to utilise the breathing techniques advised by the speech and physiotherapists
  - Advise him to pace himself
- Written
  - The person's writing will have a tendency to decrease in size and to become shaky. Specific exercises (Fig. 19.10) may help some people

- Individuals may be assisted by a variety of means, e.g. rhythmical writing exercise patterns (Fig. 19.11), fibre-tip pens, wide-lined paper, clip-boards to stabilise and angle the paper
  - The use of a word processor or electric typewriter may overcome the problem of writing
- Telephone
  - If the person experiences difficulty at this stage, push-button dialling or the 'hands free' facility allowing on-line dialling, supplied by British Telecom, can help.

Remedial activity

Specific activities, using conductive education, biomechanical, cognitive, rehabilitative *and* adaptive approaches, may be used to encourage co-ordination, and types of movement and good posture with which the individual has difficulty, for example trunk rotation, limb swing and fine movements. The therapist should encourage the person to maintain his self-care and other routines, such as getting dressed, picking up his clothes to put away and washing and drying dishes, as these activities are conducive to the maintenance of trunk rotation, general upper and lower limb mobility, and coordination.

More specific activity to improve trunk rotation and limb swing can be introduced and undertaken at home with a board game such as solitaire. As illustrated in Figure 19.12, the person sits in a dining-type chair with the board at chest height. As he removes the solitaire pieces he passes them across his body into a receptacle on the opposite side, thus moving his left arm across to his right and vice versa, simultaneously rotating his trunk.

Activity which encourages strength and coordination should be encouraged to help the individual maintain his abilities. These should relate to his interests at home, for example Do-It-Yourself, gardening, and pet care.

For the individual who has difficulty with fine movements, the therapist can scale down large activities; for example, a large chess board used in an occupational therapy department might

— storing clothing close at hand

— when undressing, preparing items to be worn again the following day by turning them right side out

— encouraging the person to assist, while ensuring he does not become overtired.

Grooming

Helping the individual to maintain a satisfactory appearance requires more effort at this stage. Increasingly, relatives will need to assist with nail care, shaving/make-up and hair-brushing/styling. Advice, particularly concerning toe-nail care, may be sought. If relatives find it increasingly difficult to manage nail clippers because of the density of their relative's toe-nails (and if soaking his feet in warm water first does not help) they should be referred to the local chiropodist, who will be able to advise and assist further. Many health service chiropodists employ foot-care assistants who are able to provide care within the home.

Eating and drinking

The effects of rigidity, bradykinesia and tremor are described on p. 539. Chewing difficulties, dribbling and an increasingly slow pace often result in reduced food and liquid intake, which is detrimental to the individual's general health. Individual needs will dictate individual solutions, but the following modifications to position, routine, crockery, cutlery, technique and food consistency may be used as a guide.

● The person should be assisted to attain and maintain the optimum sitting position so that he can continue to feed himself. This includes maintaining the head and neck in the 'natural curve' position of the spine, thereby discouraging excessive flexion, which inhibits swallowing

● It may be helpful to reduce the distance between the person's hands and mouth by raising the plate or table

● Some people will find that using the elbows as pivots facilitates hand and forearm movement (Fig. 19.13)

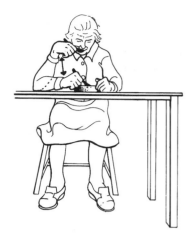

Fig. 19.13 Positioning to allow control of the upper limbs and to use one elbow as a pivot.

● The routine of three meals a day may have to be changed to five or six smaller, more regular, lighter meals, thus ensuring that the person maintains his intake. Small meals will remain hot and tire the person less

● For some people smaller, more frequent meals are not an acceptable solution as they disrupt family routine and social contact. Serving a meal on two plates, keeping one warm while the person eats the other, may be acceptable

● If he does not wish to use any of the above methods, the person may accept alternatives such as adapted cutlery or having to be fed

● Cutlery with enlarged and/or heavier grips may decrease tremor; deep spoons help to reduce spillage; sharp knives require less pressure and effort than dull ones

● Some people may find that weighted bracelets help to control movement and tremor

● Plate warmers keep food hot while it is being eaten

● Lipped plates and bowls, plate guards and non-slip mats help to optimise poverty of movement

● Two-handled and insulated mugs (which *must* be age appropriate) help to overcome the problems experienced with small, one-handled cups and mugs and help to keep drinks hot or cold

- Alternatively, providing drinking straws or half-filling a cup or mug may help
- If food spillage or dribbling poses a problem, a large table napkin or apron will protect clothing
- As swallowing difficulty increases, further advice from the speech therapist should be sought, particularly as lateral tongue movement becomes impaired
- Advice about chewing, which may be difficult due to impaired lateral tongue movement, may also be obtained from the speech therapist, and the dietitian will advise on maintaining essential nutrients and a balanced diet while the individual has to resort to softer foods which need less or no chewing
- Some people may, unknowingly, aspirate liquid during eating and drinking and this can lead to chest infection. The speech therapist will advise on methods of preventing aspiration while the physiotherapist will be able to assess lung function and help the individual to cough in order to rid his lungs of any liquid. The occupational therapist may also help if this occurs during treatment.

Washing, bathing and showering, care of teeth

Independence in these activities should be maintained for as long as possible, thus encouraging movement, coordination, dignity and a sense of well-being.

- Washing and other activities at the hand basin may need to be completed from a seated position, with required items close at hand
- Drug therapy can cause a dry mouth and mouthwashes between as well as after meals can be refreshing, although they do not replace standard dental care
- Bathing will become increasingly difficult and risky for the individual and his carers. While a bath board, seat, non-slip mat and rails may help for a time, safety should outweigh all other considerations
- A shower into which a shower chair can be

wheeled is a very satisfactory solution for many people, providing the bathroom is warm and the individual puts on a warmed towelling robe or is wrapped in a warm bath towel afterwards
- The person should be encouraged to wash independently, as far as this is possible, with a carer within calling distance for safety reasons
- In the very late stages of the disease bed baths will replace showering; assistance from a bath attendant/community nursing service is usually feasible
- Hair-washing and styling will become quite difficult, and carers or a mobile hairdresser will need to help with these tasks.

Toileting

- Constipation will be exacerbated by immobility and may cause some incontinence. Advice should be sought from the local continence service and a programme of regular toileting may help, as slowness and immobility may lead to 'urgency' and accidents.
- Most people with parkinsonism remain continent; however, in the case of the few who do not, the cause should be investigated. If the cause is environmental — linked to poor mobility or to non-medical factors — the occupational therapist can offer practical advice and assistance, such as a routine for day and/or night toileting, commodes, portable urinals and clothing modification.

Mobility

As his disease progresses the person will become less mobile and less inclined to move about his environment; this will result in his withdrawal from many activities. His environment should therefore be utilised as a stimulus to initiate and maintain mobility for as long as possible. Some people's walking is helped by vinyl or carpet patterns, or by the layout of paving in the garden or the pavement. Therapists should reinforce the relevance of maintaining existing movement and mobility to whatever degree possible in order to control any increase in rigidity.

Daily routines should be planned so that activities involving mobility are undertaken when drugs are having their maximum effect. If necessary, adaptations may need to be considered, for example a stairlift or downstairs toilet facilities.

As the later stage advances the person may eventually be confined to a wheelchair and/or to bed. His carers will need much more advice and support as his abilities decrease and the therapist will change the emphasis of her input from the individual to the carers who are managing his daily needs. Psychologically, it is vital that the family are helped to maintain their chosen routines or advised how to modify them in a way which is acceptable to them all. Advice on respite care will be invaluable.

- *Walking*. Safety is of paramount importance and the occupational therapist should work with the physiotherapist and the family to maintain the required degree of walking, standing and balance needed for transfers in particular.

- *Wheelchairs*. The person with Parkinson's disease should require a wheelchair permanently only in the very late stages of the condition, even

---

Box 19.3 Case study

Mr Y is 40. He lives with his wife. Son is away from home. He has a short Parkinson's disease history. His first admission to hospital was 18 months ago, on which occasion he was assessed and treated by the occupational therapist. The emphasis of this programme was daily living function.

On his second hospital admission he presents as totally dependent on his wife. He exists from tablet to tablet, during which time he has approximately 10 minutes when he has some function and can help his wife to assist him.

He cannot stand, walk or sit still. His gross, uncontrollable movement patterns make it exceedingly difficult for his wife to manage, for example while feeding him.

Occupational therapy

The immediate concerns are for Mrs Y. A regime of respite care has been initiated. A lightweight wheelchair with head rest has been provided for Mr Y.

Observation of Mr Y's chemotherapy regime in order to optimise the few minutes' function he acquires.

Psychological support for Mrs Y: opportunity to discuss Mr Y's care and care of herself, including her back.

---

if one has been utilised for outdoor mobility for some time. Carers should be taught how to use and care for the wheelchair and how to transfer the person from chair to car seat, from bed to chair, and so on. The environment should be modified where necessary, particularly for ease of access to and from the house.

Transfers

Carers will need to be taught back care and the techniques required for their particular circumstances. When and where the individual can still assist he should be encouraged to do so, for example by turning his head, moving his arms, and issuing instructions.

- *Chair transfers*. While the individual can still stand from sitting he should be encouraged to do so. His carer may need to offer minimal assistance, for example by applying gentle palmar pressure on the back of his head and he may find that high back and seat chairs are easier to get in and out of.

- *Bed transfers*. Increasingly the bed height will need to assist carers as well as the individual.

When turning over and getting out of bed a focal point on each side, such as a luminous clock-face or a bedside lamp, can help the person to concentrate. If relatives need to help him they should be taught to facilitate his movements with palmar pressure on the head/neck and pelvis as shown in Figure 19.14.

A grab rail attached to the wall beside the bed can be a useful aid to turning while others may find an adjustable rail on the side of the bed more helpful (Fig. 19.15).

It will become increasingly difficult for the person to raise his legs onto the bed and in order to relieve carers of constant lifting a leg lifter may be installed (Fig. 19.16).

Once he is confined to bed an electrically operated turning bed will provide a valuable adjunct to the person's care.

- *Hoists*. The need for a hoist will depend upon whether or not the individual remains at home with his relatives in the very late stages of his disease. The idea of using a hoist must be intro-

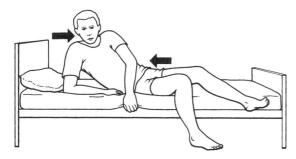

Fig. 19.14 Palmar pressure on the head/neck and pelvis will facilitate sitting up on the side of the bed.

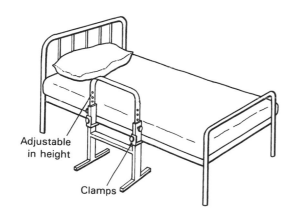

Adjustable
in height

Clamps

Fig. 19.15 An adjustable bed rail may assist turning in bed.

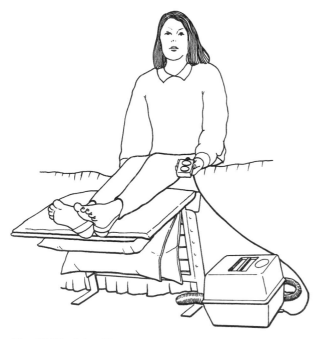

Fig. 19.16 A leg lifter.

duced tactfully. Its use must be carefully taught, as hoists require a high degree of skill to operate. Both the individual and his carers must *want* to use the hoist; this will motivate them to learn how to utilise it effectively, as its success within their home will depend on their acceptance of the equipment and the advice and support they are offered while learning how to use it.

Home-care and safety

It will become increasingly difficult for the individual to maintain all his home-care and maintenance functions but he can be involved in the decision-making within his family by being consulted about redecoration, weekly menus, and so on.

As his mobility decreases the likelihood of falls will increase; therefore, safety will assume even greater importance, and advice should be offered about lighting, floor coverings, grab rails and additional stair rails in parts of the house where he may be at risk.

In addition to the home-care suggestions made under Initial stage, above, the individual might be advised to:

- slide rather than lift kitchen appliances
- fill the kettle from a small jug
- use a trolley *if* appropriate. This particular advice needs to be considered in terms of (a) the individual's posture, i.e. will the trolley push him into an upright position or will it encourage spinal flexion because he pushes too far ahead and therefore overbalances? and (b) the environment, for example, floor surfaces, space to manoeuvre and storage.

As the person's condition deteriorates an alarm call system may become a vital lifeline. Information concerning alarm systems is included under Communication, below.

As the person's needs for care increase, his family may benefit from assistance provided by community services such as home care and meals-on-wheels. These should be introduced only if the family wish to receive them and should be seen as supporting their caring role rather than taking it over.

can only be maintained by use of flexor pollicis longus. This is known as Froment's sign.

The loss is mainly motor. Damage may occur at any level but is most common at the wrist or elbow. The intrinsic muscles of the hand, when working normally, put the fingers into a position of flexion at the MCP joints and extension at the IP joints.

When these muscles are paralysed by an ulnar nerve lesion, the fingers take up the opposite position (clawing) due to the unopposed pull of the long flexor. Sensation is absent over the little, part of the ring and possibly the middle fingers. This is very inhibiting in activities requiring stability of the ulnar border of the hand such as writing.

Lumbar and sacral plexi

The lumbar and sacral plexi are less vulnerable to injury than the brachial plexus. The femoral, sciatic and common peroneal nerves may be damaged by trauma, and the obturator nerve may be compressed by any rise in pressure in the pelvis due to enlargement of the pelvic organs. Injury to the back may compress the roots of the lumbar nerves, particularly L4 and L5.

Femoral nerve

The femoral nerve is often damaged as a result of penetrating injuries to the anterior thigh, for example with a butcher's knife. This can result in sensory impairment to the upper part of the leg which is supplied by the cutaneous branches, and can also produce a paralysis of the quadriceps, impairing standing and walking. Stairs are a particular problem, as there is difficulty in extending the knee against resistance.

Sciatic nerve

The sciatic nerve may be damaged as a result of fractures of the pelvis and femur, dislocation of the hip or gunshot wounds of buttock and thigh. The most common injury of the sciatic nerve is compression of one or more of its roots by a lumbar intervertebral disc protrusion, causing pain down the length of the leg to the foot and foot drop. Complete interruption of the sciatic nerve results in total anaesthesia and paralysis of all the muscles below the knee.

Common peroneal nerve

This is frequently traumatised by casts or tight-fitting boots as it rounds the fibular neck just deep to the skin. This results in foot drop — due to the loss of the motor nerve supply to the muscles producing dorsiflexion and eversion of the ankle — and the cutaneous supply producing anaesthesia over the dorsum. Skin care and vigilance concerning correctly fitting footwear and splints are of paramount importance due to the vasomotor and trophic changes that occur as a consequence of sympathetic and sensory loss.

ROLE OF THE OCCUPATIONAL THERAPIST

The aim of the occupational therapist is to maximise motor, sensory and sympathetic function and to help the person to compensate for any residual defects, in order that he may retain his vocational role, continue his leisure pursuits and maintain his independence in self-care.

The occupational therapist will use skills of assessment and evaluation of the injury, and will consider the psychological, social and economic factors that will affect recovery.

Liaison between the occupational therapist, physiotherapist, psychologist, social worker and rehabilitation officer is important, in order that a suitable programme of rehabilitation can be planned.

THE TREATMENT PROCESS

Treatment should be planned in three stages — the initial stage, recovery and late or chronic stage — and short-term goals will depend on the current phase of recovery.

Initial stage

The initial stage is characterised by absence of

motor, sensory and sympathetic function, and emphasis will be on the prevention of problems secondary to denervation. This stage covers the period immediately after injury and surgery until reinnervation has begun and illustrates the use of the learning, biomechanical and compensatory frames of reference and their respective approaches and techniques.

Sympathetic function

The therapist should note any signs of decreased sympathetic function such as dryness, temperature or colour changes, early soft tissue atrophy and nail changes. The person should be instructed in skin care and advised to watch out for inflammation or tissue damage. He should also be told how to cope with cold intolerance, by wearing thermal gloves and socks, until adequate sympathetic recovery occurs, an example of environment modification (adaptive approach).

Motor function

The passive range of movement should be assessed and maintained in the absence of muscle power. Active ranges need to be recorded and there should be consistent measuring by the same therapist. Treatment aims to prevent the following problems that can result from muscle imbalance:

- Overstretching of paralysed muscles by unopposed contracture of antagonistic muscles
- Shortening and eventual contracture of soft tissues
- Decreased function of intact muscle due to loss of the synergistic function of paralysed muscles.

Orthoses play an important part in the early management of nerve injuries. An orthosis can be designed to substitute for a paralysed muscle, to improve function and to help prevent overstretching and contractures by restoring the muscle balance (Lamb 1986). Figure 20.18 on page 585 shows an *orthosis* to aid *wrist extension* in radial nerve palsy.

Most people with a single nerve lesion are able to perform self-care activities independently.

Multiple, high or bilateral lesions may need provision of adaptive equipment. A functional assessment may be required and suitable advice and equipment given if the person proves to have functional difficulties.

Sensory function

Sensory loss results in a lack of protective sensation so that the person has to compensate visually. There should be an awareness of the dangers of heat, cold and sharp objects. Contact with cooker rings, heaters or lighted cigarettes often results in deep burns on the tips of fingers or the ulnar side of the hand. Insulated mugs, adequately padded oven gloves and long-handled pans should be used as a preventative measure.

Pressure and friction can cause tissue damage when tools or leisure equipment are used, and examination of the skin should be made for signs of inflammation, oedema, blisters or tissue breakdown.

Education is most important and the therapist guides her intervention with the learning frame of reference and the cognitive/behavioural approach, offering each person reasons for the various treatments he is experiencing: that muscle wasting increases in the early stages after nerve repair; that the average rate of nerve regeneration is approximately 1 mm per day; what function can ultimately be expected; that paresthesia and hyperesthesia may occur as a normal pattern of nerve regeneration diminishing with time and use of the limb.

Recovery stage

The recovery stage is characterised by progressive reinnervation — the emphasis being on the restoration of functions within the limits of regeneration — for example from the start of reinnervation to its maximisation (Lamb 1986).

Clinical evaluation of the extent of motor, sensory and sympathetic return is necessary at this stage.

The preventative measures used in the initial stage should be continued as long as reinnervation is incomplete. The protective measures utilised will enable the therapist to commence the programme to restore function.

Sympathetic function

There will still be decreased tissue nutrition and slow healing. Until sweating has returned, lanolin or similar oily products should be massaged into the skin to counteract the dryness and cracking of skin which ensues.

A simple method to test the presence or absence of sweating is to rub a plastic pen or biro over the area. If sweating is not present, the pen will slip. Comparison with the same area on the other side will demonstrate the difference, as normal skin will offer resistance to the surface of the pen.

During the recovery stage people may be resuming their former activities. Any blisters, lacerations or wounds occurring as a result of a return to normal occupations using tools and equipment should be treated with care to prevent infection and further injury. The person should continue monitoring the areas.

Motor function

The therapist should be aware of the pattern of recovery of the nerve and recognise trick movements and supplementary action by normal muscles.

Using a combination of biomechanical and rehabilitative approaches, retraining activities to increase strength, coordination and endurance can begin, but until good balance of the muscles is restored, substitution orthoses provided in the early stage will need to be worn when the person is not exercising in order to rest and support the recovering muscles.

Sensory function

Without adequate sensation the person will be unable to use his hand efficiently. Sensory stimuli are initiated as a result of excitation of sensory nerve endings of which there are two kinds:

- *exteroceptive* — occurring in skin, ears, eyes and other internal organs
- *proprioceptive* — occurring in joint capsules, muscle spindles and tendons.

Without sensory feedback from all receptors, a highly skilled and smooth performance of movement cannot be attained. At this stage treatment aims to facilitate proprioception. The therapist will utilise the developmental frame of reference, with its sensorimotor approach, to ensure appropriate biofeedback during interventions.

The stage of sensory nerve regeneration can be assessed by using the *Tinel test* (p. 578) to indicate the progression of regenerating sensory axons. The therapist may thus learn the correct time to start testing for sensory function.

The pattern of return of sensation as regeneration progresses is: protective sensation (deep pressure and pin-prick) followed by moving touch, static touch and discriminative touch.

Touch. Tactile testing is used in order that the therapist may discover whether the skin is anaesthetic, hyperanaesthetic, hypoanaesthetic or normal. This can be performed by using the light touch of the tester's finger or by using a cotton-wool ball. The person being tested is asked to identify whether the touch feels like pins and needles, is normal, or is different in any other way.

Protective sensation can be tested by using a pin-prick, or subjecting the area being assessed to the stimulus of a tube of hot water and a tube of cold water. The person indicates whether the tests are felt and whether or not the sensation is normal compared to the other limb.

After it has been shown that light touch and protective sensation are present, discriminative sensation can be tested by:

- static two-point discrimination
- moving two-point discrimination.

Two-point discrimination is the ability to recognise whether the skin is being touched by one or two points simultaneously. It is developed to a fine degree in the skin at the fingertips.

Further information will help the therapist to decide whether there is a need for sensory re-education and when it should start. This can be obtained by performing the following tests:

- localisation
- timed pick-up tests.

Localisation is the ability to recognise the exact position of a stimulus on the skin.

During the sensory recovery period the affected skin may undergo a period of hypersensitivity. This can be very distressing and may in turn hinder recovery.

Desensitisation is a programme of graded stimulation to an area to increase its tolerance for tactile input. Stimulation includes rubbing or brushing the skin with an assortment of textures which are just past the level of comfort when applied to that area. It can also include tapping or vibration. The tactile input should be followed by active use of the involved area.

Sensory re-education. The concept of improving sensory function by assessment and re-education was pioneered by Maureen Salter and Dr Wynn Parry (Wynn Parry & Salter 1976) at the Joint Services Medical Rehabilitation Unit at RAF Chessington. As a result of their work it was realised what gross disability can arise from sensory impairment. Many people who have full motor recovery claim that they are unable to work because they have impaired sensation.

The aim of re-education (Fig. 20.13) is to enable people to make the best use of their recovery by establishing a new bank of codes with which to interpret the altered sensory signals.

Chronic stage

Eventually there is a levelling off of the recovery of motor, sensory and sympathetic function and most people will have returned to their normal life-styles by this time. Those with high or multiple lesions with only a small amount of recovery will need help from the therapist, using the compensatory frame of reference with a predominantly rehabilitative approach.

The aim will be to maximise the power of normal muscles, especially those substituting for paralysed ones, and maximise the strength of muscles with return of power. For people whose proprioception is still impaired and unlikely to improve the therapist will adopt an adaptive approach to treatment, assisting the individual to modify his behaviour and environment, to help him compensate by utilising other sensorimotor functions.

It may be necessary for the surgeon to carry out tendon transfer surgery; therefore the skin and soft tissue will need to be kept soft and the maximum passive range of movement maintained. Deformities should be corrected by orthoses. Examples include thumb web spacers for tight webs (Fig. 20.14); Capener orthoses for proximal interphalangeal joint (PIP) contractures (Fig. 20.15); wrist dorsiflexion orthoses for drop wrists (see Fig. 20.18); and ankle dorsiflexion orthoses for foot drop (Fig. 20.16).

During active use of the hand, work orthoses may be needed and a work programme devised to suit the individual. Assessment may indicate the need for modification of the home or work environment; therefore liaison with community services and the person's employer is important, particularly if retraining is required.

The goal of occupational therapy must be to

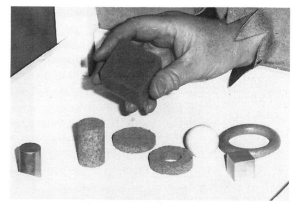

Fig. 20.13 Sensory re-education.

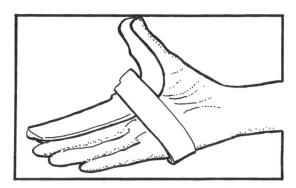

Fig. 20.14 Thumb web spacer.

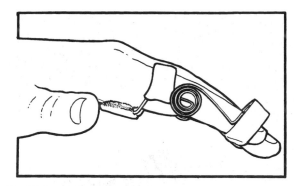

Fig. 20.15 A Capener orthosis.

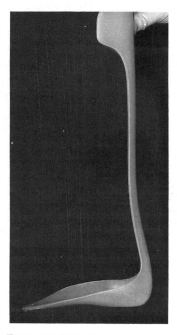

Fig. 20.16 Temporary foot raise.

restore the person to vocational, personal and leisure activities to a level which will satisfy his needs.

SPECIFIC TREATMENT FOR UPPER EXTREMITY NERVE LESIONS

Occupational therapy intervention for upper extremity nerve lesions should encompass the following:

• Provision of orthoses and adaptations appropriate to the person's needs at various stages of treatment
• Therapeutic media, for example games, computers with appropriate switches, woodwork and printing, aimed at muscle retraining and strengthening
• Education.

Brachial plexus

If the brachial plexus is ruptured, surgery will be required first, whereas an avulsion or lesion in continuity will only need rehabilitation.

Recovery, if expected, can take up to two to three years after the lesion occurs. It is important that the person is encouraged to return to his home and work environment as soon as possible. The therapist should see him at regular intervals to assess his progress, orthosis and functional levels at home and work.

Positioning the upper limb in an orthosis supports the shoulder and reduces the risk of subluxation. A wrist extension orthosis or support will stabilise the wrist and hold it in a good position. A flail arm orthosis may be provided for those whose expected recovery will be over a long period or who have total lesions (Fig. 20.17). The severe burning pain characteristic of the brachial plexus lesion can be controlled to some extent by transcutaneous nerve stimulation and anticonvulsant drugs, but distraction is also a very effective method of relief.

People should be encouraged to return to their hobbies and work and, if necessary, retrain for alternative employment. Orthosis-supported activities aimed at maintaining a range of movement throughout the upper limb and preventing subluxation of the shoulder may include:

• large draughts
• stool seating
• collating
• cooking
• computer keyboard work.

Radial nerve

The person will be unable to simultaneously ex-

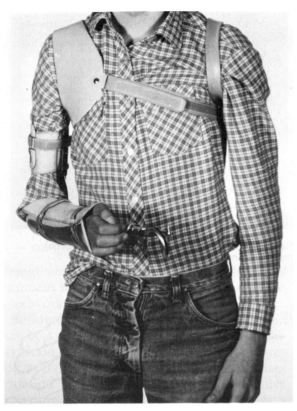

Fig. 20.17 A flail arm orthosis.

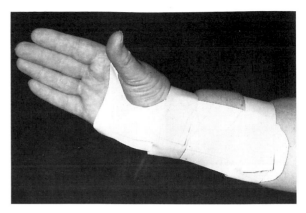

Fig. 20.18 An hand-wrist extension orthosis.

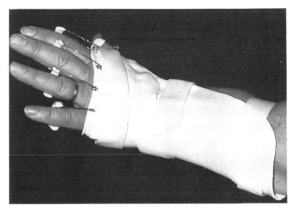

Fig. 20.19 A dynamic radial nerve orthosis.

tend the wrist and fingers and to radially abduct the extended thumb.

An orthosis is required:

- To assist grasp and enhance grasp strength by providing a stable wrist in extension
- To prevent overstretch of the wrist extensors by unopposed wrist flexion. A simple orthosis positioning the wrist in extension should be worn during all working hours (Fig. 20.18)
- To correct a wrist deformity in flexion, serial 'splinting' or a dynamic wrist extension orthosis should be worn.

A dynamic orthosis will substitute metacarpophalangeal joint extension by elastic or spring traction (Fig. 20.19).

Activities that require muscles to work in groups and therefore facilitate the development of coordination as well as strength should be selected. Those that require a stable wrist during grip, with simultaneous wrist and finger extension, are useful for radial nerve retraining and include:

- pottery — rolling out coils for coil pots
- pastry — rolling it out
- woodwork — sanding and polishing for wrist extension
- printing — an extension board on the printing press for wrist extension (Fig. 20.20)
- games — shoveboard for elbow and wrist extension, wall draughts for elbow and wrist extension
- computer — keyboard games with MULE (Microprocess Upper Limb Exerciser) and other switches should be introduced (see Fig. 20.24).

For later stages, games such as Jacks (five stones)

Box 20.1 Case study: Mr R. M., aged 35

Occupation

Cab driver (married), right handed.

Diagnosis

Laceration left wrist: (November '89)
50% division median nerve
99% division ulnar nerve
10% division flexor digitorum sublimis index finger
10% division flexor digitorum sublimis middle finger
30% division flexor digitorum sublimus ring finger
100% division flexor carpi ulnaris
100% division pollicis longus
100% division ulnar artery.

All repaired on day of injury in theatre of Plastic Surgery Unit.

- Kleinert traction to all four fingers with POP backslab.
- Pulleys fitted to produce good line of pull.
- Kleinert traction retained for 6 weeks.
- Referred to physiotherapy from day one for active extension of fingers, elastic traction producing protected flexion, with protective orthosis, monitored by OT department.
- After 6 weeks — active mobilisation under supervision.
- After 7 weeks — flexion of MCPs, but IP flexion minimal. Signs of post-traumatic sympathetic dystrophy — needing intensive exercise programme 9 weeks after operation. Improved R of M of fingers with minimal clawing of ring and little fingers.

- Complaining of sensory impairment on ulnar side of hand.
- Hypersensitivity in palm. Some poor quality sensation at tips of little and ring fingers.
- Median side of hand — feeling normal apart from palm.
- Tinel sign up to distal palmar crease on ulnar side.

Twelve weeks after operation
- Remains with no opposition of left thumb.
- Seen by Consultant who concluded that Mr R. M. would require an opponens tendon transfer to bring thumb round into opposition, although muscle power was thought to be improving in thenar eminence. EMG results after testing (L) hand median nerve produced no movement from the thenar eminence with stimulation of the median nerve, but a very small signal was recorded.
- An Electrical Sensory Threshold test produced a mixed picture of sensation.

To occupational therapy for assessment, workshop activities and orthoses as required.

Assessment

Problems (L) hand (see Table 20.1)
1. Difficulty in opposing thumb to ring and little fingers
2. Non-functional pinch grip
3. Difficulty abducting and adducting fingers
4. Reduced grasp and grip strength
5. Reduced sensation to palm, ring and little finger

Table 20.1 Activity plan using horticulture

Activity	Tool/positioning	Grading	For problem	Precaution
1. Mixing soil compounds, potting compost, sand, perlite, small gravel, pebbles, marbles	Seated at table Eyes closed/open for identification of compounds/materials	Smoother (e.g. sand) to harder (e.g. pebbles) textures Sieving increases stimulation	(5) (8) (3) (6)	Skin care * Allergy Hygiene
2. Sowing seeds	* Seated at table — Using pinch grips — Using palmar crease	Large → small sizes Using tweezers then fingers Using pinch grip easy → difficult fingers	(2) (7) (1) (5)	
3. Taking cuttings	* Seated at table Using secateurs/scissors Cutting down onto board with knife	Thin → thicker plant material Therapist assisted → independent, large → small handles on knife	(7) (4) (5) (8)	Care with sharp tools Supervision at all times
4. Watering can/mister	* Seated or standing	Amount of water Length of time Easy → difficult MCPs	(4) (1) (3) (5) (6)	Correct positioning of thumb
5. Pricking out	* Seated	Large → small leaved plants Opposing index → ring finger	(2) (3)	Avoid lateral pinch grip
6. Potting-up plants	* Seated	Large → small pots Increase	(3) (4) (5) (6) (7) (2)	As for soil compounds

NB: Concentration on thumb opposition and finger abduction/adduction where possible.
* Using dynamic opponens orthosis.

Box 20.1 (cont'd)

6. Hypersensitivity of palm
7. Difficulty flexing MCPs of ring and little finger
8. Difficulty extending PIP of ring and little finger.

Functional difficulties

Work:
Driving — handbrake, gearstick, radio controls, handling money — all necessary to job as cab driver.

Leisure:
Golf — producing a good grip.

Goal

To have increased functional ability and sensation in hand, which would enable Mr R. M. to return to work, manage activities of daily living and pursue leisure interests.

Aims

- Maintain/improve range of movement
- Maintain/improve muscle strength
- Increase grip strength
- Prevent deformity by using a dynamic opponens orthosis by day and a night-resting thumb post orthosis for opposition
- Increase ability to oppose thumb
- Increase sensibility, especially to ring and little finger
- Improve range of extension of PIP of ring and little finger
- Decrease hypersensitivity of palm
- Increase understanding of condition and precautions needed
- Increase motivation for recovery.

Treatment selected

Orthoses to deformities, and horticulture to improve dexterity and sensation (Table 20.1).
1. Capener orthosis to ring finger fully extended PIP joint within one week
2. Opponens splint worn for activities over 4 weeks.
  After one week of activities — hypersensitivity of palm diminishing, but still little sensation on ulnar border of the hand.
  After two weeks, sensation returning (tingling to ring and little finger).
  Opposition of thumb still absent, so placed on waiting list for opponens plasty.

Ten months after injury

- Excellent progress
- Almost normal sensation in median territory
- Recovering ulnar nerve sensation, with slight weakness of intrinsic muscles
- All FDS and FDP function 100% recovery
- FCU function 100%
- Now good opposition pinch, therefore does not require opponens plasty operation
- He is now working again as self-employed cab driver.

The treatment plan for this man demonstrates the benefit of purposeful activity in improving hand function and sensory return after tendon and nerve injury.

The activity plan using horticulture was devised by a since graduated London School of Occupational Therapy student, Susan Lynch.

and woodwork using tools to develop strength and stability of grip. Wall and table board draughts, printing using adapted handles and polishing to assist coordination, are other useful activities. Keyboard work is utilised for finger dexterity and adduction and abduction of fingers, as are slab and coil methods of pottery. Writing practice may be required, due to sensory involvement of the ulnar border of the hand.

Combined lesions

Lesions do not always occur singly. They may be combined median/radial or median/ulnar lesions or, very rarely, involve all three nerves. These type of lesion produce very severe disability as a result of division of the two or three nerves at wrist level. Accompanying tendon and vessel damage may cause the formation of scarring and fibrosis adhesions between the ten-

dons and nerves. There will be impairment of total hand function and a loss of all grips. The hand's appearance will be dictated by the combination of lesions present, for example the median/ulnar lesion resulting in a totally flat claw hand. Dynamic orthoses (Fig. 20.27), enabling the person to begin to use his hand functionally, should be instituted, as should vital sensory re-education. Figure 20.28 illustrates the sensory distribution of these three nerves, giving a clear indication of the very significant sensory loss of any combined lesion.

OCCUPATIONAL THERAPY SENSORY EVALUATION

A battery of tests is required in order to complete a full sensory evaluation. Sensory deficit in the hand may fit a specific pattern and can be monitored if documented efficiently.

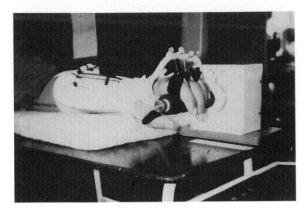

Fig. 20.27 Dynamic orthosis for a combined median and radial nerve lesion.

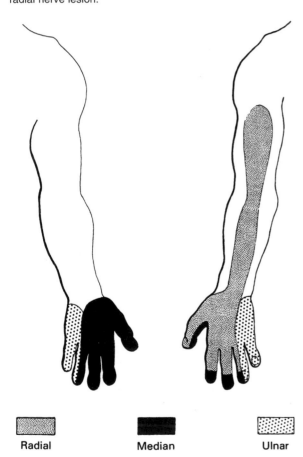

Radial Median Ulnar

Fig. 20.28 Sensory distribution in the upper limb covered by the median, ulnar and radial nerves.

The objectives are to determine whether axonal regeneration is occurring following nerve repair, to plan which sensory testing modalities should be used, to monitor this regeneration and to reduce functional deficit by sensory re-education.

The battery includes the following tests (Clark et al 1993):

1. Protective sensibility
   — Tinel
   — 0–10 subjective scale
   — hot and cold discrimination
   — light touch–pressure using monofilaments (Bell-Krotoski et al 1993)
   — pin-prick
2. Discriminative sensation
   — two-point discrimination test (Fig. 20.29)
3. Functional tests relating to sensation
   — Moberg (1958) pick-up test
   — functional assessment.

The choice of tests will depend on the stage of recovery of the nerves. Sensory evaluation must be conducted in a stimulus-free environment, where the individual can concentrate without distraction. The testing table should be covered with towels or felt to exclude noise; sensation in non-affected fingers can be excluded by using a cut-out rubber glove and sight can be excluded by using a blindfold or screen.

Localisation training

Localisation training will usually be necessary after a complete or partial division of a nerve (Salter 1987). Localisation may be altered because not all axons regenerate to their correct end-organs following surgery and so the person will receive false information from his fingertips. Training will correct this as long as he makes continual functional use of his hand.

The person is asked to close his eyes and the therapist touches an area of the volar surface of his hand, using moving finger touch, and asks him to identify the point of contact with the index finger of the other hand. A correct response can be recorded on a hand chart (Fig. 20.30) with a tick, and an incorrect response is recorded by filling in the number denoting the area which was actually touched. If the answer is incorrect the person is asked to look at the testing point to

SENSIBILITY EVALUATION FORM

Name: _____   Hosp. no:

Address: _____   Consultant:

_____   D.o.B.:

Date of test: Tester:

History of injury:

Patient subjective description:

L/R
Dorsal/volar

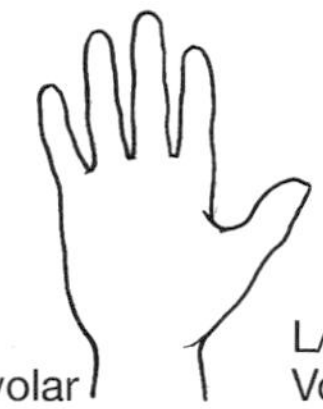

L/R
Volar/dorsal

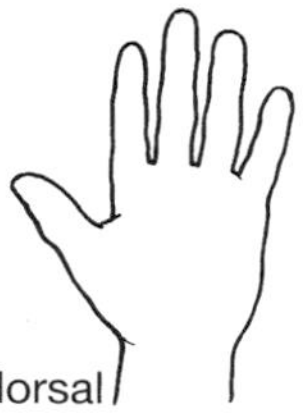

Sympathetic changes (dry skin, nail change, atrophy in pulp,
increased hair growth, skin colour,
skin temperature, sweat pattern)

Grip (kg) (average of 3)   Pinch – index to thumb
                                  Lateral   R   L
Right   Left   Pulp   R   L

0-10 Subjective scale

0   10
Anaesthetic   Normal   Hypersensitivity
hand   feeling

Fig. 20.29 Sensibility evaluation form.

relearn the location. The test should be repeated with the person's eyes open, and then with them closed. This should enable him to recognise the spot where he is being touched. Localisation training should be repeated over and over again during the subsequent weeks.

The therapist completes a functional hand assessment relating to the person's life-style, work

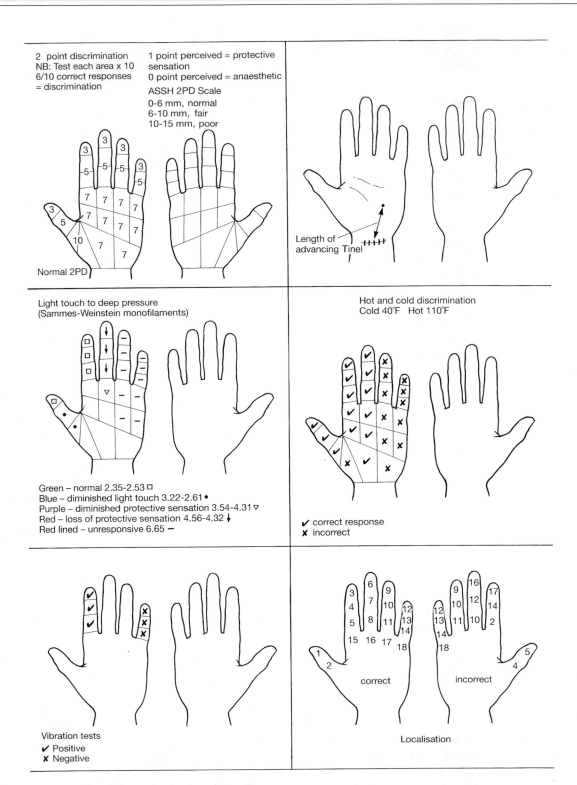

2 point discrimination
NB: Test each area x 10
6/10 correct responses
= discrimination

1 point perceived = protective
sensation
0 point perceived = anaesthetic

ASSH 2PD Scale
0-6 mm, normal
6-10 mm, fair
10-15 mm, poor

Normal 2PD

Length of
advancing Tinel

Light touch to deep pressure
(Sammes-Weinstein monofilaments)

Green – normal 2.35-2.53 □
Blue – diminished light touch 3.22-2.61 ●
Purple – diminished protective sensation 3.54-4.31 ▽
Red – loss of protective sensation 4.56-4.32 ↓
Red lined – unresponsive 6.65 —

Hot and cold discrimination
Cold 40°F   Hot 110°F

✔ correct response
✘ incorrect

Vibration tests
✔ Positive
✘ Negative

correct   incorrect

Localisation

Fig. 20.30   Sensibility evaluation form (page 2).

and hobbies, and identifies and resolves problems through provision of appropriate tools, orthoses and adaptive equipment.

Sensory re-education

Sensory re-education should commence when sensation of the palm has returned more or less to normal but the finger tips are still hyperanaesthetic. It is appropriate after division of the median nerve in particular, because the thumb, index and middle fingers are most commonly used for dexterity in pinch and prehension grips. The ring and little fingers supplied by the ulnar nerve are used mostly for power grip and so do not require the same high degree of sensitivity. The re-education programme should include specific sensory activities and activities involving functional use of the hand, for example horticulture, potting and planting, and 'Fimo' clay modelling, using rolling and pinching movements to form, for example small figures, jewellery and plaques.

Stereognosis

Stereognosis is the most appropriate means of re-educating sensation. It is recognition of objects through touch stimuli alone. A great deal of concentration is required and therefore the tests should be carried out in a quiet room, with minimum distraction. The person should be blindfolded or should keep his eyes shut during the test (Salter 1987). This is preferable to using a screen or curtain that separates hand and person. He should not see the chart or test items beforehand, in order to eliminate guessing or learning.

External stimuli can be eliminated by covering a table with a layer of foam rubber. A finger stall or cut-out glove can be used to eliminate normal sensation in ulnar-fed digits.

Method

1. The person is given one of several different shaped blocks and asked to describe it and identify as many properties as possible — for example, is it flat, smooth, cold, square? The object should be simple to identify at first. The person is then asked to open his eyes and describe the object again, adding any properties he missed. He can also repeat the test with his unaffected hand and then try again with the affected one. The time taken for correct recognition is noted.

2. The second stage involves timed recognition of textures, starting with easily identifiable contrasts such as velvet and coarse sandpaper (Fig. 20.31). As recognition improves, textures with only subtle differences can be introduced, and suitable materials include velvet, cotton wool, sandpaper, metal, cork, wool, a scouring pad and fur.

3. The final stage is the recognition of everyday objects such as a nailbrush, electric plug, matchbox or tennis ball. Once these have been mastered, fine objects such as a coin, safety pin, paper clip, button or peg can be used. This can be made more difficult by planting them in containers of rice, lentils, sand or beans (Fig. 20.32), and, additionally, speed tests can be introduced.

Trials undertaken by Salter showed normal recognition of shapes to be well under 5 seconds, and often 2 seconds. People with median nerve lesions may take over 5 seconds or not identify the object at all.

Documentation of results is important in order that regular assessment and comparison of improvement of sensory awareness is recorded and made (Fig. 20.33). Sensory re-education testing should take place regularly over a short span of time. A session should not last more than three quarters of an hour, otherwise interest and concentration diminish considerably.

Selection of participants for a stereognosis programme

- The age and experience of the person affects his ability to recognise objects and textures
- Motivation is vital
- People of different cultures and occupations will recognise familiar items at different speeds
- Expectations have to be realistic
- Functional use of the hand must be encouraged.

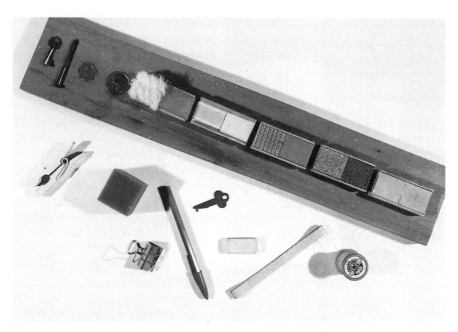

Fig. 20.31 Textures and shapes used for stereognosis.

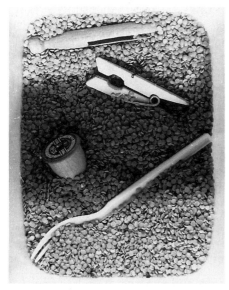

Fig. 20.32 Small objects planted in lentils can aid sensory re-education.

SPECIFIC TREATMENT FOR LOWER EXTREMITY NERVE LESIONS

After lesions of the sciatic nerve and of the common peroneal nerve (lateral popliteal) it is important to prevent foot drop and contracture of the calf muscles.

A temporary foot raise should be fitted (Fig. 20.16), and if no recovery occurs it may have to be worn permanently. Sensory loss (Fig. 20.34) demands precautionary measures and foot care. The therapist should ensure that the person understands the necessity for foot hygiene: he should wash his feet daily, carefully drying the skin, and wear clean socks or tights daily. Skin should be checked for rubbing or bruising and the cause removed before further damage occurs.

A static anti-foot-drop orthosis may be required for night use.

Activities for the lower limb should involve use of the whole leg in the early stages of treatment to maintain range of movement and muscle balance. As recovery of the common peroneal nerve occurs, activities are needed to provide active dorsiflexion and eversion of the foot. Games such as foot draughts and activities providing ankle rotation, dorsiflexion and plantarflexion, for example gardening, workshop tasks and squatting to work, can be utilised. A wobble board (Fig. 20.35)

STEREOGNOSIS TEST

Name:			**Coins** (Test 3 items)	Interpretation	Time
Date:			1p		
Shapes (Test one section only)	Interpretation	Time	2p		
			5p		
1. Square			10p		
Oblong			20p		
Triangle			50p		
Diamond			£1		
			Average time		
2. Circle					
Oval			**Objects — large** 1. (Test 3 items)		
Semi-circle			Sink plug		
Moon			Cotton reel		
			Plug		
Average time			Bottle		
			Saucer		
Texture (Test 6 items)			Soap		
Sandpaper			Egg cup		
Formica			Tea strainer		
Wood			2. (Test 3 items)		
Rubber			Pencil		
Carpet			Fork		
Leather			Metal comb		
Velvet			Ball point pen		
Fur			Screwdriver		
Cotton wool			Teaspoon		
Sheepskin			Toothbrush		
Plastic			Paintbrush		
Metal			Peg		
Average time			*Average time*		

Fig. 20.33 Chart used to record stereognosis.

is a useful piece of rehabilitation equipment, and a foot maze marble game can be incorporated to give the board's usage more purpose and interest to the user. General mobility should be encouraged at all times.

Damage of the femoral nerve requires retrain-

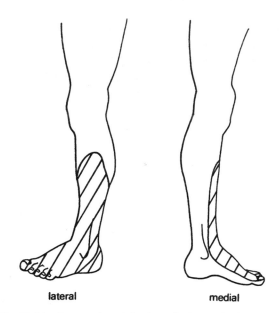

Fig. 20.34 Sensory loss following a lesion to the lateral popliteal nerve.

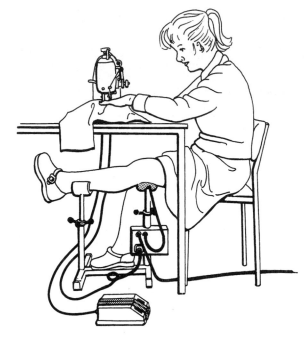

Fig. 20.36 The quadriceps switch.

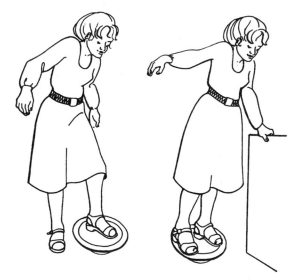

Fig. 20.35 The wobble board used to strengthen the ankles.

ing of the quadriceps muscle group. The Akron quadriceps switch (Fig. 20.36) can be harnessed to a tape recorder, computer or other electrical appliances. Computer games and biofeedback with the Myolink can also be used in lower limb muscle re-education.

After complete division of the nerves of the lower limb, recovery is often slow and sometimes incomplete. It may be necessary to continue treatment for two or three years. After a pressure neuropathy of the common peroneal nerve, a satisfactory recovery usually occurs in 6 to 12 months.

EDUCATION OF THE PERSON AND HIS FAMILY

Peripheral nerve injuries have psychological implications for the individual which may present in many ways, and reaction may not be proportionate to the extent of the physical injury. Disturbance of body image and loss of self-esteem are of major importance to some, while potential loss of function and the social factors implicated will be more important to others.

Factors that may affect the person are:

- disruption of family life due to admission to hospital of the person, whether it be father, mother or child
- temporary or permanent loss of employment
- temporary loss of personal independence

- disruption of leisure pursuits and social contact
- reaction to pain, which may be affected by the person's cultural and religious background.

Motivation can be influenced by:

- the actual degree of the injury and its effect on the person's work and leisure activities
- support provided by family and friends
- psychological state of the person before injury, for example nerve injury after attempted suicide or during clinical depression
- level of intelligence, for example the person may not be able to understand or appreciate the importance of relearning skills and their purpose
- language difficulties and cultural background
- attitude of the person to the surgeon and rehabilitation staff.

A positive working relationship between the individual and family and occupational therapist should be established. Fear and anxiety about the future may be alleviated by the provision of as much information as possible about the condition and the treatment involved. Relatives should be encouraged to participate in the rehabilitation process, and instruction about exercise regimes, orthoses and sensory training should be provided for the individual and relatives.

Photographs demonstrating the function that others have achieved with similar injuries may be helpful. A positive approach by the therapist is of paramount importance.

CONCLUSION

Working with people who have peripheral nerve lesions is challenging to the therapist because:

- the causes of lesions are numerous
- surgical intervention is increasingly inventive and skilled, particularly in the field of microscopic surgery
- conservative measures develop as people's needs dictate.

Occupational therapists' assessment, intervention and evaluation contribute practical, realistic and imaginative input into programmes, whether the individual is expected to make a maximum motor and sensory recovery or whether he has to be assisted to compensate and adapt to permanent deficits.

ACKNOWLEDGEMENT

Thanks go to Nicola Goldsmith for the inclusion of Figure 20.27.

REFERENCES

Bell-Krotoski J A, Weinstein S, Weinstein C 1993 Testing sensibility, including touch-pressure, two point discrimination, point localization and vibration. Journal of Hand Therapy 6(2): 114–123
Boscheinen Morrin J, Davey V, Connolly W B 1992 The hand: fundamentals of therapy, 2nd edn. Butterworth-Heinemann, London
Burke F D, McGrowther D A, Smith P J 1990 Principles of hand surgery. Churchill Livingstone, Edinburgh
Clark G L, Shaw E F, Igis W, Aiello B 1993 Hand rehabilitation, a practical guide. Churchill Livingstone, Edinburgh

Lamb D 1986 The paralysed hand. Churchill Livingstone, Edinburgh
Moberg E 1958 Objective methods for determining the functional value of sensibility in the hand. Journal of Bone and Joint Surgery 40B(3): 454–476
Salter M 1987 Hand injuries: a therapeutic approach. Churchill Livingstone, Edinburgh
Wynn-Parry C B, Salter M 1976 Sensory re-education after median nerve lesions. The Hand 8: 3

FURTHER READING

Barr N R, Swan D 1988 The hand: principles and techniques of splinting. Butterworth-Heinemann, London

Bell-Krotoski J A 1989 Light touch — deep pressure testing using Semmes–Weinstein monofilaments. In: Hunter J M, Schneider L H, Mackin E J, Callahan A D (eds) Rehabilitation of the hand, 3rd edn, pp 585–593. C V Mosby, St Louis

Bexon C, Greenstock M 1993 A splinting handbook. Smith & Nephew, Salisbury

Bannister R 1992 Clinical neurology, 7th edn. Oxford University Press, Oxford

Dandy D J 1993 Essential orthopaedics and trauma, 2nd edn. Churchill Livingstone, Edinburgh

Dellon A L 1981 Evaluation of sensibility and re-education of sensation in the hand. Williams & Wilkins, Baltimore

Dellon A L, Kallman C H 1983 Evaluation of functional sensation in the hand. Journal of Hand Surgery 8: 865–870

Hunter J M, Schneider L H, Mackin E J, Callahan A D 1990 Rehabilitation of the hand. Surgery and therapy. 3rd edn, Chs 42, 43 and 44. C V Mosby, St Louis

Jerosch-Herold C 1993 Measuring outcome in median nerve injuries. Journal of Hand Surgery 18B: 624–628

Malick M H, Kasch M C 1984 Manual on management of specific hand problems. Series I. American Rehabilitation Education Network, Harmaville, USA

Marsh D 1990 The validation of measures of outcome following suture of divided peripheral nerves supplying the hand. Journal of Hand Surgery 15B: 25–34

21

Spinal cord lesions

Jane Henshaw

INTRODUCTION

In 2500 BC an Egyptian physician described tetraplegia as 'a mortal condition — an ailment not to be treated'. This view of spinal lesions was held for thousands of years, extending into the early part of this century. During the 1914–1918 war 90% of all people with spinal lesions died within one year of injury but by the 1960s the mortality rate for tetraplegia was 35%.

In recent years, great strides have been made in the medical and paramedical care of people with spinal cord lesions, whose life expectancy is now virtually normal. One very important factor in the treatment of this group of people has been the establishment of centres throughout the country where the individual and his family can be given the specialist care and assistance they need (Fig. 21.1). This chapter examines the important contribution that the occupational therapist can make to the treatment of individuals who have suffered spinal cord lesions.

The first sections of the chapter describe the characteristics of spinal cord lesions, including their causes and classification as well as the complications to which they commonly give rise. The chapter then presents an overview of the kinds of treatment now available to individuals with spinal cord lesions, outlining the aims of surgical intervention, nursing care and physiotherapy as well as the significant role played by the social worker and the psychologist.

The chapter then turns in greater detail to the interventions of the occupational therapist during

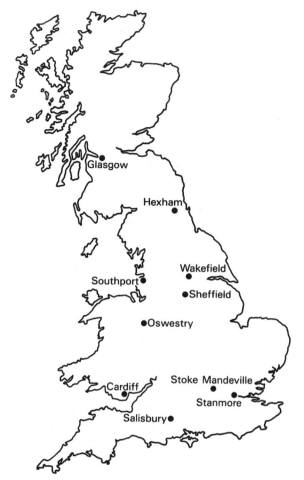

Fig. 21.1 Location of spinal units in Great Britain.

the 'acute' and 'rehabilitation' stages of treatment. First, her role in providing psychological support to the individual and his family during the acute or bedrest stage is described; this includes helping the individual to make productive use of his time while in hospital, providing therapy to maintain hand function, helping the individual to plan for his return to the community, and assessing his specific requirements in the choice of a wheelchair.

Next, the chapter describes the rehabilitation stage of treatment, during which the therapist will help the individual to regain optimum independence in self-care tasks, communication skills, domestic activities, and so on. Various transfer techniques suitable for the paraplegic or tetra-

plegic person are explained. Procedures for preparing the individual for resettlement at home and in the community are described, and practical considerations relating to work and education, leisure activities, driving and sexual function are briefly discussed.

It is evident that a spinal cord lesion can have a profound impact upon virtually all aspects of an individual's life, and that the occupational therapist's involvement in his rehabilitation will be both challenging and extensive. It is important, however, for the therapist to be aware of other sources of support for paraplegic or tetraplegic individuals, and addresses of relevant organisations are provided at the end of the chapter.

CHARACTERISTICS OF SPINAL CORD LESIONS

Causes

The causes of spinal lesion are many and varied, ranging from the bizarre to the mundane. In general, however, they may be described as either traumatic or non-traumatic.

Traumatic causes involve a direct force or impact on the spinal column causing disruption of the vertebral bodies, tearing of the ligaments and damage to the cord or, in a sudden hyperextension injury, 'pinching' of the cord in the narrowed spinal canal. Common causes of injury are: road traffic accidents; accidents at work, such as falling from heights or crush injuries; sporting accidents, for example in rugby, gymnastics, horseback riding and diving; and accidents in the home, including falling from ladders and falling downstairs — the latter being particularly common in elderly people who have spondylitic changes in the spine. At present, the annual incidence of spinal cord injuries in the United Kingdom is approximately 10–15 per million of the population.

Non-traumatic causes of spinal cord damage are: infections, such as transverse myelitis, abscess and polyneuritis; tumours which, if malignant, are usually secondary, originating from a primary focus elsewhere in the body; thrombosis in one of the spinal arteries; haemorrhage; demyelinating conditions such as multiple sclerosis; congenital deformities such as spina bifida; scoliosis; or psychological disturbance, as in hysterical paralysis.

Whatever the cause, the presenting signs and symptoms are the same and the effect on the individual concerned is equally devastating. On the whole, people find it easier to accept a disability which can be blamed on a clearly identifiable trauma than one which has resulted from a relatively obscure and difficult to understand non-traumatic cause.

Functional anatomy

The spinal cord is part of the central nervous system, which conducts messages to and from the brain. Any damage to the cord will result in the loss or disruption of messages travelling between the brain and the periphery. The spinal cord has been likened to a telephone cable joining two callers: if there is any damage to the cable the call will be either of poor quality or totally cut off.

Terminology

Damage to the cord above the level of L1 produces the symptoms of an upper motor neurone lesion. Damage below L1 results in symptoms characteristic of a lower motor neurone lesion (Fig. 21.2).

Tetraplegia/quadriplegia refers to a lesion in the cervical cord resulting in loss of motor power and sensory input in the lower limbs, trunk and upper limbs with disturbance of bowel, bladder and sexual function. The degree of upper limb involvement will depend on the level of the lesion.

Paraplegia refers to a lesion in the thoracic (dorsal), lumbar or sacral cord resulting in loss of power and sensory function in the lower limbs and trunk.

The level of injury will determine the degree of paralysis and the extent to which bowel, bladder and sexual function are disturbed.

Complete and incomplete lesions. A complete lesion results in total loss of motor power and sensation below the level of the injury. An incomplete lesion will preserve some motor power and/or sensation.

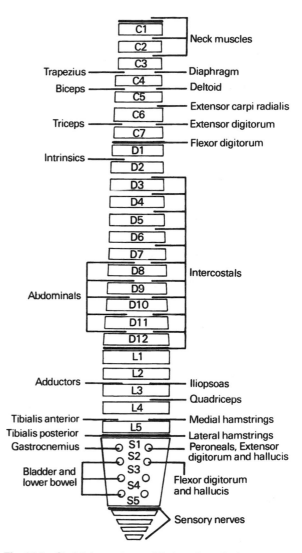

Fig. 21.2 Skeletal muscles and their major spinal segments.

Classification of lesions

The simplest method of classifying spinal lesions is to define them according to the last functioning nerve root above the injury. For example, in a complete C6 lesion all function above and including the 6th cervical nerve root is retained but functions below that level are lost. An individual with such a lesion would have the ability to move his shoulders, flex his elbows and extend his wrists. He would not, however, be able to extend his elbows, reach above his head, flex his wrists or move his fingers.

In an incomplete C6 lesion, all function innervated by the 6th cervical nerve root and above would be retained, as well as some motor and/or sensory function below that level.

It is impossible for anyone who has not suffered a spinal cord lesion to fully appreciate the devastating physical and psychological effects it has on an individual and his family. The general physical effects have already been mentioned; the psychological effects are equally profound and require at least as much attention during therapy.

Signs and symptoms

The most common clinical features of spinal lesions are:

- loss of voluntary muscle power
- loss of sensation to all modalities below the level of the lesion
- loss of sphincter control in relation to bowel and bladder function
- loss of vasomotor and temperature control
- disruption of sexual function.

Complications

Spinal shock

This condition is temporary, starting immediately after transection of the spinal cord. It can best be described as isolation of the spinal cord with total disruption of transmission between the brain and the cord. The duration of spinal shock varies; some reflex activity may appear within three days, but may take as long as eight weeks to reappear. As reflex activity returns, spasticity and increased muscle tone become evident. The full extent of the lesion and any potential recovery cannot be fully assessed until the spinal shock has subsided and bruising of the cord abated. It is usual for signs of recovery to appear fairly early if there are to be any, but there may be a delay of several weeks. Apparent late recovery may follow from the delayed repair of damaged nerve roots.

Autonomic dysreflexia

This is commonly seen in individuals with cervical lesions above the sympathetic outflow but it may be present in any lesion above T6. It may occur at any time after the spinal shock phase and is usually a response to a noxious stimulus, such as a blocked catheter resulting in a full bladder. In such a case the over-distension of the bladder results in a reflex sympathetic over-activity below the level of the lesion, causing vasoconstriction and systemic hypertension. The carotid and aortic baroreceptors are stimulated, leading to increased vagal tone and bradycardia. There is no peripheral vasodilation because of the damage to the cord, and the hypertension is therefore unrelieved.

The individual complains of a pounding headache, profuse sweating, and flushing or blotchiness of the skin above the level of the lesion. This condition should be dealt with as a medical emergency. The cause should be identified and treated and the blood pressure reduced. This may be facilitated by using vasodilators such as nifedipine tablets crushed and swallowed.

Post-traumatic syringomyelia

This is an ascending myelopathy caused by a secondary cyst forming in the cord. This condition is not uncommon, occurring in at least 2% of all people with spinal cord injury. Symptoms, which may present from two months post-injury onwards, include: pain in the arm, usually unilateral and often described as a dull ache; sensory loss, especially to pain and temperature; and, sometimes, loss of power unilaterally. The diagnosis can be confirmed by computed tomography (CT scan) or by nuclear magnetic resonance imaging (NMR scan). Treatment involves surgical drainage of the cystic cavity; although this relieves pain, there may not be any relief of sensory or motor symptoms.

Para-articular heterotopic ossification

After spinal cord lesion new bone is sometimes laid down in the soft tissue around paralysed joints, especially the hip and the knee. The cause of this is not known. It usually presents with redness and swelling near a joint and can impair movement. If surgical excision of the bone is indicated it should be delayed for about 18 months to avoid further new bone formation.

Contractures

These can result from immobilisation, spasticity or muscle tone imbalance. They may respond to conservative measures such as gentle stretching and orthoses but if this is unsuccessful surgical intervention such as tenotomy or tendon lengthening may be required.

Psychological factors

The psychological effects of a spinal cord lesion can be profound and prolonged. While on bedrest the individual will experience a wide variety of moods, including fear, anger, frustration, depression and euphoria. Sensory deprivation can result in a high level of anxiety and cause the person to become withdrawn. It is important that the individual and his family are helped and supported and given the opportunity to discuss their hopes and fears. Long-term psychological support may be necessary, as complete psychological adjustment may not be achieved for many years.

Pressure sores

Sores form as a result of ischaemia caused by unrelieved pressure. They affect the skin, subcutaneous fat and muscle as well as deeper structures. They are a major cause of readmission to hospital, yet are totally preventable by simple care routines such as suitable cushioning and mattressing, correct posture and daily skin inspections.

The general health and well-being of the individual will affect his skin tolerance. A bladder infection will make the individual more susceptible to skin breakdown.

TREATMENT APPROACH

A spinal cord lesion has a profound effect on all aspects of life for both the individual and his family. It is important that an holistic approach is taken to aid his recovery from the psychological as well as the physical trauma and to restore his confidence and self-esteem so that he can live the life that he and his family wish. The most successful way to achieve rehabilitation is to work within a multidisciplinary framework, using the resources of a doctor, nurse, physiotherapist, occupational therapist, social worker and psychologist, as well as of the individual, his family and friends.

MEDICAL AND SURGICAL CARE

The nature and extent of the individual's injuries will determine the exact course of management.

Conservative care

Depending on the level of the lesion the correct alignment of the spine is maintained by cervical traction or lumbar pillows. The individual is then nursed on bedrest for 6–16 weeks.

Internal fixation

This may be used in unstable and incomplete injuries. In the cervical area a bone graft and/or wires may be used to maintain good positioning of the fracture site. In the thoracic and lumbar regions metal rods, e.g. Harrington Distraction Rods, and wires are used. In both instances the bedrest period is significantly reduced.

Surgical intervention in the tetraplegic hand

In the longer term some tetraplegic people may benefit from surgical intervention. The tendons of fully innervated muscles are transferred to restore active elbow extension or to provide a functional grip. Although the surgery is physically possible, the selection of suitable candidates is critical and should only be done by a highly skilled multidisciplinary team. The individual must be well motivated as treatment will be difficult and time-consuming. It must not be forgotten that although surgery may improve hand and arm function, it will never restore full function or sensation to the limb.

Worldwide projects are underway assessing the feasibility of tendon transfer surgery carried out in conjunction with implanted electrical stimulation.

NURSING

The individual should be admitted to a spinal unit as soon as possible, where he will be nursed on bedrest from one to 15 or 16 weeks. Some people are nursed on electrically-operated turning beds, others on King's Fund Profiling beds with pressure-relieving mattresses supplemented by manual, regular turning.

Injuries to the cervical spine should initially be managed using skeletal traction. This will:

- reduce the fracture/dislocation
- relieve the pressure on the cord
- splint the spine.

Traction should remain in situ for six to eight weeks; at the end of this period the individual will be X-rayed again. If there is sufficient bony union the traction will be removed and a cervical collar used to provide support. Generally speaking, the individual will wear a soft collar while lying flat and sitting up to 45 degrees and a firm collar while sitting up at 45 degrees and over. The type of collar prescribed depends on the position to be maintained and on whether any other structures, such as the supporting ligaments, have been damaged. People with thoracic and lumbar lesions are nursed flat or with a pillow under the lumbar spine to preserve normal lordosis.

Initially, after injury, all systems are in shock. There may be a temporary loss of peristalsis in the intestines, which could lead to abdominal distension and vomiting. This is known as *paralytic ileus*. Until peristalsis returns and bowel sounds are heard the individual should not be given anything to eat or drink.

Skin care

Initially, turning takes place two-hourly and the individual's skin is inspected for any red marks.

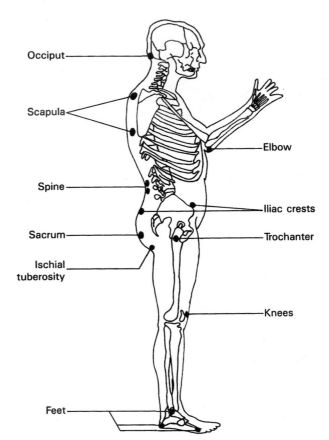

Fig. 21.3 Areas particularly likely to form pressure sores.

Subject to other injuries the turns will be supine, right lateral and left lateral. Positioning of the limbs during the bedrest period is vitally important, with care being taken to prevent contractures as well as pressure sores (Fig. 21.3). If there is no marking of the skin the length of time between turns is gradually increased. The ultimate aim is to enable the individual to sleep through the night without being disturbed.

Bladder management

The basic principle of care is that urine must be removed from the bladder efficiently and with minimum disruption to body organs or processes; an emptying routine that fits the individual's life-style must be established.

It is the advancement in the bladder management of people with spinal cord lesions that has brought about the tremendous reduction in the mortality rate.

Early care

In the newly injured person continuous catheter drainage is implemented for the first 24 hours. After this period the method of management will depend on the level of the lesion and the age and sex of the individual. A method commonly used is the passing of catheters at regular intervals (intermittent catheterisation). This is usually carried out six-hourly as an aseptic technique. Fluids are restricted until there is some return of bladder activity.

Videourodynamic investigations will show muscle and sphincter activity as well as pressure and volume during the filling and voiding stages of micturition. These investigations help staff to plan appropriate bladder training programmes.

Bladder training

Wherever possible, individuals are taught to manage their own catheterisation and general bladder care. In a lesion above L1, reflex activity returns as spinal shock subsides. The spinal micturitional reflex is intact, and an 'automatic bladder' which empties regularly and spontaneously can be developed. In lesions below L1, where the spinal micturitional reflex is disrupted, bladder function is obtained by increasing internal pressure, i.e. by filling the bladder. This stimulates the stretch reflexes in the muscles of the bladder and allows urine to flow past the sphincter by overflow incontinence. Ultimately an individual may regain continence by:

- intermittent self-catheterisation
- suprapubic catheterisation
- sacral anterior nerve root stimulation
- an artificial urinary sphincter.

Bowel management

While the person is still on bedrest his bowel is usually managed by manual evacuation and the use of suppositories if necessary. This is usually carried out every other day, and the bowel will

learn to respond to this stimulus. When the individual starts getting up from bed his bowels are managed over the toilet if at all possible; this is not only a more natural and dignified position but also makes use of gravity. Initially, nursing staff will give assistance but whenever possible the individual is taught to manage his own routine either by straining or by the continued use of suppositories. The management of the tetraplegic person's bowel is very much dependent on the care services available at home. In order to facilitate bowel management the person's diet should be high in fibre; he should be informed that changes in diet or routine could lead to faecal accidents.

PHYSIOTHERAPY

Physiotherapy commences within hours of the person's admission. During the acute phase the main aims of treatment are:

- To maintain joint range of movement. Each joint should be put through a full range of passive movement daily or, in the case of the upper limb, twice a day. This prevents contractures by maintaining muscle length. It is extremely important that the full range of movement is maintained in all joints; this will facilitate maximum independence.
- To maintain good respiratory function. Those who lie flat in bed for any length of time are at risk of developing a chest infection. All people, regardless of their level of lesion should be given prophylactic chest care, including deep breathing, percussion and coughing.
- To improve remaining muscle strength. Exercises to strengthen remaining innervated muscles may be carried out while the individual is still in bed, providing that the fracture site is not disturbed.

Once the person is out of bed for an hour or more a day his physical rehabilitation can begin. This will include the following:

- Learning basic wheelchair skills. The person is taught how to propel the chair, how to put the brakes on, position the castors, move the footplates and remove the armrests

- Retraining balance. As he has lost sensation, proprioception and motor power below the lesion, the person will be unable to balance; however, given time and practice he can learn to compensate
- Strengthening innervated muscles. Any form of exercise, including pulley work, weight-lifting, circuit training and sports can be used to strengthen muscles
- Learning transfers. This is undertaken with the assistance of the occupational therapist as well as the physiotherapist and is described fully in the section Transfers, below
- Learning advanced wheelchair skills. These include backwheel balancing, which enables the individual to manoeuvre over rough ground and to move up and down kerbs, and 'jumping' the chair sideways, which enables him to manoeuvre in tight spaces
- Standing. This is usually facilitated by a standing frame, although initially the individual who is prone to hypotension may use a tilt table that moves him into the vertical position more gradually
- Walking. People with lesions below the level of T12 may wish to walk using full-length calipers and elbow crutches. This is a slow, exhausting process and few use it as their only means of mobility.

Functional electrical stimulation

Over the years, doctors and engineers have tried to develop systems to stimulate the denervated muscles of paraplegic and tetraplegic people. With the advancement of computer technology, systems have been developed that enable individuals to stand without calipers. Other systems are being devised to give tetraplegic individuals a functional grip. All of these systems are still in their infancy and a long way from achieving their ultimate goals. Alongside functional stimulation there have been improvements in the design of walking braces. In the United States a Reciprocating Gait Orthosis (RGO) and an Advanced Reciprocating Gait Orthosis (ARGO) have been developed, while in the United Kingdom, at Oswestry, the Hip Guidance Orthosis (HGO) has

been devised. All systems offer a more normal walking pattern than conventional calipers and, consequently, conserve energy. The RGO and the ARGO have been designed to be worn under clothing, while the HGO must be worn over clothing.

THE ROLE OF THE SOCIAL WORKER

When the individual is first admitted to hospital, the social worker will make contact with him and his relatives in order to offer assistance with travelling expenses and with dealing with the many forms regarding appropriate benefits and allowances. She will also be able to offer support, a 'listening ear' and counselling. As a team member who is not directly involved in physical care and treatment, she may provide objective explanations and opportunities to discuss treatment and the future.

Contact with the person's local social services department should be made as soon as possible and a good working relationship established. This close liaison allows home resettlement to be smoother and easier for all concerned. When a return home is not possible, either because of the individual's age or the age and frailty of the carers, the social worker will make the necessary enquiries for alternative long-term living arrangements.

The social worker may also be asked to offer advice or assistance on a variety of practical issues, including local authority services, grants, local parking concessions and regarding any legal claim, including how to initiate litigation.

Compensation claims

Claims for compensation often follow a spinal cord injury. An individual with a case pending should be encouraged to contact a solicitor with proven personal injury experience as soon as he can so that as little time as possible is lost in this lengthy procedure. Solicitors ask team members, including occupational therapists, to prepare reports for the courts in support of claims for compensation. It is very important that these reports are comprehensive and thorough. The amount of a financial settlement may depend to a certain extent on the team's reports.

THE ROLE OF THE PSYCHOLOGIST

Many units now have access to the services of a clinical psychologist, who is able to offer practical help and advice to staff and carers who are trying to support individuals at a very traumatic time in their lives. Psychologists can also help by suggesting practical ways in which individuals can cope with their anxiety, anger, frustration and feelings of hopelessness.

THE ROLE OF THE OCCUPATIONAL THERAPIST

Successful rehabilitation of people with spinal cord lesions depends on a good multidisciplinary approach. Occupational therapists play a vital role within the treatment team, using their skills to assess the individual and his environment, plan a treatment programme, and facilitate the development of skills for independent living.

FRAMES OF REFERENCE

Individuals who have sustained a spinal cord lesion will present with varying degrees of paralysis. Some with a complete high cervical lesion will have minimal muscle power and grossly impaired sensation, and as a result will be totally dependent on others for many aspects of their care; others who have suffered an incomplete low lumbar lesion will have significantly more muscle power and consequently less disability, while some individuals may have no residual problems at all.

It is this diverse range of ability–disability that necessitates constant monitoring on the part of the therapist and the ability to use a number of frames of reference when planning her intervention.

Individuals with complete and incomplete lesions have a need to strengthen innervated muscle groups, and consequently a biomechanical frame of reference and its approaches would be appropriate for their management because, in the case of complete lesions, individuals have to use their fully innervated muscles to compensate for the lack of function in their paralysed limbs. A paraplegic individual needs to have very strong arms to enable him to push his wheelchair and transfer his full body weight in and out of the wheelchair, on and off the floor and in and out of the car — in fact for all the activities that would previously have been carried out by his now paralysed lower limbs.

Those with incomplete lesions equally have to strengthen their fully innervated muscles, but also have to work on maximising the strength and function in the partially innervated muscles below the level of their lesion.

Incomplete lesions also respond well to the developmental frame of reference, particularly the neurodevelopmental approach which enables the therapist to encourage normal patterns of movement where spasticity may mask apparently good isolated muscle power. This spasticity, along with poor proprioception and decreased sensation, may result in an individual reaching a lower level of independence than his lesion would suggest.

Those individuals whose level of lesion is such that they have become totally dependent on others for their care benefit from an adaptive rehabilitative approach (compensatory frame of reference) that enables them and their families to adjust to their level of disability. Such an approach helps the individual through the early hospital phase and then assists him to cope with facing the years ahead living with a spinal cord lesion. Adults who have been physically and psychologically independent will need time and help to adjust to being dependent on others for their physical needs and well-being. They will need help to express their needs to their carers, who in turn will need help to adjust to their new role. While an individual is in a spinal unit his needs change. As a consequence the frames of reference and approaches used by the therapist will need to vary and assist him to establish ongoing maintenance and any 'further progress' strategies for community living, hence the importance of continuous monitoring and evaluation of theories, approaches and treatment programme content.

The intervention discussed below is divided into 'acute' and 'rehabilitation' stages to illustrate the overall treatment of the person with a spinal lesion.

ACUTE STAGE (BEDREST)

The length of this period will vary, depending on the level of the lesion and on its conservative or surgical management. On average, the person is likely to be in bed for six to eight weeks. The aims of occupational therapy at this stage are:

- to establish a good working relationship with the individual, his family and friends
- to give psychological support to the individual and his family
- to care for the tetraplegic individual's hands
- to limit sensory deprivation and to provide the opportunity for the person to make constructive use of his time
- to make early contact with community colleagues and begin planning for resettlement at home.

These aims are described in greater detail below.

A good working relationship

It is vital that during the early stage of treatment the occupational therapist establishes a good rapport with the individual and his family and friends. This will facilitate successful rehabilitation. The therapist should learn as much as she can about the individual's life-style and the things that are important to him so that she can plan a treatment programme that is responsive to his needs and desires.

Psychological support

The therapist can do much to reassure those concerned by helping them to understand some of the difficulties which often arise and which may appear threatening at the time. For example, the home environment frequently seems daunting to a newly injured individual and his family, who may begin to panic about how they will cope at home and whether a wheelchair can be accommodated. Talking to the individual and his family about their home and what adaptations can be made may allay some of their immediate worries.

The recognition of depression, fear, boredom and aggression and their causes is of paramount importance. Any reassurance must include the relatives and friends, as should practical activity to help the individual to work through and understand the reasons for his feelings and behaviour.

Care of the 'tetraplegic hand'

Care of the individual's hands is of prime importance and in those units where orthoses are used routinely this should be undertaken as soon as possible after admission. There have been many debates over the years about the merits of splinting and although the policy differs from unit to unit the aims of care are the same:

- to maintain the functional position of his hand, i.e. to
  — support the palmar transverse arch
  — stabilise and support the thumb in abduction and opposition
  — maintain adequate web space
- to maintain good cosmetic appearance of the hand and prevent contractures
- to maintain good range of movement in all joints of the hand and wrist
- to maintain good wrist extension.

Tenodesis or *automatic grip*. This is one of the 'trick' movements which can be taught to a person with C6 tetraplegia and a functioning extensor carpi radialis longus muscle. This grip greatly increases independence, for as the wrist is extended the immobile fingers curl towards the palm (Fig. 21.4) and come into contact with the upward travelling thumb, either at the fingertips or at the side of the index finger. While wrist extension is maintained so too is this contact, which can be used as a gripping agent. Practice at picking up objects of varying shapes, weights and textures should be included in the treatment programme and the individual should be made fully aware of the utility of this grip.

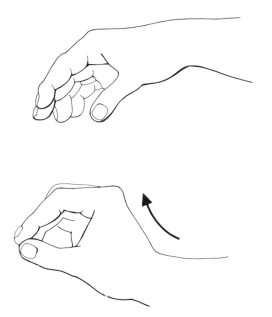

Fig. 21.4 Tenodesis grip. This action at the wrist enables the hand to provide a simple gripping function.

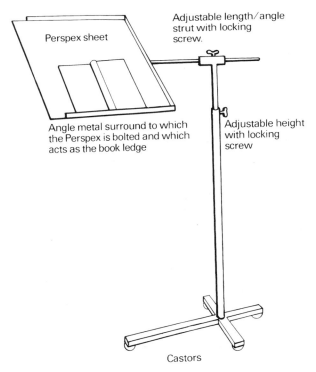

Fig. 21.5 Adjustable reading frame.

Constructive use of time

The occupational therapist can offer assistance, advice and support which may help to make enforced bedrest more bearable. She should encourage the individual to think and work through his problems. While she should discuss these with him and help him to work out solutions, the person must feel that he is still in control of his own situation, as this will help him to achieve a positive outlook and increase his self-confidence and esteem.

The following equipment may help the individual to make constructive use of time:

- Bed mirrors. One or two mirrors strategically attached to the bed and the over-bed frame will enable the person to see the ward, watch television and see those in adjacent beds.
- Prismatic spectacles. These are usually available from local opticians. The prism enables the wearer to see around the ward while looking towards the ceiling.
- Books on tape. Most libraries have an extremely good selection of books recorded on cassette tapes.
- Reading frames. A simple Perspex frame on

a height-adjustable stand will enable the person to read a daily paper. This type of frame still needs someone to turn the pages from time to time but is a relatively cheap solution to a difficult problem (Fig. 21.5).

- Electric page turners. These are not ideal while the individual is lying totally flat but do work well once he begins to sit up. Several types are available. Some turn pages forwards, others backwards and forwards; some will manage newspapers, others magazines and books.
- 'Overhead computers' enable the individual to work on the computer while lying supine. They can be used to play games such as chess, space invaders and snooker and as word processors, enabling people to write and print letters with some degree of privacy. As increasing numbers of people become computer literate, young people are now able to carry on their education lying in bed, while others may enjoy a new medium which may help to boost their self-esteem and confidence and introduce the possibility of future retraining.

Planning for resettlement

During the early stage of treatment it is important that the individual and the occupational therapist consider plans for the future. Whether the aim is to return home, live independently or move into residential care, many months of planning and negotiation will be required. An early start, therefore, is essential. The spinal unit occupational therapist and social worker should make contact with the person's local social services occupational therapist and social worker.

Home visit

The home visit should be carried out as soon as a prognosis is clear. A joint visit involving spinal unit and community staff and relatives is recommended at this stage. In some instances, when the lesion is incomplete, it may be advisable to wait until later, when the prognosis is clearer. The home visit may be very distressing psychologically for the family, as it may well reinforce the enormity of what has happened and suddenly face them with reality. It is very useful to take a wheelchair on these visits but care should be taken that introducing the chair does not cause undue distress to the family. Although this visit is carried out while the individual is still on bedrest it is imperative that he is closely involved and consulted, and that any decisions are made with his full participation.

It is always an advantage to have two members of the spinal unit staff on these visits as they can support one another, answer the family's innumerable questions and give help and support if and when the carers are distressed. The home should be assessed with a view to the following:

• Short-term measures: These will enable the individual to go home for weekend leave. Turning circles and doorway widths should be adequate. It should be decided if it is feasible to put a bed into the living/reception room in the short term. The bed height and the suitability of the mattress should be assessed.

• Interim measures. These will enable the individual to live at home before any major alterations are carried out. For example, is there access to a toilet and bath? If not, what temporary measures could be used to overcome the problem?

• Long-term measures. These will enable the individual to live independently or be cared for at home. Alterations frequently include permanent ramping, installation of a stairlift or a through-floor lift, major changes within the bathroom or a ground floor extension.

Once the home visit has been completed, the local authority staff should be invited to visit the unit to meet the individual and discuss the options available for him and his family. Younger people with cord lesions may feel that returning to the parental home is not a good idea and may wish to explore independent living before making any final decisions. The unit and community teams must be willing to discuss all options so that the individual is in a position to make an informed choice about his future.

Wheelchairs and cushions

A knowledge of the manual and electric wheelchairs supplied by the NHS will enable the occupational therapist to prescribe a suitable wheelchair for the individual. His age, size, height, weight, level of lesion and expected use of the chair will all influence the choice (see Ch. 9).

In recent years there have been great strides forward in the design and manufacture of lightweight, high-performance and powered wheelchairs. The range of chairs now available is extensive and the individual should be carefully assessed for the most suitable design to meet his needs. The choice of chairs and optional extras is so great that an individual should be advised to wait until the end of his rehabilitation before purchasing his own chair. By then, he will be better advised and more objective about his long-term requirements.

Cushions

The avoidance of pressure sores is of paramount importance and all individuals should be carefully assessed for the most suitable cushion.

Many people are able to sit on a 4″ pincore latex foam cushion with a natural fibre cover and relieve pressure on their ischii by pushing themselves up on the arms of the chair. For others, especially those with higher lesions who are unable to relieve the pressure, other cushioning needs to be investigated. Air cushions such as the Roho and gel and foam cushions such as the Jay range are very good pressure-relieving surfaces.

Pushing gloves

People with tetraplegia need some form of pushing glove when using a manual wheelchair: to prevent pressure sores from developing on their desensitised hands, to provide the necessary friction to push the chair and to protect their hands from the dirt that inevitably collects on the wheels (Fig. 21.6).

Getting out of bed

Once the person's spine is sufficiently stable he will be gradually mobilised into a wheelchair. This process may take from a day or two to one or two weeks, depending on the level of the lesion and the individual's progress and confidence. Having lain flat for a considerable length of time he will need time to adjust to the change of position and overcome hypotension. He may need to wear anti-embolism stockings and a broad elasticated waistband (abdominal binder) to help prevent the blood from pooling in the lower part of his body. If he continues with symptoms of dizziness and nausea which are not relieved by deep breathing he should be given Ephedrine approximately one hour before getting up. He can then sit up gradually on a profiling bed and, once he is in a sitting position, be transferred into a wheelchair. The length of time he is out of bed should be increased gradually from about ten minutes to all day. This may take two or three days for a low-level paraplegic or many weeks for a high-level tetraplegic.

During this period the occupational therapist, physiotherapist and nurse should work closely with the individual, helping to reassure him and build up his confidence. Initially, he will spend

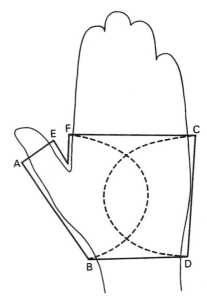

Fig. 21.6 How to make a pushing glove.
(1) Using tracing paper or greaseproof paper draw hand shape with flat palm and thumb in extension. Mark MCP heads of fingers, IP joint of the thumb and wrist joint.
(2) Allow sufficient space around the hand and thumb and draw the pattern shape as shown.
(3) Fold along line AB. Trace the shape of the thumb from A–E–F. From F draw a semicircle to the wrist at B to form an overlap of the glove on the back of the hand.
(4) Fold along line CD. From C draw a semicircle to wrist at D to form the overlap at the back of the hand.
(5) Open out the paper and cut out pattern. Try the pattern on the person's hand to ensure that the thumb width is sufficient and that the overlap at the back of the hand is adequate. Modify if necessary.
(6) Using the pattern, cut out two gloves in firm leather — cut on the bias to prevent the glove stretching when in use.
(7) Cut out palmer pieces to reinforce the palm of the glove and to give traction for pushing the chair — use leather, suede, rubber or pimple rubber.
(8) Sewing. For leather use a strong thread and a leather needle. (a) Sew reinforcement onto the palm. (b) Sew on the Velcro so that 'loop' piece overlaps 'hook' piece. (c) Sew around the thumb web space ¼″ from the edge. Try to match colours of the thread and the Velcro to blend with the leather.

the time on the ward, but when is up for about one hour at a time he will start attending the therapy departments.

THE REHABILITATION STAGE

The aim of all rehabilitation is to enable the individual to be as physically and psychologically independent as his condition will allow.

The occupational therapist's skills as a problem-solver and her ability to assess and treat an individual in an holistic manner make her a vital part of any rehabilitation team.

People with paraplegia should ultimately be totally independent, depending on factors such as age, sex, motivation and previous level of fitness. However, those with higher lesions will have greater difficulty and their final degree of independence will depend on their level of lesion (Table 21.1).

The description of intervention which follows has particular relevance to the treatment of individuals with high-level lesions.

Table 21.1 Functional expectations for a person with complete tetraplegia*

Level of injury	Functional ability
C4	Totally dependent Can use electric wheelchair with chin control Can type/use computer using a mouthstick Needs environmental control system (such as Possum) to turn on lights, open doors etc. — operated by shoulder shrug or mouthpiece
C5	Can feed with a feeding strap/universal cuff and wrist support Can wash face, comb hair, clean teeth — using feeding strap/universal cuff Can give help to dress top half Can push manual wheelchair short distances on the flat providing he uses pushing gloves and capstan rims on the wheels Electric wheelchair needed for functional mobility Unable to transfer
C6	Still needs strap to feed Still needs strap for self-care Can dress top half unaided Can assist dressing the lower half Can propel wheelchair up gentle slopes Can transfer independently into car and onto bed but rarely achieved Can drive with hand controls
C7	Can be totally independent Can transfer, feed and dress independently Can drive with hand controls
C8/T1	Totally independent from wheelchair

*It must be stressed that these expectations are general and depend on the patient's age, sex, physical proportions, physical condition prior to injury, motivation and degree of spasticity.

The following aims may be used as a framework for treatment at the rehabilitation stage:

- to encourage a positive, realistic attitude to the individual's changed circumstances
- to assist the individual to achieve his optimum independence in activities of daily living (ADL)
- to provide daily living aids, adaptations or orthoses needed for independence
- to help strengthen innervated muscles and to encourage the use of 'trick' movements where appropriate
- to help improve balance and general posture in the wheelchair
- to teach wheelchair skills to the individual and his family
- to assist with resettlement at home and advise on adaptations and equipment
- to provide information and advice for relatives, carers and friends
- to support and advise with regard to work and/or education
- to offer help and advice with regard to driving, wheelchairs and transport
- to encourage the continuation or development of hobbies, interests and leisure activities.

Personal care

After extended bedrest and dependence on others for all care, the ability to be independent in personal care activities will be very important. Initially, adaptations may be necessary but these should be re-assessed regularly and withdrawn as the individual becomes more able. The order in which these skills are attempted will vary from person to person.

Eating and drinking

Eating and drinking are both social activities and it is psychologically important that whenever possible the individual learns to manage independently. Eating can usually be facilitated by using adapted cutlery with individually moulded grips or a universal cuff with an ordinary spoon or fork (Fig. 21.7).

Box 21.1 Case study

John was a 28-year-old serviceman who at the time of his injury was on military exercise in Europe and had a water-sport accident. He was taken to the local hospital and then transferred to a spinal unit. A week later he was flown back to the United Kingdom and admitted to a spinal unit.

On examination he was found to have a fracture dislocation of C6/7 resulting in an incomplete tetraplegia below C6, complete below T4. He was a married man, living in his own three-bedroom semi-detached house.

Two weeks after admission to the unit he developed a pulmonary embolus and needed resuscitating.

He was nursed conservatively with his head in skull traction for 10 weeks. The traction was removed and two days later he began to sit up slowly, using a profiling bed. Ten days after the traction was removed he got out of bed for the first time. At this stage he was in a reclining wheelchair, his neck supported in a firm 'Philadelphia' collar. Within 10 days he was sitting in a standard wheelchair and was attending the physiotherapy and occupational therapy departments, working on balance and neck strengthening and personal ADL such as eating and teeth cleaning.

One month after John got up from bedrest the collar was removed. Over the next six months he worked at his strength and balance so that by the time he was discharged he was able to roll from side to side and sit up from lying. He could get himself in and out of bed and, using a sliding board, could get in and out of the car. He was able to wash, dress, shave and clean his teeth but found the tasks time-consuming and felt that to keep to a realistic daily schedule he would need some help.

He was able to feed himself, give himself a drink and cook a meal. He had his car adapted so that he could drive. A home visit was carried out while John was still on bedrest; the house proved to be unsuitable so John and his wife sold it and bought a bungalow which was later adapted to meet his needs.

After leaving the unit John took a computer course at a residential college and has since done work for voluntary organisations. He is still fighting a compensation claim through European courts.

He keeps fit by weight-training and swimming and has recently been on an Outward Bound course in the Lake District, where he took part in activities such as canoeing, horseback riding and abseiling.

John thoroughly enjoys cooking and has used his problem-solving skills to devise ways in which he can prepare and cook food.

Recently John and his wife have separated and although he finds it tiring he is managing to live alone, with care staff coming to help in the mornings and, occasionally, in the evenings if he feels too tired to put himself to bed.

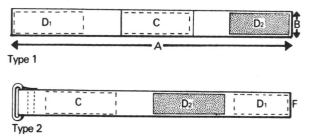

Fig. 21.7 Two types of universal cuff. (1) Straightforward Velcro overlap strap with stitched palmar pocket. (2) Strap end threads through a D-ring to fasten on to Velcro. Measurements: A=width of palm plus fastening overlap B=width (approx. 2.5 cm). C=pocket; palm width and stitched on three sides. D=Velcro 'hooks' and 'loops'.

The advantage of Type 2 is that one end F can be left threaded, enabling the tetraplegic patient to fasten and release Velcro independently with the teeth.

Initially it may be necessary to use a non-slip mat and a deep-rimmed dish or plate guard but these should be withdrawn as soon as the individual can manage without them, thus keeping specialised equipment to a minimum.

Lack of sensation in the hands and paralysis of the fingers makes drinking from an ordinary cup almost impossible. However, with practice the person may well manage a lightweight insulated mug and, in many instances, a half pint beer mug. It may be necessary for him to use a straw, in which case flexible straws will be useful. Non-return valve straws will prevent an excessive amount of air being swallowed.

Hair

Modern styles which can be maintained simply by washing and towel-drying the hair are generally to be preferred. Grooming the hair is made easier by using a round styling brush, which has a more manageable handle, rather than a comb, and a larger universal cuff will facilitate holding the brush. When necessary, handles of thermoplastic splinting material can be fitted to hair driers and other styling equipment. Individuals should be reminded about the possibility of burning anaesthetic skin with all styling equipment.

The independence achieved by a person with tetraplegia will depend upon his level of lesion as well as his age, sex and previous physical fitness. He should be verbally independent even if he cannot be independent physically, i.e. he must know how he should be dressed, fed and washed and he should be able to teach others how he wishes to be assisted.

Clothing

Advice on clothing should be kept to a minimum so that the individual is still free to express his personality. However, it is advisable that back pockets and studs are removed from jeans and other articles and that practical, natural fibres are worn. Particularly tight clothing should be avoided and care should be taken with elasticated clothing such as socks and bras so that they do not cause pressure marks. Shoes should generally be a size larger than before to accommodate oedema and prevent rubbing.

Transfers

Before the person can learn how to transfer he must learn certain standard procedures, e.g. how to position the chair with the castors forward and the brakes engaged, making the chair more stable. He will learn wheelchair transfers to and from bed, armchair, toilet, bath, car and floor. Most people with paraplegia will be independent in all of these transfers and will also be able to get their chair in and out of the car. Those with higher lesions will be more dependent upon assistance.

Bed transfers

Ideally, the bed and the wheelchair should be the same height.

There are two methods of getting on and off a bed:

1. 'Forwards on' transfer (Fig. 21.10). The wheelchair is placed at right angles to the bed and the person lifts his legs onto the bed one at a time. The footplates are swung away and the chair moved closer. The person then moves forwards, in small lifts if necessary. The procedure is reversed for transfer into the chair.

2. 'Legs down' or side transfer (Fig. 21.11). The chair is positioned and the footplates lifted and swung away if necessary. The individual moves forward on the seat to position his feet comfortably on the floor. The near-side armrest is removed and the person lifts his bottom across onto the bed, taking care to avoid the rear wheel. He then lifts his legs onto the bed. The reverse procedure is used to transfer to the chair.

Armchair transfers

These are usually achieved by positioning the wheelchair at an angle to the armchair and doing a 'legs down' transfer (Fig. 21.11).

Toilet transfers

Transferring on and off a toilet is made much easier if the toilet seat is the same height as the wheelchair seat. The toilet seat must always be padded to prevent scrapes or pressure sores. Specially padded seats are preferable to inflatable rubber seats, which tend to perish. The method of transfer will depend on the space available, but where possible the chair should be placed alongside the toilet at a slight angle and a 'legs down' transfer carried out as shown in Figure 21.11.

Rails, although useful, should be avoided if possible as the person may tend to become reliant upon them and find transferring difficult or impossible if they are not available.

Shower transfers

Ideally, the shower base should be level with the floor so that the person can either use a self-propelling shower chair or execute a 'legs down' transfer onto a free-standing shower chair. If the shower base prohibits the use of a wheelchair, then a fold-down shower seat on the wall can be used. If a free-standing seat is required it must be noted that it cannot be used with a fibreglass

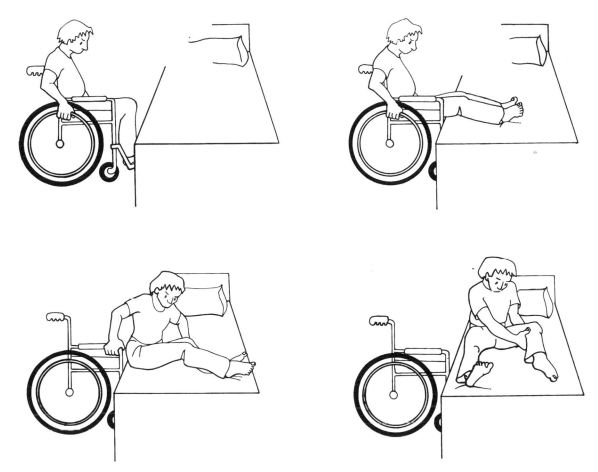

Fig. 21.10 'Forwards on' transfer onto a bed.

base. In all cases the seat must be padded to prevent pressure sores and the water thermostatically controlled to eliminate any risk of scalding.

Bath transfers

The individual may learn to transfer over the side of the bath or, if it is accessible, over the end of the bath, the same technique being used for both methods (Fig. 21.12).

Difficulty may arise if the person does not have the strength to lift himself back out of the bath. Equipment such as bath boards or seats, and electrically or battery operated bath seats which raise and lower the person may help to overcome this problem.

Safety measures are vital. The water must be run and tested before the person gets into the bath and hot water should never be added once he is in the bath.

Car transfers

The technique used to get in and out of a car will depend on the individual's ability and, to a certain extent, on the make of car being used. It is much easier to transfer into a two-door than a four-door car. Once the car door is open, the wheelchair should be pushed up as close as possible to the door sill. The footplate and the armrest nearest to the car should be removed. The person then moves himself forward on the

the best use of it. A universal or hammock sling should be used so that the individual's trunk is supported and pressure spread evenly across his back. Problems with anaesthetic skin may make it necessary to line the slings with sheepskin. A more detailed description of hoists is given in Chapter 9.

Therapeutic/remedial activity

Occupational therapy is an integral part of the treatment programme. As well as providing a welcome break from ward routine, remedial activities entail working to a timetable and encourage social interaction. Occupational therapy presents the individual with the implications of his disability by asking him to participate in normal activity. Some people may find this difficult to accept and will look for excuses to avoid participation. While an individual's choice must be respected he should, nevertheless, be encouraged to sample appropriate activities, selected to use and strengthen innervated muscles to maximum benefit and to initiate a wide and varied programme which, while being very specific, must also be enjoyable. A relaxed individual who is genuinely interested in the activities offered will participate with more enthusiasm than the individual who is tense or bored and will be able to undertake a more extensive programme of therapy, learning decision-making skills and regaining his initiative.

Workshop activities

Heavier activities such as woodwork and metalwork can provide an additional dimension to a programme designed primarily to improve balance and strengthen muscles. They may provide opportunities for the assessment of work skills and aptitude as well as practice in handling tools and equipment. Men comprise the majority of people with spinal lesions and the traditionally male-orientated working environment of the workshop can enhance self-esteem and confidence by offering the opportunity to 'roll up one's sleeves' and to participate in more male-orientated conversations. Workshop activities, of course, need not exclude women.

Communication

It is important that, regardless of the level of his injury, each person is given the opportunity to learn how to manage pen and paper so that he can communicate in writing as well as orally. Even the most uninterested person should be encouraged to relearn the mechanics of writing, even if only for the purpose of signing legal documents, cheques and greetings cards, or for doing crosswords and puzzles.

A good rapport must be established between the individual and his therapist before writing practice is introduced into the programme, as writing is difficult to perfect and requires interest, patience, practice and perseverance from them both. Gripping and controlling the pen is difficult without finger function. The pen has to be moved across the paper with movement from the shoulder, elbow and wrist instead of by the fingers.

The pen can be held between the fingers and thumb with an adapted holder or with a device that fits into the universal cuff. Alternatively, it can be held between the palms of both hands, or held between the fingers of one hand and steadied by the other. A felt-tip pen should be used initially, as it requires little pressure and can be used at any angle. The paper should be held firmly, either by non-slip matting or a clipboard. It may be more realistic for the individual to master a word processor for more efficient letter writing, in which case a typing orthosis may be needed (Fig. 21.13).

As computers are becoming more popular and an increasing number of people are computer literate, the demand for sophisticated technology is increasing. The computer technology now available is such that people with severe disabilities are able to communicate, work and run their lives at the push of a button or the blink of an eyelid. Such systems are particularly helpful for people with tetraplegia who want to live independently, or whose family are out during the day. Other practical skills related to communica-

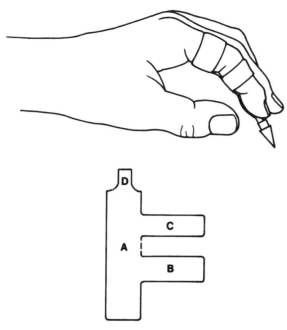

Fig. 21.13 An orthosis may make typing quicker and easier. (1) Cut the pattern out of thermoplastic material and soften in the usual way. (2) Place A along the palmar aspect of the right or left index finger so that D is beyond the fingertip. (3) Fold B and C around the index finger as shown. (4) Place a pencil-top eraser on D.

tion, mobility and independence which should be practised include operating the telephone (pushing buttons, holding the receiver, operating coin boxes and handling phonecards); handling money (coins, notes and wallets or purses); using keys (inserting and turning them and opening doors); and operating environmental control systems.

Domestic ADL

An increasing number of people with spinal cord lesions wish to live independently in their own homes. Wherever appropriate, such individuals should be given the opportunity to spend time in a domestic environment prior to resettlement at home, so that they can learn to handle equipment safely and regain confidence, strength and skill.

Practice related to food preparation should include shopping as well as making beverages, cooking snacks or meals and baking. Wherever possible, it is more appropriate to use modern labour-saving devices as opposed to equipment specifically designed for people with disabilities. Microwave ovens make cooking simpler and quicker and slow cookers enable hot meals to be prepared without lifting dishes in and out of an oven.

Bean-bag trays are useful in an environment where hot plates and cups need to be carried from one area to another.

Washing machines and tumble driers make laundering clothes relatively simple. Control knobs may need adapting to facilitate their operation. Rotary clothes-lines are simplest, providing they can be reached; alternatively, a system of lowering and raising a washing line has to be used. 'Dolly' pegs can be used by most people with weak grip. A lightweight iron and either a wall-mounted ironing board or a board with space to give knee clearance should be used. People with anaesthetic skin on their hands and arms should take great care while ironing. Day-to-day cleaning and tidying should be encouraged; while still in the ward, individuals should, wherever possible, be responsible for making their bed and keeping their 'bed space' tidy.

Resettlement at home

Most spinal units have a training flat or house which enables the individual, with or without his family, to care for himself in a domestic rather than a clinical environment. This sort of facility helps to increase the person's confidence prior to discharge. It is essential that during this stage of rehabilitation he is encouraged to interact with the local community. Trips and visits away from the hospital will help to introduce the individual to the outside world. He will probably have been in the spinal unit for between six and nine months (and in some cases longer) prior to his discharge. He will have become friends with staff and other people in the unit. Generally, he will be keen to go home and look forward to his discharge date. However, he will often need to be prepared for the 'trauma' of loneliness, boredom or frustration, as he will miss the company of the others. He may need help during the first few

Research work is being done, particularly with regard to male fertility and the collection of motile sperm.

CONCLUSION

Therapists working in the field of spinal cord lesions are given the opportunity to use all of their professional skills. During the course of treatment the therapist is likely to work within the hospital setting, out in the community, and in the work environment. She will assess and teach physical skills, help to build self-esteem and self-confidence and encourage coping skills. She will be a facilitator, a counsellor, an educator and a friend to the individual and his family.

Advances in modern technology have not only made it possible to treat people with ultra-high lesions but have dramatically improved their quality of life. This is an exciting time to be involved in the care of those with spinal cord lesions.

USEFUL ADDRESSES

Association to Aid the Sexual and Personal
Relationships of People with a Disability (SPOD)
286 Camden Road
London N7 0BJ

British Paraplegic Sports Association
Ludwig Guttman Sports Centre
Harvey Road
Aylesbury
Bucks HP21 8PP

Disabled Drivers Association
18 Creekside
London SE8 3DZ

Disabled Living Foundation
380–384 Harrow Road
London W9 2HU

Royal Association for Disability
and Rehabilitation (RADAR)
25 Mortimer Street
London W1N 8AB

Spinal Injuries Association
Newpoint House
76 St James's Lane
London N10 3DF

FURTHER READING

Bedbrook G 1981 The care and management of spinal cord injuries. Springer-Verlag, New York
Bedbrook G 1985 Lifetime care of the paraplegic patient. Churchill Livingstone, Edinburgh
Bromley I 1981 Tetraplegia and paraplegia: a guide for physiotherapists, 3rd edn. Churchill Livingstone, Edinburgh
Grundy D J, Swain A et al 1993 A.B.C. of spinal cord injury, 2nd edn. British Medical Journal, London
Malick M, Meyer C 1978 Manual on management of the upper extremity. Harmarville Rehabilitation Centre, Pittsburgh

Morris J 1989 Able lives: women's experiences of paralysis. Women's Press, London
Oliver M, Zarb G, Silver R et al 1988 Walking into darkness. Experience of spinal cord injury. Macmillan, London
Rogers M 1986 Living with paraplegia. Faber & Faber, London
Trieschmann R 1980 Spinal cord injuries: psychological, social and vocational adjustment. Pergamon Press, New York
Trombly C A 1989 Occupational therapy for physical dysfunction, 3rd edn. Williams & Wilkins, Baltimore
Whiteneck, Adler C, Carter R E et al 1989 The management of high quadriplegia. Demos Publication, New York.

Musculoskeletal and vascular problems

22

Introduction to musculoskeletal and vascular problems

Margaret Foster

INTRODUCTION

The human body is a complex mechanism which relies on the smooth interaction of a number of systems in order to function normally. The chapters in this section consider rheumatoid and osteoarthritic disorders, back problems, burns, amputations, and upper limb injuries. These disorders significantly affect the musculoskeletal and vascular systems of the body. This is not to say that other systems are not involved, but the degree of resulting impairment will generally be less from the involvement of the other systems than from the problems resulting from musculoskeletal and vascular damage.

PRINCIPLES OF OCCUPATIONAL THERAPY

The basic principles for the treatment of the conditions considered in this section do not differ from those that the occupational therapist will use in working with other kinds of disabilities or injuries. However, in a significant number of situations the aims and goals of the interventions described here may be directed towards achieving complete recovery. Following the successful clinical management of the effects of trauma resulting in burns, upper limb injuries or amputation, none of the conditions covered in this section is in itself life-threatening.

The occupational therapist is involved in helping people with any of these disorders to achieve maximum potential according to their wishes.

This may be in preparation for a total life span in the case of the person with congenital limb absence, or for a considerable number of ensuing years for many others. Where there is residual dysfunction the occupational therapist is involved in assisting the person to make positive adjustments to changed circumstances so that he can meet life-style wishes and needs.

THE ANATOMICAL AND PHYSIOLOGICAL BACKGROUND

It may be deduced from the study of the human body that the musculoskeletal system is predominantly concerned with movement and posture, the bones acting as levers and the joints as fulcrums for movement, while muscle contraction and relaxation provides the control for action to occur. Any damage to bones or muscles will therefore result in some disturbance of movement at the affected part. The effect on the person's mobility will differ according to the extent and site of the damage, but the impact on the local affected area will be the same: an alteration in the range of movement.

The vascular system is composed of the cardiovascular (heart and blood vessels) and the lymphatic systems. These are concerned with blood circulation and tissue fluid balance and are important systems in disease or injury:

- in the conveyance of nutrients and oxygen to a damaged site for tissue repair
- in the removal of waste products
- in the coagulation of blood to control fluid loss from a wound
- in the maintenance of homeostasis within the body
- in the production and transport of antibodies to combat infection.

The cardiovascular and lymphatic systems act as the transporters for the body and interlink with other systems, such as the respiratory system for oxygen and the digestive and urinary systems for waste product removal.

It is virtually impossible to damage one system in isolation. Musculoskeletal injury will have vascular implications and, similarly, a deficit in circulation may starve an area of nutrients, resulting in necrosis of tissues, which will in turn affect mobility.

In understanding health and disease it is important to consider the dependency of the body on the performance of its individual parts. The action of the major organs — the heart and the lungs — is necessary for circulation to occur, and skeletal muscle action is particularly important for venous return.

It is not possible in this text to give a detailed description of these systems, but study of human anatomy and physiology reveals the interplay of the musculoskeletal and vascular systems and their importance in the body's performance in health and disease.

It is important to consider the implications of the anatomical and physiological links between the systems for the occupational therapist's intervention. For treatment to be successful members of the rehabilitation team should understand the effects of the disease or injury on the body, as these will determine the recovery potential and the approaches chosen in the rehabilitation programme. A fracture will not heal without an adequate vascular supply. A disease or injury which reduces mobility will affect circulation, and a defect in circulation may result in secondary complications which reduce mobility. The person with arthritis may have peripheral vascular problems and the individual with peripheral vascular insufficiency may eventually require an amputation because of necrosis of tissue distally.

Occupational therapists frequently use activity as their therapeutic medium. The choice of activity will be dependent on the individual's needs, but any physical activity will obviously affect the motor function of muscles and joints and promote circulatory performance by the vascular system. This principle may form the basis for the choice of specific activities to promote physical improvement, particularly in relation to the biomechanical approach.

However, occupational therapists are primarily concerned with problem-solving and their role encompasses much more than simply addressing the anatomical and physiological implications

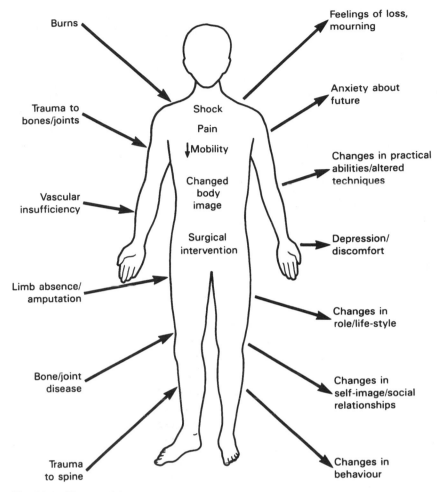

Fig. 22.1   The possible impact of musculoskeletal and vascular problems on the individual.

of various disorders. While the disorders considered in this section have certain similarities in their physical impact on the body's systems, it is the broader effects of these clinical features on a person's life-style (Fig. 22.1) — the impairments and disabilities — which form the basis for intervention. The following sections will therefore concentrate on these features of the disorders and their impact on the person, his family and his carers in terms of a changed life-style.

Psychological implications

Back injuries, amputations, upper limb injuries and burns may all be the result of an accident or injury. In these instances the impact has been sudden, leaving the individual and those close to him in a state of shock. Physical shock may need intensive specialised nursing if the person is to recover, but the impact of emotional shock may take much longer to overcome.

The stages of recovery from emotional shock may be similar to the stages of the mourning process described by Kubler-Ross and others, in which the person grieves for what is lost. The person needs to work through the stages of anger and guilt, bitterness, depression, denial and frustration if he is to come to terms with his changed circumstances. He may assign blame for the accident, or feel guilty himself at its occurrence, or be afraid of facing the future. However efficient the physical process of recovery is, unless the emotional and psychological impact of the bereavement is explored and the necessary adjustments made, the injury or accident is likely to have a long-term effect upon the person's life-style and relationships.

Numerous explanations of the stages of transition from grief to acceptance have been given by psychologists. However, it is now generally recognised that these stages may only reflect the general outline of the process and that the sequencing of the stages may fluctuate. Recovery may level off at a particular stage, causing a return of anger, depression or frustration, and creating a new hurdle to overcome in the rehabilitation process. A sudden memory of something that occurred or existed prior to the accident may trigger a return of mourning, depression or denial. Additionally, the person's response to loss and the process of adjustment is very individual and may be equally dependent on his premorbid personality, family support and security and previous life-style and on the quality of care he receives.

These factors are not unique to the traumatic conditions already identified, but may occur in any situation of loss. However, symptoms are often more dramatic where the loss has been sudden and the person has had no opportunity for gradual adjustment. Those who are affected by a rheumatoid or osteoarthritic disease, or require an amputation for peripheral vascular insufficiency may not experience the sudden initial shock. Nevertheless, many still show the symptoms of the grieving process, mourning the life that is lost or restricted by the disease. There is often a more gradual realisation of the change. In any event, the person must eventually acknowledge the reality of his condition if successful adjustments to residual dysfunction are to be achieved.

The person who has limb deficiency at birth will never have known the experience of life with limbs but in later life may express some anger or bitterness at his loss or limitation. Similarly, it is not unusual for parents to grieve for the 'normal' child they had hoped for at birth, and considerable support may be required to help them with this process.

Age distribution

When comparing or grouping the conditions discussed in this section it is interesting to consider their age distribution. Unlike many conditions seen in occupational therapy, which predominantly affect middle-aged and elderly groups, the disorders in this section have a wide age distribution, the occurrence being highest in young adulthood and early middle age. Only osteoarthritis and amputation as the result of peripheral vascular disease are most common in those over sixty years of age. With the exception of congenital limb absence, all the other disorders may occur at any age. Many result from accidental trauma, which occurs most frequently in the young adult.

Age distribution will affect the objectives and goals of therapy. The priorities of many young adults differ from those of the majority of people over sixty years of age. The potential for physical recovery is usually greater among young people, whose rehabilitation will be directed towards skills which may be actively continued for many ensuing years.

However, on the negative side, the young adult may have less life experience on which to build his rehabilitation than the older person does. This may affect work opportunities or role responsibilities as parent or breadwinner, as well as personal interactions and the social aspects of life-style.

Mobility

Inevitably, damage to the musculoskeletal system will affect movement. This may take the form of short-term loss of movement until recovery occurs, or of long-term movement deficits if there is significant damage or a systemic disorder.

The nature of the problems created by loss of mobility will vary with the area of the body affected, the extent and cause of the impairment, and the hopes and life-style of the individual. Loss of dexterity and fine finger movement may have similar effects on the life-style and hopes of a computer operator as the amputation of a lower limb may have on an elderly keen gardener. Both will have to consider management of their day-time occupation, either by finding new ways to perform the activity, or by considering alternative activities.

The emphasis on mobility in daily living will vary enormously from one individual to another. A person who is faced with compensating for loss or reduction in movement early in life may learn new techniques more quickly than an older person. However, there may be damage to other areas of the body in the long term if such techniques redistribute the stresses of mobility onto areas of the body not designed for this purpose. For example, the long-term use of crutches or walking frames may result in osteoarthritic changes in the upper limbs. Many elderly people more readily accept some reduction in mobility as part of the ageing process, but those who have prepared for an active retirement may be just as frustrated as the younger person.

Problems affecting limb movement may cause difficulty with many aspects of personal care, work and leisure skills, and may inhibit the person's communication through gesture or touch. The loss or limitation of the complex and varied functions of the hands may restrict employment opportunities or affect confidence in making relationships. The hands are highly visible parts of the body, used together in the sight of others to perform everyday tasks. If they are hidden away this may indicate embarrassment at their disfigurement or a reluctance to accept their restricted function.

The lower limbs are the tools of conveyance in the environment, allowing a person to rise from a seated position and move from room to room, level to level and place to place. A lower limb mobility problem imprisons the person in his environment and in so doing restricts social and physical contact. Studies of the physiology of exercise show that a reduction in mobility affects circulation and thereby the person's general health and potential for overcoming injury or disease.

Many members of the rehabilitation team will be involved with improving the person's mobility — most particularly the physiotherapist where physical movement techniques are affected. The occupational therapist may use activity towards furthering these physical improvements, or she may be more concerned with helping people with residual mobility problems to face the challenges of daily living.

Surgery

This may be a sudden intervention as the result of an accident or may be one of a number of techniques in a programme of treatment used to overcome a problem or to improve potential for function. A fracture may require immediate surgery following an accident in order to facilitate bony union. The person who has suffered burns may need repeated skin grafting. The joints damaged by rheumatoid arthritis or osteoarthritis may benefit from synovectomy, arthroplasty or tendon repair. Surgical amputation of a limb may be the culmination of a long period of other treatments aimed to improve distal circulation or healing.

The physical and psychological effects of surgery vary from person to person and the nature of the surgery. Many people take considerable time to overcome the physical effects of anaesthesia. The anxiety of impending surgery may be devastating for some, while others will look forward to the relief from pain and the improvement they hope will result. Advice and education regarding the surgery and the ensuing nursing care can help to relieve some of the person's fears of the unknown, thus engendering a more positive approach to the operation and the immediate post-operative care. If the person can discuss fears and anxieties about the surgery with the team, and question them on the anticipated outcome, he is likely to have a more positive, co-operative attitude, particularly in the early stages of rehabilitation, than those who are fearful and anxious of the success of the surgery and see it as a last hope when all else has failed. A joint replacement for an osteoarthritic hip may make a dramatic positive change to a person's life-style. A laminectomy may relieve pain and the limitations of spinal movement and internal fixation of a fracture will enable the person to achieve early mobilisation and thereby avoid possible complications from prolonged immobility. The surgical amputee who has suffered a long period of pain and limited mobility prior to surgery may see the post-operative stage as a new phase in his treatment which will culminate in an improved quality of life.

Obviously, when surgical intervention is sudden there is little opportunity for education and discussion of fears and anxieties, but studies have shown that where such counselling has been possible the person has been more cooperative in the early post-operative rehabilitation.

Pain

With the possible exception of the child with congenital limb deficiency, all the people with the disorders addressed in this section are likely to experience physical pain. This may be the sudden intense pain from an injury such as a fracture or burn. It may be long-term localised pain from a damaged osteoarthritic joint or from back injury, or chronic generalised pain characteristic of rheumatoid arthritis. People who have had amputations frequently suffer a phantom limb sensation which may at times be physically painful. Damaged exposed nerve endings following burns may retain hypersensitivity and be painful to touch for a considerable time after the accident.

People react differently to physical pain. Some people express the pain openly, avoiding or resisting any activity which is likely to exacerbate their discomfort. Others internalise the pain, stoically continuing activity despite intense agony. It is important for the therapist to recognise the existence and importance of pain and explore avenues of overcoming or avoiding it.

Sudden pain may be a warning. It may indicate:

- over-exertion in activity
- the possibility of infection
- further physical damage which requires investigation.

Chronic pain may destroy both the body and the mind, pressurising the person into changes in life-style, relationships and even personality. The person with chronic pain may:

- lose motivation to perform essential basic personal activities
- be unable to continue domestic, work or social roles
- put pressure on family and carers — practically, emotionally and financially
- avoid close relationships which involve any form of physical contact or other involvement which is likely to cause further pain
- alter behaviour: become withdrawn, tearful, angry, frustrated, depressed or demanding.

By recognising the pain it is hoped that the necessary measures may be taken to control it, or ensure it is of short duration or sufficiently managed to avoid gross inhibition of normal activity. Some clinical members of the treatment team may be responsible for prescribing surgical, chemotherapeutic or other ways of controlling pain, but the occupational therapist should share the responsibility for recognising the pain and encouraging the person to address it positively. In many situations the occupational therapist plays an active role in pain management through her skills in counselling, and by instructing the person in relaxation techniques and compensatory methods to avoid or overcome stressful activities. Such education should include the family or carers to ensure that a positive, understanding approach is maintained in the home environment.

It is also important to recognise psychological pain. This is not unique to people with the conditions discussed in this section, but a considerable number may be affected by it. Psychological pain may be closely linked to the bereavement process previously identified, where it presents as physical pain due to muscle tension, anxiety, fear or frustration. Relaxation and counselling may play vital roles in helping to control such pain.

Some people who have visible disfigurements also suffer emotional pain. This is frequently linked to anxieties regarding acceptance or rejection by others because of changed body image. Such situations require understanding and support to promote assertiveness and help build confidence so that the person can gradually become reintegrated into the community.

THE OCCUPATIONAL THERAPY PROCESS

The occupational therapy process as applied to musculoskeletal and vascular problems is the same as that used in other treatment areas. It consists of assessment, planning, implementation and evaluation. A variety of types of assessment may be used, but the most common are those involving physical measurement, the evaluation of daily living skills and work assessment. Planning and implementation of the intervention will vary according to the disorder, the individual and his particular needs.

As many of the disorders are the result of trauma, much of the early intervention will be clinically based. However, many people may require help on return to the community, either to assist with a short-term mobility problem or, where there is residual dysfunction, on a more long-term basis.

INTERVENTION GOALS

Unlike many areas where the occupational therapist is primarily involved in helping a person to adjust to residual deficit or progressive dysfunction, most of the conditions described in this section have the potential for functional improvement; indeed, with some there may be anticipation of almost complete recovery. Everyone, with the exception of the child with congenital limb absence, will have known normality, so rehabilitation will be a relearning rather than an initial learning process.

There will almost inevitably be some stage in all of these conditions where the person will be required to accept some form of dependency. This may be help with personal care following surgery, or assistance with mobility through the use of crutches or an orthosis. However, to avoid the downward disability spiral, where a short-term impairment becomes a long-term disability, it is important that this dependency does not extend beyond essential need and become an excuse for not making decisions or facing responsibility, or a weapon to gain attention. The treatment team should involve the person and his carers in the intervention programme. Early encouragement of the individual to accept responsibility for decision-making regarding treatment goals may help to prevent a downward dependency spiral. Therapy should aim to achieve the return of the person's maximum physical potential, but should not overlook the emotional implications of the impairment if the body and mind are to work together in unison.

In some instances total recovery will not be possible. Although advances in nursing care and surgical techniques have vastly increased the potential for the individual to return to an active life-style, residual dysfunction will result from such disorders as rheumatoid arthritis and osteo-arthritis, and following amputation and severe burns. In these situations management of the deficit is of vital importance. If, despite the impairment, the dysfunction can be minimised to enable the person to achieve his aspirations or goals, a satisfactory adjustment is more likely to occur. It is therefore important early in the intervention to ascertain the person's hopes for the future, to foster realistic objectives and prioritise the goals to achieve them.

A realistic understanding of the value of particular methods avoids later disappointments. The provision of orthoses and pressure garments will reduce the risk of serious disfigurement following burns. However, there will inevitably be scarring and it is important for the person to be aware of this from the start if he is to value these methods positively and not see the outcome as a failure. Modern prostheses, while much improved in design and movement potential over earlier models, will not truly replace the function of the limb and the person will need to accept and adjust to these limitations. A hip replacement can overcome the problems at an individual joint, but cannot directly positively affect the disease process in other parts of the body.

APPROACHES

The occupational therapist may use a number

of approaches when treating people affected by the conditions described in this section. The most commonly used approaches are humanistic, psychosocial, compensatory and biomechanical. Frequently there is overlap in the use of these approaches, particular aspects of each being used to attain specific goals at each stage of the programme. Biomechanical principles, for example, are important in the achievement of physical mobility, while the compensatory approach may be more applicable in the early stages following injury or surgery, to compensate for temporary loss of function. This may be gradually phased out in favour of biomechanical principles as recovery progresses. If the improvement is incomplete a return to the compensatory approach may be necessary to assist the person to compensate for residual dysfunction.

Humanistic and psychosocial principles are utilised in almost all areas. Occupational therapy is concerned with physical, psychological and social aspects of living and the therapist's philosophy is based in recognition of each person's volition, individuality and potential.

Occasionally, other approaches may be used. These may be specifically directed to psychological processes to facilitate recovery or promote progress. Frequently they are concerned with the acceptance of and positive adjustment to changed circumstances. For example, desensitisation techniques and assertion skills may be of assistance when coping with disfigurement following burns, limb injuries or amputation, and the use of other approaches to promote learning and adjustment may be necessary for the confused elderly amputee, or the person with depression resulting from chronic pain.

CONCLUSION

It is important for all members of the rehabilitation team to view the disorders considered in this section in context. In the past many such disorders have been seen from a predominantly physical perspective — the effects of the damage on the musculoskeletal and vascular systems of the body — and have been treated accordingly. Knowledge of these effects and their treatment is crucial to physical recovery, but equally important is the recognition of the totality of the psychosocial effects of such disorders. The understanding of the mechanics of activity and equipment, the provision of orthoses or prostheses, or the adaptation of techniques and the environment may meet the person's physical requirements, but awareness of his personality, stresses, aspirations, and life-style priorities, and of his need for education and emotional support, are equally important for successful rehabilitation.

FURTHER READING

Guyton A C 1987 Human physiology and mechanisms of disease, 4th edn. W B Saunders, Philadelpia
Hopkins H, Smith H 1988 Willard and Spackman's occupational therapy, 7th edn. J B Lippincott, Philadelphia

Kubler-Ross E 1969 On death and dying. Tavistock, London
Versluys H P 1989 Psychosocial accommodation to physical disability. In: Trombly C (ed) Occupational therapy for physical dysfunction, 3rd edn. Williams & Wilkins, Baltimore

23

Amputation

Jean Colburn*   Vivienne Ibbotson†

INTRODUCTION

Amputation may occur at any age as the result of injury, systemic disease or malformation. Occupational therapy aims to assist the affected person to attain the optimum level of function and independence following amputation. An understanding of the causes of amputation and their functional implications is necessary to explain why particular rehabilitation approaches are favoured in different situations. Physical and psychosocial problems associated with the loss of a limb and the problems associated with various prostheses are discussed. The chapter then focuses on principles of assessment and treatment, before addressing specific issues pertinent to upper and lower limb amputation.

Theoretical approaches enable the therapist to identify and focus on the specific needs of different groups in terms of physical capacity, age and prognosis. Many elderly people whose amputation results from peripheral vascular disease will be predominantly treated in a compensatory adaptive frame of reference, as wheelchair management will be essential, and wheelchair living may be indicated if the energy cost of ambulation is too high. A young traumatic amputee will need a biomechanical approach to regain maximum physical restoration, while a developmental approach is essential to meet the needs of injured children or infants with congenital limb deficiencies.

*Introduction and lower limb
†Upper limb

The occupational therapist must be sensitive to the individual needs of each person throughout intervention, bearing in mind that the partial or complete loss of a limb has profound psychological implications for the individual and those close to him.

PRINCIPLES OF REHABILITATION

Amputees require highly specialised individual treatment for continuing lifetime needs, which can only be provided through interdisciplinary collaboration. Genuine teamwork, when individuals with special knowledge work interdependently to attain a common goal, is essential. In each case the amputee is the most important member of the team.

Amputee teams are generally based in acute hospitals with outpatient and rehabilitation services, and are linked to Disablement Services Centres (DSCs) which are responsible for the provision, fabrication and fitting of prostheses. The team usually consists of the surgeon (vascular or orthopaedic), physiotherapist, occupational therapist, nurse, social worker and prosthetist, who will deal with day-to-day problems and will call on other disciplines or community-based practitioners for assistance when needed. The DSC provides ongoing prosthetic care, and may have facilities for limb training from physiotherapists, occupational therapists and prosthetists. However, the needs of each person are met more efficiently if all aspects of care (acute, rehabilitative and prosthetic) are provided by the same experienced team of health care professionals. Team members must be highly skilled in their own area of expertise and knowledgeable about every aspect of the amputee service (policy, legislation, new vascular and orthopaedic techniques, developments in prostheses and innovative therapeutic regimes).

Amputees need a continuing care regime. Many amputations result from previous medical conditions which may have necessitated earlier hospital admissions. This medical history will be important in 'setting the agenda' for acute post-surgical care and the whole rehabilitation programme. Continuing care is needed on discharge (either through outpatient clinics or community-based services) to monitor medical status and prevent secondary problems resulting from poorly fitting prostheses or inadequate self-care. Essential elements of health promotion should be reinforced to maintain active independence. This regime may be achieved through partnership with voluntary agencies, community special interest groups or support groups.

FRAMES OF REFERENCE GUIDING INTERVENTION

An understanding of the precipitating medical conditions will influence the framework of intervention, the goals of treatment and the choice of prosthesis. A thorough knowledge of the pathology and medical and surgical management of chronic circulatory conditions resulting in amputation helps the therapist to focus on the causes of functional limitations and determine a realistic baseline for treatment goals. This should be combined with a sound knowledge of biomechanics, the control mechanisms of different prostheses and the available options of prosthetic components for the individual's needs. The therapist should also be aware of the ways in which causation, post-surgical and prosthetic complications, and psychosocial or cultural background can affect the outcome of intervention.

CAUSATION AND FUNCTIONAL IMPLICATIONS OF AMPUTATION

Amputations may be acquired or congenital. Acquired amputations are secondary to chronic medical conditions or severe trauma. Congenital 'amputations' are in fact malformations of limbs at the fetal stage of development.

Peripheral vascular disease (PVD)

This systemic condition, which accounts for 80% of lower limb amputations, primarily affects people in the older age group. Arterial disease gradually impairs circulation, and if this cannot be restored by vascular surgery, amputation becomes necessary. Many people with vascular disease also have additional problems such as hypertension or diabetes, and cardiorespiratory function may also be impaired. Prognosis is poor as circulation to the other limb is usually impaired. Many people become bilateral amputees within five years.

Functional implications

People admitted for amputation as the result of PVD will have had longstanding disease. They may well have had previous vascular surgery in an attempt to save the limb, and their mobility and general health will have gradually deteriorated. Symptoms of advanced lower limb ischaemia will have been present for several weeks, causing progressive reduction in mobility, severe burning pain and frequent sleepless nights, such that the person is generally exhausted and in poor physical condition on admission to hospital. People with diabetes also frequently have a history of ischaemic ulceration and gangrene of the toes. In addition to these medical problems, many people are elderly and have reduced sensory skills, as well as other problems associated with the ageing process. Some people may be slightly confused or forgetful, due to generalised atherosclerosis, or to stress and anxiety associated with admission to hospital.

Trauma

This is the second most common cause of amputation and the principle reason for loss of an upper limb. Causes include industrial injuries, severe burns or road traffic accidents. The amputation may be immediate (the limb severed at the time of the accident) or delayed (occurring later because of deficient circulation or inadequate healing). Major trauma may have also resulted in other injuries, which will affect rehabilitation.

Functional implications

The mechanism of injury may damage the soft tissues in a number of different ways:

- Crush injuries affect all soft tissues (peripheral nerves, blood vessels, muscle tissues and ligaments) as well as causing bone fractures. Impaired circulation retards healing, and oedema may delay prosthetic fitting. Diminished cutaneous sensation or kinaesthetic awareness may also affect limb training.

- Traction injuries may tear ligaments and damage proximal joints, as well as damaging tissues at the site of amputation. Proximal joint damage or instability may limit the choice of prosthesis or its components.

- Clean 'guillotine' type severance of a limb, in which proximal joints and muscles are intact, may provide the best potential for rehabilitation, if the wound is not contaminated (for example by dirt or industrial materials) and does not become infected. Delayed healing may affect reconstructive surgery, which is particularly important for upper limb amputees, as range of movement and bilateral movement patterns are quickly lost with prolonged periods of immobility.

- Amputations as the result of burns are inevitably associated with serious tissue damage. Thermal burns may require skin grafting, and scar tissue formation may limit joint mobility and reduce the extensibility of affected muscle tissue. High-voltage electrical burns cause deep tissue damage, thus affecting other parts of the body.

If there are no other secondary factors involved, amputation as the result of trauma has the best potential for successful rehabilitation.

Malignancy and incurable bone disease

An amputation will only be performed as a life-saving measure for people with bone cancer or incurable bone disease, such as osteomyelitis, when other forms of treatment have not succeeded. Radical high-level surgery, such as hip disarticulation, hemipelvectomy or forequarter amputation of the upper limb, may be necessary.

Functional implications

Adverse side-effects of chemotherapy or radiotherapy (which may be continued as a precautionary measure following amputation) will affect rehabilitation. The amputee team should therefore work closely with the oncology team. High-level amputation radically reduces body mass, and consequently affects the centre of gravity and balance. Autonomic systems also need to adjust to the reduced skin area, so sweating is increased and maceration may lead to skin breakdown.

Congenital limb deficiency

Limb deformities occurring before birth are rare. They may be due to a number of possible causes, and may result in the partial or complete absence of one or more limbs, or multiple malformations of both upper and lower limbs.

Functional implications

A most important aspect of abnormality at birth is the effect on the family, as well as on the child's physical, psychological, emotional and social development. The child will largely be influenced by the degree of acceptance in the family, and the warmth and strength of family relationships. Care and support offered to the child and family by the amputee team through different stages of development in the formative years is extremely important. Each child is unique and has special needs. Prosthetic replacement and training is highly skilled, and active limb components are supplied only when the child is at the right stage of 'developmental readiness'.

PSYCHOSOCIAL AND CULTURAL FACTORS

Emotional reaction to amputation may be related to age, gender, culture and personality. Individuals who have good patterns of coping with stress or loss may adjust more easily, as it has been found that reactions to amputation are similar to those of bereavement (Pinzur et al 1988). Amputees may have a sense of numbness or restless pining, or be preoccupied with thoughts of loss. These may be accompanied by phantom limb sensations, which conflict with the reality of the changed body image. All amputations, even those which do not significantly affect function,

have an enormous impact on self-esteem. Individuals may project their own disgust with their change appearance onto others, becoming overly concerned about loss of sexual attractiveness or inadequate personal relationships, and may become depressed or more demanding (Blumenfield & Shoeps 1993). One study (Raphael 1984) found that adjustment was more difficult for individuals with rigid, compulsive, self-reliant personalities, or for those who had experienced prolonged illness, or a recent personal loss such as unemployment or retirement.

Family and significant others may also initially have feelings of anxiety, rejection or even disgust at the sight of deformity, and may find it difficult to cope with the 'stump' or with major deformities at birth. This may be associated with a sense of guilt in contributing to the accident, and the parent may feel personally responsible for the birth of a deformed child. Trauma then extends to the whole family.

The importance of cultural factors must also be recognised. Health beliefs and practices in different cultural groups must be understood and acknowledged, as their explanations of illness may be linked to social or group behaviours, rather than to Western biomedical perspectives. It is important that religious or cultural sensitivities are recognised at each stage of the rehabilitation process. Difficulties may occur with treatment by a member of the opposite sex, or for a Muslim upper limb amputee there may be religious and cultural problems associated with the use of the remaining hand for all activities of daily living. Appropriate rehabilitative care should be based on understanding and respect for the life-style and community values of each individual.

PROBLEMS RELATED TO AMPUTATION

PHANTOM LIMB SENSATION

Phantom limb sensation (PLS) is common and occurs in virtually all cases of amputation. The amputee has the sensation that the missing limb is still present and 'normal'. The limb often seems to move, and may feel hot, cold or sweaty, especially in highly innervated areas such as the hands and feet. In most instances this PLS is present immediately after surgery and often continues for weeks, months or even years. The phenomenon causes a great deal of anxiety, and must be clearly explained to the person before surgery (see Pre-operative stage, below) and included in assessments.

Phantom Limb Pain

This is a more serious problem. Phantom limb pain (PLP) usually affects only a small number of amputees, but has major functional implications. Sufferers experience severe pain (often described as 'stabbing', 'burning', 'squeezing' or 'crushing'), which is variable in frequency, intensity and duration. Onset may not occur for weeks or even years after the amputation. The reason why PLP occurs is uncertain, but it does seems to be linked with psychological and physiological mechanisms. It has been found that PLP can be precipitated by tiredness, minor injuries to the stump and tissue breakdown, and that it is exacerbated by emotional stress or cold weather. The condition is difficult to treat and may become chronic if pain persists for more than six months. It is vital to try to identify the pain 'triggers' for each person, and also to find ways of alleviating discomfort (such as heat, rest and distraction) when the pain occurs. Both aspects are very important in teaching the person self-management techniques in occupational therapy, and sometimes psychological counselling can also help to reduce stress and anxiety related to PLP.

PERIPHERAL NEUROPATHY

Peripheral neuropathy is often present in persons with diabetes mellitus and PVD, but may also occur in trauma. As peripheral nerves are 'mixed' nerves, sensory, motor or autonomic function may be impaired. This can cause problems such as: blunting of pain, heat and other protective sensations; weakness of muscles leading to foot deformity or maldistribution of pressure over

the soles of the feet; or dry, cracked skin. In each case there is an added risk related to breakdown of skin of the stump and of the unaffected limb. Great care must be taken with those with diabetes mellitus, as a combination of PVD and neuropathy can lead to intractible leg ulcers, infection and even gangrene (Bild et al 1989). Sensory testing of the feet should always be included in any occupational therapy assessment.

PROSTHETICS

Prosthetic choices relate to:

- active (functional) or cosmetic limbs
- components (joints, terminal devices)
- method of suspension
- method of activation.

Prostheses consist of an inner socket, an outer socket and a cosmetic cover. The inner socket is made from a plaster cast of the person's stump. Taking the cast is a highly skilled procedure; the result is designed to control the weight-bearing areas in the lower limb, and suspension and socket stability in the upper limb. The outer socket mirrors the unaffected limb as far as possible in length and contours, and contains the mechanics of joint replacements. In the lower limbs a soft cover is provided for comfort and cosmesis. Upper limb prostheses have interchangeable terminal devices and cosmetic hands.

Elderly people with lower limb loss usually need some form of auxiliary suspension (such as a waist band or shoulder strap) to keep the limb in correct alignment. Younger people, with good, muscular stumps, may not need this, and can be fitted with a total contact suction socket. This type of prosthesis gives more freedom of movement, but can also put more stress on the tissues of the residual limb. Most upper limb prostheses are held in place by a webbing 'harness' round the chest and axilla of the unaffected arm, which is also the mechanism for activating the terminal device. Self-suspension sockets may be used with a below-elbow prosthesis (such as a 'Muenster' socket which 'locks' over the olecranon process) if myoelectric controls are provided.

Community agencies (and educational services if necessary) should be notified in advance of final discharge plans and of any special needs or problems that are likely to arise.

AMPUTATIONS OF THE LOWER LIMB

LEVELS OF AMPUTATION

The level of amputation is very important in relation to prosthetic function. It is essential to preserve as much limb length as possible, as this will provide better 'leverage' and control in ambulation, and give the best options for prosthetic fitting. A short below-knee stump, for example, may not be able to tolerate the forces necessary to use the prosthesis effectively, even if the knee joint is intact, so additional suspension may be needed. Above all it is important to realise the high energy cost of walking for high-level amputees. At a normal walking pace the increased cost of energy for a below-knee amputee is 15–20%; for an above-knee amputee 50–70%, and for a bilateral amputee as much as 300%. This is very significant when making decisions about limb fitting or wheelchair living with elderly persons.

The significance of loss in relation to the level of amputation must also be understood in 'mechanical' terms. Figure 23.2 demonstrates this. Loss is cumulative, and it can be seen that even a forefoot amputation affects some very important components of gait. Key factors in addition to generalised weakness due to muscle loss are:

- loss of forefoot leverage for 'push-off', and control of balance in stance
- difficulty in accommodating to uneven ground (loss of inversion/eversion)
- loss of position sense (kinesthesia and proprioception of the knee joint)
- limited power and mechanical leverage of the leg (severely restricted with a short above-knee amputation)
- change in the centre of gravity (in relation to loss of body mass), affecting balance and righting reactions.

Normal walking is an 'automatic' learned re-

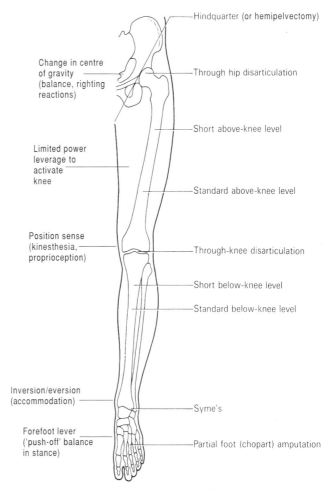

Fig. 23.2 Levels of lower limb amputation and resultant 'mechanical' loss.

sponse, based on sensory regulatory mechanisms. All amputees lose some sensory awareness as well as power, and have to relearn walking patterns and balance reactions. The loss of the knee joint is functionally very significant in this respect, and consequently every effort is made to avoid the more radical above-knee amputation. It is important to recognise that retraining postural control and righting reactions in high-level amputees requires time and effort, and because central information processing mechanisms are involved cognitive learning processes must be employed. Learning needs attention, which should initially be entirely focused on balance and control. As balance is regained, tasks in standing can gradually be introduced.

PROSTHESES

Considerable advances have been made in the design and fabrication of artificial limbs in recent years, but standard fittings are still often heavy and cumbersome. Only three of the most common types of prosthesis are illustrated here: the below-knee (BK), the above-knee (AK) and the through-hip prosthesis (THP).

It is important to note that, with the exception of Syme's and through-knee amputations (TKA) when there is no division of bone, *no weight can be taken on the end of the stump*. Designs of socket are primarily determined by the way body weight is distributed in the socket. BK amputees have patella tendon bearing (PTB) sockets in which weight is taken through the patella tendon and the medial and lateral flares of the tibia (Fig. 23.3), while AK amputees are supplied either with a quadrilateral socket, taking weight mainly through the ischial tuberosity, or with a narrow 'medial–lateral' socket in which weight is distributed over the medial and lateral aspects of the femur (Fig. 23.4). Quadrilateral sockets may

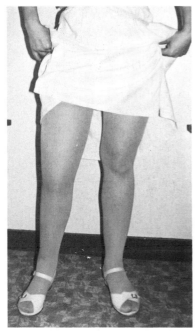

A

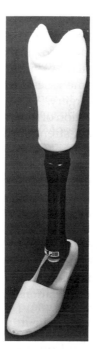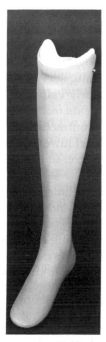

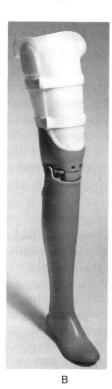

B

Fig. 23.3 Definitive below-knee prostheses. Endolite Patella Tendon Bearing limb — without and with cosmesis. (Reproduced by kind permission of Chas A. Blatchford & Sons Ltd.)

Fig. 23.4 (A) Endolite above-knee limb. (B) Above-knee prosthesis. A PRIMAP limb. (Reproduced by kind permission of Chas A. Blatchford & Sons Ltd.)

- *Toileting.* If there is a tendency toward incontinence, urgency or frequency, build in routines of regular toileting, control of fluids and regimes for bowel care, with respect to bathing and dressing.
- *Transfers.* Generally use standing pivot transfers. There must be a firm seat and mattress to avoid 'dragging', and toilet and bath aids. A high stool will be needed for the wash-basin, and one of appropriate height for the bath. Grab rails are essential.

In order to be effective, self-care routines must be habit forming and therefore carried out in a consistent, ordered manner by all members of the team. Safety is of paramount importance. Supervision is necessary while the person adjusts to poor balance and loss of position sense. If phantom limb sensations are present, it is easy for the person to forget that the limb has been amputated. To avoid the risk of falling when visiting the toilet at night, practice in the use of a bedside commode while in hospital may be advised to establish patterns for home use.

Those with lower limb amputations can cause serious problems to the stump if they knock it in the early healing stages or fall. Individuals must learn, and constantly reinforce, safe transfer techniques. A stump board will help to protect the end of the stump in a wheelchair, but the board must extend beyond the limb, and be hinged to avoid tipping the chair when the person attempts to rise.

Prosthetic stage aims are:

- *Gait training* — with temporary walking aid to evaluate potential for a permanent prosthesis.
- *Graduated weight bearing* — to increase stump and exercise tolerance.
- *Graduated standing activities in occupational therapy* — (individual or group) to develop confidence, socialisation and independence, and to promote weight transference and balance reactions.
- *Functional adaptation* — problem-solving activities related to home and community adjustment.

Early weight-bearing is important with elderly persons, to prevent loss of normal movement patterns, muscle atrophy and joint contractures.

Prosthetic training should begin as soon as possible. A temporary prosthesis may be used initially to evaluate the individual's ability to use a permanent prosthesis before a custom socket and final choice of components is made. Because of the high energy cost of walking with a 'free' knee joint, an above-knee amputee is often taught to walk with a locked knee. All amputees with PVD will need to *train* for the additional physical exertion of walking. As oxygen consumption goes up, heart rate and blood pressure will increase to accommodate the effort of ambulation, so response to effort must be monitored.

The main focus of occupational therapy should be on functional activities and safe home management techniques. Tasks in the kitchen provide an opportunity for controlled weight-bearing, problem-solving, the use of aids such as a trolley or perching stool and evaluation of the person's capacity for safely 'thinking and doing'. A visit to a local shop (using a wheelchair for outdoor mobility) may be advisable to assess problem-solving skills. The individual and the family or carer should be involved in the final stages of planning for discharge. Critical decisions have to be made on the person's capacity for independent living, on the support services needed and on a suitable regime to be followed at home. In some instances, if the home is unsuitable, alternative accommodation will have to be found. Pre-planning is therefore essential.

Trauma and malignancy

The main objective here is to *contrast* methods of management for young, active individuals with methods of management for elderly persons with PVD. In reality these categories are not quite as clear cut, as trauma and malignancy can affect people of any age.

Trauma (below-knee, above-knee)

The frame of reference in occupational therapy is primarily biomechanical, although with an injured child a developmental approach would also be needed.

Pre-prosthetic stage. The particular focus for

young people who have suffered amputation as a result of trauma is physical restoration. Treatment in physiotherapy and occupational therapy is aimed at gaining maximum strength and range of movement in the stump and proximal joints of the affected limb, and at increasing overall strength and general physical tolerance.

Treatment should be intensive, and can be rapidly progressive (unless there are complications from associated injuries). Weight-bearing can start within a few days with an early post-surgical prosthetic fitting (EPSF). Individuals may be provided with various types of prosthesis, such as a plastic air splint to control post-operative oedema and promote healing, or a pneumatic pylon (PPAM aid). This can be used five to seven days post-operatively (before sutures are removed), for partial weight-bearing with crutches.

It is most important for below-knee amputees to strengthen the quadriceps muscle and regain full extension of the knee. Resisted activities for the *unaffected* leg, with the residual limb supported in a sling (such as a treadle lathe, Fig. 23.6) will, through reciprocal innervation and static contractions of the quadriceps muscle, 'exercise' the stump. It will also strengthen the unaffected limb and trunk muscles at the same time, as strong static contractions are needed to stabilise

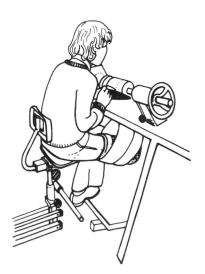

Fig. 23.6 Using the lathe to encourage static work of the quadriceps in the slung limb.

the pelvis during this activity if seated on a bicycle-type seat. The 'quadriceps switch' may also be of value at this stage, and can be used with a 'timer' to control powered equipment if required.

Prosthetic stage. Intensive treatment, carefully monitoring stump tolerance, should lead to rapid progress at this stage. Modular prostheses may be used initially (temporary standard-sized sockets, with pylon and components) to accommodate the stump until 'shrinkage' is complete and able to tolerate the custom-made limb. Workshop activities in occupational therapy provide excellent opportunities to increase standing tolerance and weight transference, and can also be used for job simulation tasks. Recreational activities that encourage spontaneous movement responses (such as table tennis, darts and bowls) will help to increase confidence. Heavy work-related skills and problem-solving tasks (such as outdoor work, managing rough ground and inclines, and general lifting and carrying) should be included in the later stages. Advice should also be given on leisure pursuits, as special components can be provided for sports activities.

Trauma or malignancy (Hip disarticulation or hemipelvectomy)

The frames of reference used in occupational therapy are primarily adaptive and compensatory.

Pre-prosthetic stage. The main difference in tissue response to injury between high-level and low-level amputations of the lower limb is that there is little, if any, post-operative oedema in high-level amputations. The pre-prosthetic stage can therefore be quite short, possibly only three or four weeks, and ends when healing is sound.

It is very important for individuals with this level of amputation to be mobile as soon as possible. In most cases of malignancy amputees are young and fit, and can stand on the sound leg two or three days after surgery. It is essential to avoid any prolonged period of immobility, as this causes generalised weakness and loss of self-confidence. Balance will in any case be affected because of the change in the centre of gravity, but most individuals can use crutches, and, as

looked. A basic opposition plate can provide a degree of function if desired.

TREATMENT
Pre-prosthetic stage

Congenital

Despite research, no reason has yet been found to account for the fact that babies are still being born with limb deficiencies. It is essential that these children and their families are referred as early as possible to a Limb Centre. A firm relationship with the rehabilitation team, comprising the doctor, prosthetist, occupational therapist and nurse, built on trust and confidence and promoting a positive attitude, can then begin. In many cases a prosthesis will not be prescribed until the baby is approximately four months old (although this varies from centre to centre). However, the parents can be supported, counselled and helped in every way possible to come to terms with what they will inevitably feel to be a failure on their part in not producing a perfect child.

The need for parents to be given the opportunity to discuss hopes and fears for the future, even at such an early stage, should be recognised. Often the best people to help with this situation are parents who are already coping with a limb-deficient baby. They will be aware of what the family is experiencing and can supply first-hand knowledge of problems and possible solutions.

Regular contact with the rehabilitation team at the centre is important, even if a limb is not to be prescribed for some months, as the family should not be left to feel isolated or uninformed. Support for the families of limb deficient children is also available through 'Reach', the Association for children with hand or arm deficiency.

Acquired

It is not always possible for the occupational therapist to be involved in the individual's pre-operative care, particularly if the amputation is an emergency procedure following trauma as opposed to elective surgery necessitated by disease. More frequently, amputees are referred to the occupational therapist after discharge from hospital, when healing has occurred and the limb is ready for the first prosthesis.

If a referral is received pre-operatively, it is necessary to assess each individual case most carefully. A realistic approach, together with a positive outlook, should be adopted, and support and counselling should be offered to both the amputee and his family. It should always be remembered that everyone close to the person is affected by the amputation and that they should therefore always be included in the management of the situation.

Surgery will try to produce an area where the skin is in good condition on the remaining part of the limb, with sensation as close to normal as possible. The scar tissue should be located in the best position available, where the prosthesis will not cause undue discomfort or pressure. The bone needs to be stable, secured by muscles, with sufficient soft tissue cover to form a protective pad. To avoid future problems from hypersensitivity, nerve endings are buried as deeply as possible. However, it must be remembered that circumstances do not always allow for all the preferred criteria to be met, particularly when the limb is severely damaged during trauma.

Following surgery, the 'stump' should be firmly bandaged to help control oedema. As the amputee is usually not able to do this for himself, the process is often abandoned on discharge from hospital because of the inconsistency in techniques used by other people. Provision of a length of Tubigrip to form a sock can be a useful alternative. The fit should be such that the sock does not roll down, forming a garter.

Mobility should be retained in the remaining part of the limb, through activity which demands a full range of movement. This will promote good circulation and assist the healing process while building up the muscle strength necessary for early acceptance of a prosthesis.

It is not always necessary to provide a temporary prosthesis or gauntlet, as it may be possible to fit a prosthesis as soon as the wound is fully healed. Should there be a prolonged period before a prosthesis is prescribed, however, the therapist should discuss this with the amputee to explain the necessity of providing a gauntlet as a temporary measure. This will enable the early return of bimanual activities and an improved level of independence.

If the dominant hand has been affected the person is usually advised to commence activity to promote a change in dominance in fine dextrous activities as soon as possible. The individual will need to develop skill in controlling his new dominant hand, as well as the artificial limb; therefore the earlier rehabilitation is initiated, the better the outcome is likely to be.

All aspects of personal ADL should be assessed. This is an important area directly related to the person's independence and one in which he can achieve early success and a boost to morale.

Prosthetic training

Congenital

When the baby is approximately four months old, many doctors recommend the fitting of the first artificial limb. This will take the form of a light plastic one-piece socket and fixed hand, fitted onto the baby's arm with an elastic cuff to prevent it slipping off easily. The fitting of this arm immediately completes the baby's body image and will encourage him to be two-handed. At this early stage he will be able to hold large toys in both hands and will begin to become accustomed to the idea of having another hand to help when playing. It will help reduce stares from strangers when away from home, as the baby will appear two-handed.

It is considered appropriate for a functional prosthesis to be introduced from approximately 18 months of age onwards, although a new development is currently being evaluated whereby younger children may learn to use a small powered hand (the Scamp hand), operated either by means of a pull switch or a single-site electrode. This provides voluntary opening with automatic spring closing. It is important to recognise that a child cannot fully operate a prosthesis until he has reached the appropriate stage of 'developmental readiness', so developmental testing is an important component of prosthetic training. For

a below-elbow absence there are two basic designs of limb, although research and development are constantly being devoted to the upgrading of these devices. The two designs are:

1. The child's version of an adult body-powered functional limb, comprising a socket, a wrist unit and a terminal device — either a small hand or a small plastic-covered split hook, both of which rotate and lock into any one of several positions on the wrist rotary.

2. The 'Child Amputee Prosthetic Program' (CAPP), which originated in the USA. Although very different in appearance, it offers the same advantages of function as the limb described above. However, it provides a better gross grip.

Both types of limb are attached and activated by a somewhat complicated strap arrangement (Fig. 23.8) which passes across the shoulders and under the opposite armpit. Once a prescription for a limb has been decided upon a cast is taken, as described on p. 639.

Objects can be picked up and dropped by using shoulder and elbow movement to open and close the hook. At this stage, several training sessions will be arranged to encourage full use of the limb and to show the family how best to supervise activities at home between sessions.

Regular appointments are recommended to monitor changes in needs, particularly as the child grows and develops.

Acquired

Once the wound has healed and most of the oedema has subsided, a referral will be made to a Limb Centre for general assessment. This will be carried out by members of the rehabilitation team. The most important team members, however, are the amputee himself and members of his family who attend the initial visit.

At this point the individual may be feeling extremely vulnerable, frightened and worried, although he will probably not admit to this until much later when recalling his initial feelings. It is therefore important to establish a relaxed, informative relationship while instilling confidence for future visits to the centre. Both the prosthetist

A

B

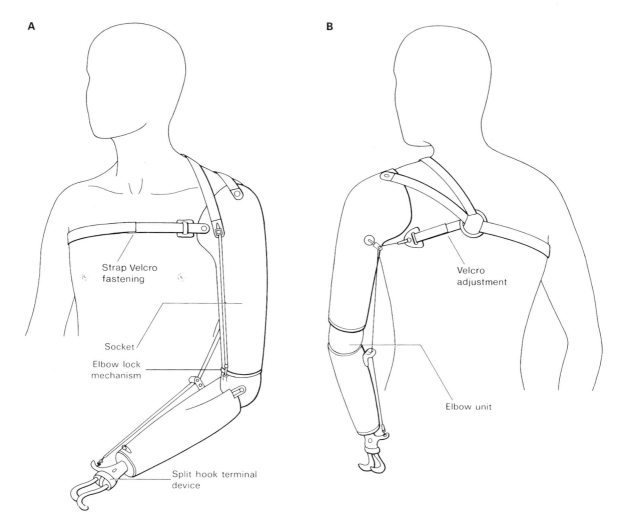

Strap Velcro
fastening

Socket

Elbow lock
mechanism

Split hook terminal
device

Velcro
adjustment

Elbow unit

Fig. 23.10 Above elbow prosthesis — alternative suspension system. (A) Front view. (B) Back view.

from two to four weeks after the first visit to the centre for the prosthesis to be delivered. From this stage the occupational therapist will take over the main part of treatment and education.

THE ROLE OF THE OCCUPATIONAL THERAPIST

The role of the occupational therapist is defined in the standards and guidelines document *Occupational Therapy in the Rehabilitation of Upper Limb Amputees and Limb Deficient Children*, produced by the College of Occupational Therapists Clinical Interest Group in Orthotics Prosthetics and

Wheelchairs (1995). As always, the occupational therapist's ultimate aim is to rehabilitate the individual to a maximum level of independence. In working towards this end the therapist will, of necessity, adopt various approaches which frequently overlap. With regard to the physical aspects of the disability, the compensatory approach is implemented throughout, although the success of this will depend considerably on how the individual's psychological and emotional stresses are overcome through the therapist's use of a humanistic approach.

Biomechanical principles may also be used to maintain or improve function in the proximal

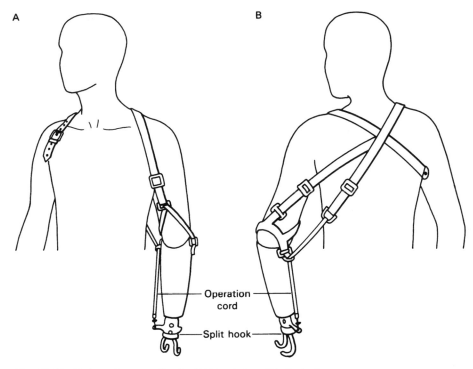

Fig. 23.11 Below-elbow prosthesis. (A) Front view. (B) Back view.

parts of the amputated limb, and developmental techniques will be used with children.

It cannot be stated too strongly that every person is an individual and should be treated as such. The amputation is only a part of the whole problem to be faced, and it is incumbent upon the therapist to take a sensitive and realistic overview of the situation.

Although this discussion has focused on the provision of functional artificial limbs, an amputee will occasionally need to achieve independence either with a purely cosmetic prosthesis or without a prosthesis at all, and it is equally important to support, counsel and advise this group of people. Congenital amputees have particular concerns at each stage of development — schooling, adolescence and vocational training — and need continuity in care and guidance.

Initially, practice in using an artificial limb aims to reinforce the information given by the prosthetist. This ensures an understanding of the limb, its parts and how they work, and the best method for the individual concerned for putting on and taking off the prosthesis. Care of the limb, particularly hygiene of the socket, is also stressed.

Once understanding of the hardware is achieved the next stage is to learn how to gain control of the limb and its terminal devices, using it effectively, naturally and appropriately. A programme of practice and learning ensues, the length of which varies considerably according to the individual, a double amputee taking considerably longer to achieve independence and prosthetic competence. In all cases, the time required will be greatly affected by motivation, home circumstances, available transport and travelling distance.

TRAINING

The therapist should be able to demonstrate the full potential of the limb and terminal devices through realistic activities. She must bear in mind throughout the programme that tolerance to the limb varies from person to person and will need to be gradually increased over a period of time.

It is advisable to utilise the arm mitts provided by the Limb Centre over the stump to improve comfort at the socket. Wearing a T-shirt can also prevent the straps rubbing on the skin during the initial stages.

It is usual to begin learning control of the limb through using a split hook. This is operated by exerting tension on a cord attachment by means of the amputee's own body power.

Whether the affected limb is the dominant or non-dominant arm, control of the prosthesis needs to be learned primarily using one-handed activities with the artificial limb. This can be gained by providing a series of objects of different dimensions to be gripped. Initially the tasks set should be easy to complete, thereby affording immediate success and building confidence.

Progression continues through activities graded from light to heavy, thick to thin, and large to small, working in different planes. Ultimately, the amputee should be capable of holding an egg or slicing a tomato without crushing the shell or skin.

Once achieved, a basic level of control can be put into practice in a project involving a variety of manipulative skills. Woodwork, for example, would require the drawing and measuring of a pattern, cutting out, sawing, planing and sanding wood, and many other tasks using both limbs in a natural, functional manner. The individual's continuation of hobbies and pastimes should be discussed, as this is as important as the maintenance of routine daily activities.

Future prospects should now be considered regarding returning to work, if this has not been previously discussed. It may be necessary to involve the Disablement Employment Advisor (DEA) for guidance on retraining possibilities. Contact with previous employers may be relevant here.

When good control has been gained and a level of confidence achieved, only perseverance in practising at home will improve speed and efficiency with the prosthesis. Provided motivation is good and there are no problems with the prosthesis and its comfort, the amputee will be well on his way to becoming a regular wearer and user.

TERMINAL DEVICES

This is the term used to describe the detachable implements which can be fitted into the wrist section of the prosthesis. A number of different grasping, manipulating and holding movements are carried out by the complicated and sophisticated mechanism of the human hand. Unfortunately these movements cannot be reproduced by any one terminal device; therefore, a large number of different devices have been devised to assist in a considerable number of activities ranging from fishing and golf to digging and driving (Fig. 23.12).

When assessing a new limb-wearer the therapist should bear in mind that the fewer devices required, the less frustrating limb-wearing will become. One device may perform several tasks, thereby necessitating fewer changes and reducing the amount of 'luggage' to carry from place to place.

The most useful terminal device by far is the split hook, and this is usually the first one to be provided. Its simplicity of design and multiplicity of uses is unsurpassed by any of the other devices. Often it is almost the only tool an amputee will use. It is made of aluminium alloy, stainless steel or carbon fibre and is comprised of two curved, rubber-lined jaws, one fixed and one movable, both tapered at the end to provide a fine grip. Grip strength is determined by the number of rubber bands attached to the hook, each one providing approximately 1½ lbs of force. (This does not apply to the carbon fibre hook.) The hook, as with other actively controlled devices, is opened by exerting tension on the operating cord and closed by relaxing that tension.

By pre-positioning the hook into any one of the 12 wrist positions, the wearer can use it for holding, carrying, pushing or picking up objects.

Assessment with and provision of tools such as quick-grip pliers, a universal tool holder or spade grip may enable a return to previous employment. Emphasis should be placed on the fact that these are tools, much the same as tools previously used in employment, even though they operate by slightly different means.

As always, assessment for terminal devices

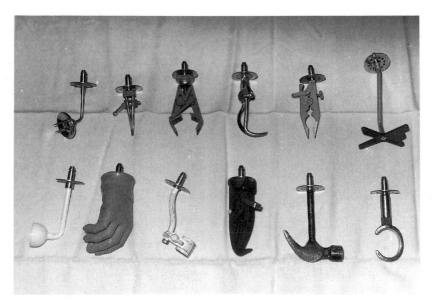

Fig. 23.12 A variety of terminal devices frequently in use. Top row: potato holder, tweezers, universal tool holder, split hook, long-nose pliers, snooker cue rest. Bottom row: driving appliance, mechanical hand, golf appliance, carbon fibre split hook, claw hammer, Williams 'C' hook.

must be geared towards provision for individual requirements (Figs 23.13 and 23.14).

PSYCHOLOGICAL ASPECTS

Although the psychological impact of amputation has already been discussed in general terms, there are certain considerations of specific relevance to upper limb amputees.

In addition to the obvious practical problems that result from being born with limb absence or from losing part of an arm, many people in these circumstances are burdened by unresolved psychological problems. These are frequently well hidden as the years pass, but are nevertheless tucked away ready to reveal themselves on unforeseen occasions.

The immediate shock and worry occasioned by the birth of a baby with a limb deficiency is taken on board by the parents. As the child grows towards adulthood there will be the inevitable questions to be answered — if answers can indeed be found — as to 'What happened?' or 'Why me?' or 'How do I cope?' However, many of these children grow up to be quite remarkable

adults, coping with everyday activities in the only way they know how, achieving independence by sometimes unconventional methods, but nevertheless achieving it.

To lose an arm or part of an arm in later life takes on a different meaning because one is losing a part of one's body that has functioned quite automatically in everyday tasks. How to carry on in the same way must seem an insurmountable problem. This may be particularly difficult when there has been, as in most cases, no time to at least try to prepare for this shattering event. Suddenly the body is noticeably incomplete; gestures of anger, frustration, caring and comforting are less easy to implement. From carrying out daily activities independently one is suddenly dependent on someone else for even the smallest task.

Allowance must be made for a period akin to grieving over the death of a close friend or relative. Support and counselling should be available to help work through this period, in which the person must feel that he has no future.

Goals should be realistically set, and a positive outlook encouraged from the beginning. It should

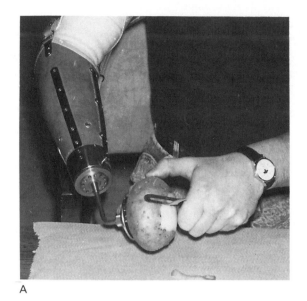

A

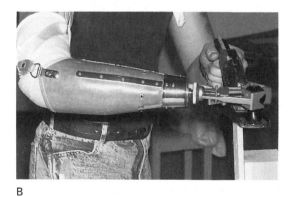

B

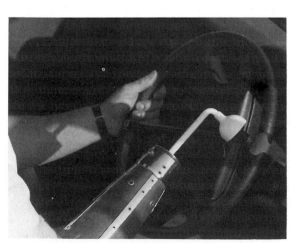

C

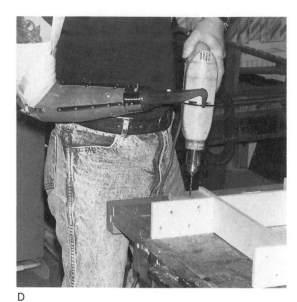

D

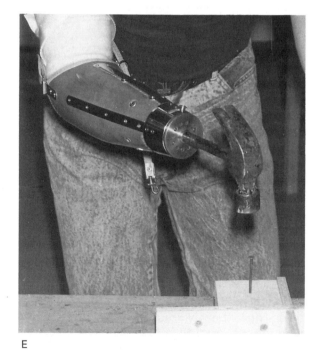

E

Fig. 23.13 Use of some of the appliances shown in Fig. 23.12. (Note: the user is wearing a heavy-duty socket, rather than the more commonly prescribed lightweight socket.) (A) Potato holder. (B) Universal tool holder. (C) Driving appliance. (D) Carbon fibre split hook. (E) Claw hammer.

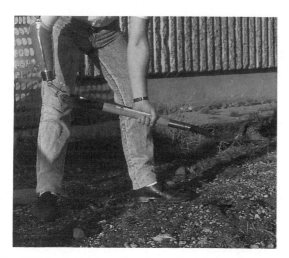

Fig. 23.14 Gardening using the spade grip attachment.

never be assumed that anyone other than the amputee knows what it is like suddenly to have lost a part of his body, or what effect this is likely to have on life in the future.

As and when necessary, the therapist should, in a sensitive manner, provide as much information as is available, together with practical help for coming to terms with the loss and subsequent use of an artificial limb.

If the situation lends itself to this, introducing the individual to another amputee with a similar background (e.g. with regard to age, sex, level of loss or circumstances leading to the loss) could be of great value. This should not be entered into lightly as it could do more harm than good if the timing is wrong or the choice of amputee is not made with care.

PHANTOM SENSATIONS

The majority of amputees will experience a degree of phantom limb sensation (PLS) and pain (PLP), as described on p. 639. The duration, severity and form of PLS and PLP vary considerably, and there is no acknowledged framework by which these feelings can be explained. Sometimes, if the amputation is due to trauma, the hand can be 'felt' in what seems to be its last position prior to the moment of impact. Other sensations range from 'pins and needles', itching

and cramp to simply a feeling that the absent part is still there.

These sensations occasionally become so extreme as to be described by the amputee as actual pains, although the pains are more likely to be felt in the stump. Care must be taken to identify the nature and extent of these feelings and, if they persist, it may be necessary to arrange for further physical or psychological treatment, after consultation with the relevant medical staff specialising in this field of work.

However, in the majority of cases where such sensations do remain, they settle to a manageable level which can be tolerated and accepted. Early exercises in stump desensitisation often help considerably in alleviating this disturbing reminder of the amputation.

MYOELECTRIC CONTROLS

Myoelectric controls are only one type of external power control unit available for operating upper limb prostheses. Available in North America and other European countries for over 25 years, trials were commissioned in Britain in 1978, when powered hands with myoelectric controls were provided for pre-school children. The trials were successful, and this type of prosthesis is now widely used for both children and adults.

Myoelectric control systems can be used to operate any device, such as a powered hand, wrist rotation unit or elbow unit. Surface electrodes embedded in the socket pick up minute electrical impulses from voluntary muscle contractions in the stump. Each signal is then amplified and processed to act as a control mechanism for a selected function. For example, with an electric hand one muscle site is needed to open the hand and another to close it. Power for all functions is provided by a battery which is either worn externally (attached to a belt with young amputees) or incorporated into the socket (Figs 23.15 and 23.16). Batteries must be regularly recharged (with continual usage this may be necessary every 24 hours).

An important advantage with this type of prosthesis is that an amputee can often have a self-suspended socket without any additional

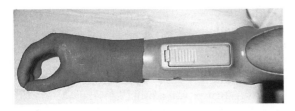

Fig. 23.15 Myoelectric controls for powered hand with battery incorporated into the socket.

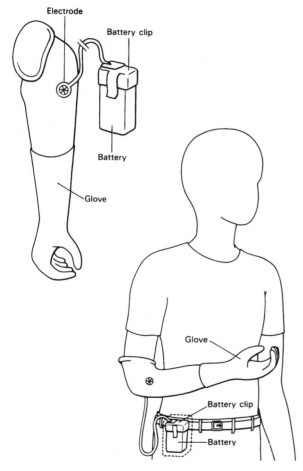

Fig. 23.16 Self-suspended below-elbow prosthesis with myoelectric controls for battery powered hand (battery is attached to belt).

crease in weight (mainly located in the powered hand), and the delayed movement response. Operation of a split hook requires only one brief movement, whereas the myoelectric hand depends on the muscle signal activating the electrode and this signal being amplified and processed before operating the mechanism of the hand. Hand movements, too, are relatively slow to give the amputee control of the grasp/release mechanism.

Developments now allow for a wrist disconnect unit to be fitted, allowing the interchange of a powered hand with a powered hook, or static appliances previously used with body powered prostheses when correctly adapted.

Myoelectric control systems are sophisticated and expensive, and with a growing child there are additional problems related to the need for continual modification of the socket. A careful team assessment of all individuals who might benefit from such a prosthesis is necessary before any decision is made. This must be based on a realistic appraisal of needs and functional potential. Unless the amputee is able to look after the prosthesis properly it can break down and require a great deal of maintenance. It is therefore important not to raise expectations too high.

ADVANTAGES AND DISADVANTAGES OF UPPER LIMB PROSTHESES

Below is a short list of some of the points to consider with regard to the wearing of an artificial arm, applicable to both congenital and acquired amputees:

Advantages

- An artificial limb completes the body image and prevents people staring
- Whichever side is affected, it will provide a non-dominant hand
- Bimanual activities can be learned or recommenced
- A return to work may be accelerated by using the limb
- If expertise is gained with an artificial arm, an amputee will still be reasonably

straps or 'harness' (Fig. 23.16), which aids freedom of movement and comfort in wearing, and the most satisfactory results have been obtained with short below-elbow amputations. The main disadvantages with this type of limb are the in-

independent should anything happen to the remaining arm

- Where a limb has been provided for a congenital absence, the child will grow up with an image of himself as being two-handed. It will also provide experience upon which he can base a later decision on whether an artificial arm is, or is not, beneficial to his life-style.

Disadvantages

- Depending on the site, important sensory feedback and sometimes movement can be impeded
- The limb and straps may be heavy, hot and uncomfortable, particularly in hot weather
- A skin reaction may arise from the materials used or an existing skin condition may be aggravated. This can usually be resolved but it takes time and perseverance to find a satisfactory solution
- Self-consciousness may be increased, especially in teenage years when many individuals are particularly sensitive concerning appearance and performance
- Frequent visits to a Limb Centre will be necessary, especially during the growth years of children and the initial stages of rehabilitation of adults. This may cause problems if there is difficulty with travelling arrangements or obtaining time off work.

One of the strongest arguments for wearing and gaining expertise with an artificial arm is the desirability of the amputee reaching a level of independence whereby he would not become totally dependent on others should he, for example, fall and fracture his remaining arm. However, account must always be taken of the amputee's feelings and aspirations before realistic intervention strategies can be put forward by the rehabilitation team.

BRACHIAL PLEXUS LESIONS

These are usually caused by trauma (often a motorcycle accident) and predominantly affect young men.

In the majority of people, the damage is irreparable because of stretching, tearing or avulsion of the roots directly from the spinal cord. Upper trunk lesions are more common than lower lesions.

At some stage when further recovery seems unlikely, a flail arm orthosis may be indicated. This appliance will enable the hand to be brought into a functional position and will supplement elbow flexion (Fig. 23.17). The ability to continue with bimanual activities will thus be maintained and, ideally, employment prospects improved.

Occasionally, where there has been complete avulsion, it may be necessary to consider amputation as an alternative option. This should, wherever possible, be discussed at length with the person affected and the implications of leaving the flail arm intact and of amputating made

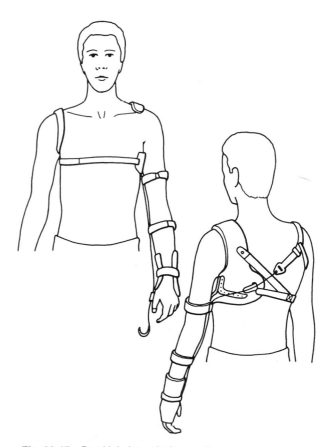

Fig. 23.17 Brachial plexus lesion appliance.

known. If surgery is decided upon, the management will be the same as for other amputees.

CONCLUSION

Information in this chapter is applicable to relatively straightforward cases of recent amputation. The main ingredient to successful rehabilitation is motivation. Without this, it is extremely difficult to encourage maximum potential with or without a prosthesis. However, in certain circumstances, motivation may not be enough. If a limb has been amputated because of disease, the type of treatment in progress for that disease may influence the timing of referral to a Limb Centre. In such cases all efforts will be focused on controlling the disease, and the amputation itself will fade into the background. The individual will still need support and encouragement, however, in gaining expertise and confidence with the remaining limb. As much information as possible should be provided regarding the future.

At times the ageing process brings with it problems such as rheumatoid arthritis, Parkinson's disease or circulatory disorders. Conditions such as these will have a bearing on the level of independence the amputee can achieve. Difficulties may also arise if the amputee has lost a partner who used to assist with some of the more difficult aspects of daily routine.

It is therefore necessary to assess the potential of the new amputee and to reassess the situation of the long-standing amputee who is facing a change in circumstances. It is essential to approach each amputee with a flexible and realistic attitude, and with an awareness of individual needs.

USEFUL ADDRESSES

British Limbless Ex-Servicemen's Association
185/187 High Road
Chadwell Heath
Essex RM6 6NA

Disabled Living Foundation
380/384 Harrow Road
London W9 2HU

Limbless Association (formerly National Association for Limbless Disabled)
31 The Mall, Ealing
London W5 2PX

Reach: Association for children
with hand or arm deficiency
(Contact the local DSC for
current details of secretary)

REMAP G.B.
'Hazeldene'
Ightham
Sevenoaks
Kent TN15 9AD

Royal Association for Disability and Rehabilitation
25 Mortimer Street
London W1N 8AB

REFERENCES

Bild D E, Selby J V, Sinnock P et al 1989 Lower-extremity amputation in people with diabetes: epidemiology and prevention. Diabetes Care 12(1): 24–31

Blumenfield M, Schoeps M M 1993 Psychological care of the burn and trauma patient. Williams & Wilkins, Baltimore

Clinical Interest Group in Orthotics, Prosthetics and Wheelchairs 1995 Occupational therapy in the rehabilitation of upper limb amputees and limb deficient children: standards and guidelines. College of Occupational Therapists, London

Colburn J 1977 Myoelectric controls — a challenge to occupational therapists? Canadian Journal of Occupational Therapy 44(1): 31–39

Collin C, Wade D T, Davies S et al 1988 The Barthel Index: a reliability study. International Disability Studies 10(2): 61–63

Derogatis L R 1983 Psychosocial adjustment to illness scale (PAIS and PAIS-SR) scoring: procedures and administration, Manual 1. Clinical Psychometric Research, Baltimore

Lerner R K, Esterhai J L, Polomono R C et al 1991 Psychosocial, functional and quality of life assessment of patients with post-traumatic fracture, nonunion, chronic refractory osteomyelitis and lower extremity amputation. Archives of Physical Medicine and Rehabilitation 72: 122–126

Malone J M, Snyder M, Anderson G et al 1989 Prevention of amputation by diabetic education. American Journal of Surgery 158: 520–524

Meenan R F, Gertman P M, Mason J H 1980 Measuring health status in arthritis: the arthritis impact measurement scales. Arthritis & Rheumatism 23(2): 146–152

Moss S E, Klein R, Klein B E K 1992 The prevalence and incidence of lower extremity amputation in a diabetic population. Archives of Internal Medicine 152: 610–616

Nissen S J, Newman W P 1992 Factors influencing reintegration to normal living after amputation. Archives of Physical Medicine and Rehabilitation 73: 548–551

Pinzur M S, Graham G, Osterman H 1988 Psychologic testing in amputation rehabilitation. Clinical Orthopaedics and Related Research 229: 236–240

Raphael B 1984 The anatomy of bereavement: a handbook for the caring professions. Hutchinson, London

White E A 1992 Wheelchair stump boards and their use with lower limb amputees. British Journal of Occupational Therapy 55(5): 174–178

Wing D C, Hittenberger D A 1989 Energy-storing prosthetic feet. Archives of Physical Medicine and Rehabilitation 70: 330–335

Wood-Dauphinee S, Williams J I 1987 Reintegration to normal living as a proxy to quality of life. Journal of Chronic Disease 40(6): 491–499

FURTHER READING

Atkin D J, Meier I I, Robert H (eds) 1989 Comprehensive management of the upper limb amputee. Springer Verlag, London

Ayoub M M, Solis M M, Rogers J J 1993 Thru-Knee Amputation: the operation of choice for non-ambulatory patients. American Surgeon 59: 619–623

Behar T A, Burnham S J, Johnson G 1991 Major stump trauma following below-knee amputation. Journal of Cardiovascular Surgery 32: 753–756

Banerjee S N (ed.) 1982 Rehabilitation management of amputees. Williams & Wilkins, Baltimore

Davidoff G N, Lampman R M, Westbury L et al 1992 Exercise testing and training of persons with dysvascular amputation: safety and efficacy of arm ergometry. Archives of Physical Medicine and Rehabilitation 73: 334–338

Day H J B, Kulkarni J R, Datta D 1994 Prescribing upper limb prostheses. Amputee Medical Rehabilitation Society, London

Department of Health and Social Security 1986 Review of Artificial Limb and Appliance Centre services, Vol I, Vol II—Annexes to. DHSS, London

Engstrom B, Van de Ven C 1985 Physiotherapy for amputees: the Roehampton approach. Churchill Livingstone, Edinburgh

Geurts A C H, Mulder T W, Nienhuis B et al 1991 Dual task assessment of reorganization of postural control in persons with lower limb amputation. Archives of Physical Medicine and Rehabilitation 72: 1059–1064

Krebs D (ed) 1987 Prehension assessment: prosthetic therapy for the upper-limb child amputee. Slack, New Jersey

Lamb D W, Law H T 1987 Upper limb deficiencies in children: prosthetic, orthotic and surgical management. Little, Brown, Boston

LoGerfo F W, Gibbons G W, Pomposelli F B et al 1992 Trends in the care of the diabetic foot. Archives of Surgery 127: 617–621

Mensch G, Ellis P M 1986 Physical therapy management of lower extremity amputations. Rockville, Aspen

Mouratoglou V M 1986 Amputees and phantom limb pain: a literature review. Physiotherapy Practice 2: 177–185

Reiber G E, Pecoraro R E, Koepsell T D 1992 Risk factors for amputation in patients with diabetes mellitus: a case-control study. Annals of Internal Medicine 117(2): 97–106

Setoguchi Y, Rosenfelder R (eds) 1982 The limb deficient child. Charles C Thomas, Illinois

Steinberg F U, Sunwoo I, Roettger R F 1985 Prosthetic rehabilitation of geriatric amputee patients: a follow-up study. Archives of Physical Medicine and Rehabilitation 66

Trevam R 1989 Peripheral vascular disease: occupational therapy in peripheral vascular disease of the lower limb. British Journal of Occupational Therapy 52(4): 132–134

Wynn Parry C B 1981 Rehabilitation of the hand. Butterworth, London

Young H 1989 Peripheral vascular disease: arterial disease of the lower limb and venous disorders of the lower limb. British Journal of Occupational Therapy 52(4): 127–132

role in family dynamics. Formal help from the psychologist or psychiatrist may assist people with serious negative responses. Pain may affect socialisation and personal relationships and sensitive counselling may be indicated for some people.

OCCUPATIONAL THERAPY INTERVENTION

ADVICE AND EDUCATION

This is by far the most important role of the occupational therapist. The aim is to inform the person about correct posture and habits and to engender awareness of the back while performing activities or when at rest — in other words, to promote a 'think back' attitude.

Posture

Correct posture should be reinforced in all stages of back care.

Posture can be loosely defined as the way one carries oneself. A good working posture is one which can be sustained with a minimum of static muscular effort, and in which it is possible to perform the task at hand most effectively with least muscular effort (Pheasant 1991). In a natural posture three curves of the spine are evident, as shown in Fig. 24.3.

Lying posture

While a firm mattress and bed base will help the person to maintain a good posture in bed, the mattress should be soft enough to accommodate the natural contours of the body. Purchase of a new, expensive 'orthopaedic' bed can be avoided by placing a firm board between the mattress and the bed base. Side-lying (Fig. 24.4) is the posture most recommended. The head pillow should be just deep enough to fill the gap between the shoulder and the back of the head, thus supporting the neck and not the head. Supine lying, with the legs raised and supported, and the hips and

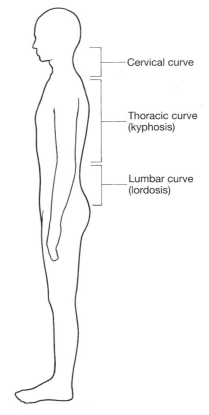

Fig. 24.3 Three natural curves of the spine.

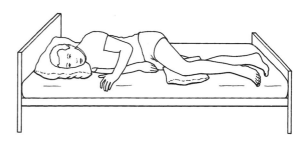

Fig. 24.4 Good lying posture. Side lying in bed with one pillow under the head and a small pillow under the forward knee.

knees flexed to approximately 45 degrees, is also considered to be a good resting position. Prone lying should be avoided as this results in a marked lordosis and extreme side twisting of the neck. Those with pain in the upper spinal region may use special orthopaedic pillows or soft cervical collars to support the neck.

Standing posture

A good standing posture is attained when an imaginary line dropped from the ear will pass through the top of the shoulder, the middle of the hip joint, the back of the patella, and the front of the malleoli of the ankle joints.

Abdominal and buttock tone should be maintained when standing. The angle of the pelvis and lordotic curve are important factors to consider. Prolonged standing can lead to exaggeration of the lumbar lordosis, putting unnecessary strain on the lower back. Obesity, pregnancy and wearing high-heeled shoes also accentuates the lumbar lordosis. When prolonged standing cannot be avoided a small footstool or block may be used to alleviate pain and postural stress, by allowing the person to flex one hip through placing the foot on the support, thereby promoting a more relaxed position (Fig. 24.5).

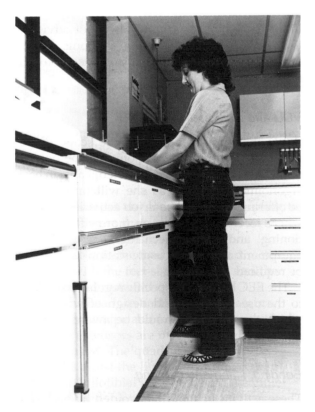

Fig. 24.5 Good standing posture: one foot forward and slightly raised to reduce lumbar lordosis.

The ideal height of a work surface when standing needs to take into account the height of the person and the specific requirements of the work itself. Generally speaking, for delicate or precision work the work surface should come just above elbow height, giving the arms some support. For light work, where space for tools, materials and containers may be required, a surface just below elbow height is recommended. For heavier work, such as woodworking or heavy assembly, a working surface below elbow height that allows for efficient use of the upper part of the body is required (Grandjean 1988).

Sitting posture

This is important for both working and resting positions. Poor sitting positions and seating are major factors contributing to low back pain and limited sitting tolerance. The ideal seat height and depth allows the person to place both feet flat on the floor when the back is fully supported. The angle of the seat and backrest will depend on the task being undertaken and the purpose of the chair. When relaxing in the chair, reclining the backrest slightly promotes a comfortable relaxed posture.

Generally speaking, a good working seat is one with an adjustable seat angle and a high backrest which is slightly concave to the front at its top end and distinctly convex in the lumbar region (Grandjean 1991). Such a seat will give support to the lumbar region when leaning forward in an active sitting position, for example when working at a desk, yet relax the back muscles while holding the spine in a natural position when leaning backwards in a resting position.

Similarly, office chairs fit the same description. The angle of the seat and angle of the backrest should be adjustable to allow for a forward or backward inclined working position. In addition, they must fulfil all the requirements of a modern seat: adjustable height, swivel, rounded front edge of the seat surface, castors or glides, five-arm base and user-friendly controls (Grandjean 1988).

A reading slope or frame on the desk may also improve the working position by overcoming

equipment or alternative techniques may overcome some of the difficulty. Kneeling to change nappies on the bed or cot rather than on the floor reduces bending. Small children may be encouraged to climb onto an armchair or the bed for assistance with dressing, and the use of simple reins enables the mother to retain contact with the small ambulant child when out shopping if stooping to hold hands or manoeuvring a pushchair causes pain.

Postnatal abdominal and pelvic floor exercises should be encouraged to counteract the onset of a prolapsed womb, which may cause long-term back strain internally.

Driving

This is frequently a very painful activity because of the limitations of car seat design, the demands made when getting in and out of the car, movements required when driving and the need to remain seated. The car seat may require modification. Except in the more expensive range of vehicles, which have lumbar adjustments, many car seats tend to encourage a forward-flexed C-shaped position which adds to stress on the lower spine. The transmission of jarring, swaying or swerving driving movements further adds to the discomfort.

The driver who suffers from back pain should be advised to relax and sit well back in the seat, adjusting the angle of the backrest to a position of comfort while retaining good vision. The seat should be positioned so that the steering wheel, gears and controls can be easily reached without stretching forwards. The legs should be comfortably flexed when using the pedals. A lumbar roll or seat insert, such as the Back Friend, may provide added seat support. Drivers should avoid long continuous periods of driving, and should adopt the habit of taking regular breaks, leaving the car and taking a short walk, at least every hour.

When getting into the car the person should commence with the seat well back, step into the car with one foot, lower himself gently into the car and onto the seat and then lift the second leg into the car. When comfortably seated he should move the seat forward into the driving position (Fig. 24.9). The procedure should be reversed when stepping out of the car. Alternatively, a person may choose to sit fully on the seat before swinging both legs round together. In either case excessive twisting and bending should be avoided.

Driving should be avoided for four to six weeks following spinal surgery, and anyone wearing a cervical collar is usually advised not to drive. If spinal range of movement is severely limited then driving, particularly reversing the car, may become impossible. Weakness of limbs, particularly that affecting the lower limbs may reduce control of pedals and reaction speeds which may affect safety, and advice should be sought from the medical officer before recommencing driving. In certain jobs which involve a significant amount of driving, special seating may be provided and financial assistance may be obtained from the employment agency where the DEA is based.

SPECIFIC TREATMENT ACTIVITIES

A wide variety of biomechanical techniques may be used to increase range of movement, strength and tolerance in the spine and limbs. Activities may be used to assess work potential and to prepare the person to return to work or the domestic role. Successful participation in purposeful, pleasurable activity may promote a sense of well-being and thus help to reduce the invasive constraint imposed by pain on activity as a whole.

All treatment activities should be based on the aims and goals identified following assessment, recognising the age and life-style of the person and his existing problems, pain-free range of movement, strength and stamina. Activities chosen may reflect domestic needs, or may be workshop based. Such equipment as the treadle lathe or rehabilitation cycle may be used to strengthen lower limbs. Bench work may be used to promote standing or sitting tolerances and may be adapted to promote particular spinal movements. Heavy activities such as outdoor gardening or sawing and planing wood may promote activity tolerance for those employed in manual work.

All activities should be perceived by the individual to be purposeful and should allow for

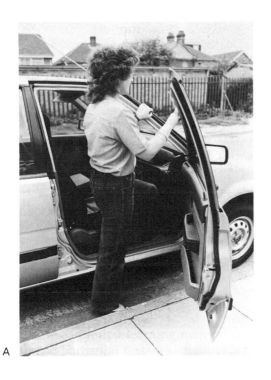

A

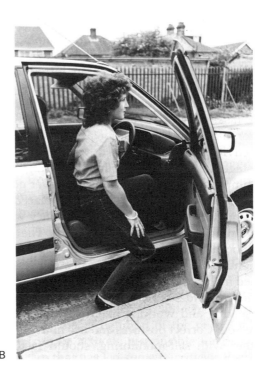

B

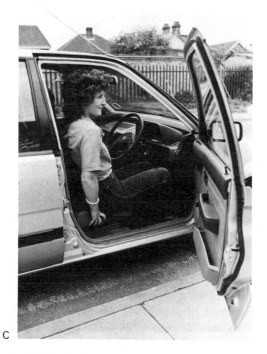

C

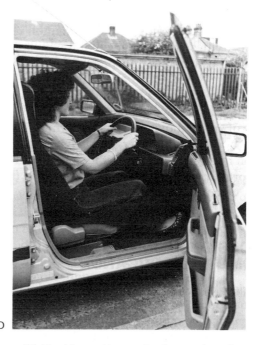

D

Fig. 24.9 Getting into a car. (A) Facing forwards, step into the car. (B) Flex hips and knees simultaneously and lower body weight onto the edge of the seat. (C) Push up on hands to move to the centre of the seat without twisting. (D) Correct driving position. Position of the arms minimises strain on the back and neck. Reverse the process for getting out.

Frederick B, Brown B E, Nelson-Allen C E et al 1980 Body mechanics, introduction manual, a guide for therapists. BAFCA Enterprises, PO Box 3192, Linwood, Washington 98036, USA

Hayne C R 1984a Ergonomics and back pain. Physiotherapy 70(1): 9–13

Hayne C R 1984b Back schools and total back care programmes — a review. Physiotherapy 70(1): 14–17

Holmes D 1985 The role of the occupational therapist — work evaluator. American Journal of Occupational Therapy 39(5): 308–313

Humphrey M 1989 Back pain. (The experience of illness series.) Routledge, London

Jayson M I V 1988 Looking after your back. British Medical Association, London

Jayson M I V 1992 Back pain. The facts. Oxford publications, London

Key S 1991 Back in action. Century, London

Liarg M H 1988 Low back pain: diagnosis and management of mechanical back pain. Primary Care 51(4): 827–847

McCauley M 1990 The effects of body mechanics instruction on work performance among young adults. American Journal of Occupational Therapy 44(5): 402–407

McKenzie R 1987 Treat your own neck. Spinal publications, Waikanae

Main C J, Waddell G 1987 Personality assessment in the management of low back pain. Clinical Rehabilitation 1(2): 139–142

Nicholas M K, Wilson P H, Goyen J 1992 Comparison of cognitive–behavioural group treatment and an alternative non-psychological treatment for chronic low back pain. Pain 48: 339–347

O'Hara P M 1992 Occupational therapy and the pain management team. British Journal of Occupational Therapy 55(1): 19–20

Place-Hayes J K 1991 Lifting: what is the best technique? Work 1(4): 75–77

Richie M H, Daines B 1992 Sexuality and low back pain: a response to patients' needs. British Journal of Occupational Therapy 55(9): 347–350

Schwed N I 1991 The back injury: acute care to employment. Work 1(4): 36–40

Sherwood P 1992 The back and beyond. The hidden effects of back problems on your health. Arrow, London

Strong J, Cramond T, Maas F 1989 The effectiveness of relaxation techniques with patients who have chronic low back pain. Occupational Therapy Journal of Research 9(3): 184–192

Sutherland R C 1991 Back to work. Work 1(4): 7–11

Tyson R, Strong J 1990 Adaptive equipment: its effectiveness for people with chronic lower back pain. Occupational Therapy Journal of Research 9(3): 184–192

Which Consumer Guides 1991 Understanding back trouble. Consumer's Association, London

25

Burns

Patricia M. Church
Rosemary Cooper

INTRODUCTION

The occupational therapist's work with people who have suffered burn injury is both demanding and challenging as it encompasses a wide range of concerns and addresses the needs of all age groups. The person who has a burn injury may need help in all spheres of life — physical, psychological and social — and in various environments, whether at home, at work or in school.

This chapter aims to illustrate the stages of occupational therapy intervention as it applies to the treatment of burn victims from hospital admission to discharge and aftercare. The first sections of the chapter explain the classification of burns by type, depth, extent and cause. The team approach to burn treatment is then outlined, followed by the application of occupational therapy theory and intervention. The specific stages of the occupational therapy process — from assessment, through early intervention, to post-grafting care — are described, along with various practical and psychosocial factors to consider in domestic and work rehabilitation. The chapter then turns to the needs of children who have suffered burn injury, with particular attention to the involvement of parents or carers.

Next, various types of orthoses that can be used to aid the healing process are described, together with their applications to various parts of the body. The use of pressure garment regimes in reducing hypertrophic scarring is also outlined.

Finally, the chapter returns to the psychosocial aspects of burn injury and the management of emotional problems that may arise during rehabilitation and reintegration into the community. Throughout, the chapter stresses the importance of the involvement of family and friends in the rehabilitation programme to its final outcome.

BURN INJURY

The skin is the body's largest organ. It is a sensory organ and acts as an environmental barrier, helping to regulate pressure and reduce loss of essential fluids. When a burn occurs the skin and some underlying structures may be damaged, thus potentially producing a life-threatening situation.

CLASSIFICATION OF BURNS

Burns may be categorised by the following criteria:

- the type of burn
- the depth of burn
- the percentage of skin surface involved.

These categories can be further subdivided according to their cause, as follows.

Type of burn

- Thermal
  — flame
  — steam
  — hot liquid
  — hot metal
- Chemical
  — acid
  — alkali
- Electrical
- Radiation
- Friction.

N.B. Exposure to extreme cold (e.g. liquid nitrogen) may produce the same effect as exposure to extreme heat. Frostbite is a type of burn.

Depth of burn

- *Superficial*. Involves the epidermis, resulting in erythema and blistering. The wound is painful but damage is minimal, healing occurring spontaneously within 7–10 days. Treatment usually consists of minor measures to relieve discomfort and prevent infection
- *Partial thickness*. May be referred to as dermal or deep dermal burn, depending on the thickness of dermis involved. The wound is painful with erythema, exudate (leakage of interstitial fluid) and subcutaneous oedema. Healing occurs from epithelium-lined skin appendages, i.e. hair follicles and sebaceous and sweat glands. Epithelialisation may take 3–4 weeks, but skin grafting is often undertaken early to minimise the amount of hypertrophic scarring. Infection can convert a partial thickness injury to one of full thickness
- *Full thickness*. Destroys the entire epidermis and dermis down to the subcutaneous tissue. This may include damage to muscle, tendon and bone. The wound is leathery and can be white or charred, with considerable subcutaneous oedema. A full thickness burn is not painful as nerve endings have been destroyed. Spontaneous healing is not possible and regeneration of the epidermis is only at the margins of the wound. Skin grafting is required to promote wound healing (Pedretti & Zoltan 1990).

It should be remembered that a burn wound is often of mixed depth. Therefore wound management is very complex and assessment of damage is a continuous process in the early stages.

Percentage of skin surface injured

Wallace's Rule of Nines is usually used to give a quick estimate of the area of the body surface affected by burn injury. This divides the body into areas of 9% or multiples of 9% (Fig. 25.1).

People who have incurred burns involving over 15% of the body surface are usually transferred immediately from Accident and Emergency to a specialised burns unit. The Lund and Browder chart for estimating the severity of the burn wound is then used to give a more accurate percentage of the body surface involved (Fig. 25.2).

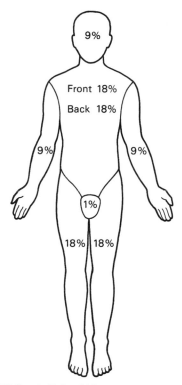

Fig. 25.1 Wallace's Rule of Nines.

Individuals who have suffered burn injuries of less than 15% are commonly treated on plastic surgery wards in general hospitals or as outpatients through Accident and Emergency departments.

Cause of burns

Most burn injuries result from accidents and the groups most likely to be at risk are the elderly (especially the frail elderly), the physically disabled, young children, those people with mental health problems and people working in potentially hazardous situations.

Over 20% of injuries are caused by bath and kettle scalds to children.

MEDICAL MANAGEMENT OF BURN INJURIES

The initial medical management of burns involves the treatment of shock following the injury.

Heat damage causes an increase in the permeability of blood vessels. Valuable electrolytes and plasma protein leak out of the circulation into the surrounding tissue space. This results in gross oedema which can be very alarming for both the individual and his relatives. Staff need to explain what is happening and provide reassurance that it is a temporary symptom. In the case of circumferential full or partial thickness burns the oedema can produce increased interstitial pressure, compromising the circulation. Escharotomy or incision of the eschar (necrotic tissue) is performed to relieve such pressure immediately. Fluids need to be replaced. The volume of fluid necessary is calculated from a formula based on the extent of the burn and the weight of the person. Primary surgical treatment involves excising or shaving the eschar and re-surfacing the area with an appropriate graft or flap. It is important to remove necrotic tissue as soon as possible and replace it with skin grafts.

Types of skin graft

- Autograft. Skin is transferred from one area of the body (donor site) to another. This should provide permanent cover
- Allograft (homograft). Skin from another human (possibly a cadaver) is used. This provides only temporary cover until an autograft is available
- Xenograft (heterograft). This uses animal, e.g. pig, skin and is also only a temporary cover.

Inhalation injuries

Damage to the respiratory system is a common complication of a burn injury, particularly in burns to the face. Inhalation of toxic fumes and smoke often necessitates ventilation and is a major cause of mortality in people with burns, irrespective of the percentage of burn injury.

The team

It is essential that all members of the team work together to ensure cohesion of the intervention programme. The consultant is responsible for

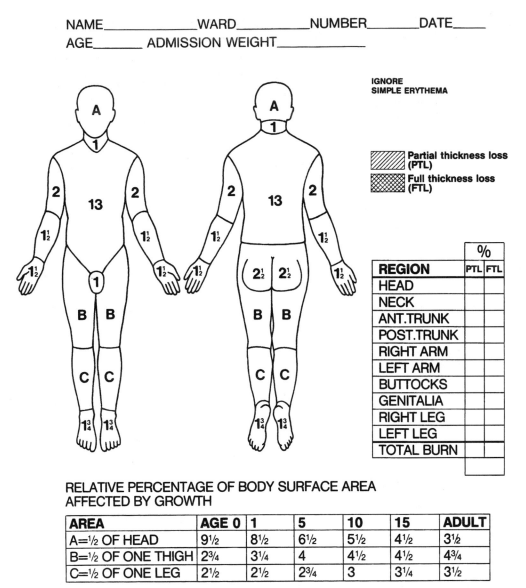

NAME_____WARD_____NUMBER_____DATE____
AGE_____ ADMISSION WEIGHT_____

IGNORE
SIMPLE ERYTHEMA

Partial thickness loss (PTL)

Full thickness loss (FTL)

REGION	%	
	PTL	FTL
HEAD		
NECK		
ANT.TRUNK		
POST.TRUNK		
RIGHT ARM		
LEFT ARM		
BUTTOCKS		
GENITALIA		
RIGHT LEG		
LEFT LEG		
TOTAL BURN		

RELATIVE PERCENTAGE OF BODY SURFACE AREA
AFFECTED BY GROWTH

AREA	AGE 0	1	5	10	15	ADULT
A=½ OF HEAD	9½	8½	6½	5½	4½	3½
B=½ OF ONE THIGH	2¾	3¼	4	4½	4½	4¾
C=½ OF ONE LEG	2½	2½	2¾	3	3¼	3½

Fig. 25.2 Lund and Browder chart for estimating severity of the burn wound. (Reproduced by kind permission of Smith & Nephew.)

medical management but relies upon specialist nurses to implement the fluid balance programme and maintain pain control. Nurses are also responsible for wound care to avoid further wound damage or infection and for the maintenance of positioning to minimise or prevent contractures. They are also frequently required to provide emotional support.

A dietitian may give advice on a high protein, high calorie diet to counteract hypermetabolism and to support tissue repair. The physiotherapist aims to encourage and maintain mobility both in the injured and non-injured areas. Exercises to promote good breathing may be beneficial for those who have inhaled hot air, smoke or other gases, or who have been ventilated. In the later stages of rehabilitation the physiotherapist is usually involved in the prevention of hypertrophic scarring and its effects.

The psychologist, psychiatrist and social worker

Box 25.1 Case study. Mr A, a 37-year-old right-handed man, sustained a 35% partial thickness flame burn. He is a motor mechanic and his injury was the result of a petrol explosion at work. He is married with a one-year-old child.

Stage	Problems observed	Treatment plan	Occupational therapy intervention
Early	Burns extending across the joints of the hands and knees Fear, anxiety, pain and shock	Provide orthoses to prevent contractures Provide reassurance	Hand orthoses Knee extension orthoses Introduce self to Mr A and his relatives. Explain procedures
Grafting	Grafts extending across joints Depressed about dependence on staff Anxious about medical procedures Passive behaviour	Provide orthoses to protect newly grafted areas ADL assessment Promote independence Provide reassurance	Hand orthoses Knee extension orthoses Teach relaxation Supportive counselling Advice and information booklets Provision of equipment: • large-handled cutlery • book rest • insulated beaker • non-slip mat Introduction to an outpatient in similar circumstances Provide opportunities in daily tasks to encourage decision-making
Post-grafting	Anxiety re: • physical function • finance • return to work • concern for relatives Lack of confidence Fear of meeting people	Explore psychological problems	Supportive counselling Liaise with: • social worker • psychologist Socialisation programme Gradual introduction of visits outside the hospital Discussions with Mr A and his wife with regard to a return to the home Discussions re work assessment and activities Introduction to support group Discussions re the need for outpatient care
	Developing signs of post-traumatic stress disorder (PTSD) with: • nightmares • intrusive flashbacks relating to the accident	Support patient through debriefing and developing coping strategies	Debriefing in conjunction with psychologist Anxiety management Cognitive restructuring
	Scarring Hyperaesthesia of scars Limited flexion at metacarpophalangeal and interphalangeal joints Slight contracture of right thumb web	Plan for scar management	Show 'before and after' pressure garment photographs Provide information booklets Provide opportunity to talk to outpatient wearing pressure garments Provide pressure garments with silicone inserts
		Assess: • hand function • ADL • work Plan activity programme	C-bar serial stretch orthosis with silicone insert Graded programme to improve hand function and reduce sensitivity Programme of work activities including a work visit and visits to petrol stations — graded exposure Introduce a work project to build sense of achievement

Box 25.1 (cont'd)

Stage	Problems observed	Treatment plan	Occupational therapy intervention
Outpatient	Fear of petrol and work situation	Explore Mr A's fears	Establish desensitisation programme
	Irritability towards wife and intolerance of young baby	Identify current problems in family relationships	One-to-one discussion with • Mr A • his wife Encourage discussion in support group Liaise with clinical psychologist
	Reluctance to return to work with less than full hand function	Reassess hand function	Upgrade activity programme including simulated work activities Project to further improve sense of achievement Reassurance as to his abilities
	Lack of energy	Education of effects after trauma	Establish home activity programme with achievable goals and monitor
	Frustration regarding use of pressure garments	Re-evaluate fit of garments Reinforce benefits More frequent outpatient appointments	Alter design of pressure garments Show 'before and after' photographs Discussion with another patient and within the support group

are frequently members of the team. Relatives and friends, whose reactions play an important part in the recovery process, should also be educated and supported in order to become positive members of the treatment team.

OCCUPATIONAL THERAPY

APPLICATION OF THEORY

Occupational therapists use a number of frames of reference and approaches to guide intervention with the person who has suffered a burn injury (Table 25.1).

As with many other areas of practice, a phenomenological frame of reference guides the humanistic, client-centred approach to intervention. Non-judgemental recognition of, and respect for individuals' wishes, values, roles and needs will assist the therapist in:

• facilitating adjustment to the accident and injury

Table 25.1 Occupational therapy frames of reference

Frame of reference	Phenomenological	Biomechanical	Compensatory	Learning	Developmental
Approach	Humanistic Client centred	Biomechanical	Rehabilitative	Cognitive/behavioural	Developmental
Techniques	Counselling Person-centred programme Respecting individuals' hierarchy of needs Developing self-esteem	Orthoses Pressure garments Graded exercise programmes to improve range of movement, muscle strength, activity tolerance, skin tolerance	Adapted tools and equipment Alternative techniques Camouflage make-up Environmental modifications Support from carers	Advice/education Developing coping strategies Problem-solving/reasoning Goal-setting	Age/stage-appropriate activities

- developing individuals' self-esteem
- guiding priorities and choices of aims and goals, and ways of achieving these.

Interventions should be determined in conjunction with the person, and where appropriate the family and carers should also be involved, and individual preferences should be respected.

In the early stages following injury, a compensatory frame of reference may be used through the provision of modified equipment to maintain some elements of independence despite mobility restrictions, surgical interventions or pain. The use of these items may be diminished as recovery occurs, but long-term compensatory techniques may be required to overcome residual impairments which threaten to restrict function, or to camouflage disfigurement.

The biomechanical frame of reference and approach is used to maintain and/or improve range of movement, muscle strength, and skin and activity tolerances, through the use of orthoses, pressure garments and graded programmes of practical activities. Where injury has affected a child or young adult, an understanding of the developmental stages is vital to determine appropriate acceptable activities and encourage developmental progress.

Within the learning frame of reference a cognitive/behavioural approach is used with almost all people who have suffered burn injuries to explore the person's understanding of, and attitude to, the injury, impairment or disfigurement. This approach may also be used with relatives and parents. Exploration of anxieties and concerns regarding the injury, the different interventions and the future prospects, and the reason for these concerns, enables the individual and the therapist to investigate and develop coping strategies for managing these issues and solving problems both in the present and for the future.

Therapists favour different models for practice, but whichever model is chosen it should be able to address the wide range of possible areas of dysfunction, and accommodate opportunities for the therapist to be eclectic in the use of a number of approaches to meet individuals' diverse needs.

INTERVENTION

The occupational therapist may be involved with the person from shortly after his admission to a burns unit or ward up to and beyond his discharge. The person may continue to attend the hospital as an outpatient for up to 18 months following the injury, and may require help in the community for some years.

The injured person and his relatives or carers should be involved with programme planning. The individual's perspective on his own needs and priorities will help to determine treatment goals.

Progression of treatment is dependent on wound recovery and the person's psychological state. Specific goals will vary from person to person, but the general aims of treatment are:

- To reduce oedema and maintain range of movement
- To prevent deformity from contractures by correct positioning and the use of orthoses
- To minimise the effects of scarring by using pressure techniques
- To maintain functional independence
- To increase tolerance to fatigue and improve muscle strength
- To assist with psychological adjustment to the injury and its after-effects
- To educate with regard to skin care, including sensory retraining following nerve involvement, desensitisation of grafted areas through graded activity, and development of a good skin care regime which includes lubrication and massage
- To resettle the person in the community and at work.

Medical management of the injured person is the priority on admission. The occupational therapist's emphasis at the early stage is to prevent deformity and to maintain range of movement by the provision of orthoses (see p. 700).

ASSESSMENT

In the acute stage background information on the person is needed. This may include:

- details of the type of burn
- an estimate of the percentage area of the burn
- knowledge of the depth and location of the injury
- any secondary factors to be considered
- the person's past medical history
- an indication of the person's functional ability prior to the injury
- the circumstances of the accident
- details of the person's family and social roles
- an indication of the person's previous psychological status.

As the person's medical condition stabilises detailed assessments should be undertaken in order to provide a baseline for further treatment planning. These may include measurements of joint range of motion, oedema, sensation, muscle strength and occupational performance.

EARLY INTERVENTION

Custom-made orthoses may be required in order to prevent deformity (see p. 700).

Assessment of independence and practice in self-care should be undertaken as early as possible. Initially this would include:

- dressing, e.g. nightwear, dressing gown
- personal grooming, e.g. combing hair
- hygiene, e.g. washing hands, cleaning teeth
- toileting — a raised toilet seat may be required
- feeding — this may require large-handled or other adapted cutlery
- drinking.

These activities often necessitate the use of a mirror. It is essential to check within the multidisciplinary team whether a mirror has been used prior to undertaking daily living activities and, where necessary, to prepare the person carefully. The occupational therapist needs to be prepared for the person's reactions and allow time for discussion, listening and counselling as appropriate.

The use of regular practice in daily living skills allows the person a level of independence and control in day-to-day activities. Decision-making should be encouraged at all times to prevent passive behaviour.

The occupational therapist may need to provide adapted or specialised equipment, e.g. large-handled cutlery, lightweight beakers, an enlarged TV switch, an alphabet communication board, etc.

Any treatment that involves providing equipment or making orthoses must be carried out with regard for the control of infection, in accordance with the policy of the burns unit and/or the hospital.

Dressing changes and wound care are very painful and traumatic procedures, thus creating enormous anxiety. Educating the person in the need for such procedures and teaching coping strategies, e.g. anxiety management and relaxation, may be beneficial.

It is important for the occupational therapist to explain her work to the person's relatives so that they understand the principles of treatment and can become actively involved. Developing rapport with the relatives at this stage is beneficial in:

- providing support and encouragement to the relatives
- helping the relatives provide support and encouragement to the person with the burn injury
- providing accurate information about long-term care, which will help to reduce anxieties about the future. Written information is particularly helpful here.

POST-GRAFTING STAGE

It is usually at this stage that a more thorough assessment can be made. Range of movement and sensation can be tested. Self-care activities can be assessed and appropriate equipment provided.

Graded purposeful activity, progressing from gentle unresisted to resisted work, can be used to improve range of movement and muscle strength using a biomechanical approach.

Desensitisation of grafted areas using activities graded from 'soft' to 'hard' may be used. Care must be taken regarding vigorous activity and shearing forces on newly healed skin, which is delicate and may break down easily.

Participation by the person in planning treatment and setting his priorities, together with his involvement in activities which require a gradual increase in the amount of decision-making and use of initiative, will help to increase self-esteem. A gradual programme of socialisation may be needed, particularly for those whose scars are visible. The burns unit or ward will have become a safe environment for the person, where staff and relatives are used to his appearance. The first visit to the occupational therapy department may need to take place at a quiet time, as the person will have to come to terms with the reactions of others gradually.

Domestic rehabilitation

The following concerns surrounding the person's return to home life may need to be explored:

- Practical considerations:
  — Safety in the home, e.g. use of fire and cooker guards, coiled safety flexes, testing of temperature of domestic hot water, storage of household fluids such as bleach and caustic soda. Leaflets on safety are available from gas and electricity boards, social services, health education departments, etc.
  — Use of specialised equipment, e.g. bath aids, electric can-openers, long-handled utensils, wheelchairs
  — Financial concerns
- Psychosocial considerations:
  — Fears associated with using appliances such as kettles, chip pans, garden mowers, barbeques; use of car — especially filling the petrol tank
  — Anxiety regarding ability to resume previous roles within the family and/or community
  — Avoidance of situations which may cause anxiety, e.g. going to the pub, sexual relationships, going swimming, lighting the gas fire
  — Over-dependency on others or inability to accept help
  — Social isolation.

The person may need to make a preliminary home visit in order to prepare for discharge. Day visits and weekend leave can assist this process.

Work rehabilitation

The person's ability to resume his previous employment will need to be assessed. Areas which may need to be considered include:

- muscle power and range of movement, e.g. ability to stand or sit for long periods or to use heavy tools or equipment
- the work environment, e.g. dust or dirt levels, exposure to chemicals
- stamina
- tolerance to noise
- anxiety, especially if the accident happened at work. Early visits to work may help to allay this
- concentration
- hand function
- access to and within the workplace.

It may be necessary to involve the Disability Employment Advisor (DEA) and the Placing, Assessment and Counselling Team (PACT), particularly if alterations to the workplace or specialised equipment are required. The DEA will also provide help with assessment, employment rehabilitation, training for new skills or sheltered employment if appropriate. Information regarding these services is available in all Job Centres.

THE BURNED CHILD

In the case of an injured child the occupational therapist will work with the child's parents/carers as well as with the child. In order to promote understanding of treatment techniques and activities and to reduce anxiety, clear explanations must always be given to both the child and the parents/carers about the importance of the procedures and what will be involved. Role play may be introduced to assist the child to accept interventions. For example, orthoses and pressure garments can be tried out on a doll or soft toy, or a parent, first.

THE CHILD IN HOSPITAL

Some regression is expected in the child during hospitalisation, but if prolonged this may necessitate the intervention of a psychologist. Regression is usually indicative of a need for love and attention in the face of anxiety, fear and pain in strange surroundings. Regression can be extremely distressing for parents who are attempting to cope with their own feelings of guilt regarding the injury. Support for the parents to provide love and care without over-indulgence is necessary to enable the child to return to his previous developmental level. Discussion with other parents, either in a support group or individually, can be very helpful.

It is useful to liaise with paediatric occupational therapists or those working in child and family psychiatry. Joint treatment sessions can be valuable and increase the help and support available to the child and parent or carer.

According to Bettelheim (1987):

Children can learn to live with a disability. But they cannot live without the conviction that their parents find them utterly loveable . . . If the parents, knowing his defect, love him now, he can believe that others will love him in the future. With this conviction, he can live well today and have faith in the years to come.

The value of play

Play is an important part of recovery for the child, and the occupational therapist can provide suitable toys which serve a therapeutic purpose. In selecting toys to use in her programme, the therapist might look for:

- toys which require and thus help to maintain upper limb range of movement and bilaterality
- toys which require different grips, thus helping to maintain hand function
- toys and floor games requiring lower limb mobility, thus helping to maintain lower limb strength and range of movement.

Parents can be actively involved in incorporating toys into the child's rehabilitation programme.

Children also use play to act out frightening experiences, for example by role-playing reactions to a fire or the incident relating to their injury. The occupational therapist, parent and any other member of the treatment team can help the child with this process. Successful re-integration to school life is dependent on the help provided to the child during the inpatient stay and to the school and teachers in preparation. Role-play will give the child the opportunity to practise coping strategies he will need in dealing with questions about the accident, scarring and so on. Liaising with the teachers and school to help them prepare for the child's return is invaluable. Providing education and training in the school environment for pupils and teachers, utilising activities such as drama, puppetry and school assemblies, can be extremely helpful for the child's re-integration.

After discharge

Parents will need support and encouragement as they implement the pressure garment regime. They often find support in talking to others in similar circumstances. If the child has been treated on a regional burns unit it may be too far for the parents to return to the unit to meet other parents, especially as travelling may involve bringing a small child and siblings. It can, therefore, be very beneficial for parents to keep in touch with other parents by telephone or through letters. The occupational therapist can often facilitate these contacts through outpatient clinic appointments and arrange face-to-face groups for those able to travel.

Liaison with the local health visitor or social worker in the community may be necessary to assist with the pursuance of prescribed treatment practices after discharge. The child will need to return to the hospital at regular intervals for replacement of the pressure garments.

ORTHOSES FOR BURNS

Orthoses are used to:

- maintain range of movement
- prevent contracture and deformity
- maintain functional position
- immobilise grafted areas.

Orthoses should be applied whenever a burn extends across a joint, taking into account the depth of the burn and the exercise regime and working practice of the unit or ward.

It is important to mould the orthosis individually on each person, as close to the skin surface as possible, and usually on the flexor aspect of the body. Areas regularly requiring orthoses include:

- joints of the forearm, wrist and hand
- the neck
- the axilla
- the elbow
- the knee
- the ankles
- joints of the feet
- planes of the face, especially around the eyes and mouth.

Static orthoses are applied unless otherwise indicated.

Joints of the forearm, wrist and hand

The hand is frequently injured because it is one of the most exposed parts of the body and is used to protect the face or extinguish a fire. Burns on the dorsum of the hand can result in a 'claw hand' deformity. This consists of hyperextension of the metacarpophalangeal (MCP) joints, flexion of the interphalangeal (IP) joints of the fingers, adduction and extension of the thumb, and radial deviation at the wrist. It also results in flattening of the palmar longitudinal and transverse arches, producing a non-functional hand.

The extensor mechanism of the hand is poorly protected, particularly across the proximal interphalangeal (PIP) joints. Any flexion, either passive or active, may be contraindicated if there is a partial thickness burn to this area. In the early days boutonnière deformity may occur due to the rupture of the central slip of the extensor tendon at the PIP joint.

Palmar burns are less common, as the palm is more protected and the skin is thicker. Burns to the palm result in tightening of the palmar fascia with flexion and adduction of the fingers and thumb; they may therefore need to be splinted in extension.

To counteract a pull towards claw hand deformity the orthosis should provide the following position:

- Wrist — 30 degrees extension
- MCP joints — 70 degrees flexion
- IP joints — full extension
- Thumb — opposed and extended
- Web space and palmar arches — maintained (Fig. 25.3).

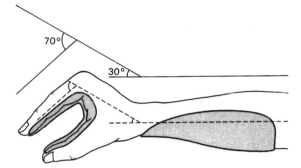

Fig. 25.3 Optimum position for the wrist and hand to prevent contracture.

Splinting a circumferential burn of the hand may need to be delayed for any necessary escharotomies to be performed, as splinting may further compromise the circulation. It may be necessary in the small child to fabricate a bivalved hand orthosis or to mould a silicone glove (Malick & Carr 1982, Walters 1987).

Dynamic orthoses may be applied if there is tendon damage.

The neck

The neck should be supported in a natural extended position contouring the anterior aspect of the neck and mandible. The collar should have a wide enough base over the clavicle and sternum to avoid pressure (Fig. 25.4).

The axilla

The axilla should be supported with the arm

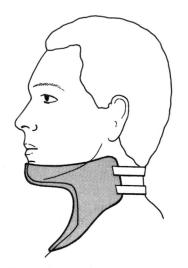

Fig. 25.4 Neck support position.

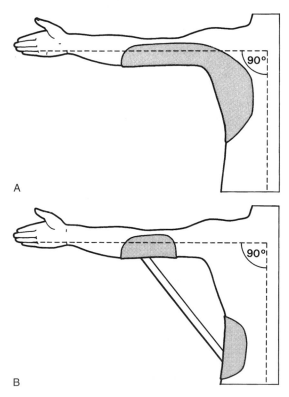

Fig. 25.5 Axilla support position. (A) Enclosed support. (B) Open support for immediate post-grafting.

abducted at 90 degrees to the body, and with a 10 degrees forward flexion at the shoulder (Fig. 25.5).

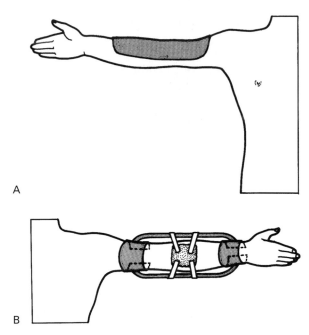

Fig. 25.6 Elbow orthoses. (A) Gutter support. (B) Three–point extension support.

The elbow

The elbow should be maintained in extension with the forearm in the neutral position between pronation and supination. Orthoses usually take the form of a gutter orthosis or a three-point extension support (Fig. 25.6).

The knee

Where possible the knee should be supported in full extension, ensuring the orthosis has a contour fit into the popliteal fossa at the back of the knee (Fig. 25.7).

The ankles and joints of the feet

The foot should be positioned in a neutral position, i.e. at a 90 degrees angle to the tibia, allowing the sole of the foot to be placed flat on the floor when mobilising. There should be no pressure on the dorsum of the heel or the medial and lateral malleoli of the ankle. Metatarsophalangeal and interphalangeal joints should be held in extension and the arches of the foot maintained (Fig. 25.8).

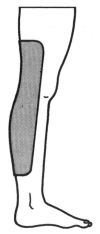

Fig. 25.7 Knee extension gutter support.

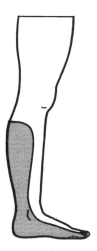

Fig. 25.8 Ankle/foot support in neutral position.

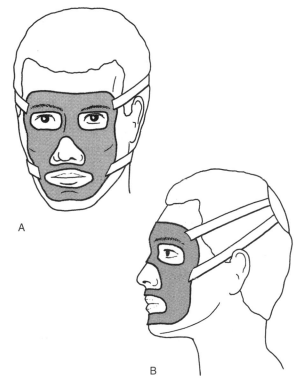

Fig. 25.9 Full face mask. (A) Front view. (B) Side view.

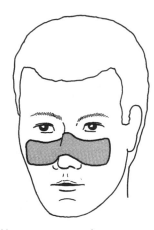

Fig. 25.10 Nose pressure conformer.

Planes of the face

The face is a complex structure which is highly mobile. Burns scarring may result in contracted tissue, particularly around the mouth and the eyes, which limits mobility and produces deformity.

Lycra, silicone or thermoplastic face masks may be used. These may be applied to the full face (Fig. 25.9) or on small areas, for example around the nose (Fig. 25.10). (Malick & Carr 1980).

Partial or full thickness circumferential burns of the mouth may contract, causing microstomia unless opposing force is applied. Full stretch of the mouth needs to be maintained by use of a microstomia splint (Fig. 25.11) (Heirle et al 1988).

Orthotic materials

The materials chosen should be easily washable, conforming, easily adjustable and suitable for bandaging on to the affected part in the early stages.

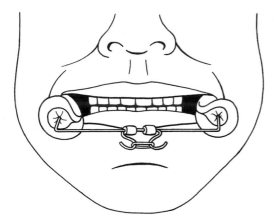

Fig. 25.11 Microstomia splint.

There is a wide range of low-temperature thermoplastic materials available on the market. Sometimes it may be necessary to increase pressure over a raised scar using one of a range of silicone materials available — Silastic foams and pastes, silicone elastomers, or silicone gel sheeting (Gollop 1988). All of these can be individually moulded to the area and taped in place, positioned in the orthosis or placed under the pressure garment.

All orthoses should be regularly re-evaluated, adjusted and, if necessary, redesigned as the person progresses. Immobilising orthoses may be necessary once grafting has taken place.

In the early stages most orthoses are bandaged on, but once oedema has been reduced straps may be applied. It is important to remember that simple alternatives to traditional orthoses may be used. For example, the person may find that a foam roll for the neck is very useful in maintaining neck extension when lying supine, particularly in the early stages. A piece of thick foam bandaged around a small child's arm may serve the same purpose as a thermoplastic elbow gutter.

If contractures do occur, serial stretch orthoses may be required, often in conjunction with the pressure garments.

The success of any orthotic regime depends on:

- appropriate prescription
- the expertise of the occupational therapist when making and fitting the orthosis
- appropriate choice of style, design and materials
- compliance of the person, his relatives and the entire treatment team.

TREATMENT OF HYPERTROPHIC SCARRING

Immediately after healing a burn wound may appear quite flat. However, over the ensuing months hypertrophic scarring may develop. The scars become cherry red, hard, lumpy and raised, and if left untreated may cause contractures and deformity.

Pressure garment regime

The application of controlled consistent pressure using pressure garments keeps the scar flat, smooth and pliable. Garments are usually required when the wound has taken longer than 2–3 weeks to heal spontaneously. For the best results the following points must be adhered to:

- The garment must be applied as soon as healing has occurred
- The garment must be worn 24 hours per day, being removed only for massage, creaming and bathing
- The person must attend regular outpatient clinics to enable progress to be monitored. Adults are usually seen every 6–8 weeks, but children are seen more frequently
- The garments should be hand-washed daily, following the manufacturer's instructions, to maintain the elasticity of garments
- The garments should be worn for 12–18 months, until scar maturation, i.e. when the scar is soft, flat and pale pink or white.

Each pressure garment is custom made, and accurate measuring is essential to ensure a good fit. The most commonly used material is Lycra. The garments are either commercially available or made in the hospital. Two or three sets of garments are usually provided and generally need to be replaced approximately every three months. Heavy use or, in the case of a child, a growth spurt may necessitate more frequent replacement. Gloves may need to be replaced every six weeks depending on the person's life-style.

In order to ensure the compliance of the burned individual and his relatives or carers it is essential to explain clearly the pressure garment regime to all concerned. 'Before and after' photographs may be used to promote a realistic understanding of the outcome. Information booklets may also assist, some of which are provided by the manufacturers.

The fitting and removal of the garments initially requires practice. Added support and encouragement are needed in the early days, particularly with parents of small children. Once the benefits can be seen or felt, the person and his family are usually self-motivated and assume an active role in the pressure garment regime.

At the end of pressure garment treatment camouflage make-up creams can be shown to the person so that he may choose if he wishes to conceal a scar; similarly, parents may wish to know what is available for their child in the future. These creams are available on prescription. It is important to be realistic about their value so that the person does not build up false expectations.

PSYCHOSOCIAL ASPECTS OF BURN INJURY

The injured person may have one or more of the following initial emotional responses to his injury.

Fear

Often accidents have occurred in places or situations which were previously considered safe. The person may be afraid to face the situation of the accident again after recovery. The actual treatment of the injury involves painful procedures which may cause fear. The person can see and feel the damage to his body and may be apprehensive about others' reactions to him. He may fear that the success of the healing will be limited. In hospital, children are frightened at the strangeness of the environment and the procedures which may be necessary; despite love and reassurance they may feel abandoned by their parents, who allow such treatment to happen.

Isolation

The person may be nursed in isolation, and this can appear to be a punishing situation, especially for children. The person is unable to see how others are reacting to pain, disfigurement and treatment techniques, and is often unsure how to react himself. He may emotionally try to isolate himself from the situation, and not see or accept the reality of his predicament.

Frustration

The person is inactive and dependent. The recovery is slow and it is difficult for him to envisage the whole of the treatment programme. Hand injuries can initially be especially frustrating and traumatic as they are clearly visible to the person concerned and they emphasise his dependence on others.

Guilt

The accident may have been the injured person's fault and others may have been hurt. The person often worries that he has caused problems for others to cope with. The parents of a child who has been burned often have deep feelings of guilt and need to be well supported throughout the whole of the rehabilitation period. Often parents tend to compensate the child for the injury by becoming over-protective and over-indulgent or by not imposing any discipline or structure on him. This tends to result in the child becoming more dependent on the parent and often causes unwillingness to participate in the treatment programme. Establishing a trusting relationship helps parents come to terms with the situation to allow the child some independence. In certain cases individual counselling or psychotherapy for the parents may be beneficial.

Loss/grief

Parents commonly grieve for the loss of their

Cahners S S 1992 Young women with breast burns: a self help 'group by mail'. Journal of Burn Care and Rehabilitation 13(1): 44–47

Carney S A, Cason C G, Gavar J P et al 1994 Cica-care gel sheeting in the management of hypertrophic scarring. Burns 20(2): 163–167

Cason J S 1981 Treatment of burns. Chapman & Hall, London

DiGregorio V R (ed.) 1984 Rehabilitation of the burn patient. Churchill Livingstone, New York

Fisher S V, Helm P A 1984 Comprehensive rehabilitation of burns. Williams & Wilkins, Baltimore

Hill C 1985 Psychosocial adjustment of adult burns patients — is it more difficult for people with visible scars? British Journal of Occupational Therapy 48(9): 281–283

Hooper W 1989 Life after a burn: how to cope at home. Available from Jobst Division of Zimmer Surgical Specialities, Swindon, Wilts

Hopkins H L, Smith H D (eds) 1993 Willard and Spackman's occupational therapy, 8th edn. J B Lippincott, Philadelphia

Kemble J V H, Lamb B E 1987 Practical burns management. Hodder and Stoughton, London

Leveridge A (ed.) 1991 Therapy for the burn patient. Chapman & Hall, London

Mason S, Forsham A 1986 Burns aftercare — a booklet for parents — your child at home after injury. Burns 12: 364–370

Mason S, Turner H, Foley A 1986 Burns aftercare — a booklet for patients at home after injury. Smith & Nephew, Welwyn Garden City

Munster A M (ed.) 1993 Severe burns: a family guide to medical and emotional recovery. The Johns Hopkins University Press, Baltimore, MD

Partridge J 1990 Changing faces: the challenge of facial disfigurement. Penguin, Harmondsworth

Porter J 1982 The therapist and the burns patient. Therapy Weekly, April 8th: 4

Quinn K J, Evans J H, Courtney J M, Gaylor J D S 1985 Non pressure treatment of scars. Burns 12: 102–108

Rivlin E, Forshaw A, Polanyj G, Woodruff B 1986 A multidisciplinary group approach to counselling the parents of burned children. Burns 12(7): 479–483

Scott M J, Stradling S G 1992 Counselling for post-traumatic stress disorder. Sage, London

Settle J A D 1986 Burns — the first five days. Smith & Nephew, Welwyn Garden City

Wallace W A, Rowles J M, Colton C L 1994 Management of disasters and their aftermath. BMJ Publishing Group, London

26

Upper limb injuries

Theresa Baxter

INTRODUCTION

Injuries to the upper limbs are extremely common, affecting people from all age groups and social classes. Young adults particularly tend to suffer severe limb injuries, which may occur at work, during sports activities or in road accidents. In the majority of instances the problems are not related to any degenerative disease process, so these individuals hope to suffer only short-term dysfunction, and intervention can be active and vigorous, aiming to return them to near normal function. However, for some people the severity of the trauma may result in permanent impairment, which necessitates adjustment to residual limitations.

This chapter examines the role of the occupational therapist in enabling people with upper limb injuries to regain maximum function and independence. The first half of the chapter is devoted to outlining the function of the upper limb, and the psychological impact of trauma to the limb, particularly that affecting the hand. This is followed by a description of the application of theoretical principles to occupational therapy intervention. The chapter then follows the occupational therapy process, commencing with assessment techniques, followed by discussion of general principles of intervention to maintain bilaterality, re-educate sensation and manage pain and oedema. Injury to particular areas of the upper limb is then discussed in detail, focusing on the shoulder, elbow and forearm, wrist and hand in turn. Management of problems related

responsibility for the limb or refuses to accept the severity of the injury. Pain may blur realistic appraisal of the situation, or dressings may hide the injury. This may be accompanied by anger or hostility to the injury, apportioning blame to self or others for the accident. Anger or hostility may also be directed at those who are attempting to enable him realistically to address the situation and take some responsibility for his future rehabilitation. For some people anger or hostility may be a disguise for anxiety about the future, fears regarding return of function, acceptance or rejection by others, and uncertainties for return to previous life-style. Others, when facing permanent impairment, however functionally minor, may suffer depression resulting from preoccupation with loss and grieving. They may feel helpless to improve the present situation and hopeless for their future.

It is important that these psychological reactions are recognised and addressed if the person is to gain maximum benefit from therapeutic intervention. Jones (1977, p. 192) supports the need for therapy to commence early, in order to enable the person to retain or regain a positive relationship with the injured part:

In the occupational therapy workshop the patient will have the first opportunity to come to terms with a disabled or disfigured hand and to re-establish that close relationship between hand and brain which will be of such importance in developing the personal destiny. The longer the period that elapses between the original accident and the first episode of re-establishing this relationship, the more difficult will be the problem.

APPLICATION OF THEORY

The ultimate aim of occupational therapy intervention for people with upper limb injuries is to maximise return of function and facilitate positive adjustment to any residual impairment. This may involve the application of a number of theoretical frames of reference and approaches, in order to achieve goals which are realistic, purposeful and meaningful to each individual. Occupational therapy intervention is directed towards maintaining and regaining range of movement at the joints, the build-up of muscle strength and

increasing endurance to activity. A biomechanical approach may be used. Application of graded activities initially aims to promote mobility, and progresses to techniques to achieve stability and stamina in line with pre-injury levels and lifestyle needs.

Identification and recognition of the unique requirements of each individual, and respect for a person's choices and preferences, reflect the application of a humanistic approach. Within the constraints of the range of resources available, the selection of activities is influenced by the lifestyle, interests, experiences and motivation of the individual, as well as the therapeutic needs of the particular injury. Activities which are familiar may have negative or positive connotations. Familiarity may engender confidence and security, allaying or overcoming the anxieties and apprehensions of the unknown. However, familiarity with an activity may also highlight present limitations when compared with previous levels of skill and competence. This may be beneficial in measuring ability to return to activity, or retrograde in accentuating a deficit to which the individual is striving to make adjustments. These factors should be addressed and explored prior to commencing the activity.

A compensatory frame of reference may be necessary where there is residual impairment, or in some instances during the early stages following injury, before recovery commences. In the latter case a compensatory approach is favoured. Equipment or other compensatory means can be gradually withdrawn as recovery occurs, whereas some adaptive skills may become established as 'trick movements' which are more difficult to discard. Adaptive skills should be encouraged for the person with residual impairment, and, where these are not adequate to meet individual needs, compensatory techniques and equipment may be beneficial.

When treating people with upper limb injuries, some aspects of the learning frame of reference are frequently used by occupational therapists in order to promote individuals' understanding of the injury, and to highlight the importance of commitment and active participation in rehabilitation. An educational approach is an important technique in facilitating individuals' cooperation and compliance with their own rehabilitation programme. This may include an outline of the anatomical and physiological effects of the injury, and discussion of the implications of pain, oedema, diminished sensation, wound care and scar management on the overall intervention strategy. Cognitive techniques may be used to promote insight into feelings regarding the injury and explore attitudes towards treatment and future prospects. Some behavioural techniques may also be used to promote bilaterality, assist with desensitisation of particularly sensitive areas, or develop positive patterns of management and use of the limb.

The occupational therapist should be aware of the natural process of human development, and the stages of acquisition of hand function. When working with all age groups, but particularly with children and the elderly, activities must be chosen which are age and developmentally appropriate. It is not uncommon for individuals to regress following trauma, so awareness of previous stages of development is important in order to recognise regression, and help the individual to return to these former levels of achievement.

ASSESSMENT

Comprehensive assessment of individuals who have suffered injury to the upper limb should be carried out prior to commencement of intervention, and specific assessments are necessary at regular intervals during treatment to measure progress.

Assessment should include interview, observation, specific tests and measurement, as well as reference to records of previous treatments.

Interview

Interview may be used to ascertain the history of the injury, the individual's life-style needs, and the person's level of knowledge regarding treatment.

Observation

The therapist's observations should commence at the first contact with the individual. Clues to the individual's psychological attitude to the injury may be gained by watching how he holds and handles the limb. These may also provide an indication of levels of pain and discomfort. Observations of behaviours during treatment may reflect the person's motivation, knowledge and general psychological state. The therapist should also use skills of observation to support measurements of specific aspects of the injury. This may include observations of levels of oedema, the state of the wound and scar tissue, skin condition and colouration, and the comparison of range of movement with that of the other limb.

Specific tests

Many departments use specific tests of function which have been devised locally, often in conjunction with other professions within the treatment team. While these may provide valuable means of measuring a range of skills, few have been standardised.

McPhee (1987, p. 163) evaluated a number of specific hand function tests and concluded that 'the clinician should not use one particular type of test exclusively to evaluate all disabilities, but should study and analyse each test to understand its appropriate use. Clinicians should have a number of functional hand tests at their disposal'.

Some occupational therapists also use sections of standardised assessments of function, which are designed in total to assess a wider range of skills; for example, the stereognosis box and the coathanger construction test of the COTNAB may be used to assess sensory awareness or manual strength and dexterity.

Measurement

Areas such as range of joint movement, muscle strength, oedema, sensation, coordination and dexterity should be measured regularly to determine the levels and rates of progress. Details of measurement techniques are covered in detail in

MAINTAINING BILATERALITY

Where a person has injured an upper limb it is important to counteract any tendency to become one-handed. The inclination to favour the affected part should be offset by encouraging functional use, with or without the help of equipment, as early as possible. The person's natural protective tendencies need to be overcome in order to maintain a bilateral body image and facilitate function of the injured part.

TOLERANCE TO ACTIVITY

Activity tolerance must be developed by gradually increasing the duration and frequency of an activity. This applies to both tolerance to certain movements and skin tolerance. If skin has been extensively scarred, grafted or has simply lost its normal toughness during the time the individual has been off work, time will be required to harden the tissues. Progress should be closely monitored so that there is no risk of skin breakdown. Increasingly tough materials can be used for progressively longer periods of time in therapy.

COMPLIANCE

When treating individuals with upper limb injuries the therapist needs to be aware that the individual is the most important member of the treatment team. The therapist needs to be able to gain his cooperation and trust, because the individual's commitment in following through the treatment regime, both during treatment sessions and at home, is essential to the success and recovery of the injury.

There are many factors which affect an individual's compliance to treatment, including fear of pain and lack of motivation. Motivation seldom affects the aetiology directly, but it can influence both the pathological progress and the individual's response to that process (Bear-Lehman 1983). Success of treatment is therefore dependent on not only the therapist's technical skill, but also her understanding of all the aspects of the injury. Another factor which may influence an individual's compliance to his treatment is lack of understanding. The therapist needs to explain clearly what commitment is required of the individual, and the general outline of the proposed treatment programme and the duration of attendance. It needs to be remembered that, nowadays, more and more people are self-employed or are on short-term contracts, and commitment to a four-month treatment programme may be incompatible to their work situation and threatening to their economic security.

Pending litigation claims also affect compliance and many believe that financial reimbursement of work-related accidents inhibits recovery in some individuals (Moran 1986). Also, factors such as cultural and religious beliefs, occupational development, family history and educational level may all have an influence upon an individual's compliance to treatment. Research has shown (Bear-Lehman 1983) that the therapist can contribute considerably to the individual's ultimate recovery and performance by addressing his sociopsychological needs alongside the technical requirements of the injury.

TREATMENT PLANNING

Treatment planning for an individual with an upper limb injury needs to take many factors into account. A full assessment needs to be carried out, consideration being given to the clinical aspects and prognosis of the condition or injury. A functional assessment of all aspects of the individual's daily activities in home, work and leisure is valuable, and a psychosocial assessment with regard to the individual's attitude to his injury and the disruption to his work and family life is advisable.

The individual needs to be involved in the planning process as his commitment to the programme is essential to the successful recovery of the injury.

Regular reassessment should be carried out so that the treatment programme can be adjusted to meet the individual's requirements. Close contact should be maintained by the therapist with others involved in the care of the individual to ensure that everyone is working towards the same outcomes.

In the early stages of treatment the therapist may need to provide adaptive equipment to encourage use of the injured limb, and in some cases it may be necessary to carry out a home visit and to liaise with social services.

In the latter stages of treatment liaison with the individual's employers may be appropriate, although this should only be done in consultation with the individual concerned. A work-hardening programme may then be initiated.

The therapist needs to remember to provide a home programme of activity for the individual to follow, which will require upgrading at regular intervals.

THE SHOULDER

The shoulder is one of the most mobile joints in the body. Its wide range of mobility helps to position the arm and hand for the many prehensile activities the individual may perform. The shoulder can move through almost a full arc in the frontal and sagittal planes, a facility used by the swimmer. Most activities of daily living do not require full range of movement at the shoulder, and an individual can often compensate for reduced mobility by increased motion of the cervical spine and distal upper extremity joints (Donatelli 1991).

Treatment is directed towards restoring mobility and providing stability. A clear understanding of the mechanics of this complex structure is necessary in order to aid the restoration of function. The therapist needs to carry out an in-depth evaluation of the individual's injury, to enable them together to develop a personalised treatment programme. Most activities are performed with the shoulder in some degree of flexion and abduction, the maintenance of which is the goal of the early stages of treatment unless the nature of the injury contraindicates this approach.

A common condition that may be encountered by the therapist is the frozen shoulder, which tends to be a 'catch all' diagnosis for a wide variety of shoulder problems. It has an insidious onset, beginning with pain and tenderness. Move-ment aggravates the pain, and gradually the individual experiences limitation of both passive and active movement. This results in hampering of activity and disturbed sleep. The latter stages of the condition can result in a stiff, useless but painless shoulder which only hurts when forcibly moved (Cailliet 1991).

Other conditions of the shoulder that may be seen are associated with individuals who have a hemiplegia resulting from a cerebrovascular accident (see Chapter 14), brachial plexus lesions (see Chapter 23), sports injuries and shoulder girdle fractures.

Treatment of the shoulder is dictated by diagnosis, assessment, treatment protocols and the needs of the individual. The occupational therapist will usually work in close cooperation with the physiotherapist. The occupational therapist may encourage the use of bilateral activities to encourage controlled use of the injured shoulder. Care must be taken that the individual does not allow the injured part to become a 'passenger' in these types of activity. In initial stages of treatment the activities should be lightweight and positioned so that the individual stretches but does not stress the joint. In some cases a suspended sling may be used to minimise the effects of gravity.

An adjustable height table is an invaluable piece of equipment when treating an individual with a shoulder injury. The height can be adjusted to accommodate the individual's needs, and various remedial activities can be positioned on the table to facilitate movement at the shoulder. Activities that may be used include therapeutic putty, sliding puzzles, span games with varying height poles (Fig. 26.1) and light woodwork projects such as varnishing and pyrography.

As the shoulder strength and range of movement improves, treatment can be upgraded by reducing the support, lengthening the treatment sessions and increasing the resistance and complexity of the activity. Heights of activities can be increased, and the position of the individual in relation to the activity can be changed so that a particular movement can be isolated.

The therapist needs to be alerted to 'trick' movements by the individual in using trunk and elbow

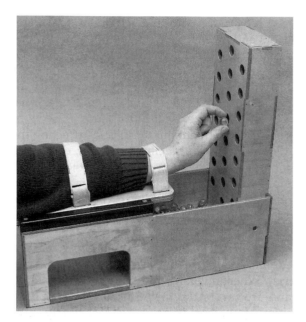

Fig. 26.3 Marble game.

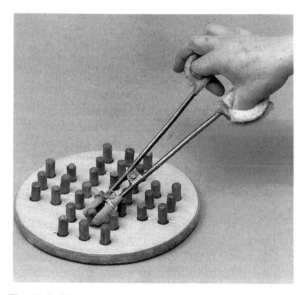

Fig. 26.4 Flexion tongs used to promote PIP joint flexion.

THE HAND

The hand is a complex, delicately balanced structure capable of the strongest grip and the most delicate touch and it has a rich and complex sensory innervation (Wynn Parry 1981). The ability to use the hand requires sensation, mobility, sta-

bility and freedom from disabling pain or anxiety (Moran 1986). The hand is a highly integrated structure, so injury to one part always affects the others. For this reason a detailed and accurate assessment is necessary (see Chapter 7). The therapist's assessment should start as soon as the individual walks through the door: how is he holding the injured hand, and what is his general attitude towards the injury and treatment? On occasions the individual may disassociate himself from the injured hand, and in these cases the sooner the programme of activity is initiated, the easier it will be to help the individual come to terms with his injury. Consideration should be given to the history of the injury, and detailed examination of the hand should be completed. A standardised assessment should preferably be carried out to provide a baseline for treatment and evaluation of treatment.

Reduction in oedema around the small joints of the hand is of particular concern. Swelling in the hand causes characteristic positioning, with the thumb adducted, the metacarpophalangeal (MCP) joints extended and the interphalangeal (IP) joints flexed. This position must be corrected if mobility is to be restored to the hand.

Good hand function depends on three components of the human anatomical system working correctly (Spaulding 1989): the muscle fibres must produce tension or force; the bones, tendons and ligaments must transmit this force; and the skin must indicate the point of force application. Therapists need to have an awareness of the mechanical principles of hand movement to assist individuals with injured hands to resume purposeful and functional activities.

Flexion

The aim of treatment is to achieve both gross grip and individual digit flexion. The two are inextricably linked — as IP joint flexion improves, so does grip — and the two must be developed in tandem so that the maximum potential improvement is made. Many treatment activities will enhance both flexion and grip, but the therapist should ensure that specific rehabilitation of individual digital flexion is not overlooked.

Remedial games may be used to isolate specific movements. MCP and IP joint flexion of fingers and thumb may be encouraged through the use of tongs or an isolation splint with remedial games or fine pincer activities. The tongs or splint, if positioned just proximal to the joint to be mobilised, will promote specific movements. The goal is to flex the digit to pick up an object that is just a millimetre or two smaller than the digital flexion range. For example, the person may start with 2 cm pegs and eventually upgrade to nails or pins in remedial games such as solitaire. MCP and PIP flexion may also be encouraged using remedial games in which pieces are picked up between the fingertip and the heel of the hand.

Other activities that may prove helpful are woodwork with adapted tools, gardening and therapeutic putty exercises. Grip activities are usually graded to progress from gross hand grip to finer grip. Power grip is primarily a function of the ulnar side of the hand. Precision handling involves the radial side of the hand, where fine manipulative movements are carried out between the thumb and the tip of the index and middle fingers (Boscheinen-Morrin et al 1985). Again remedial games in a variety of sizes may be valuable, as may adapted computer devices, woodwork, gardening and domestic tasks.

Handles on tools and aids can be modified to obtain the specific grip size required or to promote a particular joint movement. With imagination the therapist can find many and varied activities to maintain the person's interest and motivation in accordance with his individual needs.

Therapeutic putty may be used very effectively in warm-up exercises to promote grip strength and isolate specific joint motion. Suppliers produce a booklet illustrating its application.

Orthoses have a vital role to play in restoring flexion but can never replace specific treatment by the physiotherapist and occupational therapist. Although their styles and applications are too numerous to describe comprehensively here, some basic orthoses are illustrated in Figures 26.5–26.7.

Extension

Although the general tendency is for therapists

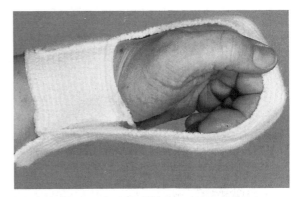

Fig. 26.5 Flexion orthosis. Elastic bandage with Velcro fastenings provides semi-dynamic pull to encourage MCP and PIP flexion.

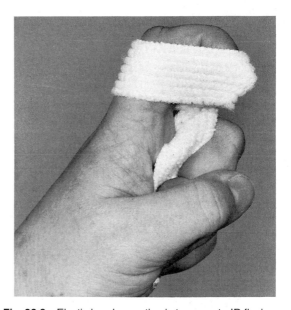

Fig. 26.6 Elastic bandage orthosis to promote IP flexion.

to focus on flexion in the early stages of treatment, maximum extension is also vital for function. Extension is required to release objects, in manipulative work and for everyday hand dexterity. Given the anatomy of the extensor muscles, it is more difficult to isolate specific digit extension than specific digit flexion. Therapeutic putty exercises are useful here as warm-up activities (Fig. 26.8).

Remedial games with increasingly larger size pieces, woodwork with adapted tools, and adapted

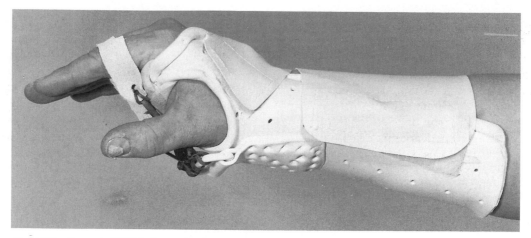

Fig. 26.7 Dynamic MCP flexion orthosis.

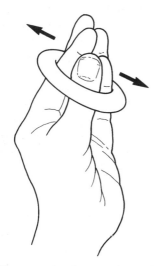

Fig. 26.8 Warm-up extension exercises using therapeutic putty.

computer activities may be useful in encouraging extension of the hand.

Orthoses, including serial night extension orthoses to stretch joint contractures or adhesions, may be used. Dynamic orthoses may be required to achieve improved specific joint extension.

Adduction and abduction

Many of the activities suggested above for use in promoting pronation and supination will also encourage adduction and abduction. The 'intrinsic

frame' may also be used. This is a wooden frame with interwoven elastic bands which allows the person to exercise his intrinsic muscles. (The intrinsic frame may also be useful in improving flexion, extension and opposition.)

Opposition

While this movement is encouraged in the treatment already outlined, specific attention should be paid to its return to ensure that good thumb-to-fingertip pinch is realised. Serial C-bar orthoses may be required to stretch a contracted first web space. Any activity which facilitates pad-to-pad pinch can be used to gain opposition.

Manipulative skills

As range of motion improves the person will need to be given practice in manipulative skills, especially if his job involves fine, detailed work. The person's normal work activities should be simulated as closely as possible.

SPECIFIC INJURIES

BASIC PRINCIPLES OF FRACTURE MANAGEMENT

Diagnosis is usually through history of the injury, clinical examination and X-ray. Symptoms such as deformity, swelling, bruising, tenderness, localised pain, impaired function and crepitus may indicate a fracture. Fractures heal through callus formation but reduction and support may be necessary to facilitate healing. This may take the form of casting or orthoses to support the fracture site in a good anatomical position and protect other structures, such as nerves or blood vessels, which may be at risk if bone movement occurs. Fractures may also be immobilised by internal or external fixation.

Rehabilitation falls into two categories:

- maintenance of movement of all uninvolved joints to preserve their function throughout fracture healing
- mobilisation of joints proximal and distal to the fracture after union has occurred, together with restoration of maximum function of the whole limb.

The occupational therapist may be involved in applying orthotic techniques for immobilisation or rehabilitation. Practical activities are important in enhancing the healing process and preventing or reducing the risk of permanent disability. Since any fractures interfere with everyday function, attention must be given to independence in daily living activities throughout the rehabilitation programme, most particularly in the early stages. However, it is equally important that as treatment progresses and more active movement is encouraged, any superfluous compensatory equipment is gradually withdrawn.

Clavicle, scapula and upper part of the humerus

The precise nature of the occupational therapist's intervention will depend upon the mode of support or immobilisation for the fracture and the age and needs of the person. These fractures are usually treated by means of a sling to support the weight of the arm, but some may be reduced by means of a figure-of-eight bandage or an abduction orthosis. All will affect the use of the arm in daily living activities, and the individual will need to learn techniques for maintaining independence while he has the use of only one hand. Following the removal of the support, gentle active exercise to promote shoulder movement should be encouraged and the use of any compensatory equipment for daily living activities re-evaluated. Therapeutic activities chosen should be relevant to the needs of the individual, and gradually upgraded to increase range of movement at the shoulder joint and gradual return of strength to the whole limb. The elderly may need practice with domestic duties to regain confidence in their bilaterality.

Shaft of the humerus

The type of fracture incurred at this site often depends on the nature of the accident. A fall on the outstretched hand frequently results in a spiral fracture, whereas direct force or a fall on the elbow is more likely to cause a transverse fracture. If the person is upright and the arm is supported in a sling, the effects of gravity will usually reduce the fracture. A plaster U-slab is often applied to the upper arm to prevent angulation when the person is sitting or lying. After one week the initial oedema will usually have been reduced; the fracture can then be held more effectively in a functional brace. If the occupational therapist is involved at this stage she should encourage the individual to use the arm for light activities involving a pendular movement of the shoulder. Abduction of the arm, however, should be avoided. The support provided by the brace should be checked regularly as the oedema subsides.

After six weeks, it is usual for the brace to be discarded and for active shoulder mobilising activities to be introduced. Some fractures are internally fixed by plating or intermedullary nailing, and active shoulder mobilising may usually commence at three weeks post-fixation. It is not unusual for the radial nerve to be compromised by the fracture. A dynamic orthosis is usually supplied, and wrist and hand function are encouraged alongside shoulder mobilisation. In some elderly people, particularly those with pathological fractures, bracing may be used for long-term support.

Forearm

There are a number of different fractures which may occur in the forearm, but almost all are treated by reduction and immobilisation in a plaster support. Depending on the type and site of the injury, the plaster may enclose the wrist joint and forearm and, in the case of fractures to the upper part of the radius and/or ulnar the elbow joint may also be immobilised. Internal fixation with plates and screws may also be used, and in some cases external fixation may be applied.

The support may be worn for a period of four to eight weeks, depending on the injury and the method of fixation. In some cases the plaster may be replaced with a functional brace after two weeks.

The therapist's role is to maintain mobility in the non-immobilised joints of the whole limb, to reduce any oedema in the hand and to retain maximum independence in personal care activities. The therapist should also be alert for any signs of median or ulnar nerve involvement.

Following removal of the immobilisation, treatment aims to restore mobility to the elbow, forearm and wrist joints. Extension of the wrist is particularly important for grip, and restrictions in forearm pronation and supination will affect many everyday activities.

Scaphoid bone

Scaphoid fractures are relatively common and may take six to eight months to heal. Fractures of the middle one-third or waist of the scaphoid are notorious for delayed or non-union. If the fracture is displaced, open reduction with a screw is preferable; otherwise the wrist is immobilised from the upper forearm to the proximal phalanges, incorporating the proximal phalanx of the thumb. The plaster may be replaced after 8–12 weeks with a closely moulded thermoplastic support to allow full finger flexion but retain thumb immobilisation. This support will be required for a further six weeks, and may be used even longer for protection in the work situation. To reduce the risk of further stress to the fracture

site, power grip should be discouraged until X-ray confirms healing.

Metacarpus and phalanges

Metacarpal and phalangeal fractures may be the result of direct violence, a crush injury or a fall. Reduction and immobilisation are obtained through application of plaster or a thermoplastic support, with or without internal fixation by wiring or small plates and screws. Reducing angulation is particularly important in regaining alignment of the digits for functional grip and finger dexterity.

Rehabilitation should concentrate on regaining full mobility and dexterity of the whole hand, but individual finger movements may be obtained through remedial games or specific therapeutic activities involving precision or hook grip, opposition or extensor movements.

TENDON INJURIES

Tendon injuries occur most frequently in the hand and lower forearm. Often only one or two digits are affected, but damage is occasionally widespread, with tendon injuries to all the digits and at several levels. A sound knowledge of the principles of wound healing and the anatomy of the flexor and extensor system is essential in assessing and treating an individual with tendon injuries.

Numerous management methods have arisen for tendon injuries, owing to the controversy concerning tendon healing (Moran 1986). Both static and dynamic therapeutic approaches are used, depending on the area of the injury and the protocols of the unit. Successful management depends on close liaison with the surgeon, the therapist and the individual concerned.

All treatment protocols aim to restore full function to the injured tendons by:

- reducing adhesions
- preventing joint stiffness or contractures
- restoring tendon glide.

Flexor tendon injuries

There are numerous variations in the postoperative management of flexor tendon injuries; all, however, have a common goal of preventing the formation of adhesions.

The therapist will usually see the individual one to three days postoperatively to remove the bulky dressings, commence an exercise programme and apply a thermoplastic orthosis. The orthosis is usually fitted dorsally with the wrist in 20–30 degrees of flexion, the MCP joints in 70 degrees of flexion and the IP joints in full extension. This position is important because it keeps the collateral ligaments out to length and so prevents secondary joint contracture caused by prolonged immobilisation with the ligaments relaxed.

Kleinert elastic band traction may be added. The injured digit is maintained in a position of almost full passive flexion by tension on the elastic band. The orthosis should permit full active IP joint extension, and the elasticity of the band should permit such action without excessive tension. As the resting posture of the PIP joint is flexion, great care should be taken to avoid PIP joint contracture by ensuring that full extension is achieved regularly.

Whatever the orthotic technique employed, the therapist will be involved in supervising a regime of exercise specific to the injured tendon and to all affected joints. Once the person is familiar with the regime, supervision can be gradually reduced to periodic checks that progress goals are being achieved.

The therapist also needs to consider oedema control, wound care and scar management as part of the treatment regime. The treatment protocol for flexor tendon injuries lasts approximately 12 weeks, and a graded programme of exercise and splinting is recommended throughout this period.

The individual's compliance is of utmost importance throughout the rehabilitation process, as non-compliance can jeopardise the functional results of the tendon grafts. The therapist therefore needs to remain flexible in her approach and work with the individual to consider feasible alternatives to treatment programmes (Dovelle et al 1988).

Extensor tendon injuries

Extensor tendon injuries of the hand are common.

Without correct surgical and therapeutic intervention these injuries may result in permanent functional limitations of the hand (Dovelle et al 1988). Rehabilitation of extensor tendon injuries tends to be less complex than that of the flexor system.

The hand is generally supported in an extended position according to the site of the injury, and is mobilised to regain active movement according to the treatment protocols of the unit.

Treatment goals will be to promote tendon healing, restoration of function, oedema and pain control and scar management. Extension lag (a deficit between passive and active extension) is most commonly caused by the tendon healing in slight attenuation. Night splinting in full extension and activities to encourage full extension will help eliminate the lag.

A dynamic extension orthosis may be supplied to allow active flexion against traction, while the extensor system is rested and allowed to heal in a satisfactory position.

LIGAMENT INJURIES

The collateral ligaments of the MCP joint of the thumb and the PIP joints of the fingers are those most often damaged. Primary treatment may be conservative or surgical, depending on the severity of the problem, and is followed by the use of orthoses to protect the joint from lateral movement for several weeks (Fig. 26.9). An orthosis which allows some movement in acceptable directions will help to reduce potential joint stiffness (Fig. 26.10).

The lengthy immobilisation necessary to achieve a stable and therefore functional digit may result in joint stiffness. Passive stretching of the joint is not usually recommended until the later stages of treatment so that the healing ligament is not jeopardised. Likewise, care must be taken at all stages in treatment not to use an activity which will stress an injured ligament by stretching it. Treatment should aim to restore full active range of movement to the affected joint. However, there may be some residual deficit in flexion/extension.

Injuries to the volar plate of the PIP joint frequently occur as the result of sports injuries in

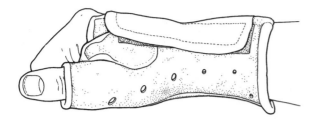

Fig. 26.9 Orthosis to protect MCP joint ligaments of thumb.

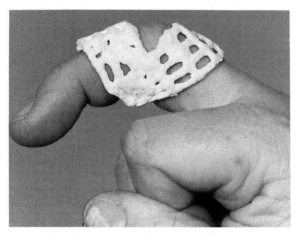

Fig. 26.10 Orthosis to protect PIP joint ligaments allows 75% normal joint range while achieving lateral stability.

which the end of the finger is struck by a ball and the joint hyperextended. Treatment involves protection from full PIP joint extension for approximately six weeks using an orthosis similar to that shown in Figure 26.10, while allowing maximal PIP joint flexion and full distal interphalangeal (DIP) joint movement.

It is not unusual for volar plate injury to occur in association with damage to the collateral ligaments. The same orthosis can be used in both instances, with slight loading towards the injured side to hold the ligament in a relaxed position.

Frozen shoulder or capsulitis of the joint often has its origin in a trivial accident in which the shoulder is suddenly stressed. The person may be unaware of the incident which precipitated the painful and stiff joint. Treatment should be gentle and rhythmic; care should be taken not to cause further insult to the inflamed capsule.

CRUSH INJURIES

These can be sustained to a single digit or the whole of a limb. Even where there is no fracture, rupture of tendons or injury to neurovascular structures, soft tissue damage will lead to gross oedema and considerable pain. Scar tissue will form, with the consequent danger of adhesions causing profound limitation of movement.

It is sometimes tempting to regard a person with no specific diagnosis beyond a soft tissue crush injury as poorly motivated when he presents with a painful, stiff hand and fails to make a swift response to rehabilitation. In fact such injuries often take more hard work and commitment on the part of the individual and therapist than those with a specific diagnosis or in which surgical intervention is required. Damage to soft tissues is frequently widespread, involving all systems. The person will need encouragement and support, especially in the early stages when progress is slow and hard-won and pain rules the tolerance to activity.

In major crush injuries fractures, amputations and severe damage to tendon and neurovascular systems may occur. There may be skin and muscle loss. A person involved in such a mutilating accident will be shocked and may well go through a bereavement reaction. While surgeons are able to revascularise and reconstruct a severely damaged digit or limb, the decision to do so must be balanced against the likely functional outcome and the person's own agenda and priorities.

Compartment syndrome may occur following a severe crush injury, particularly in the lower limb. To relieve the pressure in the muscle compartments a fasciotomy is performed. Skin grafting is usually necessary. The therapist is involved from the early stages in applying orthoses, facilitating sensory adaptation, increasing range of movement and muscle bulk and aiding mobilisation. Provision of pressure garments may be particularly valuable in some cases.

The psychological 'backlash' of losing part or all of a limb and any disfiguring scarring is as vital a symptom for treatment as physical dysfunction. Both the individual and his relatives will need care, support and a listening ear if they are to adjust well to a new body image and its implications. It is important to remember that people's reactions and ability to cope vary greatly and while one person may hide a whole hand from view, having lost only a fingertip, another may lose a whole hand or live with terrible scarring and cope amazingly well, both functionally and emotionally.

Early orthoses are aimed at resting the injured part in a good position for recovery. Shoulder and elbow injuries are rested with the forearm supported in a sling, while those to the wrist or hand are immobilised in the 'safe' position with collateral ligaments out to length to reduce the risk of joint contractures.

In any crush injury the first aim is to reduce oedema and encourage active movement. The two are inextricably linked: as oedema is reduced, active movement is facilitated; as range of motion improves, oedema is pumped out.

Assessment of daily living skills and provision of help as necessary is particularly appropriate for people who have suffered severe crush injuries which will incapacitate them for some time. The benefits of assistive equipment should be carefully weighed against the need to encourage bilaterality and controlled use of the injured part. The therapist should bear in mind that early facilitation of a degree of independence can be a considerable boost to the injured person's confidence.

THE STIFF HAND

An acutely stiff hand is characterised by oedema, pain and decreased range of movement, and may be a result of minor or major trauma to the hand. Early intervention by the therapist is essential to prevent the development of a chronically stiff hand. The main goal of treatment is the restoration of function, and the treatment programme will consist of assessment and evaluation, oedema control, therapeutic activity and splinting.

Exercise should be carried out within the individual's limits, and encouragement should be given to use the hand as much as possible in everyday activities. The therapist will need to educate the individual about the importance of carrying out his exercises, but will need to warn against over-zealous continuous exercising which may cause further pain and oedema. With the acutely stiff hand, improvement of the range of movement and reduction in oedema should be evident within the first week of treatment.

REFLEX SYMPATHETIC DYSTROPHY

Reflex sympathetic dystrophy (RSD) is a vasomotor dysfunction that can be localised to one area of the limb or can involve the whole limb. Pain is the most outstanding complaint, and swelling is the most outstanding feature. RSD is characterised by pain that is disproportionate to the original injury and has three intrinsic phases:

- *Acute phase* (first three months). Disabling, disproportionate pain is the outstanding symptom and is accompanied by gross pitting oedema. Joint stiffness becomes progressively worse, with locally increased temperature, sweating and hyperaemia.
- *Sub-acute phase* (three to nine months). Pain becomes progressively worse, and the swelling becomes firm, fixed and brawny, with periarticular fibrosis. The traumatised part becomes dry and cyanotic.
- *Chronic phase* In this phase pain levels out and swelling subsides, leaving the affected part stiff, atrophied, shiny, pale and cool, with osteoporosis clearly visible on X-rays.

RSD may follow any trivial or major insult — accidental or surgical — and occurs most commonly in the upper limb. It is important to recognise the condition early and, in consultation with medical staff, to begin intensive treatment immediately.

The possible connection between susceptibility to RSD and personality traits or psychological factors continues to be debated. While a number of people will undoubtedly be affected by these influences there are others who suffer from RSD yet have no apparent negative personality factors and are not achieving any secondary gain.

The keys to successful rehabilitation of RSD whether in the lower or upper limb, are:

- early recognition and intervention

- establishing good, supportive rapport with the person involved.

Close teamwork with medical and physiotherapy staff is essential, but good communication with the individual is even more vital. Part of the therapist's role is to help the person understand the need to push himself to use the limb actively despite intense pain. The doctor may prescribe pain-killing drugs or TENS to facilitate the return of function. Interesting, purposeful activities are particularly helpful in distracting the person and encouraging concentration on the activity rather than on the pain of movement.

Rehabilitation may continue for many months. Initially, daily attendance at therapy sessions may be advised in order to prevent a return to the vicious circle of pain and disuse. Orthoses to improve passive and active ranges of movement and maintain a good resting position have an important role, but should not be allowed to substitute for hard work by the person and his therapist.

DUPUYTREN'S CONTRACTURE

In Dupuytren's contracture there is fibrosis and shortening of the palmar aponeurosis, leading to a flexion contracture of the digital joints and an adduction soft tissue contracture (Boscheinen-Morrin 1985). Many methods of surgical treatment are reported, and postoperative treatment also varies, although the common goal is to promote wound healing, minimise scarring and maximise mobility (Clark 1993).

The therapist will be involved in the provision of splinting where required, wound care management, oedema control, scar management, therapeutic activity and the promotion of independence. Recurrence of the contractures may occur and require further surgery.

CUMULATIVE TRAUMA DISORDERS

Cumulative trauma disorders (CTDs) are disorders of the soft tissue caused by repeated exertions and movements of the body. The structure of the upper limb is particularly vulnerable to soft tissue injury (Putz-Anderson 1988), nerves, tendons, tendon sheaths and muscles being the most frequently reported sites (Hunter et al 1990).

Many other terms, such as repetitive strain injuries, repetitive trauma disorders and regional musculoskeletal disorders, are used to describe this range of disorders. CTD belongs to a collection of health problems which are work-related, and there is often a long time between beginning work and the onset of the disorder. There are few distinctive or dramatic features relating to the onset of CTD; hence an individual may be exposed for many years to the source of the microtrauma without being aware of the potential hazard.

Repetitiveness of work is one of the common risk factors in CTD, and it has been shown that the risk of such disorders as tendinitis and carpal tunnel syndrome increase with increasing force and repetitiveness (Hunter et al 1990).

It is widely recognised that all the disorders principally result from cumulative overuse (although in the case of carpal tunnel syndrome, systemic factors may also play a part) (Pheasant 1991). The causative factors most commonly implicated are:

- fixed work posture
- repetitive motions
- psychological stress.

Disorders of the upper limb are associated with repetitive, short-cycle tasks, and CTD is most common in jobs in which repetition rates are high and forceful gripping activities are required.

Conditions associated with CTD include De Quervain's tendonitis, lateral epicondylitis (tennis elbow), trigger finger, medial epicondylitis (golfer's elbow), gamekeeper's thumb and many more. Not all CTDs are associated with an individual's workplace; in some cases they result from sport and recreational activities.

For simple cases of tenosynovitis, rest of the aggravated tendons in an orthosis for several weeks followed by gradual return to use of the affected part is effective. It is, however, common for the problem to recur.

When treating the individual with CTD the therapist needs a thorough understanding of the principles of ergonomics, so that this knowledge can be incorporated into the assessment and evaluation of the affected limb and the possible cause of the trauma. Treatment and advice can then be offered to the individual on how he may adapt his working and leisure practices to reduce the effects of the stress on the upper limb.

There is much medicolegal debate over the diagnosis of CTD, and although legislation is coming into force in the workplace related to CTD, through European Directives, more research and education is needed in this area.

Whether or not there is a sound pathological basis for a diagnosis of CTD, those who suffer from it can become substantially disabled. Sensitive treatment and counselling may enable people with this diagnosis to come to terms with their discomfort and expand their functional horizon.

CONCLUSION

When treating upper limb injuries the occupational therapist employs a number of approaches. The use of the biomechanical approach predominates in specific techniques to overcome physical impairments. However, the therapist should equally address the needs and wishes of the individual, and the use of the limbs in the fuller context of living. The objectives of rehabilitation are to minimise the long-term effects of the injury and to promote maximum functional activity, along with adjustment to any residual dysfunction. In the upper limbs, mobility and dexterity are particularly important for everyday tasks, and the psychological impact of injury may have a significant effect on rehabilitation. Elements of learning, compensation and humanism all play an important part in the occupational therapist's theoretical repertoire when treating upper limb injuries.

Any trauma will have psychological implications for the individual and his close relatives, and these should be respected and addressed to help the person to attain a realistic and positive approach to therapy. Activities should be purposeful and appropriate to the needs and wishes of the individual, and should provide specific anatomical exercise for the injured part and the limb as a whole. As recovery occurs regular assessment and evaluation of the limb will enable the individual and the therapist to measure change and adjust activities accordingly. In the later stages of treatment, activities should particularly aim to promote return to role duties and leisure pursuits. For many people physical recovery from a limb injury may be almost total. Where this is not possible the therapist should aim to help the person to attain his maximum functional potential and to adjust both physically and psychologically to any residual deficit.

ACKNOWLEDGEMENTS

Thanks to Glenys Crooks, Kate Abbott and Ruth Sampson at the Derbyshire Royal Infirmary NHS Trust, whose original text in the previous edition provided a valuable basis for this chapter.

REFERENCES

American Society for Surgery of the Hand 1990 The hand — primary care of common problems. Churchill Livingstone, New York
Bear-Lehman J 1983 Factors affecting return to work after hand injury. American Journal of Occupational Therapy 37(3): 188–194
Blumenfield M, Schoeps M M 1993 Psychological care of the burn and trauma patient. Williams & Wilkins, Baltimore
Boschcinen-Morrin J, Davey V, Conolley W B 1985 The hand — fundamentals of therapy. Butterworth, London
Cailliet R 1982 Hand pain and impairment. F A Davis, Philadelphia
Cailliet R 1991 Shoulder pain. F A Davis, Philadelphia
Cason J S 1981 Treatment of burns. Chapman & Hall, London
Clark G L, Shaw-Wilgis E F, Aiello B, Eckhaus D, Eddington L V 1993 Hand rehabilitation — a practical guide. Churchill Livingstone, New York
Donatelli R A 1991 Physical therapy of the shoulder, 2nd edn. Churchill Livingstone, New York

Dovelle S, Heeter P K, Fischer D R, Chow J A 1988 Early controlled motion following flexor tendon graft. American Journal of Occupational Therapy 44(7): 457–463

Dovelle S, Heeter P K, Fischer D R, Chow J A 1989 Rehabilitation of extensor tendon injury of the hand by means of early controlled motion. American Journal of Occupational Therapy 43(2): 115–119

Giudice M L 1990 Effects of continuous passive motion and elevation on hand oedema. American Journal of Occupational Therapy 44(3): 189–194

Hunter J M, Schneider L E, Mackin E J, Callahan A D 1990 Rehabilitation of the hand, 3rd edn. C V Mosby, St Louis

Jones M 1977 An approach to occupational therapy. Butterworth, London

Miles W 1989 Cited in Mackin E (ed.) 1986 Hand clinics. W B Saunders, Philadelphia

McPhee S D 1987 Functional hand evaluations: a review. American Journal of Occupational Therapy 41(3): 158–163

Moran C A (ed.) 1986 Hand rehabilitation. Churchill Livingstone, London

Pedretti L W, Zoltan B 1990 Occupational therapy. Practice skills for physical dysfunction. C V Mosby, St Louis

Pheasant S 1991 Ergonomics, work and health. Macmillan, London

Putz-Anderson V (ed.) 1988 Cumulative trauma disorders — a manual for musculoskeletal diseases of the upper limbs. Taylor and Francis, London

Spaulding S J 1989 The biomechanics of prehension. American Journal of Occupational Therapy 43(5): 302–307

Wynn Parry C B 1981 Rehabilitation of the hand. Butterworth, London

Yerxa E J 1983 Development of a hand sensitivity test for the hypersensitive hand. American Journal of Occupational Therapy 3(3): 176–181

FURTHER READING

Adams J C, Hamblen D L 1990 Outline of orthopaedics, 11th edn. Churchill Livingstone, Edinburgh

Beasley R W 1981 Hand injuries. W B Saunders, Philadelphia

Bowker P, Condie D N, Bader D L, Pratt D J 1993 Biomechanical basis of orthotic management. Butterworth-Heinemann, Oxford

Burke F D, McGrouther D A, Smith P J 1990 Principles of hand surgery. Churchill Livingstone, Edinburgh

Cailliet R 1976 Neck and arm pain. F A Davis, Philadelphia

Conolly W B, Kilgore E S 1979 Hand injuries and infections. Edward Arnold, London

Dandy D J 1989 Essential orthopaedics and trauma. Churchill Livingstone, Edinburgh

Lamb D W, Hooper G 1984 Hand conditions. Colour aids series. Churchill Livingstone, Edinburgh

Lister G 1983 The hand: diagnosis and indications. Churchill Livingstone, London

Macnicol M F, Lamb D W 1984 Basic care of the injured hand. Churchill Livingstone, Edinburgh

Macnicol M F, Lamb D W 1990 American Society for Surgery of the Hand — primary care of common problems. Churchill Livingstone, Edinburgh

McRae R 1989 Practical fracture treatment, 2nd edn. Churchill Livingstone, Edinburgh

Pashley J 1989 Grip strengthening with adapted computer switches. American Journal of Occupational Therapy 43(2): 121–123

Penrose D 1993 Occupational therapy for orthopaedic conditions. Chapman & Hall, London

Salter M I 1987 Hand injuries. A therapeutic approach. Churchill Livingstone, Edinburgh

27

Osteoarthritis

Jane James

INTRODUCTION

Osteoarthritis affects the majority of people by the age of 55. It is the most common form of arthritis, affecting men and women equally, except for primary generalised osteoarthritis, which is ten times more common in women. For some people, osteoarthritis is a severely disabling condition, causing considerable functional impairment; for others, it never reaches a stage where treatment is required.

Osteoarthritis is a degenerative disease which causes the normally smooth articular surface of the joints to become damaged. This in turn restricts the range of movement of the joints and causes pain and stiffness. Osteoarthritis can affect any joint. However, the large weight-bearing joints in the hips, knees and spine are particularly at risk. Primary generalised osteoarthritis most commonly affects the first carpometacarpal and metatarsophalangeal joints.

Osteoarthritis cannot be cured but the restrictions it causes can be minimised or reduced in various ways to enable the person to continue living an independent and fulfillng life and to cope emotionally with any remaining impairment. Surgical intervention is becoming more effective as new techniques evolve; however, people treated surgically require further rehabilitation to ensure maximum potential is reached. The occupational therapist, along with other members of the primary health care team, has a vital part to play in encouraging people to reach their goals for independence. Her role includes

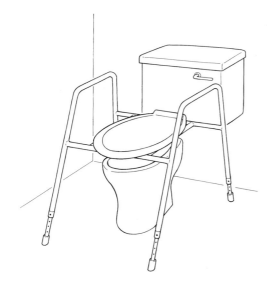

Fig. 27.7 Toilet with combined raise and frame.

is a separate cubicle the therapist may suggest a seat. This may be a free-standing chair or stool (providing the shower base is strong enough to withstand the pressure from the legs) or may be a wall-mounted seat.

Using the toilet

This poses difficulty if the toilet is low but various means can be taken to raise the seat height and provide assistance in rising. An example of a combined raised toilet seat with rails is shown in Figure 27.7. This can be free-standing or fixed to the floor. A separate seat raise can be provided and should be fitted to the toilet securely. A grab rail or frame might also be required.

Dressing

The therapist may advise the person to be seated at a comfortable height while dressing and to make use of long-handled equipment and easy fastenings.

Other equipment

For the person with osteoarthritis in the lower limbs, standing to carry out kitchen tasks may be painful; provision of a high perching stool

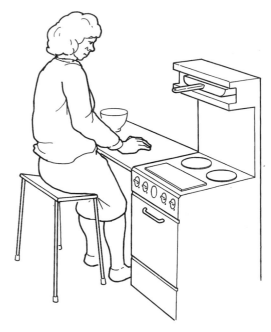

Fig. 27.8 Use of perching stool for kitchen tasks.

(Fig. 27.8) can help ease pain and reduce dependency on carers.

More complex equipment may be relevant for those people with greater impairment, particularly if surgical treatment is not possible or has not succeeded. Hoists can greatly assist transfer of a wheelchair-bound person and help to relieve his carer (see p. 240). Special beds can greatly assist in easing the pain caused through immobility, by enabling the person to change his own position during the night. Such beds can also contribute towards reducing any swelling by elevating the legs, and may assist nursing care by raising the person's height. As beds tend to be fairly expensive items, and since the features offered in different models vary, careful choice should be made before purchase.

Hand function

Generalised osteoarthritis may affect upper limb function, particularly the power grip, where the carpometacarpal joints are affected. Strong gripping activities such as turning taps, opening containers or holding heavy objects may pose problems. These may be overcome by the provision of small equipment such as tap turners, jar openers or teapot tippers. Where hand function is severely affected a comprehensive assessment of everyday activities will highlight areas of difficulty, and consideration of alternative techniques or the use of labour-saving equipment to avoid lifting or strong hand movements may be advised.

Orthoses, particularly to support and stabilise the base of the thumb, may prove beneficial to maintaining hand function.

Surgical intervention for the osteoarthritic hand is less common than for the hand affected by rheumatoid arthritis, but where surgery has been necessary the occupational therapist may be involved in treatment to improve hand function following surgery.

Diet and exercise

An overweight person will put greater strain on the joints and so will possibly experience more pain than a person of normal weight. Advice about healthy diet for weight loss and maintenance will be valuable and may be provided by the occupational therapist or the dietitian. The therapist may help the person to plan regular rhythmical exercise such as swimming. Diet and exercise may be more successful if pursued as a group activity with others who have similar problems. The person will usually be able to undertake exercise of this kind without attending a hospital or centre for a formal programme, and the therapist should encourage participation in normal activities to work toward improved strength and range of movement with a reduction of pain as the muscles become stronger.

Joint protection

The person and his carer should be given advice and information about the condition so that they know what precautions are needed. The occupational therapist may be requested to provide resting orthoses for joints of the knees, wrists and hands or may provide working orthoses for hands. Spinal supports may also be requested to assist posture.

Principles of joint protection and the advan-

tages of different teaching methods are covered extensively in Chapter 28. Methods of altering movement patterns when performing activities, and guidance on energy conservation and exercise, are particularly important for people with osteoarthritis to help to alleviate stress on the affected joints.

Work and leisure

Many people with osteoarthritis who are still in employment find problems at work, particularly with mobility or hand function. The occupational therapist should discuss these and identify whether any changes may reduce strain. Alterations to machinery, provision of a supportive chair and assistance with mobility to and from work may all reduce demands on joints and enable the person to continue his job. The Disability Employment Advisor (DEA) may be able to help with these or other modifications. If the job is not adaptable, or the impairment is too significant to continue in the present job, the DEA can provide advice on assessments for retraining and future employment prospects (see Ch. 8).

The therapist should also discuss leisure activities, and may make suggestions regarding equipment or other alternatives to enable the person to continue these. Alternatively she may suggest a new interest which accommodates his disability.

The occupational therapist also needs a knowledge of the welfare rights system in order to advise people on claiming benefits. This is a complex area, but a general knowledge of the system and whom to refer to for expert guidance will prove invaluable, particularly when advising people who have to leave work or whose impairment deteriorates such that they require further assistance.

The occupational therapist should also be aware of other sources of support and information, for example details of local support groups or access to services such as home care. The NHS and Community Care Act 1990 and Section 9 of the Disabled Persons (Services Consultation and Representation) Act 1986 describe the requirements of authorities to provide relevant information to disabled people. Therapists should

Physiotherapy

The main aims of physiotherapy are relief of pain, improving muscle strength, increasing mobility of joints, and prevention or correction of deformity. Pain relief can be aided with a number of physical modalities:

- Electrotherapy (e.g. infrared radiation, shortwave diathermy and ultrasound)
- Heat therapy, usually provided in the form of wax baths (commonly for the hands)
- Cold therapy.

Mobility is improved through:

- teaching correct performance of an appropriate daily exercise programme to maintain joints' range of movement
- individual or group intensive rehabilitation programmes, using isometric and progressive resistive exercise to improve muscle strength and stamina
- hydrotherapy — warm water (34–37°C) provides muscle relaxation and the buoyancy effect further aids mobilisation and exercise
- assessment and provision of walking equipment and teaching correct gait patterns
- teaching correct posture, resting and lifting techniques
- provision of static and serial splinting (particularly for the lower limb), traction and stretch techniques to reduce contractures.

Social work

The social worker can provide advice and assistance with claiming benefits and other financial advice; liaising with employers and employment services; advising on voluntary work and appropriate community leisure facilities for people taking early retirement; and liaising with social services to provide support systems such as home care, Meals-on-Wheels and day centre placement for people with more severe disease. As counsellors they can also provide psychological support to aid individuals and families in adjusting to the disease, and some may be trained in sexual counselling.

OCCUPATIONAL THERAPY INTERVENTION

ASSESSMENT

As RA is a chronic disease, assessment is ongoing. Increasingly, hospital rheumatology departments include regular functional assessments in the medical notes to monitor disease progress. Two assessments are commonly used, both having potential to be more widely used in occupational therapy as progress and outcome measures, and for use as initial assessments to aid in identifying individuals' perceptions of their major problems. These are:

- the HAQ (Health Assessment Questionnaire: anglicized version, Kirwan & Reeback 1986), including 24 functional activities with additional scales to measure individuals' satisfaction with ADL, perceptions of functional change and pain on functional activity
- the AIMS (Arthritis Impact Measurement Scale: anglicized version, Hill et al 1990) which evaluates mobility, walking and bending, self-care, household tasks, arm function, hand and finger function, social support, work, social activities, pain, level of tension and mood, along with scales for individuals' satisfaction with their abilities in these and for identifying in which areas they would like most improvement.

Both questionnaires are self-administered, the HAQ taking five minutes and the AIMS 20 minutes to complete. These can be completed prior to initial assessment (being posted to the outpatients department in advance) and can then form the basis of interview. Rheumatology occupational therapists often have contact with individuals over many years. These assessments can facilitate individuals in: identifying their own needs more readily; actively participating in the decision-making process of treatment planning so that this is a collaborative partnership; and increasing their perceptions of control. The breadth of the AIMS, in particular, can assist occupational therapists to ensure that the wide range of arthritis problems is addressed in treatment (if resources allow). It also provides an opportunity formally to assess psychological state and to discuss this during interview, supplemented by observation.

Functional assessments

Reliable, valid rheumatology assessments include:

- the Robinson–Bashall Functional Assessment for Arthritis Patients (McCloy & Jongbloed 1987) of 41 items on four scales (self-care, ambulation, transport and activity tolerance), using timed tests
- the Functional Status Index (Jette 1987), measuring dependence, pain and difficulty in 45 activities (mobility, hand, personal care, home and social/role activities). These may be supplemented with non-standardised checklists to ensure that all ADL problems are identified, for example the St Albans City Hospital ADL Checklist (developed by Marion Ferguson at St Albans, Hertfordshire) or an ADL Checklist described by Melvin (1989), or generic occupational therapy assessments such as the Canadian Occupational Performance measure and Functional Independence Measure.

For people with more severe disease, a home assessment should be considered to obtain a clear picture of their ADL ability at home, and the techniques, equipment and adaptations currently used. In addition an evaluation of how realistic the individual and carers are about their current and future needs, and to what degree the person is relying on others' assistance, can be made. Information about the local environment, facilities and social support can also be identified.

Hand assessments

A number of functional and anatomical hand assessments are available (see Chs 7 and 10). Hand measurements may include:

- grip and pinch strength (using the Jamar dynamometer)

- joint range of movement, hand span and deformities, using for example the method described by Treuhaft et al (1971)
- pain, using for example visual analogue scales
- hand and grip function, during simulated ADL using the Quantitative Test of Upper Extremity Function, Jebsen–Taylor Test or Smith Hand Function Test
- dexterity, using for example the Purdue Pegboard test.

These, and other hand assessments, are described in Melvin (1989). Assessment choice will be influenced by the reason for conducting the test. Hand and grip function tests help in determining the need for splinting and in evaluating its effectiveness. These, plus more detailed hand measurements, aid decision-making, pre-surgery on to the most appropriate operation, and post-surgery to evaluate outcome.

Compliance with hand joint protection education can be assessed using the Joint Protection Behaviour Assessment (Hammond 1994a).

Daily activity patterns

The NIH Activity Record (Gerber & Furst 1992) is a daily log self-report measure requiring individuals to record their main activity (e.g. rest, housework, watch TV, work, sleep) during half-hour periods throughout a week and a weekend day. Each activity is rated for: pain and fatigue; meaningfulness, enjoyment and difficulty; and whether they rested during it. This can be used to:

- identify which tasks cause most pain and fatigue and to evaluate rest patterns during the day, which assists in planning individualised joint protection and energy conservation education and evaluating their outcomes
- evaluate individuals' daily life patterns and balance of activities, which can be used to help explore a more enjoyable, balanced life-style and in developing goals and programmes to enable this to be achieved.

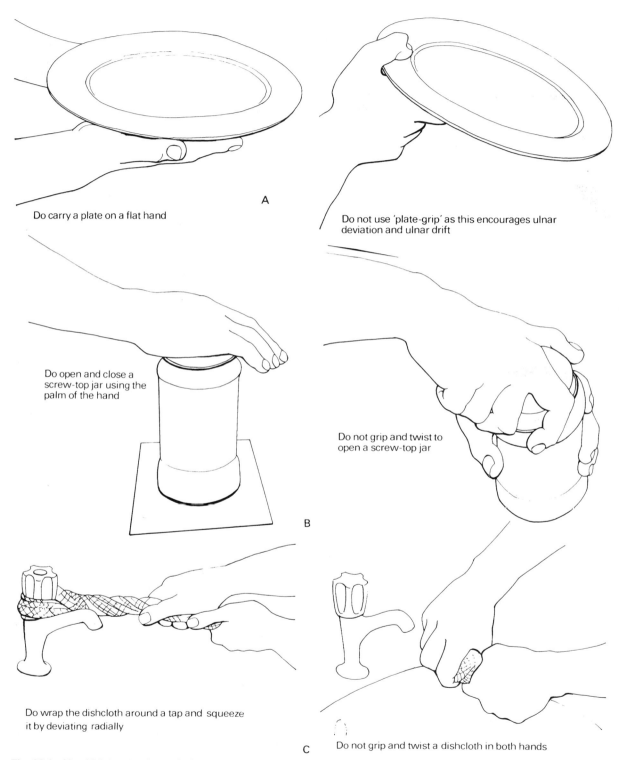

Do carry a plate on a flat hand

A

Do not use 'plate-grip' as this encourages ulnar deviation and ulnar drift

Do open and close a screw-top jar using the palm of the hand

Do not grip and twist to open a screw-top jar

B

Do wrap the dishcloth around a tap and squeeze it by deviating radially

Do not grip and twist a dishcloth in both hands

C

Fig. 28.1 Hand joint protection techniques in rheumatoid arthritis. (A) Carrying a plate. (B) Opening a jar. (C) Squeezing a dishcloth.

4. *Reduce effort.* Using less muscular effort to perform daily tasks reduces internal joint stress. Examples include:

- Using technical devices. Most commonly used in the kitchen are the jar opener, tap turner, easy vegetable peeler, Stirex knife and dycem mat. Apart from the Stirex knife these are relatively inexpensive. Padded cutlery, sharp knife and cooking utensil handles are other, inexpensive aids
- Labour-saving devices. The most popular and useful purchases seem to be: electric can openers (preferably table-top rather than hand-held models), food processors, dishwashers, tumble driers and, for some, electric knives
- Employing leverage, e.g. by extending handles or using a knife to flip off ring-pulls
- Avoiding lifting and carrying, e.g.:
  — using wheels (e.g. a small hostess trolley to move items round the house, a laundry basket on castors, a shopping trolley)
  — sliding objects along work surfaces or the floor
  — tipping (e.g. placing a jug kettle on a 2–3 inch block of wood and tipping to pour rather than lifting, or using a kettle tipper).

It is better to recommend a few, well-selected pieces of equipment, as these are far more likely to be afforded, used and accepted, than to present a wide range of options, which may be seen as too many visible reminders of dysfunction. Recommending equipment and labour-saving gadgets commonly found in kitchen shops and household sections of department stores is less 'labelling'. Other equipment may be necessary as more joints become more severely affected. Evidence exists that use of some technical equipment (e.g. electric can openers and vegetable peelers) reduces pain. However, a substantial proportion of technical equipment (between 18 and 59%) is not used. This is again indicative of the need to ensure appropriate prescription.

People with arthritis are often valuable sources of information on alternative methods and gadgets, as they are experiencing day-to-day living with the disease. It may be useful to collate this information in a resource file, a copy of which could be kept in clinic waiting areas for reference by others.

5. *Avoid positions of deformity.* Stresses contributing to common patterns of deformity should be avoided. These may be external pressures, e.g. pushing joints sideways or downwards when lifting objects, or internal stresses from muscular compressive forces. For example:

- Strong power, pinch and tripod grips promote anterior subluxation at the MCP joints, and strong pinch promotes IP joint deformities. Handles, pens, etc. can be enlarged and padded
- Finger twisting actions promote ulnar deviation. The palm should be used to turn taps and open jars, with the fingers held straight
- Lifting heavy items with a flexed wrist promotes wrist anterior subluxation. The wrist should be extended.

Effectiveness of joint protection has not been evaluated. Anecdotally, using different movement patterns to perform painful tasks can immediately reduce pain on activity and, with continued use, can reduce joint stress and inflammation over a several day period (Melvin 1989). Two pilot studies have evaluated whether or not pain and reduction of joint stress occur as a result of using joint protection. Campbell & Schkade (1991) and Agnew (1987) identified that some subjects had more pain and used more, rather than less, wrist muscle activity when using joint protection methods. Compliance with joint protection is also questionable. A study evaluating standard joint protection education demonstrated that, following education, no significant change in the use of hand joint protection occurred (Hammond 1994a,b). Most subjects reported that they believed it very beneficial and were pleased to have received the education. However, joint protection methods were used only occasionally in response to pain and many already spontaneously used these techniques. Major barriers to behaviour change were difficulty in recalling methods sufficiently and in making these changes habitual. Careful attention to the patient education techniques used is essential.

Rest, positioning and sleep

Acutely inflamed and painful joints should be rested. However, research shows prolonged rest can have deleterious effects, with up to 3% of muscle strength lost per day. Remaining in bed should not be encouraged unless prescribed by the doctor, but people should rest for 10–12 hours per day (unless in remission), including one hour or more during the afternoon, to assist natural recovery processes, improve overall endurance for activity and enhance muscle function (Melvin 1989). Increased daily rest should be accompanied by a regular exercise programme. Too much inactivity can cause muscle wasting, osteopenia, boredom and depressed mood, with worsening of symptoms. People may also see this as emphasising dysfunction, thus reinforcing illness and the sick role. Careful education on the benefits of rest and its contribution to the package of life-style changes is necessary.

Advice should be given on correct resting positions. Joints should be well supported when sitting and lying. Chairs should have adequate seat depth to support the upper legs; allow the hips, knees and ankles to be positioned at 90 degrees; have a supportive back, which may include a lumbar back support, and support the head; and have firm arms to assist with rising.

Beds should be flat and firm, providing even support. This can be assisted by providing bedboards. Positioning should support and preserve the anatomical curves of the spine. A neck pillow (or soft towel) is more supportive than a regular pillow, which causes neck flexion and tension. This should correctly support the neck with the occipital bone touching the mattress. People should spend part of the night on their back, maintaining hips and knees in extension. A pillow should not be used to support the knees as this can encourage flexion contractures in more severely affected joints. Beds with foot boards, or bed cradles, can help to keep the weight of the bedclothes from dragging on the feet, which can contribute to foot drop in people with weak leg muscles. If there are nodules and skin involvement, sheepskin pads and foam protectors help to reduce pressure. Duvets are often easier to

pull up during the night than are sheets and blankets. For those wearing night resting orthoses, a shorter design, extending just beyond the finger and thumb PIP joints, leaves the finger tips free to pull up bedclothes, switch the beside light and radio on or off and turn the pages of bedtime reading. Orthoses limiting ability to perform these tasks can cause sleep disturbance and annoyance, resulting in them not being worn as recommended.

Sleep problems are common, because of pain, stiffness, mood changes and stress, and can contribute to fatigue and reduce function. Sedatives, sleeping pills and alcohol may be used by some, but are not suitable solutions as they suppress certain stages of sleep, causing sleep disturbance. Advice and discussion is useful on:

- ensuring that the bedroom is a comfortable environment (with reference to the bed, noise level, temperature and lighting)
- avoiding drinks containing caffeine (which acts as a stimulant) several hours before bedtime
- setting aside a relaxing period, e.g. by using relaxation methods or a warm bath
- an electric underblanket (on a low setting), which can, in some people, assist with pain relief
- a regular sleep schedule for going to bed and rising. As people get older, they require less sleep. Rest need not be equated with sleep
- taking medication as prescribed before bedtime — the doctor or pharmacist can advise on the best time to take these to minimise nocturnal pain, if this is the cause of sleep problems
- a few gentle range of movement exercises in bed before sleeping to help reduce pain and discomfort.

For those with early morning stiffness, it may be helpful to set the alarm to wake up early to take medication and rise later when this has had an effect. This should be discussed with the doctor as certain drugs must be taken with food.

Energy conservation

This can assist in reducing fatigue. These techniques enable the person to save energy during daily tasks, enabling greater control of how energy is distributed to activities which are meaningful throughout the day. The main principles of energy conservation are:

- Balance rest and work. Regular short breaks during prolonged periods of activity (e.g. five minutes every 20–30 minutes) increase the total duration over which individuals continue to have enough energy to perform activities. This may be difficult for some to adjust to, particularly if they consider resting to be a sign of 'giving in' to arthritis. It may be helpful to ask them to compare energy levels (by completing the NIH Activity Record) during their normal activity patterns with those when using regular rest periods.
- Use correct body positions. Good posture balances the weight of the head and limbs on the bony framework so that the force of gravity helps to keep a correct joint position. More energy is used to maintain poor postures as muscles have to work against the effect of gravity to maintain position. Hunched shoulders, craned necks and bent backs cause muscle tension, pain and tiredness. Standing requires approximately 25% more energy than sitting, so tasks should be performed seated if possible.
- Avoid staying in one position for long periods, which can lead to stiffness. It is recommended to change position every 20–30 minutes, for example taking a short walk round the house rather than remaining seated for the whole evening, or stretching the hands out regularly rather than continuing writing.
- Have correct work heights, which are those that allow the head and neck to be held as straight as possible while sitting or standing. Work surfaces should be approximately two inches below the elbow when the shoulders are relaxed. Work surfaces can be altered (by reducing their height or raising them with stable blocks), or a high stool with a back support may be used (ensuring that the feet are supported).
- Avoid activities that cannot be stopped if they become too stressful, i.e. cause sudden or severe pain. Some tasks, for example carrying a heavy package along a corridor, cannot be readily

---

Box 28.1 Work simplification: task analysis
<ul><li>How many trips were made between two points?</li><li>Could the number of trips be reduced?</li><li>Could the order of performing different parts of the job be reduced?</li><li>Are the materials and needed equipment within easy reach? Can storage areas be reorganised?</li><li>Do storage areas contain only the needed equipment or are they cluttered with seldomly used things?</li><li>Can any part of the task be omitted or changed and still produce the desired results?</li><li>Are good body mechanics used in posture, sitting, standing and lifting?</li><li>Are two hands used to the best advantage?</li><li>Would the use of wheels be helpful?</li><li>Are sitting facilities comfortable? Are these and work surfaces of the proper height?</li><li>Are the materials pre-positioned and ready for use?</li><li>Is the rate of work too fast?</li><li>Should someone else do part of the task?</li></ul>

stopped and could therefore strain weakened ligaments.

It is helpful to train people in work simplification analysis so that they can apply these principles themselves to functional problems at home. Wilden (cited in Melvin 1989) suggests questions that can be used to assist in making changes (Box 28.1).

Not all activities can be changed to reduce energy consumption, but altering some will lead to a reduction in fatigue. Evaluation of the effectiveness of energy conservation by Furst et al (1987) have demonstrated that using regular rest periods during the day to prevent fatigue increases the duration of daily physical activity. However, no reported difference in self-reported pain, functional disability or fatigue occurred in their short follow-up period, meaning that this study is inconclusive.

Exercise

Muscle strength and joint range of movement should be maintained through exercise and full ranging of joints during daily activities. Exercise programmes are prescribed by physiotherapists. The occupational therapist may be concerned with reinforcing information on when and how

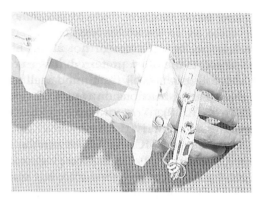

Fig. 28.5   Dynamic extensor orthosis.

deviation. These may also be used following extensor tendon repair to overcome MCP extension lag.

● Foot orthoses are important as foot problems can easily be overlooked. Provision of insoles with metatarsal pads, bars or domes, toe spacers and hallux valgus orthoses can reduce foot pain and increase mobility. Commercially manufactured shock-absorbing insoles (as used for sports shoes) can also reduce foot joint stress. Foot orthoses should always be provided, with advice on footwear. Flat, well-cushioned, supportive (over the fore- and mid-foot, and round the ankle) shoes should be worn. If insoles are fitted, shoes may need to have greater depth to accommodate the foot adequately without excess joint pressure developing.

● Other orthoses include cervical collars, knee supports and long-leg resting orthoses.

Particular attention should always be paid to orthoses' strapping systems, as people with poor reach or poor manual dexterity may not wear these if they are difficult to manipulate. Regular review is essential, especially within the first week, to ensure correct fit and application and that function is being improved. If hand deformities progress, orthoses may no longer fit adequately, and repeat review is beneficial when people attend for routine clinic appointments. People should be taught to be aware of pressure points, and any increase in redness, heat or swelling at enclosed joints should be checked to ensure that the orthosis is not the cause.

ADL training

As the disease progresses, function is increasingly impaired. Common problems as lower limb joints are affected are: getting on and off the toilet, chairs and bed; climbing stairs; getting in and out of cars; and bending to put on socks, tights and shoes. Common upper limb difficulties as shoulder, elbow and hand joints are increasingly affected include: doing up bras behind the back; adjusting collars and fastening ties; pulling clothes (particularly heavy coats) over the shoulders; hair care; peroneal care and adjusting clothing when toileting; reaching for items above shoulder level; clothes fastenings; turning keys and knobs; and writing. Alternative techniques, along with joint protection advice and energy conservation, may enable the person to complete tasks independently. Technical devices, such as bath boards, toilet aids, chair raises or lifting seats, dressing sticks, long-handled shoe horns, adapted longer-length handles, universal turning aids and Velcro fastenings, may become necessary. Care should be taken to prescribe them appropriately, and over a period of time if necessary, to assist the person gradually to adjust to the need for using them. Environmental adaptations, such as altering knobs on kitchen equipment, door handles, plugs, switches, heating controls and taps, may be needed. Disabled Living Centres are useful sources of advice, and it may be beneficial for individuals to visit these to try different models of equipment and be aware of what is available to help, if further difficulties develop.

Home adaptations may also be necessary for those more severely affected. Kitchen work surfaces may need raising or lowering. Toilet rails, other hand rails and an additional stair rail may need fitting. Steps may be ramped or reduced, or indoor lifts or stair lifts may be provided. Alternatively, it may be necessary for support services to consider aiding the person in moving to adapted, one-level housing, with ergonomically designed fixtures.

Leisure and work counselling

People continuing to work may experience increasing difficulties. For those in sedentary jobs, work heights may need adjusting and supportive seating may need to be provided. Those operating VDUs may experience hand and upper limb pain and should be provided with supportive orthoses. Health and Safety recommendations should be applied. Appropriate equipment should be made available (e.g. wrist support pads) and the work station ergonomically assessed and altered to reduce neck and upper limb strain. For those in manual jobs, work task analysis can help to identify how to apply joint protection principles and correct lifting techniques to reduce strain. The person may, however, need to consider changing to lighter work in the long term. The Disablement Employment Advisor (DEA) can explore, with the person and the employer, providing adaptations to the work environment, lighter or part-time work, or alternative employment. The social worker can help to identify the financial implications of this. Home-based employment may be another realistic possibility.

Referral to a Disability Driving Centre may be appropriate, for advice on Motability, easier cars to drive (e.g. those with power steering) and car adaptations. Leisure and social activities are affected early in the disease. Interest Checklists may be used to explore alternative hobbies and interests and to give advice on adapting current hobbies.

Patient education and treatment compliance

People are encouraged by therapists to use multiple self-management strategies: joint protection, energy conservation, rest, exercise and relaxation. These require time to perform and many changes to normal routine. It has been estimated that at least 50% of people with RA are non-compliant, irrespective of the intervention. Between 35 and 65% do not follow home exercise regimes provided by physiotherapists; between 35 and 75% do not wear orthoses as recommended; and people receiving standard energy conservation (Furst et al 1987) and standard joint protection education (Hammond 1994a,b) demonstrate either no or very limited increase in the use of these behaviours, despite considering these beneficial.

This is perhaps not surprising given Eberhardt et al's (1993) findings that many do not consider, two years post-diagnosis that they have a chronic disease. A major challenge to all rheumatology team members is to educate people with RA, motivate them to perceive that the treatments offered are beneficial and provide treatment and education using techniques proven to promote compliance.

Research has demonstrated that the best way to achieve these changes is by using cognitive–behavioural approaches, utilising teaching and learning principles to aid recall of information given, and using motor learning strategies to aid learning of motor skills, e.g. joint protection and exercise (Hammond 1994a, Furst et al 1987). Small group programmes (e.g. of two hours per week over a 4–6 week period, with 4–8 people attending) enable time to be used more efficiently in group treatment, allow people with RA to gain additional support from meeting others with RA, and increase compliance by enabling people to learn through modelling and peer support to use self-management methods at home. Methods proven effective in achieving behavioural change (Hammond 1994a, Furst et al 1987, Lorig 1992) include:

- regular repetition of information (verbal and written)
- repeat demonstration of behaviours
- repeat practice of techniques (for longer and in more complex sequences as the programme progresses)
- weekly goal-setting to practise strategies
- weekly review of this practice with repeat demonstrations by patients.

Inviting a relative or friend to attend also helps to increase practice and support at home. Arthritis education programmes incorporating teaching multiple self-management strategies not using these approaches have been shown to be ineffective in changing behaviour (Hammond 1994a). It is more effective to encourage people to attend separate short education programmes, each targeting one self-management strategy (e.g. joint protection, energy conservation, exercise, relaxation or pain management) at a time. This enables the person slowly to build up a repertoire of habitually adopted skills. Verbal information should always be supported by written information. The Arthritis and Rheumatism Council and Arthritis Care provide a wide range of high-quality patient education materials (written and video), either free of charge or at low cost, and run local support groups.

CONCLUSION

RA cannot be cured, but people can be helped to adopt self-management techniques and lifestyles which will reduce disease symptoms to some extent, help them to adjust psychologically to the changes the disease can impose, and maximise quality of life. Education is an important component of therapy to enable people to make informed decisions on how to manage their disease most effectively. Many people develop their own methods of coping with the disease, which should be respected. Clinical trials have shown that comprehensive team care leads to better functional outcome. Multidisciplinary teams coordinating effectively, planning education and treatment to dovetail, with regular monitoring, review and re-referral to therapy, give rise to better outcomes than do *ad hoc* referral systems with irregular review. All team members should aim to provide coordinated and comprehensive care.

REFERENCES

Agnew P J 1987 Joint protection in arthritis: fact or fiction? British Journal of Occupational Therapy 50: 227–230

Bishop A T, Hench P K, La Croix E, Millender L H, Opitz J L 1991 Keeping the rheumatoid hand working. Patient Care 25: 74–111

Blalock S J, DeVellis R F 1992 Rheumatoid arthritis and depression: an overview. Bulletin on the Rheumatic Diseases 41: 6–8

Blalock S J, DeVellis M B, Holt K, Hahn P 1993 Coping with arthritis: is one problem the same as another? Health Education Quarterly 20: 119–132

Campbell R M, Schkade J 1991 Clinical investigation into the efficacy of joint protection education. Arthritis Care and Research 4: S26

Dieppe P A, Doherty M, McFarlane D, Maddison P 1985 Rheumatological Medicine. Churchill Livingstone, Edinburgh

Eberhardt K B, Rydgren L C, Pettersson H, Wollheim F A 1990 Early rheumatoid arthritis — onset, course and outcome over 2 years. Rheumatology International 10: 135–142

Eberhardt K, Larsson B-M, Nived K 1993 Psychological reactions in patients with early rheumatoid arthritis. Patient Education and Counselling 20: 93–100

Furst G P, Gerber L H, Smith C, Fisher S, Shulman B 1987 A program for improving energy conservation behaviors in adults with rheumatoid arthritis. American Journal of Occupational Therapy 41: 102–111

Gerber L H, Furst G P 1992 Validation of the NIH Activity Record: a quantitative measure of life activities. Arthritis Care and Research 5: 81–86

Hammond A 1994a Evaluating joint protection for people with rheumatoid arthritis. Unpublished PhD thesis, University of Nottingham

Hammond A 1994b Joint protection behavior in patients with rheumatoid arthritis following an education program: a pilot study. Arthritis Care and Research 7: 5–9

Helewa A, Goldsmith C, Lee P et al 1991 Effects of occupational therapy home service on patients with rheumatoid arthritis. The Lancet 337: 1453–1456

Hill J, Bird H A, Lawton C A, Wright V 1990 The Arthritis Impact Measurement Scales: an anglicized version to assess the outcome of British patients with rheumatoid arthritis. British Journal of Rheumatology 29: 193–196

Jette A M 1987 The Functional Status Index: reliability and validity of a self-report functional disability measure. Journal of Rheumatology 14 (suppl. 15): 15–19

Kirwan J R, Reeback J S 1986 Stanford Health Assessment Questionnaire modified to assess disability in British patients with rheumatoid arthritis. British Journal of Rheumatology 25: 206–209

Lineker S, Badley E, Hughes A, Bell M 1994 Development of an instrument to measure knowledge in individuals with rheumatoid arthritis: the ACREU Rheumatoid Arthritis Knowledge Questionnaire. Arthritis Care and Research 7: S16

Lorig K 1992 Patient education: a practical approach. C V Mosby, St Louis

Lorig K, Fries J 1980 The arthritis helpbook: what you can do for your arthritis. Sovereign Press, London

McCloy L, Jongbloed L 1987 Robinson–Bashall Functional Assessment for arthritis patients; reliability and validity. Archives of Physical Medicine and Rehabilitation 68: 486–489

Melvin J L 1989 Rheumatic disease in the adult and child: occupational therapy and rehabilitation, 3rd edn. F A Davis, Philadelphia

O'Leary A, Shoor S, Lorig K, Holman H 1988 A cognitive behavioural treatment for rheumatoid arthritis. Health Psychology 7: 527–544

Reisine S T, Goodenow C, Grady K E 1987 The impact of rheumatoid arthritis on the homemaker. Social Sciences and Medicine 25: 89–95

Treuhaft P S, Lewis M R, McCarty D J 1971 A rapid method

for evaluating the structure and function of the
rheumatoid hand. Arthritis and Rheumatism 14: 75–87

Unsworth H 1986 Coping with rheumatoid arthritis.
Chambers, Edinburgh

FURTHER READING

Brattstrom M 1987 Joint protection — rehabilitation in
chronic rheumatic disorders. Wolfe Medical, London

Palmer P, Simons J 1991 Joint protection — a critical review.
British Journal of Occupational Therapy 54: 453–458

in the hands of any rascal who chooses to annoy or tease me', before he proved his point by dying suddenly when he permitted himself to get involved in a heated boardroom debate (Tuke 1872).

Without evidence of proof many scientists expressed profound scepticism about the value of these anecdotes, but the rapid development of techniques for measuring changes in the internal systems now makes it possible to shift many of the anecdotes from the realms of supposition to the category of fact.

Studies of maladaptive behaviour patterns that dispose to cardiovascular ill-health suggest that drive, coping ability and information processing are extremely important factors.

DRIVE

In 1896 an eminent physician, William Osler, observed that patients with coronary heart disease were ambitious and aggressive and had no ability to relax: their engines were set at full steam ahead. Since Osler's time many descriptions have appeared in the literature and the portrait of the competitive, aggressive, irritable, achievement-oriented, over-extended, hostile individual, unwilling or unable to relax, is nowadays familiar both to health professionals and lay persons.

One of the first attempts to study these behaviours systematically was made by two Californian cardiologists, Meyer Friedman and Ray Rosenman (1974), who proposed that the constellation of behaviours be called type A.

In recent years research has been carried out to identify the pathogenic component of these behaviours, and hostility is emerging as the important 'toxic' element. Glass (1977) has suggested that the hostility and overdrive which foster cardiovascular disorder and disease originate in childhood, possibly through a lack of unconditional love and a need to strive for the achievements that might bring them the reward of the love they need.

A second explanation for the excessive drive is that endlessly keeping busy enables the person to avoid facing up to deep anxiety or insecurity. Behind the workaholic's ceaseless activity there may lie a need to anaesthetise the mind against

some underlying pain or feeling of emptiness. It is equally possible that the 'adrenaline' generated by deadline challenges, risk-taking and conflict is just as addictive as the better known forms of addiction to external substances such as alcohol and nicotine. If the work addict is ordered to take a break and to rest, he may become extremely disturbed and feel imprisoned by the inactivity: after a heart attack it can be extremely difficult to persuade him to rest well enough to achieve his heart's potential for recovery.

COPING ABILITY

Wolf (1958) observed that the coronary-prone individual responds to increasing challenges by making greater and greater effort until he is exhausted, joyless and vulnerable to cardiovascular ill-health. He called this response Sisyphean after the legendary King of Corinth (Fig. 29.2).

In exhaustion performance deteriorates through loss of energy and stamina. Responses lose speed and accuracy. The individual struggles to carry the same load as he did when 'fighting fit', but this exhausts him further, frustrates him and reduces his ability to cope with his burdens.

Characteristically the exhausted individual fails to secure the sleep and rest required for becoming unexhausted. More often than not he will 'burn the midnight oil' to accomplish tasks. Indeed he may take on extra tasks and further overload himself through the inability to say 'no',

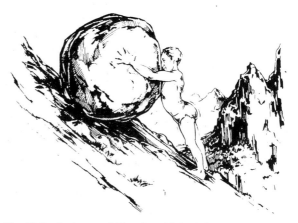

Fig. 29.2 A picture of Sisyphus, King of Corinth, who was condemned to spend his life rolling a boulder up a mountain.

and the more exhausted he becomes the greater becomes the difficulty of saying 'no'. Other maladaptive behaviours in exhaustion include the tendency to sit around talking, eating, drinking and smoking too much instead of resting or getting on with the job in hand; living with seemingly endless deadlines through poor planning; taking up displacement activity; and procrastinating – putting off tasks until the last minute of the eleventh hour.

INFORMATION PROCESSING

Evidence suggests that the brain's capacity for processing information can have a profound effect upon behaviour and health (Lipowski 1975). In exhaustion, for example, the brain's ability to handle information is reduced. Concentration and memory are impaired. The 'automatic pilots' solve fewer problems and off-load more on to the exhausted mind. The ability to reason diminishes, and the person becomes more resentful and emotional, and more hot and bothered about things. He stops listening to others and loses the ability to discriminate between important problems and secondary or peripheral matters. He is less capable of managing his time and resources efficiently: molehills become mountains. Ultimately he may feel overwhelmed by effort and distress, and trapped in his predicament (Fig. 29.3).

When the information coming from the internal systems of the body to the brain is not presented to consciousness in a recognisable way, the individual cannot guard himself effectively against fatigue, strain and excessive emotionalism. The condition is called alexithymia (Greek: a = lack; lexis = word; thymia = emotion). Alexithymia can cause great clinical difficulties because the individual who does not recognise the levels of physical and emotional overloading that make him ill is likely to become confused and irascible when the problems raised by his difficulties of perception are discussed with the therapist.

Another anomaly of information processing is denial, an unconscious or conscious inability to face up to the reality of a threatening situation or one's own inadequacies. Displacement activity

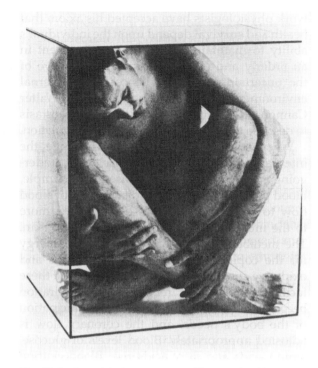

Fig. 29.3 A model of a man trapped in an unhealthy predicament without the energy and/or information required for him to escape. (Reproduced from Levi 1975 *Emotions, their Parameters and Measurement*)

is a form of denial: many make themselves too busy with exhausting tasks to pause, examine their options and deal with the crucial problem. False attribution is another way of denying the unacceptable. For example one person might rationalise and persuade himself that his pain cannot be cardiac because he is too young or has no family history of heart disease. Another might choose to exercise in an attempt to prove that his pain is benign, evidence of indigestion perhaps, and, in doing so, bring a cardiac catastrophe upon himself.

The maladaptive behaviours discussed here are important because they can exhaust the individual and outstrip the ability of his homoeostasis to maintain an orderly and stable internal environment.

HOMOEOSTASIS

Ever since Claude Bernard's (1855–6) pioneering

cardiac surgeons whose practices are guided by this model focus on changing the person's internal environment by interventions such as:

1. Reducing the heart's burdens by opposing overactivity with the use of drugs such as sedatives and hypnotics or beta-blockers. Angiotensin-converting enzyme (ACE) inhibitors appear to improve the mechanical functions of the injured or overloaded (e.g. hypertensive) heart
2. Improving coronary blood flow by the use of drugs such as coronary vasodilators and by surgery such as angioplasty and coronary artery bypass grafting
3. Opposing clot formation by the use of aspirin, heparin or anticoagulants
4. Treating acute thrombotic occlusion with thrombolytic drugs (the 'clot busters')
5. Reducing the volume of the blood, and consequently the back pressure exerted upon the lungs, by the use of drugs such as diuretics
6. Transplanting a donor heart into the person with severe heart disease.

In recent years there has been a growing acknowledgement of the inadequacy of the reductionist approach: its technical wizardry is not enough when it is applied without due attention to the personality of the individual patient and his needs and aspirations. Chandra Patel (1987), a general practitioner, emphasised this disquiet when she wrote that the concept of the heart as a purely mechanical pump is falling out of favour. Doctors as well as the general public are increasingly aware of the influence of the brain and mind upon the heart.

For many years Peter Nixon (1982, 1984), a cardiologist, has argued that a comprehensive approach to rehabilitation should integrate the reductionist medical and surgical treatments with skills drawn from the enabling professions who can promote anabolic restorative processes by paying close attention to the relationships between the external environment, the mind of the person and his internal *milieu*, and enable the person to succeed in his adaptation to cardiac impairment.

THE ROLE OF THE OCCUPATIONAL THERAPIST

The occupational therapist is especially well equipped to contribute to the comprehensive approach: her conceptual frameworks acknowledge that emotional, psychosocial and spiritual dimensions of life are important determinants of behaviour and health. Moreover she understands the reductionist perspective and the philosophies of other health care workers, and endeavours to integrate her work with theirs.

The occupational therapist's role in cardiac rehabilitation is to enable individuals to increase their competence at coping and adapting, and thereby influence the internal processes in such a way as to foster recovery and prevention, the development of hardiness and the improvement of the quality of life.

CONCLUSION

The next two chapters describe different aspects of the occupational therapist's role. The first chapter considers her responses to those individuals who have acute cardiovascular disorder and disease potentially amenable to restoration and prevention through the processes of rehabilitation. The second chapter is concerned largely with the adaptation and modification of the environment which might be required in chronic heart conditions.

REFERENCES

Adam K, Oswald I 1984 Sleep helps healing. British Medical Journal 289: 1400–1401

Barker D J P, Osmond C 1986 Infant mortality, childhood nutrition, and ischaemic heart disease in England and Wales. Lancet 1: 1077–1081

Bernard C 1855–6 Leçons de physiologie experimentale appliqué à la medicine. J B Baillère, Paris

Brindley D N, Rolland Y 1989 Possible connections between

stress, diabetes, obesity, hypertension and altered lipoprotein metabolism that may result in atherosclerosis. Clinical Science 77: 453–461

Cannon W B 1932 Wisdom of the body. W W Norton, New York

Cassel J 1976 The contribution of the social environment to host resistance. American Journal of Epidemiology 104: 107–123

Forsdahl A 1977 Are poor living conditions in childhood and adolescence an important risk factor for arteriosclerotic heart disease? British Journal of Preventive and Social Medicine 31: 91–95

Friedman M, Rosenman R H 1974 Type A behaviour and your heart. Wildwood House, London

Glass D C 1977 Behaviour patterns, stress and coronary disease. John Wiley, New Jersey

Helsung H J, Szklo M, Comstock G W 1981 Factors associated with mortality after widowhood. American Journal of Public Health 71: 802–809

Jenkins D C 1978 Low education: a risk factor for death. New England Journal of Medicine 299: 95–97

Kobasa S C, Maddi S R, Kahn S 1982 Hardiness and health: a prospective study. Journal of Personality and Social Psychology 42: 168–177

Levi L 1975 Parameters of emotion: an evolutionary and ecological approach. In: Levi L (ed) Emotions, their parameters and measurement. Raven Press, New York, pp 705–711

Lipowski Z J 1975 Sensory and information inputs overload: behavioural effects. Comprehensive Psychiatry 16: 199–221

Nixon P G F 1982 Stress and the cardiovascular system. Practitioner 226: 1589–1598

Nixon P G F 1984 Stress, life style and cardiovascular disease: a cardiological odyssey. British Journal of Holistic Medicine 1: 20–29

Osler W 1896 Lectures on angina pectoris and allied states. New York Medical Journal 64: 177

Patel C 1987 Fighting heart disease. Dorling Kindersley, London

Rees W D, Lutkins S G 1967 Mortality of bereavement. British Medical Journal 4: 13–16

Rose G, Marmot M G 1981 Social class and coronary heart disease. British Heart Journal 45: 13–19

Tuke H D 1872 The mind upon the body in health and disease. J & A Churchill, London, p 245

Wolf S G 1958 Cardiovascular reactions to symbolic stimuli. Circulation 18: 287–292

trials led to the realisation that the ability to perform well in a gym might not make much difference to the individual's ability to cope with the emotional and social problems of everyday life. Furthermore, psychological and social factors began to be seen as possibly more important determinants of the illness and its outcome than the physical damage of the myocardial infarction.

Today there is no consensus upon policy for cardiac rehabilitation. Methods vary from hospital to hospital and centre to centre. Some — for example, 'Heartbeat Wales' — emphasise risk-factor advice about diet and smoking (Catford & Parish 1989) whereas others stress the physical, psychological and social aspects of rehabilitation. The emphasis usually depends upon the particular philosophy and professional background of the staff who have set up the service.

In some areas cardiac rehabilitation is approached through the formation of a group which attends a programme of talks and videos, and discussions with members of staff. However, the information and education provided by the members of staff from the different philosophical and professional backgrounds (e.g. medical, nursing, occupational therapy, physiotherapy, counselling and dietetic) is not necessarily congruous and coordinated.

In other areas staff have integrated their knowledge and core skills to evolve a comprehensive rehabilitation service that is flexible, adaptable and focused upon the need of the individual. Most importantly the provision of information and education is consistent and coordinated. This teamwork both enables and depends upon its disparate members transcending the conceptual boundaries and core skills which they carry with them into the team. It is a simple example of the systems approach to practice.

Systems theory, the conceptual framework which enables the diversity of team members to function as a whole, also accommodates the interrelationships between the systems of the person's external environment and those of his internal *milieu*, and sees their outcome as an important determinant of health.

Many outstanding accounts of systems theory have been published and the reader is referred to the work of Barris et al (1988), Capra (1982), Cunningham (1986) and Engel (1980, 1982) for more information.

This chapter applies systems theory to the field of acute cardiovascular disorder and disease. It begins by describing the state of an orderly cardiovascular system enjoyed by the healthy person; the processes by which disorder and disease can occur; and the occupational therapist's role in the restoration of health through modification of the relationships between the external environment and the internal *milieu*. This modification depends upon support, assessment, information and education; the therapists' professional knowledge of occupation; and the effects of sleep, arousal, breathing, rest, effort and self-esteem (SABRES, see below) upon performance.

Models are provided in the chapter to clarify relationships between various elements of the systems involved in the genesis of cardiovascular disorder and disease, and the processes of restoration.

CARDIOVASCULAR ORDER

The treadwheel depicted in Figure 30.1 is a useful starting point for considering cardiovascular order and disorder (Nixon 1989). The figure on

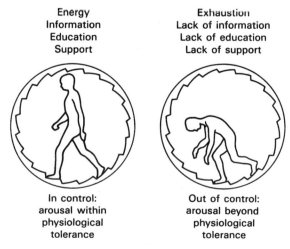

Energy	Exhaustion
Information	Lack of information
Education	Lack of education
Support	Lack of support

In control: arousal within physiological tolerance

Out of control: arousal beyond physiological tolerance

Fig. 30.1 The treadwheel: a model for considering the requirements for cardiovascular order (figure on the left) and disorder (figure on the right).

the left of the diagram represents the healthy, well-balanced person. By either good fortune or good management he has enough energy, information, education (in its broadest sense) and support to satisfy his needs, to cope and to adapt to change. His level of arousal — a reflection of what he is doing, the stress to which he is exposed and how he perceives this stress — is within the boundaries of physiological tolerance and allows his homoeostatic self-regulatory processes to maintain an orderly and stable internal *milieu*. In particular:

• The autonomic nervous system (sympathetic and parasympathetic) is functioning smoothly and suffering neither from overstimulation nor understimulation.

• The levels of the neuroendocrine agents, particularly adrenaline and noradrenaline (catecholamines) from sympathetic and adrenal medullary activity, and cortisol from pituitary stimulation of the adrenal cortex, are within tolerable levels. The acronym S-AM is used for the combination of sympathetic and adrenal medullary activity, and P-AC for the pituitary stimulation of adrenal cortical activity.

• The linings of the arteries are not a battleground suffering damage or excessive wear and tear from undamped and excessive S-AM and P-AC activity.

• The breathing pattern is appropriate: it provides oxygen for the tasks in hand and regulates the level of carbon dioxide in the blood.

• The provision of sleep is adequate for the person's anabolic needs, i.e. the restorative processes of tissue maintenance, repair and growth that offset the effects of the day's wear and tear upon his internal *milieu*. He wakens refreshed, and eager for the activities of the new day.

• During the day high levels of activity might be demanded or chosen. Arousal rises and the internal systems adjust to accommodate the increase of performance (Fig. 30.2; up-slope). Once the activity has been accomplished arousal falls and the body's homoeostatic self-regulatory processes return the internal environment to the restorative state. The optimal conditions for this are relaxation and sleep.

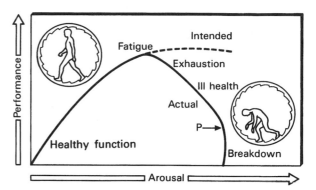

Fig. 30.2 The human function curve: a model illustrating the relationships between performance, arousal and health. On the up-slope, performance increases with arousal; the cardiovascular system is in an orderly state and the metabolism anabolic. On the down-slope, every increment of arousal reduces performance. The cardiovascular system is disordered and the metabolism catabolic. Some individuals are hardy and have high curves which permit great performance, whereas others have low curves and are vulnerable to exhaustion, ill-health and coronary breakdown (P = breakdown point). The dotted line indicates the intended level of activity and the solid line the actual level of performance. The more the individual struggles to close the gap between what he can do and what he thinks he ought to achieve, the further down he moves and the worse he becomes (Nixon 1976).

CARDIOVASCULAR DISORDER AND DISEASE

The person on the right of Figure 30.1 represents the individual who has gone over the top of his performance–arousal curve (Fig. 30.2). He has carried himself there by unhealthy levels of effort and emotional arousal (e.g. anger and hostility) or has allowed himself to be driven there by circumstances, perhaps by stuggling and failing to cope and adapt to large and frequent life changes.

The person in this position instinctively struggles to close the gap between what he can do and what he intends to achieve (Fig. 30.2) but the effort is self-defeating. It moves him downwards and causes him to become more hot and bothered about more things. Vigilance and restlessness increase. Discriminative powers deteriorate and the management of time and resources becomes less efficient. Exhausting displacement activity — such as furiously digging the garden to avoid confrontation within the home — might be taken

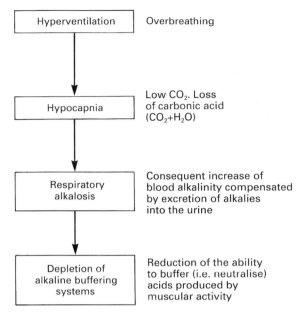

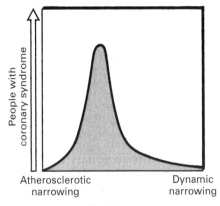

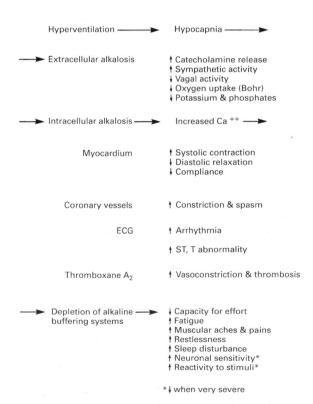

Fig. 30.5 Acid–base changes induced by hyperventilation.

Fig. 30.6 Hyperventilation-related disorders.

atherosclerotic coronary disease might be unaware that anything is amiss until his disease reaches a critical level for obstruction.

When the coronary arteries are narrowed by severe atherosclerosis the angina tends to occur at more or less the same level of effort on every occasion (fixed onset angina), given the usual fluctuation with cold winds, hot tempers and over-filled stomachs.

When the dynamic factors of constriction or spasm are predominant there is a great variation of capacity for effort (variable onset angina): the individual may speak of good days when he can walk for miles and climb hills, and of bad days when it might be difficult to walk from the car park to the office (King & Nixon 1988, Nixon 1989, King 1992). Most people presenting with a coronary syndrome have both atherosclerotic and dynamic causes of impairment. The spectrum is illustrated in Figure 30.7.

Occupational therapists work with those at both ends of the spectrum, that is to say with those who have severe atherosclerotic narrowings requiring surgical treatment and with those who have dynamic factors as well as with the majority who suffer from a mixture of atherosclerotic and dynamic factors.

The occupational therapist should be aware

Fig. 30.7 A model illustrating the distribution of arterial appearances in angina pectoris. At one extreme a few patients have overwhelming, rigid atherosclerotic factors and at the other end a few have purely dynamic factors in arteries with relatively little or no disease. The majority of patients have both atherosclerotic and dynamic factors.

that the left ventricle becomes more vulnerable to adverse influences when it is damaged by fibrosis and scarring from repeated ischaemic injury, as in angina pectoris, and poorly nourished as a result of severe coronary disease. These adverse influences include myocardial stiffening and tachycardia.

Myocardial stiffening can be produced by influences such as cold, isometric effort (static muscle strain) and anger, which raise the blood pressure sharply. The rise of blood pressure makes it more difficult for the heart to empty its contents adequately, so the left ventricle becomes over-distended and, rather like an over-inflated football, stiffened. In this condition its oxygen requirements increase, but the stiffening opposes coronary blood flow through the myocardium and thereby fosters damage by ischaemia. Stiffening can also be produced by changes in calcium and magnesium ions brought about by hyperventilation combined with high S-AM and P-AC activity from struggling and failing to cope.

Tachycardia is a common consequence of emotional arousal and physical effort. It can create problems by reducing the coronary filling time, i.e. the period between beats during which the coronary flow reaches the myocardium, and thereby produce ischaemia and anginal pain even where the radiological appearance of the coronary arteries is within normal limits for age.

It is not the purpose of this chapter to discuss the various medical conditions which can cause angina in the presence of normal coronary arteries, but it should be noted that they include severe anaemia and thyrotoxicosis.

RESTORATION OF HEALTH

Successful restoration of health depends upon both the recovery of an orderly and stable state of the internal *milieu* and the ability of the individual to learn to maintain this state while returning to his daily activities and carrying them out at a fitting level.

In the acute stage of illness the person may be out of control and unable to manage the crisis in a calm and sensible way. He will rarely have enough information to dispose of anxiety and to dispel fear. He can behave in maladaptive ways. For example, he might:

- deny there is a problem and feel he has nothing to learn
- feel trapped in an unacceptable position without options, and hyperventilate as a displacement activity
- be driven by anxiety and frustration to struggle onwards beyond the boundaries of his heart's tolerance and make his condition worse
- adopt a passive role of resignation
- give up and fall into a mode of overwhelming despair, which largely, through P-AC mechanisms, encourages fluid retention and heart failure.

When these forms of maladaptive behaviour are dominant it is not possible to teach the person the skills he needs to cope: learning new skills requires a receptive mind and a great deal of energy, but he is already exhausted by effort (Fig. 30.1, figure on the right). The additional struggles to learn or conform will only increase his arousal, reduce his performance (Fig. 30.2) and create greater internal disorder (Fig. 30.4).

The first stage, therefore, is to stop the struggling and to get the person off the treadwheel (Fig. 30.1). The management of this acute stage is usually carried out by nurses. Their skills enable the person to withdraw from effort and reduce arousal. Sleep, rest, a sense of well-being — security, confidence and dignity — and relaxation (Fig. 30.4) permit the disturbed homoeostatic self-regulatory mechanisms to recover. An abdominal pattern of breathing is a useful clinical sign of recovery (King 1988, King & Nixon 1988, Nixon 1989).

THE ROLE OF THE OCCUPATIONAL THERAPIST

This is to foster, through the processes of support, information and education, each individual's

more, adequate sleep enables emotion and effort to be handled in a much less demanding way. Consequently the general arousal level falls, reducing fatigue and easing the performance of daily activity (Fig. 30.2).

The occupational therapist can take two steps to help. The first is to teach the individual to be aware of the difference in well-being produced by good sleep and bad sleep. The second step is to provide tips and tactics for promoting good sleep, such as unwinding during the evening, setting an 'activity deadline' ninety minutes before bedtime, listening to music, taking a nightcap, avoiding caffeine drinks such as coffee, using a relaxation technique or practising self-hypnosis. With such tuition most people soon appreciate that the quality of sleep reflects the quality of the day and come to learn that good sleep is a reward for organising the other elements of SABRES (Fig. 30.8).

Arousal

Each person needs to be able to recognise his arousal level and keep his emotional reactions within tolerable limits. Methods for increasing awareness of arousal include the occupational therapist drawing the person's attention to muscular tension and posture, such as grinding the teeth or hunching the shoulders. Once the person is aware of excessive tension he needs to be encouraged to talk about his feelings of anger (S-AM activity) and despair (P-AC activity) instead of bottling them up. Communication can reduce emotional arousal and modulate its physiological disturbances, and so the creation of a therapeutic relationship for this purpose is invaluable.

Arousal can also be modulated through the use of relaxation techniques and of guided mental imagery conducive to relaxation and well-being (Fig. 30.4). In teaching relaxation to individuals or groups the occupational therapist needs to be aware that those with buffer depletion (Fig. 30.5) can become restless or feel unwell (Fig. 30.6) if the delicately balanced acid–base equilibrium is disturbed by a reduction of either muscular tension or respiration. Individuals with hyperventilation commonly constrict their peripheral blood vessels and cool their hands if they struggle to relax. The cooling is caused by vasoconstriction, an indicator of the fact that the struggle is self-defeating.

Those who are overwhelmed by their burdens of coping and adapting can become 'depressed' (P-AC activity) if they are encouraged to relax, and they should not be jollied into fatiguing displacement activities. They need the occupational therapist to work with them, to provide unconditional support, to help them reduce their guilt and to show them how to achieve their goals with less effort and emotion. The quality of their social support can be improved through the use of community resources such as adult education classes, church groups or local clubs. Some districts have 'coronary clubs' or 'coronary self-help groups' which may be of benefit provided they do not extend the 'coronary role' beyond the period of need.

Once the general level of arousal has been lowered to a tolerable level it is usual for the person to find that he can think more clearly, identify coping strategies with greater ease and put them into use with greater effect.

Breathing

Each person needs to become aware of his breathing disorder and be able to control it if he is to outwit the morbid consequences of hyperventilation (Fig. 30.6). Success in this requires the occupational therapist to inform the person that she is focusing on an inappropriate pattern of breathing, referred to as hyperventilation (Figs 30.5 and 30.6). Here respiration is linked with emotional arousal, uncoupled from the body's physical needs, and is excessive. It is not breathlessness due to heart and lung disease, nor is it hysterical overbreathing (King 1988).

Methods for increasing awareness include encouraging each person to observe his pattern of breathing. In both sitting and lying positions he should note whether it is upper thoracic, irregular in rate and depth, punctuated by sighs and sniffs, or whether it is predominantly abdominal and rhythmical in rate and depth. The rate can be counted. The use of mirrors, the placement of hands — one on the chest and the other on the abdomen — or the use of a light object such as a box of tissues on the abdomen can all sharpen awareness.

During this observation phase the occupational therapist should remember that the increase of rate and depth which is sufficient to precipitate cardiovascular disorder might not be obvious to the untrained eye. In some the hyperventilation is episodic, and occurs only when they encounter or think about personally relevant stressors (Nixon & Freeman 1988).

Once the fact of his hyperventilation has been perceived each person needs to learn how to outwit the influences that cause the inappropriate pattern of breathing, and to recover the predominantly abdominal pattern that meets the needs of the body for making effort and orchestrating the internal systems.

Having learnt to do this at rest in a therapeutic setting, the person needs to practise at home and learn to go about his daily activity with a well-fitting respiratory pattern. It is important for him to be wary of stressors that might whip up a surge of emotional arousal and carry the breathing away from the needs of the body.

Rest and effort

Each person needs to understand that rest is

> **Box 30.2** Case study
>
> Sarah, a 26-year-old architecture student who complained of chest pain, was referred by her general practitioner to the cardiologist's outpatient clinic. While having an electrocardiogram (ECG) she talked to the cardiac technician about her boyfriend leaving her. She was observed to become agitated with anger and to hyperventilate. Her heart rate rose from 120 to 210 beats per minute, at which level the ECG showed ischaemic changes sufficient to cause her chest pain. Her chest pain disappeared when the occupational therapist discussed her problem with her and taught her not to hyperventilate when emotionally upset.

---

the condition of stillness and calmness required to offset the effects of effort, and to learn what amount of rest is needed to sustain the varying levels and intensities of effort encountered in daily life.

This can be achieved through discussion, but most people only acknowledge the value of rest once they have incorporated periods of it into their programme of daily activity, and experienced the great increase of well-being and performance that comes from becoming untired. The length and timing of the rest periods must be adjusted and readjusted to accommodate the ups and downs of effort and arousal during recovery. The contingencies of life and psychosocial burdens can reduce the heart's capacity for making and sustaining effort and need to be taken into account.

A useful starting-point is to discuss three levels of performance: the level when the individual was last well (100%), the present level, and the level he wants to achieve with the occupational therapist's help. The therapist must be prepared to draw upon her experience and say whether the intended level is realistic. In this way both the person and the occupational therapist can look at the gap between the actual and the intended levels (Fig. 30.2) and work out strategies for closing it as well as possible and accepting reasonable compromises.

Points that often crop up and need to be incorporated into the programme of activity include the need:

- to be realistic about functional capabilities,

to have a healthy respect for fatigue, to recognise when to go forward, and when to change course or back off.

● to build on good days and back off on bad days, to conserve energy and eradicate unnecessary effort, to learn to say no, to eliminate extravagant and time-wasting habits and emotionalism, and to avoid the demoralising effects of procrastination.

● to avoid producing symptoms of excessive effort, to become familiar with the cost of becoming emotionally drained, and to weigh up the burdens of different sorts of mental and physical activities.

Isometric activity, i.e. physical activity which involves straining to pull, push, carry and lift, and interferes with the breathing, puts a heavy demand upon the heart by increasing left ventricular distension, systolic blood pressure and myocardial oxygen demand. It is therefore important for the occupational therapist to emphasise the importance of easing off before fatigue interferes with the performance of the activity, particularly when working against the clock. Teaching the person to make a whistling sound during isometric effort often helps him to remember not to hold his breath. It is also wise for isometric effort to be broken up into short stretches and alternated with periods of rest or isotonic (easy, mobile) effort. This ensures that the associated blood pressure rises are brief and not allowed to surge to great heights for prolonged periods.

Some occupational therapists may choose to arrange a programme of activity within their department in order to let the person understand the practical differences between isometric and isotonic effort, recognise his functional ability, and develop stamina. This knowledge dispels fear and thereby encourages the arousal level to fall.

Self-esteem

By learning to outwit dynamic influences and minimise the impact of disease on his life through the various elements of SABRES (Fig. 30.8), the individual can do more of what he wants, meet more of his goals, fulfil more of his needs, and adopt a healthier set of compromises. His sense of being back in control and his increasing confidence in his abilities reduces arousal and restores a feeling of worth.

It is only when a person is well on the road to recovery that he can look back and say how he felt at the bottom of the pit of despair when he was bereft of self-esteem. Ultimately a well-guided and successful person might say that the crisis was the best thing that could have happened at that period of life because it enabled him to stop, to think, to take stock and to make changes for success and endurance.

BIOFEEDBACK

Biofeedback provides information about the body's function and responses which can help the person to monitor his progress.

Body awareness and appearance

It is important to teach the person and his family to become aware of the changes in appearance and behaviour that mark the passage over the top into exhaustion and ill-health (Fig. 30.2). By doing so the person becomes aware of the warnings his body gives before its systems break down. Recognising these warnings reduces anxiety about the possibility of sudden and unexpected relapse. Increasing self-awareness also enables the person to understand and estimate his reserves for coping with burdens in the future.

It is thought that recovery is quickest in 'pink time' when the person is warm to the touch, untired and cheerful, and slowest in 'grey time' when he is cold, tired and harassed.

Heart rate and blood pressure

Some people find it helpful to learn to take their heart rate in order to gain information about the physiological costs of emotional and physical effort.

Many of those with a diagnosis of hypertension can be taught to use a sphygmomanometer and keep annotated charts in order to identify and overcome the influences which might appear to be slight but prove with measurement to have potent hypertensive consequences. This information can then be discussed and incorporated within the person's daily activity programme.

Skin temperature

In teaching the person to relax, a simple biofeedback machine for registering the temperature of the skin of the fingers and toes may be useful. Efficient relaxation combined with abdominal breathing warms the fingers and toes within minutes.

Biofeedback and drug therapy

Heart rate, blood pressure and skin temperature measurements can be misleading when drug therapies interfere with the person's physiological responsivity.

RESUMING NORMAL ACTIVITIES

At some point in the individual's recovery, questions and issues regarding specific activities crop up. These frequently include:

Return to sexual activity

Sexual activity is an embarrassing topic for those who are shy about discussing fears and anxieties related to loss of libido and potency, or fear the provocation of another heart attack. The occupational therapist should be sensitive to these personal concerns and use her skills in such a way as to make the person feel comfortable about discussing his fears and anxieties.

It is generally considered that sexual intercourse with a familiar partner is equivalent in effort to climbing two flights of stairs. The timing of the return to sexual activity depends upon the individual, but by four weeks after a myocardial infarction or heart surgery most people can climb two flights of stairs and have enough confidence for sex. Comfort is important and positions which require heavy isometric effort should be avoided at first. Physical closeness and caring touch can do much for morale and the recovery of confidence.

Certain cardiovascular drugs such as beta blockers and diuretics can oppose the recovery of sexual performance. If the person is unaware of this he might blame himself and not think about asking his doctor to consider a change of medication.

Return to driving

The recommended time for returning to driving is one month from myocardial infarction or coronary artery bypass grafting, and one week from coronary angioplasty in straightforward cases.

It is desirable for the return to driving to take place in conditions of little stress and hazard, beginning with short quiet drives in daylight, keeping off the motorways and avoiding heavy town or rush hour traffic. Racing against time should always be avoided. Power steering helps to avoid angina from isometric effort.

It is advisable for the person to notify his insurance company of his illness, since failure of disclosure might invalidate his policy. There is usually no difficulty in maintaining cover, and most insurance companies will merely require a medical certificate stating that the person is fit to drive.

Provided that the recovery has been uncomplicated drivers do not need to inform the Drivers and Vehicle Licensing Agency (DVLA, Medical Advisory Branch, Oldway Centre, Orchard Street, Swansea SA99 1TU) about the onset of a coronary condition. If angina occurs during driving the person should stop driving thereafter and inform the DVLA: driving will be permitted once a satisfactory control of symptoms has been achieved.

The law relating to vocational driving, as in the case of drivers of large goods and passenger-carrying vehicles, is more stringent: licences are usually withdrawn if the person has angina or heart failure. Following successful recovery from myocardial infarction, coronary artery bypass grafting and coronary angioplasty the driver may apply for re-licensing three months after the event (Medical Advisory Branch 1993).

Going on holiday and flying

Many consider a holiday as a useful agent of recovery. Both the location and the type of holiday require consideration. The terrain should not be too hilly, nor the climate too hot or cold. The altitude should be below 6600 feet (2000 metres) in order to avoid hyperventilation, a physiological response to an increase of altitude. Alcohol may be taken in moderation, but its effects will be increased by altitude and hyperventilation.

Travelling by coach or train is often less tiring than driving long distances. Car driving should be delegated or shared. Certainly the journey should be broken into easy stages and overnight stops planned to avoid fatigue.

Flying in a pressurised aircraft should not create any problems if the person is not put into anxiety or hyperventilation. The most common hazards are arriving late at the airport, carrying too much baggage (as judged by being unable to walk and talk at the same time), anxiety, hyperventilation (particularly during queuing), and loss of temper. Careful organisation is the best defence.

Airline staff are willing to do all they can to make the person's journey as hassle-free as possible, for example by providing wheelchair transport at airports if notice is given when the flight is booked. If the flight is made within eight weeks of the myocardial infarction a certificate of fitness to fly from the family doctor might be demanded.

It is always wise to obtain adequate insurance cover against illness and cancellation and important to check the small print for exclusion criteria based on pre-existing illness, such as myocardial infarction.

Return to recreation and sport

Well-chosen physical exercise promotes a feeling of well-being, increases general mobility and stamina and serves to obtain the level of fitness required for reasonable recreation and sport as well as work.

For those who enjoy it, walking is a good choice of exercise. There is no 'correct' distance: it is what is right for each person on a given day that is important. The aim should be quietly to increase distance, promoting stamina rather than speed. Speed can be increased when distance has been achieved.

Common sense should prevail, for example:

- The person should not expect to be able to increase his capacity for physical effort if he neglects other elements of SABRES (Fig. 30.8).
- He should remember that there is always a return journey and not to wait for fatigue before deciding to turn back. About 60–70% of what he thinks is his maximum — the level of activity that might be limited by symptoms — is the right distance for the journey there and back. Observing the 60—70% rule also ensures that the person has enough reserves to cope with contingencies.
- On a bad day, when he is grey and tired, or faced by adverse weather, he should accept the wisdom of backing off, i.e. staying in and resting or restricting exercise to a few gentle mobility exercises.
- Exercise should not be taken after a large meal.
- The vasoconstrictive effect of cold weather should be outwitted by appropriate clothing, breathing through a scarf and wearing gloves. A hat is important because about 25% of body heat is lost through the uncovered head.

Fitness training can be organised for those who wish to return to sport. The warming-up phase should never be neglected.

The desirable training level of 60—70% of the person's maximum can be gauged from the pulse rate. A formula commonly used soon after myocardial infarction is to subtract 40 plus the person's age in years from 220. The result is called the 'target' or 'training heart rate'. This should be taken as the ceiling for 20 minutes of exercise 3 times per week (Nixon et al 1976).

The fit of this formula in the individual case should be checked by the doctor, who might exercise the person on a treadmill or bicycle ergometer to ensure that it does not create the risk of myocardial ischaemia.

Recreational activities or sports that put sudden severe demands upon the left ventricle, such as squash, should be discouraged, as well as those that depend upon isometric effort, particularly with exposure to cold, as in water-skiing. Going for 'the burn' as encouraged in some forms of aerobics is also inadvisable.

It is important for the person to be aware of the fact that to compete with himself or with others invites defeat.

Those who enjoy sitting in a sauna should know that the heart rate will suddenly rise after a period and that they should move out before the onset of tachycardia.

Return to work

About 10 to 12 weeks from the time of the infarction or surgery most people begin to return to work.

Adapting to going back to work is most easily accomplished by returning to a three-day week, i.e. Mondays, Wednesdays and Fridays during the first month, keeping Tuesdays and Thursdays for rest and exercise. Going back every day even when the hours are reduced is less effective.

Important influences upon the success of the return to work are the degree of control the person has over the effort of his work, and its effects upon the recreational, social and domestic needs of his life.

The place of work, the performance required, the travelling entailed and the psychological factors involved must all be taken into account when the occupational therapist and the person plan strategies and consider whether it is the work itself or personality clashes that require attention.

Being compelled by the heart condition to change career puts a much heavier demand upon a person than going back to a familiar job with old workmates and support groups.

FOLLOW-UP

It should be anticipated that at some point in his recovery the person will overtire himself, become anxious, hyperventilate and induce chest pain. When this occurs he should make an audit of his use of SABRES (Fig. 30.8) by asking himself if he is:

- *sleeping* properly?
- too wound up *(aroused)* for his own good?
- *breathing* properly?
- keeping too busy, not balancing *rest* with *effort*, doing more than 60–70% maximum?
- feeling down and losing his *self-esteem* because he is taking on too much to be successful?

From the start of the illness to the time when she is no longer needed the occupational therapist should remain friendly and approachable, ready to give advice either formally by appointment or informally by telephone. This liaison provides not only continuous assessment and audit but also a valuable channel for communication between the members of the cardiac rehabilitation team, the general practitioner and the providers of community resources. Through the occupational therapist's support and provision of information and education the individual learns how to recover healthy function and minimise the need for drugs and surgery.

Surgical intervention

It is taken as axiomatic that the occupational therapist will promote anabolic conditions, and encourage the person in urgent need of surgical intervention to maintain an optimal level of sleep and rest and avoid effort.

There are many cases where indications and contraindications for surgery are not clear cut. Here the occupational therapist might well be asked to use full remedial measures against the dynamic factors. If the severity of the atherosclerotic factors precludes satisfactory progress the physician is likely to carry out angiography to obtain information about the coronary arterial anatomy and the state of the left ventricle, with a view to angioplasty or coronary artery bypass surgery. This does not mean that the period of training with the occupational therapist is wasted: if surgery is recommended the surgeon is only too glad to find the person in a stable and orderly condition and well prepared. The informed occupational therapist knows that coronary artery bypass grafting and angioplasty do not in them-

- the 'Access to Work' scheme (June 1994) that provides equipment and aids in the workplace to enable employees to continue to work
- retraining, in which case contact with the Disablement Employment Advisor (DEA) may be appropriate
- working part time
- working from home
- early retirement.

Finlayson & McEwen (1977) found that the chance of men returning to work one year after myocardial infarction was significantly higher where their wives named multiple sources of social support during and after the crisis.

Alternatively, if the person does not return to work at all, the occupational therapist can discuss the purposeful use of time, such as attendance at day courses or involvement in voluntary organisations. It is important in these circumstances to try to maintain a balance of self-care, leisure and productivity activities, even where the nature of productivity has changed from paid employment. A person can still be 'productive' in terms of output, for example writing letters, growing tomatoes or baking, even if he is not, strictly speaking, 'employed'.

Social outings and entertaining

The relaxing, enjoyable social side of life can be the first to suffer when impairments such as heart failure affect the energy level and capacity for activity. When feeling generally unwell or less capable through weakness and fatigue, the individual may find that the effort required to socialise becomes too much. Another reason for reduction in social contact can be the fear of other people's reactions and their natural tendency to over-protect, thereby preventing full participation in activities. Maintenance of contacts with friends and neighbours can be a little easier, whereas meeting new acquaintances and explaining one's situation to them may at first be awkward. The more people who understand the situation, the easier future events will become. It is important to try to have some regular events that provide a pattern and focus in the week to prevent drifting into lethargy or depression, which can exacerbate the potential isolation and make it harder to maintain a social life.

Use of free time

New hobbies can be taken up or old ones modified. Participation in clubs, committees and organisations of interest will provide a useful set of contacts and help to fill free time in a satisfying manner. Some examples of leisure activities, together with some ideas for their modifications, are given below.

Gardening. Planting seeds, taking cuttings, growing indoor plants and bulbs, and cultivating tray or bottle gardens can provide a rewarding alternative to the strenuous job of tending a garden or allotment. Salad growing can be encouraged as an alternative to the heavy work involved in root vegetables.

Music. Listening to music or learning and playing a musical instrument can be very relaxing and enjoyable, particularly when playing with others. Any musical activity can be modified according to the personal resources available.

Dance. Dancing can be good exercise and provide opportunities for socialisation, tea dances being popular events. Dancing can be modified to a suitable level according to physical tolerance; ballroom dancing, for example, is less strenuous than styles such as Latin American or disco.

Pets. Taking responsibility for a pet can ensure that the owner also takes responsibility for himself. For example, shopping for the pet's food will entail an outing to get essential groceries, while walking a dog provides vital exercise. The choice of a new pet should obviously be made very carefully, taking into consideration food and care costs, the type of property the individual lives in, and the space and exercise that the pet will need. Cats often make good pets as they are independent. It is believed that stroking an animal can be beneficial, leading to a general feeling of well-being.

Public houses and social clubs. Pubs and social clubs provide opportunities to meet and mix with people and some elements of exercise to travel to and from the pub or club. Pub games such as bowls, darts or pool provide some level of exercise, while less physically strenuous activities include playing cards, chess and cribbage.

Sport. Numerous sports activities provide a suitable level of exercise, as well as social contacts, if carefully chosen and monitored for stress and energy levels. Competitive sports are generally more stressful and may be avoided, but activities such as swimming and walking can be retained as long as the length of time spent doing them is appropriate to the tolerance level of the person concerned.

Walking. When walking any distance, it is good practice for the individual to take the local taxi firm's telephone number and money for the return journey, just in case it is needed. Other suggestions are to plan a route via friends' houses in case a rest stop is needed, or to take transport out to a destination and walk back home. If a walk is planned along a bus route, it is easy to catch a bus the rest of the way to the destination, or home. A voluntary driver or 'dial-a-ride' scheme operates in some areas and can be used for lifts into shopping areas or to visit family and friends.

Arts. Activities such as painting, writing, crafts, photography, video camera work and sewing can be rewarding and productive when more strenuous hobbies have to be given up. Attending evening classes can be a good way of learning or continuing with an arts subject, and of refreshing or renewing skills. As well as the social benefit of meeting with a group of people, there is the advantage of being able to continue the activity at home.

Voluntary work. Libraries and Citizens Advice Bureaux are a good source of information about local voluntary societies, and most high streets have charity shops. The amount of time and effort given in voluntary work can be tailored to meet the ability, interest, energy levels and needs of the individual.

Holidays. Restful periods away from home are essential to revitalise as well as to provide a natural break from the usual routine. With regard to the person with heart disease, the only precaution is that air travel should not be undertaken until at least three months after an acute myocardial infarction, as the oxygen level in pressurised cabins is too low. Separate holidays for couples may not seem appropriate, but a few days spent with another relative or friend may give the spouse a break from the strain of feeling responsible for someone with a heart condition. The degree of stress experienced by the carer if the correct amount of appropriate assistance is not available cannot be overlooked, and if respite is the only form of relief in a given situation, the whole process should be handled tactfully to prevent any feelings of rejection or being a burden.

Travel agents will usually respond to any particular needs if requested, and access to facilities guides are now available for many cities and towns, and for other countries. These will give the reader an idea of places to stay that are accessible for wheelchair users and therefore likely to have lifts to rooms and services.

The Winged Fellowship Trust provides a holiday service that includes the family. Its address, along with other ideas for holidays for people with particular needs, can be found in a number of books produced by RADAR, 25 Mortimer Street, London W1N 8AB, and also available from major bookshops.

John Grooms Holidays also cater for all disabled people's requirements, and in some of the hotels personal assistance can be arranged.

The family. For many elderly people the additional free time available may be valuably used in extending their role as grandparent, aunt or uncle (either real or social). For a busy family with school-aged children the presence of a responsible adult to babysit, attend school concerts and open days, be available when the child (or parent) is sick, do the school run, help at parties, knit sweaters, and be involved in many other activities required by the children, can be invaluable. The relationship between old and young is often rewarding for both. Where families live some distance away, offering to have children to stay for a few days in the holidays, writing regular letters, making phone calls to the child or dressmaking is usually much appreciated. For those without this role, it may be possible to join an

THE EXPERIENCE OF LOSS

Throughout life we experience loss. Some losses may be of things that assume great importance to us — as in the loss of a job, the failure of a relationship, a divorce, the thwarting of an ambition because of exam failure, the loss of freedom through a prison sentence or of independence through the demands of a young family. Other losses may assume less importance, as in the case of a lost or stolen item, the loss of daily contact with a friend or community because of moving house, or the loss of money through a 'bad' buy. All these occasions involve change and adjustment to a new situation. The experience of loss brings with it memories of old ways and forces us to begin again with the new. It has many similarities to the situation in which the terminally ill person may find himself and, while he may have no direct experience of death, he may well benefit from the opportunity to draw similarities between previous occasions of loss and his present situation. To realise that he has experience, even if it is limited, of losing a familiar situation and having to face a new one may help him draw on past strategies and use them to his advantage.

A FRAMEWORK FOR THINKING

When working in such circumstances the occupational therapist should bear in mind that she, too, has needs. Work with the terminally ill can be emotionally draining and at times even harrowing. While this work is not without its joys and successes the therapist must examine the effect it has on her and create a system of support for herself and any assistants. Similarly, because of the diverse and sometimes physically intangible nature of the work it is vital that the therapist base her intervention on sound theoretical principles. These will provide guidance for her own input and will help her, as part of a team, to recognise the boundaries within which she is functioning.

The occupational therapist's needs may be summarised as follows:

- A sound knowledge of the process of dying and bereavement and of the medical procedures and philosophical viewpoints applied by the unit/team in which she is working
- A support system for herself and other members of the occupational therapy team in which there is the opportunity to express feelings, discuss ideas and gain emotional support
- A knowledge of the services, both voluntary and statutory, which are available in her area
- Self-knowledge: an awareness of her own attitudes, prejudices, fears, strengths and weaknesses and a clear view of her own areas of experience and inexperience
- An ability to work as part of a team and to listen and communicate well within it
- A conceptual framework on which to base her intervention.

With regard to this last point, many 'conceptual frameworks' could be used (see Ch. 2). The therapist must use the framework that she is most comfortable with — the one that she feels is the most meaningful and that best meets the individual's needs. This framework should also fit in with the philosophy of the unit/team in which she is working. The Reed & Sanderson model (1980), for example, has provided a framework for one unit working in the field of HIV/AIDS (see Ch. 33). This introduction, however, will use Abraham Maslow's 'hierarchy of needs' as a basis for thinking.

MASLOW'S HIERARCHY OF NEEDS

In 1954 Abraham Maslow (1970) postulated a hierarchy of human needs that he felt motivated human action. He saw our basic needs as physiological ones and felt that these were the strongest drives that had to be satisfied before other, higher needs could be fulfilled (Fig. 32.1) Thus, higher needs, such as fulfilling one's ambitions, can be interfered with by disturbances of needs at lower levels. For example, one might argue that a person is unlikely to feel good about himself (self-esteem) if he does not feel loved by others (love and belonging) or, on a more vernacular note, that he will not be able to concentrate on

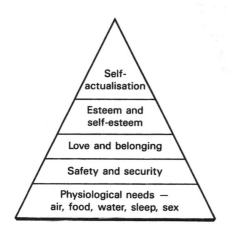

Fig. 32.1 Maslow's hierarchy of needs. (After Dworetzky 1988.)

an exquisite piece of music at a concert if he needs to visit the toilet.

While Maslow's hierarchy has been developed since it was first postulated, this chapter will use the five-layer version (Dworetzky 1988) as a basis for illustration. In using this version of the hierarchy as a background the occupational therapist could consider her intervention within the categories described below.

Physiological needs

These are seen as the strongest drives and the ones that need fulfilment before an individual can consider other needs. These physiological needs encompass basic bodily drives such as for food, drink, air, sleep and sex.

The ability to meet these independently is a basic need for most people. The loss of dignity and control which comes from being fed or taken to the toilet can increase feelings of helplessness and non-worth. The occupational therapist can discuss and explain methods, techniques and equipment available to enable the person to continue to look after himself for as long as is feasible. Establishing priorities, however, is equally important in enabling both physical and emotional energy to be used most effectively. Looking at standards and discussing how some things cannot be as they have always been may help allieviate feelings of guilt about not coping.

Thus, the role of the occupational therapist at this stage is to help the person accept that some tasks will gradually have to be given over to others. This may be done by encouraging the individual and his family to talk about and organise such tasks. Issues related to helping the person maintain roles and decision-making while devolving functions to others can be addressed. By helping to create an environment that allows the person to conserve energy, the therapist helps to ensure that he will be able to care for his basic needs for as long as possible. Assisting with mobility problems through the provision of a wheelchair, chair raises, grab rails, a hoist or other equipment or methods, will also help the person in this way.

People who experience difficulties with breathing and/or sleeping, as a direct result of their condition and/or because of increased anxiety related to their diagnosis, may benefit from the use of relaxation techniques, yoga, anxiety management skills or biofeedback techniques. People who are relaxed are more likely to be able to reduce or cope with pain, which is often a feature of cancer, and to fall asleep more easily.

Other physical symptoms such as vomiting and incontinence can cause great distress to both the individual and his carers and the persistence of these can make progress in other areas impossible. They also draw attention to the increasing lack of control the person has over his body. While control of these symptoms is not within the province of the therapist, she may be involved in helping the person to cope practically with them by arranging for the provision of laundry services and/or equipment, and by offering the person and his carers the opportunity to express their feelings of guilt, disgust and despair.

Sexual needs may be overlooked, either because of embarrassment or, in times of high emotion and distress, a reduction of libido. The person (or his partner) may find his body unattractive because of the physical changes brought about by the illness. Expressions of love through hugs, kisses, presents and treats, rather than full sexual activity, can provide comfort and give great support. Morris (1979) found that a year after surgery 25–33% of women who had had a simple mastectomy still had sexual and relationship problems as well as disrupted working lives and depression. He found that people suffer high levels of anxiety and depression during their illness and that these feelings were often exacerbated by such treatment as chemotherapy and radiotherapy, which made them feel extremely ill, affecting their self-image, confidence and relationships. In other words, because of their illness and its treatment people found difficulty in fulfilling even their most basic needs; the fulfilment of higher needs was consequently disrupted.

Safety and security

According to Maslow, the need for safety and security is, after physiological needs, the strongest basic motivator. A feeling of safety derives from being able to operate from a firm, stable base. This can be seen both as a 'physical' base, e.g. one's familiar home and surroundings, as well as a 'psychological' base, that is, the security gained from familiar people, roles, routines and customs.

When familiar routines and roles are disrupted for whatever reason there is strain on both the individual and those close to him. Where illness causes an inability to perform familiar roles and routines, the person may need help to adjust to this changed situation (see Chs 1, 2 and 8). The occupational therapist's knowledge of the individual's roles and duties within the home and family, at work and during leisure time can provide a basis for helping to reduce stress. By assisting him to prioritise routines, in terms of role demands, perceived needs and leisure interests, she can help him retain those that are most important to him. Familiar routines such as coping with a daily shower and styling hair are vital to some people's self-image and form a high priority in their need to be 'themselves'. For others such activities may be less important; while walking the dog, attending church, writing letters, going to work or meeting friends for a drink on Friday night may be the ones they are reluctant to relinquish. By helping the individual to explore and prioritise his activities, relinquishing those that are less personally important and maintain-

ing the others for as long as possible, the occupational therapist can help him 'to feel himself' for as long as possible.

It is also important to discuss the need to give a structure to the days and weeks as old and familiar routines disappear. Loss of habits that give a framework to a person's life can leave him feeling unmotivated to undertake even the smallest task. Setting a focus to each day, be it a regular phonecall to a friend, a trip to the hairdresser or attending an evening class, helps the individual plan his time purposefully around the event and to look forward to it the next time. Establishing new routines in place of those which have gone can also bring satisfaction. The person may find that he now has time to do things that he could not do before, such as embarking on a course of study or attending local community meetings, and may gain much pleasure from doing so.

Maintaining his role, and role duties, also helps the person to retain a feeling of security in that which is familiar. Too much change all at once can increase anxiety and insecurity, especially when accompanied by changes to the body brought about by the condition. The individual needs to consider how he will maintain those roles that are most important to him. The therapist can help him reflect on how he sees his roles, and the importance they hold for him. His role as a breadwinner may assume great importance. Discussion with his employer as to the possibility of viable alternative arrangements, negotiations with his bank and other financial institutions to rationalise his financial situation and make practical arrangements, and making a will or paying off his mortgage may help him feel he has done the best for his dependents for the future.

In his role as a homemaker the person should be encouraged to learn energy-saving techniques, to continue to make decisions about how the home is run, and to relinquish those role duties that can be taken over by others.

The person may be tempted to relinquish social and leisure roles very early in order to continue with others that seem more important, but remaining in contact with friends and acquaintances will help him to keep as many aspects of his life intact as possible. If he is no longer able to bowl for his local cricket team or play a game of football, his knowledge and experience may be of use in keeping club books or helping to organise social events.

A person's role as a partner should not be overlooked. His ability to give support and pleasure remains important if the relationship is not to become one of constant giving by one person and receiving by the other. While an imbalance of this kind may be to a certain extent inevitable during the course of the illness, the person's ability to fulfil the physical and emotional needs of his relationship is vital both to himself and to his partner. Similarly, the person may see his role as a parent as one of the most important parts of his life and he may need help in working through how he will remain a parent to his children even though he can no longer do with them those things he has done before.

Safety, the other element of this level of Maslow's hierarchy, is also found in working within one's physical and emotional capacity. Safety within the home environment can be enhanced by adaptations and equipment and by working within one's physical capacity. 'Tricks of the trade' are useful, and remembering well-tried advice (e.g. 'If the bedroom's a mess, make the bed; if the kitchen's a mess, wash up; if the garden's a mess, mow the lawn; If you're a mess, take a bath') can save much energy and worry.

In reflecting that safety stems, to an extent, from remaining in control it is clear that the individual may need help to accept the changes that are happening to him. He should be encouraged not to pretend that nothing has happened, or that nothing will change, but should address these changes and make positive decisions *around* them, rather than reluctant changes *because* of them.

Love and belonging

In Maslow's view, when the two previous basic needs are satisfied, the need for love, affection and belonging becomes the strongest drive. A person will feel the need to be part of a group or family and, without this, will feel lonely, rootless and ostracised. He may also feel an especial need to regain or strengthen ties with a wider group — his home town and old school friends for example, if he has moved away from these, or his religious, cultural or ethnic roots if he is apart from them.

All human beings have a need to love and be loved and to belong within a family and social group, and many anxieties and sadnesses can be created for an individual and his family when they fear they will lose this love.

People also have the need to actively 'let go', to say goodbye and 'to put their house in order' when faced with the possibility that life will not continue as anticipated. Much anxiety can be reduced by sorting out what will happen and how things will change. Putting one's house in order may mean different things to different people. Some may need help and information to make a will; others may wish to discuss their faith and the afterlife if this is important to them. To be able to teach carers new skills and to watch these being acquired can bring comfort during this period of letting go and may also lessen guilt and help the person to relinquish his roles more positively.

Some people may need encouragement to seek help for problems they cannot overcome themselves. For example, a man relinquishing his role as a father, breadwinner and husband may feel enormous guilt at the stress and burden he is causing his partner, and despair at not seeing his children grow up. The opportunity to express these feelings along with other deep emotions may help him let go of some of the emotional luggage which he might feel is overwhelming him at times. The inability to express fears, either because of concern for the worry and distress this may cause his family, or because such fears may betray weakness or seem trivial, can greatly hinder communication between loved ones at a time when this is extremely important. Fears often revolve around the unknown and may relate to the process of dying or of losing one's identity and body image as the illness progresses. The individual may also have fears of loneliness, pain, suffering, loss of dignity and self-control,

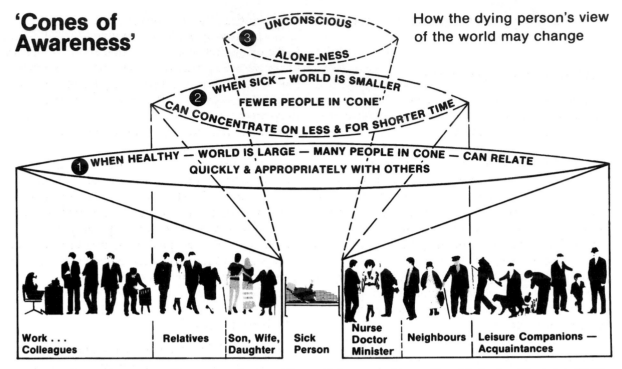

Fig. 32.2 Cones of awareness. How a person's view of the world changes as his condition deteriorates. (Reproduced from Ainsworth-Smith & Speck 1982, Letting Go, with kind permission.)

and, as his illness progresses and his world diminishes, he may fear isolation and rejection as he becomes physically and emotionally less able (Fig. 32.2).

The opportunity and encouragement to express these fears can help reduce the person's anxieties about them. He may need 'permission' to be frightened and sad. To facilitate communication, partners and families need to make conscious opportunities to talk. Wining and dining with each other, going for walks together, reviewing family albums, reminiscing on anniversaries, taking away-days and second honeymoons may all be ways in which these opportunities can be created. The occupational therapist may encourage the person's expression of feelings through the use of reminiscence, art, and other creative and expressive techniques. Education and understanding of the processes of bereavement and dying and an understanding of the disease and treatment processes and their consequences can help reduce fear of the unknown.

Anticipatory grief, which follows from the awareness of what is to come, affords the individual and his family the opportunity to reminisce on both good and bad aspects of the past, to bury the hatchet or clear the air if need be, and to express disappointment about what will not be. Garfield (1980) and Worden (1986) consider that gradual loss is easier for relatives to accept than sudden bereavement. However, such a process can cause problems if the family or individual withdraws from one another in anticipation of the event. The maximum period during which the anticipation of loss may have some benefit is seen as six months; after this time problems such as withdrawal begin to occur.

Making the most of the present with those he loves, within the circles to which he belongs, should be a goal for the person at this time. Where changes and illness bring unsolvable problems, seeking a viable, albeit imperfect, alternative rather than dwelling on the unattainable will help reduce stress and enhance a feeling of belonging and caring.

Esteem and self-esteem

All people, according to Maslow, have a need or desire for a stable, firmly based and (usually) positive evaluation of themselves. This need is, first, a desire for achievement, competence, independence and freedom and, secondly, a desire for status, recognition and dignity. Those who satisfy their self-esteem needs feel confident and useful. These positive feelings are of particular importance to a person who is terminally ill in order that he can see personal purpose and worth in his remaining life. When such needs are thwarted, feelings of inferiority and helplessness result; this will particularly impede the person's ability to cope with his condition and its often unpleasant side-effects.

Loss of normal appearance and familiar bodily functions can lead to diminishing self-esteem, loss of ability, energy and roles, and increased feelings of helplessness and uselessness.

The individual should be encouraged to pursue activities and goals that help him to feel more positive about himself. Opportunities to give to others, especially through articles related to the person himself, will help him feel that something of himself can still give lasting pleasure to others. Creating a life history album for children or grandchildren, researching and producing an illustrated family tree, passing on a skill, growing a cutting from a prized plant, or making a gift of home-made preserves, wine or confectionery can give the person a long- or short-term project which will result in an end product that he feels is very much part of himself.

The individual should be encouraged to continue to make decisions and to be in control. He should be listened to and consulted and should not be made to feel that he is being written off because he is no longer physically able to carry decisions through. Taking part in everyday decisions as he has always done — for example: what to eat for lunch, and when and where to eat it; what to watch on television; whether to turn on the central heating; what vegetables to plant in

the allotment — is all-important in maintaining one's self-worth. Being involved in long-term decisions that will affect events in the future is equally important. Which model of car to buy, which wallpaper to use, and whether or not to have the house painted outside this year or to wait until next year are decisions for which the person's experience, opinion and knowledge can still be sought.

Help with improving or maintaining personal appearance is also important, as is support in retaining special skills which particularly reflect the individual's self-image. If a person has always enjoyed and been good at playing the piano or taking photographs, for example, continuing these skills for as long as possible will help him feel good about himself.

Self-actualisation

Maslow (1970) describes self-actualisation as 'a tendency toward fulfilment, toward actualisation, toward the maintenance and enhancement of the organism'. Self-actualisation entails developing one's potential to the fullest. It involves the quest to do what one is fitted for. Maslow writes:

A musician must make music, an artist must paint, a poet must write, if he is to be ultimately at peace with himself. What a man *can* be, he *must* be. He must be true to his own nature.

As this is the highest level of the hierarchy, Maslow considers it to be somewhat fragile and easily interfered with by lower needs. He also describes the experience of 'transient self-actualisation' which, he considers, is felt by many people during 'peak experiences' — times of happiness and fulfilment that may occur in a variety of contexts. Transient self-actualisation may indeed be the state that a terminally ill person should seek if true self-actualisation eludes him.

According to Owens and Naylor (1989), coming to terms with oneself and getting on with living are two gains that the terminally ill person might derive from his situation.

The ability to retain control of one's physical self for as long as possible has been discussed

experienced only by the family and friends of a person when he has died. With HIV and AIDS, bereavement begins as soon as diagnosis is made. A person given a positive HIV antibody status experiences a sense of great loss of life, control, health, relationships, sexuality, job, income, support, friends and life expectancy. This list is by no means complete. Other areas and aspects may become evident once the therapist works with and gets to know the person.

Around 60% of people with AIDS become aware of their AIDS diagnosis after admission to hospital following a period of ill health. Having an AIDS diagnosis, as one would expect, presents a profound set of psychosocial difficulties which have to be dealt with and reviewed by a person and his partner, relatives, friends and colleagues. It demands straight talking and 'no-jargon' explanations by the health care team, who, at the same time, must show sensitivity and care. As yet there is no cure for AIDS; therefore, having an AIDS diagnosis may present the person with the realisation of what lies ahead. Commonly, the person has had a partner or friends who have died of an AIDS-related illness, or been in an environment where others are very ill with AIDS. A person may experience extreme isolation and stigmatisation because of the disease and its implications. His self-esteem may completely collapse under the strain of rejection by family and friends and their complete denial of the issues raised.

Quite often, this is the first time the person has revealed his homosexuality to friends and family, and this may be greeted with shock, denial and anger. Even though a person may have been unwell for a period of time, and may have had his suspicions, such a diagnosis will still be a shock, no matter how well prepared he is thought to be. It may, however, come as a relief to some to have their suspicions confirmed, so that they know what they are up against. People with AIDS usually experience overwhelming changes, both psychologically and physically. A person's life may alter considerably; health, social life, leisure, income and finances may all be affected.

Once an AIDS diagnosis is given, it will take time for its implications to be digested and for the person to feel able to question or respond. It is therefore important for the team to visit regularly following diagnosis so that the questions that will inevitably be asked can be responded to, and so that support can be given at this difficult stage. Some people may not have known their HIV antibody status prior to becoming unwell; for them, receiving such a diagnosis will have been a great shock, causing denial and numbness. A person may be heard to say 'I just can't believe it, it can't be me.' The person's reaction may be overlaid with anger and guilt; the anger may be directed towards himself, his partners or his close friends. One of the greatest difficulties in coming to terms with an AIDS diagnosis is the uncertainty — uncertainty about the course of the disease, about how people will react, and about how the individual's sexuality, life-style and independence will be affected. The reaction to the AIDS diagnosis may well mirror the mourning process as the person will be grieving for the loss of his previous healthy life and will be coming to terms with a new state of uncertainty and ill health. The reaction may be shown in the following ways (Parkes 1972):

- *shock* at the diagnosis and the possibility of death
- *anxiety* related to uncertainty about the
  — prognosis and course of illness
  — effects of medication and treatment
  — status of lovers and the lovers' ability to cope
  — reactions of others (family, friends, etc.)
  — loss of cognitive, physical, social and occupational abilities
  — risk of infection from others and to others
- *depression* stemming from
  — feelings of helplessness in the face of changed circumstances
  — the perception that the virus is in control
  — reduced quality of life in all spheres
  — the prospect of a gloomy and possibly a painful, uncomfortable and disfiguring future
  — self-blame and recriminations for past 'indiscretions'

— reduced social and sexual acceptability and isolation
- *anger* about
  — past, high-risk life-style and activities
  — the inability to overcome the virus
  — new and involuntary life-style restrictions
- *guilt* about
  — being homosexual
  — being a drug user
  — having the 'unacceptability' of homosexuality confirmed via illness
- *obsessions*. These may show as over-activity related to:
  — a relentless searching for explanations
  — a relentless searching for new diagnostic evidence on one's body
  — the inevitability of decline and death
  — fads over health and diets.

The length of time needed for an individual to adjust to an AIDS diagnosis and its implications ranges from days to months. At this time follow-up by the counsellor or health care worker may be needed to monitor, support and assist the person in resolving issues and solving problems.

THE CONTINUING MANAGEMENT OF AIDS

In the continuing care of a person with AIDS it may be important to introduce him to a counsellor or long-term support network, to continue discussion with partners and friends, and to give information about support agencies, both voluntary and statutory. The occupational therapist is but one part of a multidisciplinary team (Fig. 33.3).

It will be up to the individual how involved he wishes his partner, carer or family to be in this process. However, it would be usual to involve the partner at the earliest opportunity, as he or she too will experience the bereavement process and will need to adjust. Commonly counselling time is offered to partners either alone or with the individual.

It is at this time that spouses, brothers and sisters, other relatives, lovers and friends become far more important than perhaps ever before. Many people, in the absence of parents or family, develop a very close network of friends who

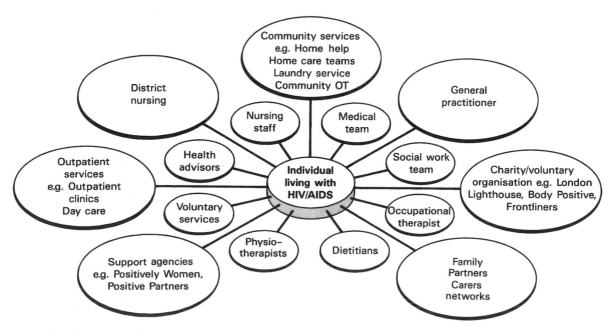

Fig. 33.3 The multidisciplinary team.

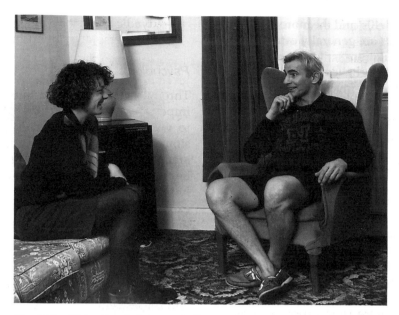

Fig. 33.8 Giving time to listen and offer support.

Groups are often a useful forum in which to involve carers, partners or families, perhaps through the establishment of a carers' support group. These provide a forum to increase awareness and understanding and often restore confidence in caring. They may also teach new skills, or build on existing ones and overall provide a better supportive network.

There are many useful texts in which the process of group work and its development are well documented, for example *The Red Book of Groups and how to lead them better* (Houston 1990), and it is essential that the therapist becomes familiar with these.

ADAPTING TO AND WITH THE ENVIRONMENT

With Reed & Sanderson's Human Occupation Model, not only the physical environment needs to be considered but also the person's biopsychological and sociocultural environments. The non-physical aspect will include the various components which go together to make up the identity of the person and the differing groups of people with whom he may have common values, social structures and expectations. These may include age, gender, class, ethnic background, religious beliefs and rituals, economic status and political beliefs. In planning to meet a person's needs effectively in the future (for example post-discharge from hospital or from a treatment programme) these issues should be borne in mind. The person may, for example, have to relate effectively to new care workers or people not previously known, as well as maintain his self-identity and relationships within his existing social spheres. This will be not only within his home setting but also wherever he had links in the past, possibly social venues, parents groups and neighbourhood or church groups.

Within the physical aspects of the environment an occupational therapist may be asked to assess the person's home, work environment, college or other place of study. During all stages of treatment a person's wishes must be respected. This applies, for example, to the person's preference on where he is to be cared for in the future or after hospital admission. If a person chooses to return to, or die, at home, this avenue must be fully explored and the resources to enable him to do so must be researched and discussed. With the advent of the Community Care Act (1993) additional care can be bought in by the local

Box 33.1 Case study

Richard is a 37-year-old Caucasian, married man.

He lives with his wife and seven-year-old son. They have recently moved down from Scotland and for the last six months have been living in London. While in Scotland Richard was a chef but now does not work. His wife has a part-time job as a secretary and cleaner. They live in a two-bedroomed, first-floor flat which they purchased on moving down to London. They do not know the neighbours, although they see them pass in the joint entrance porch. Most of their friends and all their family live in Scotland and since being in London they have made few friends.

The son is at school locally and is unaware of his father's illness.

Reason for occupational therapy referral

Richard was first diagnosed HIV-positive by his GP in Scotland in January 1986, complaining of 'flu-like symptoms and general tiredness and fatigue. For two years he remained well and his main complaint was tiredness.

In February 1988 he had a short admission to hospital with pneumocystic cariniipneumonia (PCP), a common opportunistic infection. Up until December 1993 he remained well and continued to work. Towards the end of the year the family decided to move to London. While plans were being made, Richard had another episode of PCP, resulting in admission to hospital. He lost a great deal of weight and his mobility became more difficult.

In February 1994 the family moved to London to avoid prying questions from family and to remain anonymous. After six months in London Richard attended a treatment centre with his wife. He presented unsteady on his feet, with some loss of vision, fatigue and poor mobility. After several clinical investigations, he was diagnosed as having CMV retinitis and concern was expressed about his ability to manage at home. His wife also expressed her anxiety about coping and how she should care for Richard.

After assessment it was felt that the occupational therapist would be of most assistance in dealing with the following problems:

Performance components

- Sensorimotor:
  — Lack of mobility (difficulty with stairs, transfers)
  — Decreased endurance and strength
  — Increased pain
  — Loss of sight and blurred vision
  — Increased fatigue
- Psychological:
  — Confusion because of visual problems
  — Determination to be self-reliant
  — Diminished self-concept (from provider to dependent)
  — Changed self-identity (from capable to helpless)
  — Wife concerned for husband and child

  — Changed levels of responsibility
  — Poor coping skills
  — Difficulty with relationships
- Social:
  — Friends deceased and limited social contact
  — Unfamiliar with new neighbourhood
  — Withdrawal
  — Few interests
  — Potential conflict with the family.

Occupational components

- Self-maintenance:
  — Difficulty performing self-maintenance activities such as bathing, dressing, medication routine
- Productivity:
  — Difficulty with reading/writing
  — Difficulty with performing home management tasks such as meal preparation and cleaning
- Leisure:
  — Inability to engage in leisure activities.

Action plan

Performance components

- To assess and assist limited mobility and aid safety through the provision of daily living equipment such as grab rails and a pill mill dispenser.
- To teach manual handling techniques to Richard's wife and other carers.
- To refer to specialist services such as the Terrence Higgins Trust for additional support at home for the whole family.
- To make a joint referral with the GP to a local hospice for periodic respite care.
- Support was offered to the whole family via practical strategies, as above, and via counselling and support groups.
- Richard's wife was put in touch with her local carers' association, although she chose not to engage this service.

Occupational components

- To refer to community agencies for community care, such as home help and care assistants.
- To liaise with GP and refer to district nurses for medical and nursing management at home.
- To teach energy conservation techniques.

Conclusion

This highlights the complex needs of an individual as well as associated others in the care and provision of services. It also demonstrates that services need to be integrated between both statutory and voluntary services.

It is important to realise that care should be truly multidisciplinary in order to meet the needs of Richard and his family.

National AIDS Helpline
Tel: (0800) 567123
This is a free 24-hour national helpline which offers advice and information on any aspect of HIV infection to anyone calling.

The Patrick House
17 Rivercourt Road
London W6 9LD
Tel: 0181–846 9117
Patrick House is a residential nursing home for people with brain impairment related to HIV and AIDS. It is the first such institution of its kind in Europe.

Positively Women
5 Sebastian Street
London EC1V 0HE
Tel: 0171–490 5515
A wide range of free and strictly confidential counselling and support services are provided to women with AIDS and HIV. These include support groups, telephone and/or face-to-face counselling and a buddying service.

The Terrence Higgins Trust
52/54 Grays Inn Road
London WC1 8LT
Tel: 0171–831 0330
    0171–242 1010 (Helpline)
The Terrence Higgins Trust is the largest AIDS/HIV charity in Britain. Services which it provides include a helpline, buddying, counselling, a legal helpline, welfare advice, hardship grants, prison visits and support groups.

Threshold Housing Advice Centre
91–99 Tooting High Street   126 Uxbridge Road
London SW17 0SU   London W12
Tel: 0181–682 0322   Tel: 0181–749 2925
This group will provide help for anyone with HIV infection who is facing any sort of housing problem.

REFERENCES

Barter G, Barton S, Gazzard B 1993 HIV and AIDS: your questions answered. Churchill Livingstone, London

Catalan J 1988 Psychosocial and neuropsychiatric aspects of HIV infection: review of their extent and implications for psychiatry. Journal of Psychosomatic Research 32(3): 237–248

Houston G 1990 The Red Book of groups and how to lead them better. Rochester Foundation

Kubler-Ross, E (ed.) 1986 Death: the final stage of growth. Simon & Schuster, New York

Parkes C M 1972 Studies of grief in adult life: bereavement. Tavistock Publications, London

Reed K, Sanderson S 1992 Concepts of occupational therapy, 3rd edn. Williams & Wilkins, Baltimore

Saunders C (ed.) 1978 The management of terminal disease. Edward Arnold, London

Seidl O, Goebel F D 1987 Psychosomatic reactions of homosexuals and drug addicts to the knowledge of a positive HIV test result. AIDS-Forschung 2(4): 181–187

FURTHER READING

Adler M W 1987 ABC of AIDS. BMA, Taylor & Francis, UK

AIDS Project Los Angeles 1987 AIDS: a self care manual. IBS Press, Santa Monica

BMA Foundation For AIDS 1990 The management of HIV infection in primary care. BMA Foundation for AIDS, London

Bury J, Morrison V, McLachlan S (eds) 1992 Working with women and AIDS. Routledge, London

Cusack L, Phillips L, Singh S 1990 The role of the occupational therapist in HIV disease and AIDS. British Journal of Occupational Therapy 53(5): 181–183

Cusack L, Singh S (eds) 1994 HIV and AIDS: practical approaches. Chapman & Hall, London

Daniels V J 1987 AIDS: the acquired immune deficiency syndrome, 4th edn. MTP Press, Lancaster

Farthing C F 1986 A colour atlas of AIDS. Wolfe Medical Publications, London

Green J, McCreaner A 1989 Counselling in HIV infection and AIDS. Blackwell Scientific Publications, Oxford

King M 1993 AIDS, HIV and mental health. Cambridge University Press, Cambridge

Kirkpatrick B 1988 AIDS — sharing the pain. Darton, Longman & Todd, London

Kubler-Ross E 1970 On death and dying. Tavistock Publications, London

Lancet 1989 Latest AIDS figures. 11: 1055

Miller C 1987 Living with AIDS and HIV. Macmillan, London

Miller D, Webber J, Green J 1986 The Management of AIDS patients. Macmillan, London

Miller R, Bar R 1987 AIDS — a guide to clinical counselling. Science Press, London

Pratt R 1991 AIDS — A strategy for nursing care, 3rd edn. Edward Arnold, London

Richardson D 1987 Women and the AIDS crisis. Pandora Press, Routledge, Chapman & Hall, New York

Scott P 1989 National AIDS manual. National AIDS Manual, London

Shilis R 1988 And the band played on. Penguin Books, Harmondsworth

Tatchell P 1987 AIDS — A guide to survival. Gay Men's Press, London

Wells N, Taylor D 1988 HIV and AIDS in the United Kingdom. OHE briefing, 1988(23) Office of Health Economics, London

Willard M S, Spackman C S, Hoplans H L, Smith M D 1993 Willard and Spackman's occupational therapy, 8th edn. J B Lippincott, Philadelphia

Youle M, Clarbour J, Wade P et al 1988 AIDS: therapeutics in HIV disease. Churchill Livingstone, Edinburgh

34

Cancer

Sue Beresford

INTRODUCTION

Having cancer is a very lonely and frightening position to be in, people are embarrassed and frightened if you talk about it. It is far easier to say you feel well and are coping, than to tell the truth about how frightened you are, about the pain and dying and all the fears that beset you.
    (Maggie Hoult, quoted in Foreman & Hobbs 1988)

Despite an increasing awareness of the disease and its treatments, cancer is still perceived by most people to be a terrifying illness. It requires people to think about many feelings with which they are uncomfortable and which they would rather ignore. It is, however, a subject that most health care professionals will have to consider at some point in their working lives.

Oncology can be defined as the study or science of cancer, a disease that has been known about for over 2000 years. More money is spent on research into causes of and cures for cancer than on research into any other medical condition, but sufferers still have to deal with the misguided attitudes of family and friends.

This chapter discusses the role of the occupational therapist in helping the cancer sufferer to cope with his illness, to maintain the maximum independence possible and to gain satisfaction from life regardless of the prognosis of his disease. The chapter begins with an introduction into the causes, pathology and clinical features of cancer, and describes the physical and psychological problems that are likely to be faced by the person with cancer. The various forms of medical treatment that are available for cancer are also outlined.

The chapter then turns to the philosophy of care adopted by many professionals in their intervention with cancer sufferers. Based on hospice philosophy it recognises the unique needs of each individual and his family and uses a multi-disciplinary team approach to address these needs.

The chapter next turns to more specific aspects of the therapist's role with cancer sufferers, describing her approach, whether the individual has responded to active treatment or is receiving palliative care. Suggestions are made on how the therapist may address assessment and intervention for people with cancer wherever they receive treatment.

The final section of the chapter describes the occupational therapist's role in the individual's resettlement at home following treatment in hospital. As always, her support will extend to family members, and her intervention will be carried out in cooperation with the other members of the rehabilitation team.

'Cancer' is a general term that refers to a malignant growth of tissue in any part of the body. The growth is parasitic, non-functional and invasive.

One in three people is likely to develop cancer at some stage in their lives, and one in five will die as a result of the disease. Much is now known about the disease. Many of the 200 or more of its forms respond to treatment, and 40% of sufferers can expect to be cured. It is thought that cancer can be caused by external agents which, in some susceptible people, result in malignant disease. The list of implicated agents grows as new carcinogens are discovered through research. Many forms of cancer (up to 70%) are known to be preventable, and emphasis is now being placed on health education in an effort to encourage people to adopt a healthier way of life (Fig. 34.1).

PATHOLOGY

A tumour or neoplasm is an abnormal overgrowth of cells. Tumours fall into two main categories: benign and malignant.

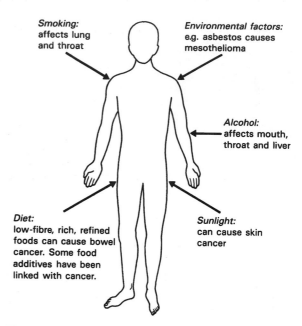

Smoking: affects lung and throat

Environmental factors: e.g. asbestos causes mesothelioma

Alcohol: affects mouth, throat and liver

Diet: low-fibre, rich, refined foods can cause bowel cancer. Some food additives have been linked with cancer.

Sunlight: can cause skin cancer

Fig. 34.1 Some causes of cancer.

Benign

These tumours are made up of normal cells which resemble the host tissue. They are slow growing, encapsulated and do not produce secondary deposits (metastases). They may be cysts (filled with fluid), adenomata (glandular tissue), fibromata (fibrous tissue) or lipomata (fatty tissue). While they are not usually life threatening, they may encroach upon and compress other tissue, thus potentially causing very serious problems and, if left untreated, may develop into something more grave.

Malignant

These tumours are fast-growing cells, abnormal to the host area which spread, if left untreated, via the lymphatic and circulatory systems. This spread results in metastases forming away from the primary tumour. Many primary tumours have a predictable line of spread (Fig. 34.2), and since many of them have few initial signs and symptoms, they may not be detected until they have formed metastases. There has been an increase in health education in this area to encourage

Primary site	Risk of metastases	Common sites of spread	Favourable prognostic factors	Poor prognostic factors	Appropriate investigations
Gynaecological Ovary	* * *	Peritoneal cavity Direct extension Lung Liver	Stage 1 Low grade histology	Advanced stage High grade histology	Abdominal CT scan or ultrasound
Uterus	*	Direct extension Lymph nodes Lung	Stage 1 (tumour confined to corpus) Low grade No myometrial invasion	Tumour spread beyond corpus Large uterine cavity High grade histology Myometrial invasion	Chest x-ray
Cervix	* *	Direct extension Lymph nodes	No parametrial/pelvic extension	Advanced stage	IVP Lymphogram
Urological Kidney	* *	Direct extension Lymph nodes Lung Bone	Tumour confined to kidney – capsule intact	Extra-renal spread Positive lymph nodes Renal vein invasion	Chest x-ray Abdominal CT scan or ultrasound Bone scan
Bladder	* *	Direct extension Lymph nodes	Low grade Papillary tumour Early stage	High grade Deep muscle invasion Squamous histology	IVP Lymphogram CT scan
Prostate	* * *	Direct extension Lymph nodes Bone	Small nodule Low grade histology	Extracapsular spread High grade histology	Acid phosphatase IVP Lymphogram Bone scan
Head and neck	*	Direct extension Lymph nodes	Localised tumour	Advanced stage Bulky nodes	CT scan/x-ray tomography Skull x-rays (special projections) e.g. SMV
Melanoma	* *	Direct extension Lymph nodes Liver Lung Brain	Superficial lesions (Clark I and II) Negative nodes	Large primary Infiltrating lesions (Clark III-V) Positive nodes	Chest x-ray Liver scan/ultrasound Bone scan Brain scan
Thyroid Papillary and follicular	*	Lymph nodes Lung	Young patients Primary < 5cm Negative nodes	Older patients Large primary	Chest x-ray ^{131}I Body scan
Medullary	* * *	Lymph nodes Lung Liver Bone	Normal calcitonin following surgery Negative nodes	Persistently raised calcitonin Positive nodes	Chest x-ray Bone scan Liver scan Serum calcitonin
Anaplastic	* * *	Lymph nodes Lung Liver Bone		Any anaplastic histology	Chest x-ray Liver scan Bone scan

Fig. 34.2 Caption see overleaf

Primary site	Risk of metastases	Common sites of spread	Favourable prognostic factors	Poor prognostic factors	Appropriate investigations
Breast	***	Lymph nodes Bone Liver Lung	Small primary tumour Low grade histology Negative axillary nodes	Large primary tumour High grade histology Positive nodes Family history	Chest x-ray Bone scan Liver scan/ultrasound (contralateral mammogram)
Bronchus	***	Lymph nodes Liver Brain Bone/bone marrow	Resectable lesion (except small cell type) Negative nodes	Non-small cell history Lymph node/blood vessel invasion Extra-thoracic spread	Liver scan/ultrasound Bone scan Brain scan
Gastro-intestinal Stomach	***	Direct extension Lymph nodes Liver Lung Bone	Small lesion Low grade histology Confined to muscularis mucosa Negative nodes	High grade histology Extension through wall Positive nodes	Gastroscopy Barium studies Liver scan/ultrasound
Pancreas	***	Direct extension Lymph nodes Head lesion – liver Tail lesion – liver, lungs, bone		Any pancreatic cancer	CT scan/ultrasound of abdomen
Colon and rectum	**	Direct extension Lymph nodes Liver	Duke's stage A and B Low grade histology	Dukes C_1 and C_2 Positive nodes High grade histology	Liver scan/ultrasound
Hodgkins disease	**	Contiguous nodes Spleen Liver/Bone marrow	Early stage < 4 node groups involved No 'B' symptoms	Advanced stage Mediastinal involvement 'B' symptoms Lymphocyte depletion	Chest x-ray + tomography Lymphogram + IVP CT scan abdomen Bone marrow trephine Exploratory laparotomy
Non-Hodgkins lymphoma	***	Non-contiguous lymph nodes Liver Bone marrow CNS Extranodal sites	Nodular histology (all stages) Stage I disease (diffuse/mixed histology)	Diffuse histology Advanced stage	Chest x-ray ENT examination Lymphogram Bone marrow trephine Liver ultrasound/biopsy CSF cytology (diffuse)

Fig. 34.2 Patterns of metastases. (Reproduced by kind permission of Farmitalia Carlo Erba Ltd.)

people to have any unusual lumps investigated promptly.

CLINICAL FEATURES

Many tumours have very few initial signs and symptoms but are detected at routine examinations, which include self-examination and body scanning techniques such as mammography. Certain symptoms, described below, are common to many types of tumour.

Fatigue and weight loss

These symptoms will often prompt a person to see his general practitioner. They are insidious in onset, and the person tends to feel foolish about bothering his physician with something so trivial. By the time he has sought advice, however, it is not unusual for a person to have lost up to 2 stone (13 kg) in weight. The general practitioner is unlikely to make a diagnosis of cancer on these symptoms alone, but will refer the person to a specialist so that further investigation can be made.

Pain

Seventy per cent of people suffering from cancer experience some form of pain. The chronic pain of cancer differs from the acute pain that accompanies a fracture or infection such as appendicitis. Whereas the individual will expect acute pain to decrease as health is restored, he may see chronic pain as meaningless and unending. The treatment of chronic pain is complex and requires accurate diagnosis and specialist knowledge. Regular analgesia, of the correct strength, should be provided to prevent the pain returning before the next dose is due, and should be closely monitored and adjusted according to the severity of the pain.

In addition to the cognitive aspect (actual perception of pain), there is also an affective aspect (how the person responds emotionally to the pain). This can vary, not only from one person to another, but in the same person from day to day or even hour to hour. Medication is only part of the overall management of pain; consideration of the psychological aspect of pain is also needed. This is an area in which occupational therapy can make a valuable contribution.

Besides medication, there are other forms of pain control that may be considered; these include nerve blocks, transcutaneous electrical nerve stimulation (TENS) and radiotherapy. Some surgical procedures are also useful and may be indicated.

Nerve stimulation (acupuncture) has been used to relieve pain for thousands of years. Its effectiveness in relieving the pain of cancer has not been proven, but it may be helpful for some individuals.

Constipation

This may be drug induced, a symptom of bowel cancer or a combination of the two. Opiate medication, often used in the treatment of cancer pain, has a constipating effect which, if left untreated, can cause pain and discomfort, anorexia, vomiting or confusion. Aperients should be prescribed routinely for people taking this type of medication.

Respiratory symptoms

Dyspnoea is experienced by about 40% of people who are admitted to a hospice (Kaye 1991), but is usually less common in the early stages of cancer, unless related to a chest infection. It brings a fear of suffocation; consequently it is important to attend to environmental factors by providing good ventilation or a cooling fan. Anxiety often accompanies breathing problems, and this should be treated along with any physical causes such as pleural effusion or chest infection. Physiotherapy can reduce dyspnoea by encouraging the use of breathing exercises and relaxation techniques to reduce anxiety.

Lymphoedema

When this occurs in conjunction with cancer it is caused by a blockage in the lymphatic system, usually as a result of surgery or radiotherapy damage. The build-up of fluids in the affected area causes the limb to swell, reducing mobility and increasing pain. Lymphoedema often occurs in the arm following mastectomy.

The condition is treatable, in most cases, by massage, the use of compression pumps, and in some cases, a course of compression bandaging. Following this treatment, it will be necessary for the person to wear a pressure garment on the affected limb to prevent return of the swelling.

The reduction of lymphoedema is usually the province of the physiotherapist; however, any loss of mobility and strength resulting from the condition can be treated by occupational therapy.

Neurological symptoms

Mood changes, confusion, hemiparesis, headaches, ataxia and dysphagia can all be symptomatic of cerebral tumours. As intracranial pressure fluctuates, these symptoms can vary in severity. Tumours growing close to the spinal cord can result in cord compression, which may cause paraplegia and incontinence.

People who develop paraplegia and hemiplegia will almost certainly be referred to the occupational therapist for help with activities of daily living. In this situation it is important to remember that their medical condition is unstable and that physical symptoms will fluctuate.

The control and management of symptoms is important, whether a person is receiving treatment and can be expected to recover or whether the disease has progressed beyond this stage. It can mean the difference between living and existing. Most symptoms can now be controlled, not only by medication but also by a variety of other means.

MEDICAL TREATMENT

Certain tumours respond well to specific interventions. The three main types of treatment offered to people who have been diagnosed as having cancer are:

1. surgery — most often indicated if there are no signs that the tumour has spread

2. radiotherapy — which can be effective in the treatment of well-differentiated tumours, e.g. Hodgkin's disease

3. chemotherapy — efficient in the treatment of poorly differentiated tumours, e.g. leukaemia and lymphoma.

Surgical intervention

There are three main types of surgical treatment in cancer care: explorative, curative and palliative.

Explorative

Much diagnostic work is now done using X-rays and body scanners. However, these machines cannot tell whether a tumour is malignant. This still requires the removal of part or all of the tumour for subjection to pathological tests.

Curative

Surgery is usually performed if the tumour is small, well defined and sited away from any vital organs. Such surgery may necessitate the use of deep X-ray treatment (DXT) and chemotherapy to ensure that all the malignant cells have been removed. For example, when a breast tumour is removed, the use of DXT and/or chemotherapy can eliminate the need to perform a complete mastectomy.

Palliative

Removal of part of a tumour may be necessary if the tumour is threatening one or more of the vital organs. This type of surgery may involve procedures such as forming a colostomy to bypass an intestinal obstruction.

Radiotherapy

Radiotherapy aims to shrink the tumour by killing the cancer cells using gamma or X-rays. Cancer cells are more sensitive than normal cells, and are less able to repair damage. Since normal cells can be affected by radiotherapy, courses of this type of treatment are carefully planned to give maximum exposure to the tumour and cause minimum damage to normal tissue.

The skin over the treated area may become red and sore. Since DXT affects the fast-dividing tissue of a tumour, it can also affect normal fast-dividing tissue, as in the alimentary tract. If the radiation is close to this type of sensitive tissue, it can give rise to more common side-effects, such as tiredness, mouth ulcers, nausea, vomiting and loss of appetite.

Chemotherapy

This form of treatment uses cytotoxic drugs, which are very toxic (poisonous) to cancer cells but, fortunately, are not so toxic to normal cells. There are many different drugs used, in combination, during chemotherapy. Four of the main group are:

- alkylating agents
- cytotoxic antibiotics
- antimetabolites
- Vinca alkaloids.

The choice of drug depends on the nature of the tumour. It may be necessary to use three, four or five drugs in combination to attack some tumours.

Administration may be by:

- mouth
- subcutaneous or intramuscular injection
- intravenous drip.

Chemotherapy is usually given for several days, followed by a rest period before the next course is started. Treatment usually continues while a response is gained and the tumour shrinks, and may last many months.

As with DXT, chemotherapy affects the cells which reproduce rapidly. These include the cells of the alimentary tract, the mouth and the bone marrow. Side-effects, if any, are likely to be nausea, vomiting and mouth ulcers; if the first two are severe and troublesome, antiemetic drugs can be prescribed. As the blood cells are produced in the bone marrow, tiredness may occur as a result of decreased production of red blood cells. Moreover, the decreased production of white blood cells can lead to the loss of immunity to infection. Sometimes the cells of the scalp are affected, resulting in hair loss, but the hair will re-grow after treatment has ceased.

At the time of diagnosis, it is often hoped that the malignant disease can be cured, and while acute medical treatment is vital at this stage, attention also needs to be given to the psychological care of the individual. If at the time of diagnosis it is felt that the disease is incurable, attention to psychological support is even more important. The philosophy of care outlined below provides ideas on how treatment can be offered to the individual, maintaining his dignity and autonomy throughout the treatment process, whether this be curative or palliative.

A PHILOSOPHY OF CARE

You matter because you are you. You matter to the last moment of your life and we will do all we can, not only to help you die peacefully, but also to live until you die.

(Dame Cicely Saunders, cited in Zora & Zora 1981)

This philosophy of care is based upon the hospice philosophy, a set of ideas and attitudes on the care of a person suffering from a potentially life-threatening disease such as cancer. The practice of hospice care need not be confined to an institute, and is just as relevant in the home as in the hospital setting.

While it would be inappropriate to recreate the total hospice philosophy in a hospital setting, many of its features could and should be incorporated into the care of cancer sufferers wherever they receive treatment. The principles of this philosophy are summarised below.

CARE AND EMPATHY

These qualities underpin this type of work. Even if the disease is curable, a diagnosis of cancer can be very frightening, and brings the person face to face with his own mortality. This is an area that many people avoid, so any health care professional working in this field must be able to listen to these fears and not be afraid of them.

She may not have all the answers, but to care is often enough. Although this type of care requires the therapist to give of herself, its rewards can be immense.

THREE-DIMENSIONAL PERSPECTIVE

People are 'three dimensional'; that is to say, they have needs which can be identified as physical, emotional and spiritual, and, as Figure 34.3 shows, these needs are interconnected. In order that a person remains healthy, all these aspects need attention. The person who suffers pain that no amount of analgesia can control often has deep anxieties and fears which need consideration. While most people accept that they have physical and emotional needs, many are reluctant to accept their spirituality and often deny its existence. Coping with a potentially life-threatening situation can necessitate consideration of a person's spirituality. The chaplain or other spiritual minister is an important member of the multidisciplinary team, and people receiving treatment should be aware of his or her availability.

The acknowledgement of physical, emotional and spiritual needs is equally important for the members of the treatment team. They should give consideration to their own needs if they are to remain effective in helping others to identify theirs.

It is important to identify concerns of the individual, since a problem which appears insurmountable to one person may be unimportant to another. It is necessary to take time to listen to each individual and gain a sensitive understanding of his priorities and needs.

UNIT OF CARE (Fig. 34.4)

People do not live in isolation. When a disease like cancer affects an individual it also affects the family or others with whom the person lives. Close family members will probably become the main carers and will need help and support in their task. Family involvement and support should begin at the time of diagnosis and continue throughout the course of the illness.

GRIEF REACTION

Kubler-Ross (1970) has described the five emotional stages through which people pass on being told they have a potentially life-threatening disease: denial and isolation, anger, bargaining, depression and acceptance. Although not all people pass through these stages in order, and many shift back and forth between two stages for a while, Kubler-Ross's model is generally accepted. Throughout this emotional journey, it is important to preserve a sense of hope, which must be distinguished from denial. Hope is demonstrated, for example, by the usually realistic person who talks openly of his prognosis but also talks about the future. This is the kind of optimism that keeps life bearable.

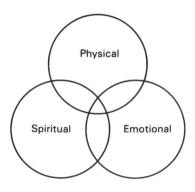

Fig. 34.3 Needs of people.

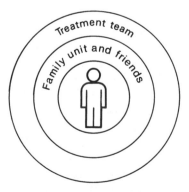

Fig. 34.4 The unit of care. The treatment team must consider the needs of the individual and his family unit.

COMMUNICATION

This is a skill that can be learned. The heart of good communication lies in the ability to listen creatively, hear what is being said and respond accordingly.

By listening attentively to the person as he expresses his needs, the therapist affirms that he is important and deserving of respect. She helps to restore his self-esteem and supports him in solving some of his own problems, as well as providing a solid foundation for her relationship with the individual. Careful listening may offer the therapist insight into how she might help with the other problems.

TEAM WORK

Just as people do not live in isolation, neither do they work in isolation. A good team, working together, cannot be bettered. The team of people working in this field can be quite extensive. The roles of individual members frequently overlap, and boundaries of responsibilities may become blurred. It may be helpful for each member of the team to have his or her own exclusive care responsibility. This helps to identify each member's role and affords him or her the freedom to operate with maximum effectiveness in the other areas of work.

An occupational therapist working predominantly within the field of oncology must be mature and secure. It can be very lonely to be the only member of a particular professional group in a team, without the back-up of other occupational therapy staff.

The team usually comprises a consultant, ward doctor, physiotherapist, occupational therapist, chaplain, social worker, dietitian, speech therapist and radiographer, as well as nurses (including Macmillan nurses). Other disciplines may be represented as necessary.

Macmillan nurses are Registered General Nurses with a district nursing qualification who have been specially trained to advise on pain relief and symptom control. They work as members of the primary health care team with general practitioners, district nurses and hospital and hospice staff. They provide emotional support to cancer sufferers and their families, which continues through bereavement. They are an education and teaching resource for the district in which they work and enable many people who would otherwise be hospitalised to remain at home.

In some instances, the number of people involved in caring for a family can become very large. It can be advantageous to nominate a key worker within the team to coordinate the different services. This role often falls to the Macmillan nurse, but may equally be undertaken by any other member of the team if he or she is better acquainted with the family and their needs.

STAFF SUPPORT

Working with people who suffer from life-threatening illness can be emotionally as well as physically draining. Staff support varies widely. Some people favour formal support groups, run by a member of the team, while others see the need to employ a counsellor, who is not directly involved or working within the team, to provide support. It is necessary that all team members are supported by each other on a daily basis, in addition to having access to formal support.

CARE OF THE BEREAVED

Grieving is a normal process and accompanies any life change. It is a usual reaction to loss and begins when an individual is told that he has an illness from which he will not recover. It is important, therefore, having been told the prognosis, that a person be given the opportunity to return and discuss his worries and feelings as they occur. Since the unit of care is identified as the whole family, there needs to be provision for bereavement counselling, both before and after death, which may be on an individual or group basis. Bereaved people often find group support by other people in the same position most effective.

It is important to help the person to live his life as fully as possible throughout the duration of his illness, whether his life expectancy is ten days or ten years.

CANCER REHABILITATION

The overall aim of cancer rehabilitation can be defined as 'endeavouring to improve the quality of survival of cancer patients so that during their period of survival they will be able to lead as independent and productive a life as possible at the minimum level of dependency, regardless of life expectancy' (Dietz 1981). Dietz further identifies four stages on the way to rehabilitation:

- *Prevention.* Potential disability is lessened by training and education (i.e. people learn about causes of cancer and how they can adjust their life-style to prevent this).
- *Restoration.* The disease is reduced or eliminated by treatment.
- *Support.* The disease cannot be eliminated, but treatment can reduce the impact of disability.
- *Palliation.* The progress of the disease causes increasing problems, but treatment can improve the quality of life.

At present oncology rehabilitation is carried out in the community, in district general hospitals, in oncology/radiotherapy units and in hospices. Fig. 34.5 shows these settings in relation to Dietz's stages of cancer readaption.

Hammond (1988) shows that more work with cancer sufferers is undertaken by occupational therapists working in radiotherapy units and hospices than by those working in other settings. It is felt that this may be either because of the doctor's reluctance to refer patients, from a lack of awareness of the scope of the occupational therapy service, or because of a shortage of staff with sufficient training to carry out this work in general hospitals or the community.

REFERRAL

The method of referral depends largely on the area in which the work is carried out. Ideally a blanket referral system should be adopted, as this has the benefit of allowing the occupational therapist to screen her case load and provide appropriate intervention at the right time. Clearly such a system can only be successful in a defined area such as a unit or ward. Where this is not possible, for example in the community, problems may arise when referrals arrive too late for a good service to be provided. In such circumstances the therapist may consider instituting an education programme for staff, to increase the number of appropriate referrals.

THE ROLE OF THE OCCUPATIONAL THERAPIST

THEORETICAL FRAMEWORKS

The contribution by occupational therapists to oncology rehabilitation is still developing. It is a new and exciting area of work that requires the blending of traditional skills and new ideas to form a complete concept of care.

Hospice philosophy, outlined earlier in the chapter, emphasises the importance of various aspects of care for the individual and his family.

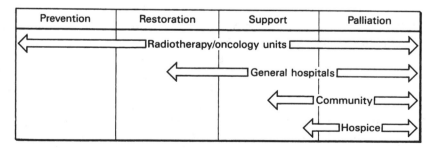

Fig. 34.5 Involvement of adult oncology settings in relation to Dietz 1980. Stages of cancer re-adaptation. (Reproduced by kind permission of Weston Park Hospital, Sheffield.)

Many of these areas are also encompassed by the philosophy of occupational therapy. The humanistic approach to care based on unconditional positive regard and the belief that a person can achieve his potential, is fundamental to both, as is the belief that adaptation of the individual physically and psychologically can be encouraged by his active participation in treatment.

Of the various conceptual models available to the occupational therapist, Keilhofner's Model of Human Occupation will be used as the model of choice to provide a basis for assessment. This model has been chosen because it aligns to hospice philosophy and humanism, and because it emphasises the importance of self-motivated treatment and the individual's ability to grow towards self-actualisation. A person who has been diagnosed as having cancer will need to learn to internalise new information and alter his thoughts and actions accordingly. In this way he will be able to adapt his life-style to compensate for the physical, emotional and psychological changes he will encounter.

The Model of Human Occupation suggests that humans learn to adapt their behaviour through positive reinforcement of their actions as they aim for self-actualisation. Conversely, negative experiences reinforce failure and lack of ability, which discourages forward movement. Within this system, the structure of human occupational behaviour is arranged in a hierarchy of three sub-systems known as volition, habituation and performance (see Ch. 2). A diagnosis of cancer can affect any or all of the sub-systems and cause the balance of the benign cycle to be disrupted (vicious cycle). Despite the severity of the diagnosis, it is possible, through carefully planned intervention, to enable balance to be restored. Important factors in enabling this to happen are described below.

Volition

Most people live their lives knowing that at some time in the future they will die. Few people give thought to how or when this will be unless a crisis occurs which brings their mortality into question. People exercise control over their lives at the level they feel able and appropriate, but a diagnosis of cancer, regardless of whether it is terminal or not, reinforces the fact that ultimate control lies elsewhere. This can lead to the individual feeling out of control, a situation which can be compounded by well-meaning health professionals who, by their attitude, reinforce powerlessness.

Generalised weakness or specific disability caused by this illness can affect the type of activity in which the individual feels able to participate and the level to which he can become involved. This area is one in which the therapist, through careful assessment, can improve quality of survival for the individual.

At the time of diagnosis, a person may experience shock, disbelief and denial, and may need more care. As reality returns, issues of personal causation, values and interests are more important than ever if the individual is to regain any quality of life. Despite living with a life-threatening illness many people wish and are able to achieve and fulfil their potential (see also Ch. 32).

Habituation

People suffering from cancer need to identify and examine the depth and number of roles they perform, and decide which are important to them. It may be that functions within these roles need to be delegated or reorganised if the person becomes weaker, and some functions may have to be handed over completely to another person while still maintaining the locus of control over the content. Where this occurs, the therapist will need to help the individual and his family to maintain a balance in the roles they undertake.

This can be illustrated where a mother is diagnosed as having cancer. Curative radiotherapy or chemotherapy may be suggested which may make her feel unwell and reduce her levels of function. It may be necessary for her husband and children to take over the shopping and other domestic tasks, but in order that she maintain her role as mother, she may still wish to write the shopping list, and may become critical of the way in which the housework is carried out. If this creates a problem within the family, the therapist may be required to discuss with them ways in which the mother can still maintain her role, even though some of its functions have been given away.

Adaptation to living with a terminal illness will require that thought be given to organisation of time and energy. For example, a wheelchair may be needed to go shopping, to enable the person to enjoy looking round the shops on arrival. Careful prioritisation by the individual is vital.

Performance

Many people with cancer have few symptoms which impair function, unless the disease is advanced, or where the tumour affects a vital centre such as the spinal cord, or causes secondary dysfunction such as a lymphoedematous arm. Assessment will require attention to the psychological adjustment attached to living in a wheelchair for example, in addition to any physical problems which this may present.

ASSESSMENT

Assessment takes the form of helping the individual to identify areas of dysfunction which cause him problems and establish functions that he needs and wishes to preserve. It is important to note that cancer can cause progressive disability, and the individual will require regular re-evaluation to maintain the best level of independence.

Approaches most frequently used in this type of work relate to humanistic philosophy and the learning and compensatory frames of reference. Belief in the ability of the individual to change and develop through the media of learned techniques and compensation for disability form the basis of cancer rehabilitation.

INTERVENTION

The following section identifies areas of need that are common to many people with cancer. Some of these fall directly within the sphere of occupational therapy, while others may equally be performed by a physiotherapist, social worker or Macmillan nurse. In any event it is important

that each task is undertaken by the person best qualified to perform it.

The treatment programme begins to be formulated during assessment, and the direction it takes will depend on the stage at which the person is referred. Someone referred following successful medical treatment, for example, will require different kinds of help from the person who has been told that his condition can be controlled for the moment, but not cured. As with all treatment planning it is important for the therapist and the individual to consider treatment aims together, in order that a meaningful series of priorities can be worked out.

Generally, however, the treatment plan must be flexible and capable of frequent alteration if the person's needs change. It is important in planning treatment to remember that the person's medical condition will not remain stable. A series of short-term goals should enable the person to achieve good results, thus improving morale and increasing self-esteem.

Some areas of intervention can be directly related to humanism through the occupational therapy and hospice philosophy. Others rely on individuals' ability to learn new techniques from information given and compensate for their lack of ability by adapting their thinking and actions in the light of the changing circumstances. Areas of intervention will include both physical and psychological issues and may include the following.

THE USE OF BELIEF IN THE INDIVIDUAL
Body image adjustment

Some medical treatments used in cancer management can lead to disfigurement and can dramatically alter a person's physical appearance. A mastectomy, for example, which results in the physical removal of a woman's breast, can also lower her self-esteem. In her eyes the alteration to her body reduces her physical and sexual desirability: she becomes less of a woman. Where this occurs the holistic approach of the occupational therapist not only addresses the physical aspects — provision of a prosthesis and adapted clothing — but also allows time for the individual to discuss her feelings about herself and the new situation, and helps her to work towards resolution of negative emotions.

When a person suffers physical disfigurement the attitudes of people around him are very important. Acceptance of a person as he is, however he may look, can prove difficult if disfigurement is severe, and some individuals may need help just to come out of their room and meet others if they feel they are physically unacceptable. Tact and sensitivity are vital in such situations, and helping the person initially to simply be in the same room as others, without having to interact with them, can help to build his self-esteem. As confidence grows, activities that involve communication with one, then later several others, can be used, before the person is helped to meet people outside the unit, perhaps through a trip to the hospital shop and then outside the confines of the institution.

Support

People who have cancer will obviously suffer considerable emotional stress. While the degree of this may fluctuate, an individual will find it very difficult to pursue an active and productive life if he is continuously hampered by negative emotions. In these circumstances the therapist can do much to help him and his carers, by acknowledging the presence of these feelings and offering techniques and strategies which may help him come to terms with them.

The amount of support required by cancer sufferers and their carers varies widely and will, therefore, have to be tailored to suit the individual. Support may be given by anyone on the team; often each member contributes in his or her own way. Support can take many forms, which may include the following:

Emotional support

In order for the occupational therapist to offer professional counselling it will be necessary for her to undertake post-graduate training to de-velop her skills. However, it is quite possible for her to help in complementary ways using skills she has already learned during her training.

The occupational therapist's skill in problem-solving can be helpful, both emotionally and physically. When a person has developed a major physical problem, for example, the occupational therapist may be involved in assessing his future needs. This will involve working with both the person and his carers, who may need a great deal of emotional support as they consider various options and come to terms with the fact that solutions may not suit everyone or, indeed, that a satisfactory solution is not possible.

If the disease has progressed past the restoration stage, carers will need both physical and emotional support. Many people want to care for their loved one at home for as long as possible, and may indeed wish for them to die at home rather than in hospital. In order for this to be possible, practical help, in the form of equipment, advice on lifting and general nursing care, will be essential. The individual may also need respite care, possibly for a week or two, or perhaps just for an afternoon to enable his carers to go shopping.

Self-help groups

Many cancer sufferers have much to offer in the way of support. Self-help groups are run locally throughout the country by cancer sufferers for others in the same position. There may be input from professionals such as Macmillan nurses, but these professionals are not the key figures within the group. Groups offer a meeting place for the individual and his carers where they can discuss problems and help each other find solutions.

The occupational therapist should be aware of self-help groups in her area. She may indeed be asked by such for help and advice.

Charities

Many national and local charities have been established to help people who are suffering from cancer. Some of these offer financial assistance while others offer practical help. It is important for the therapist to be aware of these charities and of the type of help they offer.

Carers' support groups

While emotional support for carers can be offered on an individual basis by team members, it may be appropriate for the occupational therapist and/or social worker to establish a support group for carers, where they can meet and draw support from others in the same situation, as well as gaining further access to professional advice.

Bereavement support

Bereavement counselling is another area in which, if the occupational therapist wishes to become involved, she must first seek further training. It is, however, possible to offer support to people coping with grief through the relationship that has been developed between the therapist and the individual's carers. The opportunity to talk to someone who has known their loved one, and the occasion to share information, can be very comforting at this time.

Grieving is a normal process and most people, if allowed, will cope well with bereavement, with the sensitive help of friends and relatives. It is helpful, however, for the occupational therapist to be able to spot the development of any problems and to be aware of counselling facilities in her area.

Anyone offering support needs to achieve a warm, friendly relationship with the individual and his carers while retaining a measure of objectivity and professionalism. It is important not to take personally the unpleasant feelings that may be exhibited during and after a long, distressing illness, and to maintain a sense of proportion at all times.

Specific therapeutic activity

While there has been an apparent move away from the use of certain therapeutic activities by occupational therapists in recent years, such activities have a place in the treatment of people suffering from cancer, particularly in the later stages of the illness.

Although it would be arrogant to presume to divert the person's attention from his situation, a person suffering from cancer, especially in the later stages, is facing events and circumstances with which he has to come to terms. As it is neither possible nor desirable for him to dwell continuously upon these, time set aside for discussion of these worries can be interspersed with activities and hobbies which provide much-needed light relief and interest.

If a person is in pain and possibly waiting for medication to take effect, concentrating on an activity in which he is interested can relieve tension and shift his focus of attention away from his pain.

The later stages of the disease may also be the time for the person to participate in hobbies he has previously not had time for. Activities should be easy to start and put down, to be completed later, and should also be quick to finish.

When a person suffers from a disease such as cancer, there is a temptation to think he needs to have a lot done for him. While this may be so, it is also important for him to feel useful and productive; activities can be selected with this in mind. For example, articles can be made for fund-raising events or as presents to give away. Such presents are especially important as they serve as a lasting reminder of a person even after his death. While it may be tempting to encourage a person to continue with an interest he has had in the past, this can prove unsatisfactory as he may no longer be able to perform it as well as he used to. For this reason, it may be wiser to encourage a totally new interest.

Reminiscence work

The importance of reminiscence work is discussed in Chapter 32. While such work may take various forms, either in a group or on a one-to-one basis, this section will outline the format used in Cynthia Spencer House, Northampton. This is a Macmillan Continuing Care Unit built with locally raised funds and staffed by NHS and voluntary personnel. In this unit one element of reminiscence work takes the form of a tape-recorded interview which is later transcribed and given to the interviewee to keep. While this technique is not strictly a therapy, those who choose to be interviewed find the experience worth while and rewarding. It can be pleasant to talk to an interested listener and to reflect upon the past.

A project based on work of this type has been running in Northampton since 1987, and three booklets of excerpts from these transcriptions have been published to date. Examples are given in Box 34.1.

People facing an uncertain life expectancy may also wish to write diaries or letters to loved ones, or help their families to create scrapbooks about their lives together. In this way, the individual feels he has contributed to the future of his family and will not be forgotten by those he loves.

Creative writing forms another part of this work. The writer Jane Eisenhaur (1989) has used

---

Box 34.1 ILLUSTRATIONS OF CREATIVE WRITING BY PEOPLE WITH CANCER. (Reproduced from *Slices of Life* [Foreman & Hobbs 1988] and *Life at Work* [Foreman 1989])

I sold my business, retired and bought a small van and done a little bit of, not wholesaling like I done before, but retailing, I used to do bags of potatoes, polythene bags, and I used to go up the club or the pub or anywhere and get rid of thirty or forty bags. I was always doing something. I kept that up until... almost 'til this [present illness] come along.

Well, I've enjoyed life. That's one good thing. And I've made a fair bit of cash. That's another thing. So I've got nothing to grumble at, have I?

Harry Saunders (born 1900)

Beauty can be found
In oh, so many things.
Amongst the most amazing:
A pair of insect wings.

A filigree of colour
Of every shade and hue,
And movements quite
Incredible to folks
Like me and you.

Pat Groot

We used to go to Harlestone Firs. We used to go up there and take a bottle of drink with us. Usually I ended up with cold tea! (laughs) And some sandwiches. We used to eat that then go back for tea. Just friends like, several friends. It was a happy childhood really.

June Baucutt (born 1925)

---

this activity in her work at St Joseph's Hospice in London. Because it takes some effort to put pen to paper, a person who is less well may need a scribe to put his ideas onto paper for him.

LEARNING FRAME OF REFERENCE
Provision of information

While team members may have concerns regarding the amount of information a person can accept about his condition, the individual will often be quite clear about the level he can accept. One man, for example, on being asked how much he knew about his condition replied, 'I know as much as I want to know and I will learn the rest as I go along'. Another woman arrived for her clinic appointment saying, 'Don't you go telling me anything I don't want to hear!' Both these people made their feelings quite obvious, and clearly such feelings must be respected.

If, however, the signals are not so clear, it is important to answer questions accurately without giving too much detail, thus leaving the way open for further questions. In this way the person can find out the information he requires at the time, and can control the amount he has to cope with.

Some of the information a person requires will be painful for him to hear and will take time to assimilate. For this reason a person may ask the same question many times of different team members before he is able to accept the implications of the answer. It is important to remember this so that team members can be sure that the answers are consistent and that they do not become irritated by being asked the same question many times.

In this field of work, the information available is vast; clearly no one person can know all the answers. While it is essential to admit this, it is also vital to know where to look, or who to ask, to get information. For example, the therapist should be aware of national and local organisations with information and education resources.

Relaxation

Tension can both increase pain and decrease the

effects of medication. One way of helping to dispel tension is through the use of relaxation techniques. People who teach relaxation often develop preferred methods, most of which evolve from one of the following techniques. However, while the therapist may have a preference for a particular method, she must be flexible in her use of different techniques to suit varying needs:

- *Progressive relaxation*. This approach involves the individual becoming aware of different muscle groups and areas of the body in turn, and learning to tense and relax them.
- *Autogenic training*. This involves relaxation of each part of the body in turn, e.g. hand, wrist, forearm, while imagining each part becoming warm and heavy.
- *Imaging*. Here the power of imagination is used to visualise a story or an activity, for example walking through a warm, sunny meadow or along a peaceful beach.

These and any other techniques can be used in conjunction with breathing exercises to help the person gain maximum benefit.

While relaxation sessions are normally initiated by the therapist, it is possible to obtain taped cassettes of exercises for those who wish to continue relaxation at home. In this way the person can learn to reduce tension as and when it occurs, rather than just during therapy sessions.

When considering different relaxation methods, the therapist should remember that the method should be as simple and short as possible, while still being effective, especially to begin with. As the person becomes more proficient, it may be possible to increase sessions in length and complexity.

COMPENSATORY FRAME OF REFERENCE

Life skills

Although the emphasis will depend on the level at which the person is functioning, this area of intervention will need to include self-care and home care advice and practice, as well as the provision of equipment to help overcome dis-ability. Equipment, where necessary, should be loaned if at all possible, so that it may be easily changed if the need arises.

In cases in which dramatic changes have occurred, such as amputation of a limb or compression of nervous tissue resulting in paraplegia, the presenting condition will obviously require practical consideration, along with the other concerns of particular relevance to the individual. Attention to body image changes will also be necessary (see above), as will regard to the instability of the condition. Where the individual becomes severely disabled as a result of his illness, external help in the form of district nurses, social services or voluntary agencies may be necessary to enable the family to care for the individual at home.

If the condition is well advanced, it may be necessary to teach energy conservation techniques (see Ch. 31). The therapist may also need to work with the person and his carers in helping the former to come to terms with being cared for, especially in circumstances in which the individual has been the key homemaker.

Enabling a person to become independent in daily living activities following a period of dependency can improve self-esteem and achieve goals far in excess of those expected.

Mobility

Encouraging purposeful activity to improve mobility can increase stamina and generally enable a person to lead a more active life. A person who has been inactive through fear of exacerbating symptoms, such as pain, can often regain high levels of activity once his symptoms are controlled by correct medication and he has gained the confidence to begin activities again.

In some cases it may become obvious that full mobility will not be achievable. However, the person may be reluctant to entertain the idea of using a wheelchair, and it will be necessary to introduce the subject with sensitivity. Where stamina is low, the use of a wheelchair can greatly improve a person's sphere of activity. It may, for example, enable him to visit the shops or a club after he has been confined to the house for some time. The ultimate decision of whether or not to use a wheelchair must, however, remain with the individual, as he may still prefer to remain less mobile rather than use a wheelchair, even after all the advantages of the latter have been explained.

If the disease has progressed to the point at which extensive metastases have weakened bone tissue, pathological fractures may occur. In such instances, and in others in which mobility is not possible, full assessment for a permanent wheelchair, appropriate seating and other accessories will be necessary. The person will then require training in the use of the chair and in transfer techniques (see Ch. 9).

Social and leisure activities

People's attitudes to cancer can vary enormously; consequently it can be a daunting prospect for a person suffering from cancer to get out and about following treatment for his disease. He may feel rejected by his friends who find his condition hard to cope with or talk about, or he may feel that he wishes to tell everyone about his experiences, thus creating fears and barriers within relationships. Alternatively he may feel he cannot cope with an excessive curiosity on the part of colleagues and friends, or with their apparent lack of interest, which may stem from their discomfort at not knowing what to say. Allowing time for discussion of these feelings, therefore, may be valuable.

Large gatherings and crowds may be equally daunting for a person who does not feel very well. Keeping outings short and restricting them to places where the person feels comfortable, and which he can leave early if he feels the need, can help him to retain his social life.

Where the disease has reached an advanced stage, it may be difficult for the person to get out. In some areas units have access to adapted vehicles; alternatively charities and local organisations may offer to help. Where this cannot be arranged, it is important to 'take the mountain to Mohammed' by encouraging visitors, phone calls and letters so that the person does not feel isolated from his family, friends and colleagues.

Where a day centre facility is available for cancer sufferers, this can provide not only company and support for the individual but also support and relief for his carers.

Resettlement

While a person is being cared for in hospital, it is hoped that he will regain much of his independence. However, until he returns home he still relies on physical and emotional support from the staff. Most skills involved in helping a person with cancer to return home are no different from those used in resettling any other person being discharged from hospital, but there are one or two points that need particular consideration, especially if the person concerned is quite unwell.

As has been stated, most people suffering from cancer are not medically stable; consequently consideration needs to be given to each individual's expectations. If it is felt that the person will continue to improve following treatment and discharge, any action to be taken is usually reasonably easy to determine on a home visit. However, if expectations are not so high it may be necessary for two or more members of the team to undertake a home visit. This will afford the opportunity for team members and carers to talk in the carers' own environment and to bring to light the carer's areas of concern. There may also be times when the health care team have reservations about the appropriateness of a person returning home; while they clearly do not have the right to prevent him from doing so, observing him in his own home can give them a basis for open discussion about their concerns.

There will often be discussion concerning whether the carers, as well as the individual, feel they can cope once the person is at home. Sometimes this may serve to crystallise feelings of fear and anxiety and can lead to the realisation that, no matter how much help and support is provided, the carers will be unable to cope, and a different solution must be sought. In fact it is not unknown for a home visit to be necessary in order to allow a person to come to this conclusion and to give him permission not to return home.

Following the home visit there will often be

problems to solve before discharge. Solutions need to be realistic, and if alterations are to be made it will be necessary to choose those which take the least time while affording maximum benefit to the person. Prognosis is often very difficult to assess, and it is essential to keep a positive attitude once a decision has been taken to help a person to return home.

Once the person has returned home he and his carers may encounter further difficulties. It is important to encourage carers to accept help before they reach a state of exhaustion. If a day care facility is available, this can provide time off for carers, as well as new interests, social contact and support for the individual. If this is not available, or in some cases of severe illness, agencies such as Crossroads can offer a sitting service to allow carers to take a break.

In some areas the occupational therapist may be the main link between the hospital and the community. In such cases it is important for her to arrange for the continuation of support links in accordance with the person's needs.

The case study in Box 34.2 illustrates how principles and concepts within the Model of Human Occupation, the compensatory frame of reference and the use of belief in the individual can be used to assess, plan and implement care for a young man living with severe malignant disease.

COMPLEMENTARY THERAPIES

Many people with cancer wish to explore the alternative therapies available to help them cope

---

Box 34.2 Case study

Neil, a 39-year-old ex-publican, was diagnosed as having an advanced spinal tumour when admitted to hospital following episodes of intractable pain and weakness in his legs. He underwent emergency surgery to remove as much of the tumour as possible, and although he was unable to walk, he was determined to go home.

The initial occupational therapy assessment identified that extensive alterations to the home in the form of ramps and a shower/toilet/downstairs bedroom would be necessary, and relevant equipment would be needed to enable him to be independent in activities of daily living at home. In addition Neil was reluctant to delegate any of the functions within the roles he fulfilled. He was sad not to be able to return to work as a driver but was keen to maintain his roles as husband and father within his family. Adjusting to life in a wheelchair was difficult and painful for him emotionally, and he concentrated hard on exercising his legs in the hope that some functional mobility would return.

At this stage he was referred to the local hospice for day care, physiotherapy to maximise the movement in his legs and continued occupational therapy support as necessary to enable him to be cared for at home. Care was provided mainly by his 37-year-old wife, helped by his two stepchildren, all of whom needed to use considerable skill in helping Neil to compensate for the losses he had experienced.

Although little improvement in mobility was noticed, Neil was determined to live life as fully as possible. He continued to go out socially and participated in activity sessions at the day unit, making many articles which he then bought and gave to friends as presents. As he

became weaker, nursing support was needed at home to help with personal care and transfers, and frequent visits were made by the occupational therapist to advise on different equipment necessary to maintain independence.

Neil was reluctant to accept the limitations placed upon him by his illness and the likely outcome, and while his wife was more realistic about the future, she wished to preserve hope. Emotional support was required to help them both to maintain realistic hope yet enable them to look at the difficulties that arose. Support centred on both Neil and his wife, who were encouraged to use their own resources to meet the emotional demands placed on them by the illness.

As his wife's birthday approached (five months from Neil's first attendance at the day unit), Neil's condition began to deteriorate. Despite severe pain and discomfort, he refused admission to the hospice because he had planned and organised a surprise party for his wife, and was determined to attend it.

Neil was admitted to the hospice during the weekend following the party and died peacefully there three weeks later. Throughout his final few months of life, the occupational therapist had become close to the family and it was therefore appropriate that she continued to see Neil's wife and offer bereavement support.

Neil and his wife needed support to adjust to their new, unwelcome situation, and fought hard to maintain normality within their lives. Despite severe physical disability, Neil became a valued member of the day unit, offering support and friendship to others in a position similar to his own. He was greatly missed by everyone at the hospice after his death.

with their illness. A person with cancer may feel the need to find a way of complementing the treatment he is receiving through orthodox medicine. He may, indeed, feel that the conventional treatment he is receiving does not meet his needs and might, therefore, look to alternative therapy. Aromatherapy (use of aromatic oils), homeopathy and visualisation (relaxation combined with visualising the growth as being weak as it is attacked and destroyed by the body's immune system) are some of the therapies available.

The basis of many of these therapies is positive thinking and attitude, and realisation that the effort to get better has to come from within. There has been little documented work on the effectiveness of these therapies, but many people who have used them feel they have derived benefit from doing so. However, the person may feel a failure if he is not cured, as he may feel that he did not work hard enough at his treatment.

CONCLUSION

Oncology rehabilitation is an area that has been developing rapidly in recent years. There is much that can be done to help a person and his carers cope with the possibility of a devastating crisis in their lives. There is no magical formula for this help, only the implementation of good, caring practice. Neither are there any right or wrong answers; what must be sought are the solutions that seem best for a particular person at a particular time. The occupational therapist working in this field will find herself having to call on nearly all the skills learned in her basic training as she helps the person and his carers in the physical, emotional and social aspects of their lives. However, her practice will also be enriched by additional training in specific areas such as counselling and relaxation techniques.

ACKNOWLEDGEMENTS

Grateful acknowledgement is made to: Dr Nigel Bird, Clinical Assistant, Cynthia Spencer House; Jackie Phillips, Senior Clinical Nurse, Cynthia Spencer House; Mr A W Ross, Pharmacia Ltd, Milton Keynes; Alison Hammond, Occupational Therapist, Derby School of Occupational Therapy; Dr Peter Kaye, Dr John Smith and all the staff of Cynthia Spencer House, Northampton; and our patients, past and present, who are a constant source of inspiration to us all.

USEFUL ADDRESSES

BACUP (British Association of Cancer United Patients)
3 Bath Place
London EC2A 3RJ

British Association for Counselling
1 Regent Place
Rugby
Warwickshire CV21 2PJ

Cancer Care Society (CARE)
21 Zetland Road
Redland
Bristol BS6 7AH

Cancer Relief (National Society for Cancer Relief)
Anchor House
15/19 Britten Street
London SW3 3TZ

Cancer Research Campaign
10 Cambridge Terrace
London NW1 4JL

Crossroads (Association of Crossroads Care Attendant Scheme)
10 Regent Place
Rugby
Warwickshire CV21 2PN

CRUSE (National Organisation for Bereaved People)
Cruse House
126 Sheen Road,
Richmond TW9 1UR

Disabled Living Foundation,
360–384 Harrow Road
London W9 2HU

Help the Hospices
BMA House
Tavistock Square
London WC1H 9JP

Hospice Information Service
St Christopher's Hospice
51–59 Lawrie Park Road
London SE26 6DZ

Lisa Sainsbury Foundation
8–10 Crown Hill
Croydon
Surrey CR0 1RY
(Provides videos, tapes and book references, and organises workshops.)

Marie Curie Cancer Care
28 Belgrave Square
London SW1X 8OQ

There are many more relevant charities, some set up to help people suffering from particular forms of cancer. Their addresses are published annually by:

Family Welfare Association
501–503 Kingsland Road
Dalston
London E8 4UA

REFERENCES

Dietz J H 1981 Rehabilitation Oncology. John Wiley, New York

Eisenhaur J (ed.) 1989 Traveller's tales: poetry from hospice. Marshall Pickering, London

Foreman R (ed.) 1989 Life at work. (Compilation of reminiscences.) Available from Cynthia Spencer House, Manfield Hospital, Kettering Road, Northampton NN3 1AD

Foreman R, Hobbs L (eds) 1988 Slices of life. (Compilation of reminiscences.) Available from Cynthia Spencer House, Manfield Hospital, Kettering Road, Northampton NN3 1AD

Hammond A 1988 The role of the occupational therapist in oncology. Unpublished report. Available from the author at Derby School of Occupational Therapy, Highfield, 403 Burton Road, Derby DE3 6AN

Kaye P 1991 Symptom control in hospice and palliative care. Hospice Education Insititute, Connecticut

Kubler-Ross E 1970 On death and dying. Tavistock, London

Zora R, Zora V 1981 A way to die. Sphere, London

FURTHER READING

Boston S, Trezise R 1987 Merely mortal. Methuen, London

Du Boulay S 1984 Cicely Saunders. Hodder Christian Paperbacks, London

Brearley G, Birchley P 1986 Introducing counselling skills and techniques. Faber & Faber, London

Bryan J, Lyall J 1987 Living with cancer. Penguin, Harmondsworth

Buckman R 1988 I don't know what to say. Papermac, London

Chave-Jones M 1982 The gift of helping. Intervarsity Press, Leicester

Disability Rights Handbook, 19th edn (April 1994 – April 1995). Available from Universal House, 88–94 Wentworth Street, London E1 7SA

Downie P 1975 Cancer rehabilitation. Faber & Faber, London

Hagedorn R 1992 Occupational therapy: foundations for practice. Models, frames of reference and core skills. Churchill Livingstone, Edinburgh

Hinton J 1967 Dying. Pelican, Harmondsworth

Kopp R 1980 Encounter with terminal illness. Lion Publishing, Tring

Kopp R 1986 When someone you love is dying. Lion Publishing, Tring

Kushner H 1981 When bad things happen to good people. Pan Books, London

Kushner H 1986 When all you've ever wanted isn't enough. Pan Books, London

Lamerton R 1985 Care of the dying. Pelican, Harmondsworth

Lewis C S 1940 The problem of pain. Collins, Glasgow

Lewis C S 1966 A grief observed. Faber & Faber, London

Lewis M 1989 Tears and smiles; the hospice handbook. O'Mara Press, London

Munro E, Manthei R, Small J 1975 Counselling: a skills approach. Methuen, New Zealand

Parkes C M 1976 Bereavement. Penguin, Harmondsworth

Regnard C, Davies A 1986 A guide to symptom relief in advanced cancer, 2nd edn. Haigh & Hochland, Manchester

Sampson J 1987 The courage to hope. Scripture Union, London

Souhami J, Tobias J 1986 Cancer and its management. Blackwell, Oxford

Strong J 1987 Occupational therapy and cancer rehabilitation. British Journal of Occupational Therapy 50(1): 4–6

Tigges K 1980 Occupational therapy for the person with terminal cancer. Unpublished sabbatical report to the Department of Occupational Therapy, State of New York at Buffalo

Whithouse J M A 1986 Chemotherapy: a guide for patients. Farmitalia, St Albans

Worden J W 1991 Grief counselling and grief therapy. Routledge, London

Glossary